The Differential Diagnosis of Chorea

The Differential Diagnosis of Chorea

Edited by

Ruth H. Walker, MB, ChB, PhD
Department of Neurology
James J. Peters Veterans Affairs Medical Center
Bronx, NY; and
Mount Sinai School of Medicine
New York, NY

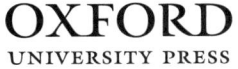

OXFORD
UNIVERSITY PRESS

2011

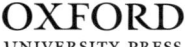
OXFORD
UNIVERSITY PRESS

Oxford University Press, Inc., publishes works that further
Oxford University's objective of excellence
in research, scholarship, and education.

Oxford   New York
Auckland   Cape Town   Dar es Salaam   Hong Kong   Karachi
Kuala Lumpur   Madrid   Melbourne   Mexico City   Nairobi
New Delhi   Shanghai   Taipei   Toronto

With offices in
Argentina   Austria   Brazil   Chile   Czech Republic   France   Greece
Guatemala   Hungary   Italy   Japan   Poland   Portugal   Singapore
South Korea   Switzerland   Thailand   Turkey   Ukraine   Vietnam

Published by Oxford University Press, Inc.
198 Madison Avenue, New York, New York 10016
www.oup.com

Oxford is a registered trademark of Oxford University Press

About the cover image: **Edges in Eternity** is a contemporary forum to examine
the boundaries of our shared existence. These paintings orientate through atmospheric storms.
The intention is bring the viewer to the edges of natural power to encourage ethical reflection.
The artist, Noreen Dean Dresser invites individual participants whose life experience mirrors
the storms to reflect. This body of work re-examines the confrontation with the sublime in
nature and corporately as stewards of the earth.
www.parlour153.com

Library of Congress Cataloging-in-Publication Data

The differential diagnosis of chorea / edited by Ruth H. Walker.
 p. ; cm.
Includes bibliographical references and index.
ISBN 978-0-19-539351-4 (alk. paper)
1. Chorea—Diagnosis.   2. Diagnosis, Differential.   I. Walker, Ruth H.
[DNLM: 1. Chorea—diagnosis.   2. Chorea—complications.
3. Chorea—etiology. WL 390 D5695 2011]
RC389.D54 2011
616.8'3—dc22
2010003463

The science of medicine is a rapidly changing field. As new research and clinical experience broaden our
knowledge, changes in treatment and drug therapy occur. The author and publisher of this work have checked with
sources believed to be reliable in their efforts to provide information that is accurate and complete, and in
accordance with the standards accepted at the time of publication. However, in light of the possibility of human
error or changes in the practice of medicine, neither the author, nor the publisher, nor any other party who has been
involved in the preparation or publication of this work warrants that the information contained herein is in every
respect accurate or complete. Readers are encouraged to confirm the information contained herein with other
reliable sources, and are strongly advised to check the product information sheet provided by the pharmaceutical
company for each drug they plan to administer.

9   8   7   6   5   4   3   2   1

Printed in the United States of America
on acid-free paper

To all those affected by chorea, as individuals, family members and care-givers. Special appreciation is extended to those who have supported and participated in the study of these disorders, without whom this work would not have been possible

Foreword

The basal ganglia, the brain, and life itself are comprised of multiple pathways that interconnect and in the best of circumstances function with relative balance. Destabilizing forces, both physical and emotional, routinely perturb the system; and in most situations the dynamic brain reequilibrates, adapts, or compensates. In medicine, we call these destabilizing forces "disease" or "illness." In life, these forces can become new directions or "opportunities."

While a fellow, Ruth studied a family suffering from chorea and combined medical excellence and a background in neuroanatomy to systematically investigate the complex constellation of symptoms associated with the motor phenomenology of chorea. Clinicians and scientists recognize symptoms and signs, form a differential diagnosis, conduct reasonable diagnostic studies, and initiate treatment when possible, while forming new hypotheses and researching the disorder. The exchange of new information through publications, such as this volume, extends our base of information and creates new opportunities, thus enabling the next series of clinical and laboratory experiments.

Ruth embraced these principles, and it is fitting that she brought together an impressive multinational group of authorities who collectively provide knowledge needed for the scientist and clinician interested in choreas. The pathophysiology of chorea touches multiple medical disciplines, and this volume provides a reference for those interested in understanding, treating, and ultimately curing these often challenging disorders. With each scientific advance, the future will hopefully supersede the present.

Rarely, a cure is identified in medicine; more commonly, for most of the neurodegenerative choreas, physicians are shepherds in ameliorating suffering. The patients, their families, and their loved ones need better treatments and ultimate cures. They are waiting, urgently.

Mitchell F. Brin, MD
Irvine, California, USA

The Family's Perspective

Most of us walk and move our limbs in a fluid, coordinated, and easy manner. For some, however, an insignificant twitch does not go away but slowly becomes an uncontrollable flailing of limbs. A slightly stumbling gait develops into an awkward jumble of jerks and exaggerated effort to retain balance.

Our daughter's early movement problems seemed to be easily corrected. "Don't let your left toe point inward when you walk." "Keep your hands on the banister when you climb the stairs." But within months the chorea took over her movement and left her, at age 26, unable to lead the independent, productive, adult life she had just begun.

We then learned firsthand how difficult diagnosis can be. Office visits to specialist neurologists produced many biopsies and tests that led to wrong provisional diagnoses including Wilson disease, multiple sclerosis, and motor neuron disease. It was only when she stayed in the National Hospital for Neurology and Neurosurgery, Queen Square, London, that the coordination of a number of specialists including hematologists and geneticists correctly identified chorea-acanthocytosis as the disease that produced the chorea.

The further development of such a coordinated approach to diagnosis will be encouraged and aided by Dr. Walker's book. This book combines an algorithm for the diagnosis of chorea with detailed descriptions of the natural history of the diseases associated with chorea and documents a systematic approach to finding the cause of these rare, troubling, and costly chronic diseases.

What use is a diagnosis of a condition for which there is no cure? When it is acknowledged that the problems are not psychiatric, there is much that can be accomplished by patients with the help of speech and occupational therapists. There are drugs developed for epilepsy that may control seizures. Treatments used for other movement disorders such as Parkinson disease, including levodopa and deep brain stimulation, have brought some relief of symptoms.

Perhaps more important are the social and psychological benefits of a diagnosis. Within our memories, people with severe chorea and speech impairment were seen to be "mad" and locked away out of sight. With a diagnosis, we can understand that the patient is not an oddity but a person afflicted by a contorting loss of movement control. As a friend with chorea-acanthocytosis nobly said, "I have the disease; the disease does not have me."

We can also see Dr. Walker's valuable contribution as an important step toward exploring the pathogenic pathways that may be common to the onset of chorea and related to neurodegeneration.

Ginger and Glenn Irvine
Advocacy for Neuroacanthocytosis Patients
London, UK

The Patient's Perspective

In 1979 I started working at E. R. Squibb's (now Bristol-Myers Squibb) in the Analytical Research and Development department (AR&D) labs. In AR&D, I performed physical characterization on bulk pharmaceuticals prior to their incorporation into a formulation, as well as testing a myriad of materials for stability for various lengths of time. Every 12–18 months, all the chemical-handling personnel were give a complete blood panel.

My blood results came back quite elevated for bilirubin. My liver enzymes were out of range, as was the level of the muscle enzyme creatine kinase. However, my hemoglobin was surprisingly normal—no anemia. The Squibb company physician told me that I could have Gilbert syndrome (a benign liver condition) and, probably, "not to worry"! I pursued this on my own.

Somehow, in 1981 a sample of my blood got to a hematologist–oncologist named Dr. Edward Schnipper. He was aware of certain researchers at the New York Blood Center who were screening for rare and unusual blood types. Hence, my blood was sent to Dr. W. Laurence Marsh; and within a short period of time, my brother and I were diagnosed with McLeod syndrome (documented cases 25 and 26 at the time). We were informed that it was a syndrome at the time, not a disease. I could not donate blood, nor could I receive any, except my own. My brother and I began to donate our own blood to be stored at the New York Blood

Center in case we ever needed a transfusion. We were also told that we may expect some muscle fatigue later in life . . . the rest is history!

At present (28 years later), I exhibit involuntary movements of my jaw, lips, and tongue. Personally, I am aware that my fingers move erratically and are not very controllable, especially when I type on the computer. Thank goodness for the "spell checker"! My wife says that I do a lot of finger tapping, whereby I connect the top of my index finger to the top of the thumb on the same hand . . . news to me! I also am quite aware that I repeatedly tap my feet, as well as rotate my ankles while seated in a chair. My wife says that this movement occurs in one foot or both feet; however, it appears to happen more often with my right foot. Besides the limb movements, my wife says I move my mouth, lips, and especially my tongue quite a bit. I am completely unaware of the latter. I'm aware that I make vocalizations. It's hard to explain, but I constantly purse my lips and then let out a very subtle "pop." It's quite hard for me to describe.

There are also all my other symptoms, maladies, etc. and the complications that have resulted from them. These include muscle atrophy, loss of balance, and seizures, which resulted in the suspension of my driver's license, again. However, I think you can tell that chorea is not a major factor in my daily routines. It's all of the other complications. Then there's my scleroderma with the accompanying Raynaud phenomenon (more severe now), difficulty swallowing, and the stomach problems.

I tell myself often that there are those much worse off than myself, but I confess that there are many times that "I don't want to hear about it." I have become more depressed and find myself obsessing about it. The eating difficulties are more upsetting than the chorea. My wife has always been there for me and constantly offers encouragement. I get lots of compliments on how well I cope. However, there are those "bad days" when I don't agree with them and, of course, there the "good days" when I can agree.

My older brother Felix, who also had McLeod syndrome in addition to other medical problems, recently passed away unexpectedly. Despite his limitations and increasing mobility problems, Felix continued to pursue his interests. At family functions we could always count on Felix to document these events through photography. He was a loving husband to his wife, a devoted father to his daughters, and a caring brother me. He will be sorely missed.

Joseph DeVincentis,
Polonia, New Jersey, USA

The Genetic Counselor's Perspective

K. was a young woman with concerns regarding her desire to possibly have children and the potential risks given her family history of her father with a neurological disorder (undiagnosed) and brothers with unexplained mental retardation. Her father was at a nursing home, and she had two brothers in adult facilities on Long Island. The family history on her father's side revealed several generations of a "shaking" condition. After obtaining medical records, the most likely diagnosis suspected was Huntington disease. K.'s father was brought from his nursing home for an examination and to have blood drawn for DNA testing for this condition. I spoke with K. at length about the psychological ramifications of possibly learning that she may be at 50% risk of developing this late-onset condition. K. was steadfast in her desire to finally know the diagnosis in the family and have the ability to determine if this condition was something she would have to plan for in her reproductive choices as well as in her other life decisions.

We were both surprised when her father was negative for this condition. While in the midst of trying to diagnose her father we still had to deal with the mental retardation affecting her brothers. Getting the brothers evaluated proved difficult. I spoke with K. about testing her for the most common form of inherited mental retardation in males, fragile X syndrome. K. consented to the testing after we discussed the X-linked inheritance of the condition and the potential risk for her offspring if she were found to be a carrier. The testing demonstrated that K. was indeed a carrier of this gene. Now, she had the extremely bad luck of dealing with two inherited disorders in the family. K. took the news well; in retrospect, I think she had already assumed that she would not have children due to her family history.

Both K. and I were focused on trying to find out what disorder was affecting her father and his side of the family. I reviewed her father's chart again and noticed a single comment about seeing acanthocytosis in one of his blood tests. I hit the books (this all occurred before I would automatically hit the Internet) and found a listing for chorea with acanthocytosis, which was dominantly inherited. I thought, "Eureka! I have found the answer," and now I needed to find a physician to confirm this probable diagnosis.

I contacted Columbia Presbyterian and spoke to a genetic counselor whose husband was a neurologist at Mount Sinai who did research with movement disorders. K. and I arranged an appointment with Dr. Brin at Mount Sinai and brought her father for an evaluation.

K. was also in contact with her paternal cousins and found out that one of these cousins was also starting to have behavioral as well as physical symptoms similar to those seen before in the family. This cousin was also brought in for evaluation and testing, as was one of his brothers who was not symptomatic. Samples were tested and data collected, but no specific diagnosis was yet made.

We discussed with K. the possibility of donating her father's brain for research after he died. Initially, K. was understandably unsure if this was something she could do, but she took the necessary papers and thought it over.

Once I brought the patients and all the paperwork I had amassed to Mount Sinai, I took a back seat, getting involved mainly at the request of Dr. Brin, Dr. Walker, and K. I did accompany Dr. Walker and K. to visit her brother, who was living in an adult center. K. had informed Dr. Walker that he was reportedly having unusual movements and losing function beyond his disabilities due to fragile X syndrome. Unbelievably, her brother had a genetic double whammy and appeared to have both conditions. With K.'s help I also spoke with her cousins in Texas, explaining to them their link to this history and encouraging them to be involved.

After K.'s father died, she was amazingly brave and signed the forms to have her father's brain donated for research. That step led to the eventual discovery that his diagnosis was of a very rare, newly described disorder called "Huntington disease-like 2."

K.'s dedication to her family and the desire to solve the family's mystery was truly unbelievable. Although stretches of time would pass in between, I would occasionally get a call keeping me up to date on the study's progress from K. and Dr. Walker. My involvement with this family was certainly one of my most memorable cases, and the satisfaction I felt at helping this family solve a multigenerational puzzle will never fade.

Barbara Feldman, MS, CGC
Madonna Perinatal Services
Mineola, New York, USA

Preface

WHY A BOOK ON CHOREA?

Chorea is one of the most common forms of hyperkinetic movement disorders and can have a multitude of etiologies. Phenomenologically, there is not much to learn about the diagnosis by observing the patient with chorea, with a couple of exceptions. In contrast to neurosyphilis, which is classically known to mimic a panoply of neurological disorders, the single symptom of chorea can result from an ever-expanding list of metabolic, structural, and genetic causes. However, there can be many clues in the family and medical history and the neurological exam before the examiner embarks upon an often expensive, and sometimes unrewarding, work-up.

Personal connections have led many of us in medicine to our areas of specialization. My introduction to the topic of chorea came during my fellowship in movement disorders with Mitchell F. Brin, MD, and C. Warren Olanow, MD, at the Mount Sinai School of Medicine, New York. We consulted on a family who carried an autosomal dominantly inherited neurodegenerative disorder in which acanthocytes had been found. This family came to us via a rather circuitous route, spurred on by the young woman whose father was affected and who wanted to know the diagnosis to find out if she was a carrier as she wanted to have children. Her father's mother, grandmother, and great-aunts and her cousin had suffered from a similar condition; and there was family lore that it was bad to have children. The genetic counselor involved with the family knew Mitchell's wife, who was also a genetic counselor, and she knew of Mitchell's interest in neuroacanthocytosis due to his biochemist father's knowledge of vitamin E malabsorption disorders. Although the neuroacanthocytosis syndromes associated with vitamin E deficiency due to the inherited conditions of abetalipoproteinemia and hypolipoproteinemia are quite distinct from the neuroacanthocytosis syndromes affecting the basal ganglia, Mitchell had become interested in them and had written up the pathology of a case during his time at Columbia-Presbyterian Hospital. After the death of her father from this unknown neurodegenerative disorder, the young woman ensured that his brain came to autopsy; and eventually we were able to make the diagnosis of Huntington disease-like 2, a rare autosomal dominantly inherited disorder found only in people of African ancestry.

Advances in molecular medicine in the past two decades have led to advances in the genetic diagnosis of disorders which were previously assumed to be Huntington disease. In the absence of a family history, older patients were given the diagnosis of "senile chorea." In this volume I have tried to gather together what I hope to be a relatively comprehensive collection of descriptions of known causes of chorea. I hope that this will facilitate the diagnosis and, ultimately, with further advances in molecular medicine, the treatment of patients with these disorders.

Ruth H. Walker

Contents

Contributors

Octavian R. Adam, MD
The Parkinson Disease Center and
    Movement Disorders Clinic
Department of Neurology
Baylor College of Medicine
Houston, TX

Benedikt Bader, MD
Neurologische Klinik und Poliklinik
Ludwig-Maximilians-Universität
Munich, Germany

Brandon Barton, MD
Department of Neurological Sciences
Movement Disorders Section
Rush University Medical Center
Chicago, IL

Nora L. Chan, MD
Department of Neurology
Mount Sinai School of Medicine
New York, NY

**Patrick F. Chinnery, PhD,
FRCPath, FRCP, FMedSci**
Department of Neurogenetics
Mitochondrial Research Group
University of Newcastle-Upon-Tyne
Newcastle-Upon-Tyne, UK

Esther Cubo, MD, PhD
Department of Neurology
Hospital General Yagüe
Burgos, Spain

Adrian Danek, MD
Neurologische Klinik und
    Poliklinik
Ludwig-Maximilians-Universität
Munich, Germany

Andrew Evans, MBBS, MD, FRACP
Neuropsychiatry Unit
Royal Melbourne Hospital
Melbourne, Australia

Steven Frucht, MD
Department of Neurology
Columbia University Medical Center
New York, NY

Donald L. Gilbert, MD, MS
Movement Disorders Clinics
Cincinnati Children's Hospital
    Medical Center
Cincinnati, OH

Rebecca M. Gilbert, MD, PhD
Department of Neurology
New York University Langone
    Medical Center
New York, NY

Jennifer G. Goldman, MD, MS
Department of Neurological Sciences
Section of Movement Disorders
Rush University Medical Center
Chicago, IL

Susan Hayflick, MD
Departments of Neurology and
    Molecular & Medical Genetics
Oregon Health & Science University
Portland, OR

Penelope Hogarth, MD
Departments of Neurology and
    Molecular & Medical Genetics
Oregon Health & Science University
Portland, OR

Hans H. Jung, MD
Department of Neurology
University Hospital Zurich
Zurich, Switzerland

Joseph Jankovic, MD
The Parkinson Disease Center and
    Movement Disorders Clinic
Department of Neurology
Baylor College of Medicine
Houston, TX

Camilla Kilbane, MD
Department of Neurology
Mount Sinai School of Medicine
New York, NY

Katie Kompoliti, MD
Department of Neurological Sciences
Rush University Medical Center
Chicago, IL

Nayana Lahiri, BSc, MBBS, MRCP
Institute of Neurology
MRC Prion Unit
University College London
London, UK

Russell L. Margolis, MD
Department of Psychiatry
Division of Neurobiology
Laboratory of Genetic Neurobiology
Johns Hopkins University
    School of Medicine
Baltimore, MD

Alisdair McNeill, MRCP
Clinical Genetics Unit,
Birmingham Women's Hospital
Birmingham, UK

**Simon Mead, BMBChir,
MRCP, PhD**
Institute of Neurology
MRC Prion Unit
University College London
London, UK

Shyamal H. Mehta, MD, PhD
Movement Disorders Program
Department of Neurology
Medical College of Georgia
Augusta, GA

Jonathan W. Mink, MD, PhD
Child Neurology
Department of Neurology
University of Rochester
Rochester, NY

John C. Morgan, MD, PhD
Neurological Service
Charlie Norwood VA Medical Center and
Movement Disorders Program
Department of Neurology
Medical College of Georgia
Augusta, GA

Michael H. Pourfar, MD
Department of Neurology
Northshore University Hospital
Manhasset, NY

**Guilherme G. Riccioppo
Rodrigues, MD, MSc**
Department of Neuroscience and
Behavioral Sciences
School of Medicine of Ribeirão Preto
University of São Paulo
São Paulo, Brazil

Dobrila D. Rudnicki, PhD
Department of Psychiatry
Division of Neurobiology
Laboratory of Genetic Neurobiology
Johns Hopkins University
School of Medicine
Baltimore, MD

Marta San Luciano, MD
Department of Neurology
Beth Israel Medical Center
New York, NY, and
Department of Neurology
Albert Einstein College of Medicine
Bronx, NY

**Rachel Saunders-Pullman,
MD, MPH**
Department of Neurology
Beth Israel Medical Center
New York, NY, and
Department of Neurology
Albert Einstein College of Medicine
Bronx, NY

Kapil D. Sethi, MD, FRCP
Movement Disorders Program
Department of Neurology
Medical College of Georgia
Augusta, GA

Kathleen M. Shannon, MD
Department of Neurological
Sciences
Movement Disorders Section
Rush University Medical Center
Chicago, IL

Frank Skidmore, MD
Department of Neurology
University of Florida
Gainesville, FL

**Sarah J. Tabrizi, BSc, MBChB,
FRCP, PhD**
Institute of Neurology
MRC Prion Unit
University College London
London, UK

Winona Tse, MD
Department of Neurology
Mount Sinai School of Medicine
New York, NY

**Dennis Velakoulis, MBBS, MPM,
FRANZCP, DipCrim**
Neuropsychiatry Unit
Royal Melbourne Hospital
Melbourne, Australia

**Mark Walterfang, MBBS,
Hons, FRANZCP**
Neuropsychiatry Unit
Royal Melbourne Hospital
Melbourne, Australia

S. Elizabeth Zauber, MD
Department of Neurology
Indiana University School of Medicine
Indianapolis, IN

The Differential Diagnosis of Chorea

1

Introduction: An Approach to the Patient with Chorea

Ruth H. Walker, MB, ChB, PhD

INTRODUCTION

"Chorea" is the term used for involuntary movements of the limbs, trunk, neck, or face which rapidly flit from region to region in an irregular pattern. Derived from the Greek term for "dance" (*choros*, χορος), the term suggests the fluidity of the movements but not their arrhythmicity. Movements are not repetitive and involve different muscle groups in an unpredictable manner.

This movement disorder can be due to a large number of neurological disorders, and diagnosis can be challenging. However, the etiology may be suggested by features of the patient's family and medical history as well as medical and neurological examination (Table 1–1). The work-up of the patient with chorea can be extensive (Table 1–2), expanding every year; and yet some patients remain undiagnosed. There are a number of well-characterized genetic disorders which typically cause this movement disorder and others where it may occur less often, for example, as part of a mixed movement disorder (Tables 1–3 and 1–4). Advances in molecular medicine have facilitated the recognition of atypical presentations of genetically defined disorders, often with a later age at onset than is typical.

Chorea may also be a feature of metabolic disturbances which affect neurotransmission in an apparently identical manner to that seen in neurodegenerative diseases. Similarly, structural lesions can physically disrupt neuronal pathways

TABLE I–I. History and Clinical Features in the Evaluation of the Patient with Chorea

KEY ELEMENT	DIAGNOSIS SUGGESTED
Time course	Stroke, metabolic disorder, neurodegenerative disease, paroxysmal dyskinesia, etc.
Drug (prescription or nonprescription)	Drug effect or tardive syndrome
General medical condition	Metabolic effect (e.g., thyroid disease, diabetes, pregnancy), central nervous system involvement (e.g., paraneoplastic syndrome, autoimmune disease, metastatic disease)
Family history	Genetic disorder, suggested by pattern of inheritance
Psychiatric features, cognitive impairment	Frontal cortical or subcortical involvement
Unilateral chorea, localizing neurological features	Structural lesion

TABLE I–2. Laboratory Evaluation of the Patient with Chorea

TEST	POSSIBLE DIAGNOSIS
Serum glucose and electrolytes	Hyper-/hypoglycemia, hyper-/hyponatremia, hypomagnesemia, hyper-/hypocalcemia
Uric acid	Lesch-Nyhan syndrome
CBC with smear	Neuroacanthocytosis syndrome (ChAc, MLS, HDL2, PKAN)
Liver function tests	Wilson disease, ChAc, MLS, acquired hepatocerebral degeneration
Thyroid function tests	Hypo-/hyperthyroidism
Parathyroid levels	Hypo-/hyperparathyroidism
Pregnancy test	*Chorea gravidarum*
Creatine phosphokinase	ChAc, MLS
Ceruloplasmin	Wilson disease, aceruloplasminemia
Ferritin	Neuroferritinopathy
Sedimentation rate, antinuclear antibodies, anti-DNA, anti-SSA, anti-SSB, anti-Ro, anti-La, etc.	Autoimmune disease
Lupus anticoagulant	Systemic lupus erythematosus
Antiphospholipid antibodies	Antiphospholipid syndrome

TABLE 1–2. (continued)

TEST	POSSIBLE DIAGNOSIS
Anti-streptolysin O, anti-DNase B titers	Sydenham chorea
HIV test	HIV-/AIDS-related infection
Antigliadin antibodies	Celiac disease
Antineuronal antibodies (anti-CRMP-5/CV2, anti-Hu, anti-NMDA receptor, anti-Yo)	Paraneoplastic syndromes
Alpha-fetoprotein	Ataxia-telangiectasia, ataxia with oculomotor apraxia 2
Cholesterol	Ataxia with oculomotor apraxia 1, 2
Plasma/CSF lactate/pyruvate	Mitochondrial and other energy metabolism disorders
Erythrocyte Kx and Kell antigens	MLS
Genetic testing	(see Tables 1–3 and 1–4)
MRI (including gradient echo sequence for iron)/CT + contrast	Structural lesions, iron deposition, calcification
EEG	Seizure-related syndrome, Creutzfeldt-Jakob disease
Lumbar puncture	Creutzfeldt-Jakob disease, chronic infection, lactate/pyruvate for mitochondrial and other energy metabolism disorders
Urinary and serum organic and amino acids	Organic/aminoacidopathies

AIDS, acquired immunodeficiency virus; CBC, complete blood count; ChAc, chorea-acanthocytosis; CSF, cerebrospinal fluid; CT, computed tomography; EEG, electroencephalography; HDL2, Huntington disease-like 2; HIV, human immunodeficiency virus; MLS, McLeod syndrome; MRI, magnetic resonance imaging; PKAN, pantothenate kinase–associated neurodegeneration; SSA/SSB, Sjögren syndrome antigens A and B.

with the same clinical outcome. This vulnerability to a multiplicity of causes suggests a delicate balance of neuronal inputs from direct and indirect pathways to basal ganglia output pathways (Chapter 2).

Several years ago I was invited to give a talk on chorea by Dr. Kathleen Shannon as part of the movement disorders course at the American Academy of Neurology annual meeting and was given the title "How Can We Know the Dancer from the Dance?" (from W. B. Yeats, "Among School Children"). I realized that the dance in this case reveals relatively little information about the dancer or, more specifically, the cause of the dance. However, knowing more

TABLE 1–3. Molecular Features of Autosomal Dominant Genetic Choreiform Disorders

DIAGNOSIS	GENE	LOCATION	PROTEIN PRODUCT	MUTATION	USEFUL BLOOD TESTS	MOVEMENT DISORDER	OTHER NEUROLOGICAL FEATURES	USUAL AGE AT ONSET
HD	*HTT/IT15*	4p15	Huntingtin	Expanded CAG repeats	—	Chorea, dystonia, parkinsonism	Ataxia, seizures (juvenile onset)	Inv. related to repeats
HDL1	*PRNP*	20p12	Prion protein	192 nucleotide insertion	—	Chorea, rigidity	Seizures (variable)	20–40 years
HDL2	*JPH3*	16q24.3	Junctophilin-3	Expanded CAG/CTG repeats	Acanth. +/–	Chorea, dystonia parkinsonism	Hyperreflexia	Inv. related to repeats
Spinocerebellar ataxia 1	*ATXN1*	6p23	Ataxin-1	Expanded CAG repeats	—	Chorea, dystonia	Ataxia, supranuclear ophthalmoplegia	Inv. related to repeats
Spinocerebellar ataxia 2	*ATXN2*	12q24	Ataxin-2	Expanded CAG repeats	—	Chorea, dystonia, parkinsonism, tremor	Ataxia, supranuclear ophthalmoplegia	Inv. related to repeats
Spinocerebellar ataxia 3	*ATXN3*	14q32.1	Ataxin-3	Expanded CAG repeats	—	Chorea, dystonia parkinsonism	Ataxia	Inv. related to repeats
Spinocerebellar ataxia 17	*TBP*	6q.27	TATA-binding protein	Expanded CAA/CAG repeats	—	Chorea, dystonia parkinsonism	Ataxia, hyperreflexia	Inv. related to repeats
DRPLA	*DRPLA/ATN1*	12p13.31	Atrophin-1	Expanded CAG repeats	—	Chorea, myoclonus	Ataxia, seizures	Inv. related to repeats

Disease	Gene	Locus	Protein	Mutation	Biomarker	Movement disorder	Other features	Age of onset
Benign hereditary chorea	TITF-1 (NKX2.1), other	14q13.1	Thyroid transcription factor 1, other	Transversions, deletions, substitutions	—	Chorea	Mild ataxia	Childhood
Neuroferritin-opathy	FTL	19q13.3	Ferritin light chain	Adenine insertion	Serum ferritin	Chorea, dystonia, parkinsonism	Spasticity, rigidity	40–55 years
Paroxysmal kinesogenic dyskinesia	EKD1, EKD2, EKD3	16p11-q12 16q13-22.1 other	—	—	—	Chorea, dystonia	(seizures in ICCA)	Childhood
Paroxysmal nonkinesogenic dyskinesia	MR-1	2q33	Myofibrillogenesis regulator	Missense	—	Chorea, dystonia	—	Childhood
Paroxysmal exertional dyskinesia	SLC2A1	1p34.2	Glucose transporter GLUT1	Deletion, missense	Low CSF glucose	Chorea, dystonia	Seizures	Childhood
Paroxysmal choreoathetosis/ episodic ataxia	KCNA1	12p13, other	Potassium channel	Point mutation	—	Chorea, dystonia	Ataxia, myokymia, dysarthria	Childhood
Paroxysmal choreoathetosis/ spasticity	—	1p.21-p13.3	Potassium channels?	—	—	Chorea, dystonia	Spasticity, dysarthria	Childhood

Acanth., acanthocytosis; CSF, cerebrospinal fluid; DPRLA, dentatorubropallidoluysian atrophy; HD, Huntington disease; HDL1, Huntington disease-like 1; HDL2, Huntington disease-like 2; ICCA, benign infantile convulsions and paroxysmal choreoathetosis; inv. inversely.

TABLE 1–4. Molecular Features of Autosomal Recessive, X-Linked, and Mitochondrial Choreiform Disorders

DIAGNOSIS	MODE OF INHERITANCE	GENE	LOCATION	PROTEIN PRODUCT	MUTATION	USEFUL BLOOD TESTS	MOVEMENT DISORDER	OTHER NEUROLOGICAL FEATURES	USUAL AGE AT ONSET
Chorea-acanthocytosis	AR	VPS13A	9q21	Chorein	Many	Acanth., CK, LFTs	Chorea, dystonia, parkin-sonism, od	Seizures, pn, self-mutilation	20–50 years
PKAN	AR	PANK2	20p.13	Pantothenate kinase 2	Deletions, missense mutations	Acanth. +/-	Chorea, dystonia	Spasticity, rigidity, retinal degeneration	Childhood (occ. older)
Infantile neuroaxonal dystrophy	AR	PLA2G6	22q12-q13	Phospho-lipase A	Many	—	Chorea, dystonia	Ataxia	Childhood
Acerulo-plasminemia	AR	CP	3q23	Ceruloplasmin	Nonsense	Ceruloplasmin, glucose	Chorea, dystonia	Ataxia, retinal degeneration	30–50 years
Wilson disease	AR	ATP7B	13q14.3	Copper-transporting ATPase 2	Many	Ceruloplasmin	Coarse tremor, parkinsonism, dystonia	Psychiatric disease	6–55 years
HDL3	AR	NK	4p15.3	NK	NK	—	Chorea, dystonia	Seizures, spasticity, ataxia	Childhood
Infantile bilateral striatal necrosis	AR, mito-chondrial	NK	19q13.32-13.41, mito-chondrial	—	—	—	Chorea	Dysarthria, pendular nystagmus, oa	Infancy

Ataxia-telangiectasia	AR	*ATM*	11q22.3	Serine-protein kinase ATM	Many	Alpha-fetoprotein	Chorea	Ataxia, oculomotor apraxia, dysarthria	Early childhood
Ataxia with oculomotor apraxia 1	AR	*APTX*	9p13.3	Aprataxin	Many	Hypoalbuminemia, high cholesterol	Chorea, dystonia	Ataxia, oculomotor apraxia, pn	Childhood
Ataxia with oculomotor apraxia 2	AR	*SETX*	9q34	Senataxin	Truncation	Alpha-fetoprotein, high cholesterol	Chorea, dystonia	Ataxia, oculomotor apraxia, pn	Childhood
Friedreich ataxia	AR	*frataxin*	9p13	Frataxin	Trinucleotide expansion, deletion	—	Dystonia, chorea	Ataxia, spasticity, myoclonus	Childhood
Nonketotic hyperglycinemia	AR	Various	Various	Glycine cleavage enzymes	Many	Glycine	Encephalopathy, chorea	Ataxia, ophthalmoplegia	Child/adult
Recessive hereditary methemoglobinemia type II	AR	*DIA1*	22q13-qter	NADPH-cytochrome b_5 reductase	Many	Methemoglobin	Chorea, dystonia	Encephalopathy	Child/adult
Pyruvate dehydrogenase deficiency	AR/X-linked	Various	Various	PDH, various subunits	Many	Lactate, pyruvate	Chorea, dystonia, parkinsonism	Encephalopathy, seizures, pn, ataxia	Child/adult

(continued)

Table 1-4. (continued)

DIAGNOSIS	MODE OF INHERITANCE	GENE	LOCATION	PROTEIN PRODUCT	MUTATION	USEFUL BLOOD TESTS	MOVEMENT DISORDER	OTHER NEUROLOGICAL FEATURES	USUAL AGE AT ONSET
McLeod syndrome	X-linked recessive	*XK*	Xp21	XK	Deletions, missense, insertions	Acanth., Kx/Kell antigens, CK, LFTs	Chorea, dystonia, parkinsonism, od	Seizures, pn, myopathy	40–70 years
Lubag	X-linked recessive	*DYT3*	Xq13.1	Multiple transcript system	Missense, deletions	—	Dystonia, chorea parkinsonism, tremor, myoclonus	—	10–40 years
Lesch-Nyhan syndrome	X-linked recessive	*HPRT*	Xq26-27	Hypoxanthine phospho-ribosyl transferase	Many	Hyperuricemia	Chorea, dystonia	Spasticity, self-mutilation	Infancy
Leigh syndrome	Mitochondrial	Many	Many	Many	Many	Elevated lactate/pyruvate	Chorea, dystonia	Hypotonia, cn, ataxia, seizures	Infancy

Acanth, acanthocytosis; AR, autosomal recessive; CK, creatine kinase; cn, cranial neuropathy; HDL3, Huntington disease-like 3; LFTs, liver function tests; NADPH, nicotinamide adenine dinucleotide phosphate; NK, not known; oa, optic atrophy; od, orofacial dyskinesias; PDH, pyruvate dehydrogenase; PKAN, pantothenate kinase–associated neurodegeneration; pn, peripheral neuropathy.

about the dancer may lead us to the cause of the dance. At present, our therapies focus only upon the dance; but with advances in molecular medicine and in the understanding of basal ganglia physiology, we will ultimately be able to treat the dancer.

Here, I discuss the approach to the patient with chorea, with an emphasis upon the features of the family and medical history, as well as the clinical examination and evaluation, which can lead us to the correct diagnosis. A similar approach specifically directed toward the pediatric patient with chorea is described in Chapter 13. The features of each disease are summarized in each relevant section, with a reference to the chapter where more detail can be found.

In relatively few cases can treatment be directed toward the underlying causes. Our therapies at present are aimed primarily at reducing the involuntary movements (Chapter 22) and other distressing associated features, such as dystonia or psychiatric symptoms (Chapter 20).

FAMILY HISTORY

Inheritance

If present, a positive family history can be very informative in diagnosing the patient with chorea. A clear, or even suggestive, history of autosomal dominant (AD), autosomal recessive (AR), or X-linked recessive inheritance limits the number of disorders which need to be considered.

However, the absence of a family history does not exclude any inherited disorder. In the case of an AD disorder, the family history may be confounded by the death of the carrier parent before disease manifestation. This is especially true of disorders in which there is anticipation, that is, earlier onset with successive generations due to expansion of a trinucleotide repeat, where the symptoms may have been minimal or absent in the parent prior to death. Trinucleotide repeat disorders such as Huntington disease (HD, Chapter 3) may be partially penetrant in subjects with a repeat expansion in the intermediate range. Alternatively, the disorder may not have been recognized in the parent, for example, if there is significant phenotypic variation. A prominent psychiatric component which is often seen in these disorders due to basal ganglia involvement (Chapter 20) may have resulted in long-term care in a setting in which other neurological features were not recognized or were attributed to medications, specifically, tardive dyskinesia.

The issue of nonpaternity should be considered in every genetic counseling situation, including the possibility that this might be unmasked by genetic testing.

De novo mutations are unlikely to cause disorders due to trinucleotide repeat expansions, but other types of mutations, such as deletions or missense mutations, can occur in patients without a family history.

Autosomal Dominant Inheritance

The prototypical AD chorea is HD (Chapter 3). Now that genetic confirmation is available for this diagnosis, it has become apparent that a number of patients with this phenotype, who were previously labeled as having HD, have another disease. A number of disorders are now described (with greater or lesser degrees of accuracy) as being "HD-like (HDL)." Of these, HDL1, HDL2 (Chapter 5), and HDL4 show AD inheritance. HDL1 (Xiang et al., 1998) has been identified as a prion disease (Moore et al., 2001) (Chapter 11), and HDL4 (Richfield et al., 2002) is known to be spinocerebellar ataxia 17 (Chapter 12).

The phenotypes of the AD spinocerebellar ataxias (SCAs) can involve movement disorders attributable to basal ganglia dysfunction in addition to cerebellar neurodegeneration (Chapter 12). These neurodegenerative disorders are in most cases due to expanded trinucleotide repeats involving various proteins. The size of the expansion, however, does not in general appear to correlate with the phenotype. The most common SCA in most populations, SCA3 (Machado-Joseph disease), can present with parkinsonism, dystonia, and chorea, usually in association with the typical cerebellar signs and eye findings. Patients with SCA1, along with the cerebellar findings, may rarely present with or develop chorea during the evolution of the disease (Geschwind et al., 1997; Namekawa et al., 2001). Patients with SCA2 may occasionally develop chorea (Rottnek et al., 2008). A variety of movement disorders may be seen in SCA17, including parkinsonism, dystonia, and chorea (Schneider et al., 2006; Stevanin et al., 2003; Toyoshima et al., 2004; Zuhlke et al., 2003; Zuhlke and Burk, 2007), in addition to the more typical phenotype of ataxia, dementia, and hyperreflexia.

Dentatorubropallidoluysian atrophy (DRPLA) is also a trinucleotide repeat expansion disorder and is found more often in Japanese populations but relatively rarely in Caucasian (Le Ber et al., 2003a; Martins et al., 2003; Wardle et al., 2008; Wardle et al., 2009) or African American (Burke et al., 1994) families (Chapter 12). DRPLA may present with movement disorders, including chorea and myoclonus, although more usual features are ataxia and dementia.

AD inheritance of a disorder with brain iron accumulation on magnetic resonance imaging (MRI) is indicative of neuroferritinopathy (Chapter 9). AD inheritance without progression and minimal cognitive or psychiatric impairment suggests benign hereditary chorea (Chapter 4).

Autosomal Recessive Inheritance

In AR disorders, siblings from the same parents may be affected; however, small family size reduces the chance of there being an affected sibling. Known or possible consanguinity, for example, in geographically or socially isolated communities, guides the investigation toward AR inheritance.

The majority of the inherited pediatric metabolic disorders are due to AR inheritance (Chapters 8, 13) as in most metabolic pathways enzyme levels have to be significantly reduced or absent to result in substrate or by-product accumulation. Atypical forms in which there may be partial residual enzyme activity may present later in life and with different phenotypes from the typical childhood or infantile forms. The clinical presentation is dependent upon the stage of brain maturation and myelination (Chapter 13).

Glutaric aciduria typically presents with generalized dystonia, although chorea is sometimes seen in addition to the other features of encephalopathy (Friedman et al., 2006; Ojwang et al., 2001; Voll et al., 1993) (Chapter 13). Chorea, typically mild, can be seen in propionic acidemia, due to propionic coenzyme A carboxylase deficiency (Sethi et al., 1989; Surtees et al., 1992). Other aminoacidopathies in which chorea may occasionally be seen include 3-methylglutaconic acidemia (Gascon et al., 1994) and succinic semialdehyde dehydrogenase deficiency (Chapter 13).

Pantothenate kinase–associated neurodegeneration (PKAN) (Hartig et al., 2006; Hayflick et al., 2003; Zhou et al., 2001) (Chapter 8) results in a progressive hyperkinetic syndrome due to mutations of pantothenate kinase 2 (*PANK2)* (Zhou et al., 2001). In typical cases the disorder presents during childhood with dystonia, choreoathetosis, and spasticity, and progresses rapidly over the next 10 years (Hayflick et al., 2003).

Chorea has been occasionally reported in Niemann-Pick C (Josephs et al., 2003; Shulman et al., 1995), chronic GM_2 (Oates et al., 1986) and late-onset GM_1 gangliosidoses, neuronal intranuclear inclusion disease, and metachromatic leukodystrophy (Chapter 13).

HDL3 has been reported in a single consanguineous family, where siblings were affected, suggesting AR inheritance (Kambouris et al., 2000). Linkage localized the mutant gene to chromosome 4p15.3, distinct from the HD locus; however, no further studies have been reported.

Friedreich ataxia is a common inherited AR ataxia (Chapter 12) and is usually characterized by onset during childhood and areflexia. Rarely, chorea can be a presenting symptom prior to the development of other features (Hanna et al., 1998; Spacey et al., 2004; Zhu et al., 2002).

The other childhood-onset ataxias, ataxia-telangiectasia (AT), and the ataxias with oculomotor apraxia (AOA) 1 and 2 can result in chorea (Chapter 12). Atypical, later-onset forms of AT have recently been reported (Verhagen et al., 2009), suggesting that this diagnosis should be considered in adults with unusual movement disorders. There is increased risk for malignancy, particularly leukemia and lymphoma, due to impaired DNA repair and to infection due to immunodeficiency. AOA1 (Chapter 12) is the commonest AR ataxia in some populations (Le Ber et al., 2003b; Shahwan et al., 2006). AOA2 is similar in presentation to AOA1.

X-Linked Inheritance

For an X-linked pattern of inheritance to be recognized, the carrier mother needs to have an affected father and possibly affected brothers. Additionally, there should be no transmission of disease from father to son. Female carriers can occasionally be symptomatic for X-linked disorders, due to X-chromosome inactivation.

There are relatively few X-linked causes of chorea. These include McLeod neuroacanthocytosis syndrome (Danek et al., 2001; Symmans et al., 1979) (Chapter 7) and Lesch-Nyhan syndrome (Chapter 13). These should be clearly distinguished from each other by the age of onset and additional neurological features. Rarely, X-linked Filipino dystonia-parkinsonism (lubag) (Lee et al., 1976) can present with chorea.

Pyruvate dehydrogenase deficiency is an X-linked disorder which typically presents in the neonatal period with episodes of hypotonia, encephalopathy, and seizures and later with peripheral and central demyelination (Debray et al., 2008). When symptoms develop at a later age, movement disorders are more likely to be seen, specifically dystonia or chorea (Mellick et al., 2004) (Chapter 13).

Mitochondrial Disorders

Leigh syndrome can be caused by a number of different mutations of mitochondrial DNA and presents in early childhood, although adult-onset presentation has been reported (Goldenberg et al., 2003). In addition to dystonia and chorea, a variety of different neurological signs may be present, including acute encephalopathy, seizures, psychomotor retardation, hypotonia or spasticity, myopathy, and dysarthria. An overlap with mitochondrial encephalopathy with stroke-like episodes (MELAS) may occur (Crimi et al., 2003). Other mitochondrial disorders may also present with chorea (Caer et al., 2005; Morimoto et al., 2004).

Ethnic Background

There are a small number of disorders where the patient's racial and ethnic background can be informative.

Lubag is found solely among Filipinos from the province of Capiz on the island of Panay (Lee et al., 1976). Although parkinsonism and dystonia are typical, chorea can occasionally be seen (Evidente et al., 2002). The typical presentation is in the teens until the mid-40s with focal dystonia (*lubag*, describing the twisting movements, and *wa-eg*, the abnormal sustained postures, in the local Illongo dialect) and parkinsonism (*sud-sud*, named for the shuffling gait) (Evidente et al., 2002). Although mostly males are affected, affected carrier females have occasionally been reported, one of whom had chorea (Evidente et al., 2002, 2004; Waters et al., 1993). Thus, this diagnosis should be considered in any Filipino with any movement disorder so that genetic testing and appropriate counseling can be undertaken (Evidente et al., 2002). The causative gene has been identified as coding for a multiple transcript system whose function is not yet known (Nolte et al., 2003).

HDL2 (Chapter 5) is similar to HD in that it is a trinucleotide expansion disease (Holmes et al., 2001), but it has been reported to date only in people of black

African ancestry (Holmes et al., 2001; Margolis et al., 2001; Rodrigues et al., 2008; Santos et al., 2008; Stevanin et al., 2003). No patients of Caucasian or Asian ancestry have yet been reported (Bauer et al., 2002; Stevanin et al., 2002, 2003). The presence of African ancestry may be obscured by the family and may require haplotype studies to be evident (Santos et al., 2008). The data suggest either a rare common ancestral mutation or a population skewed toward longer alleles prone to expansion in Africans (Bardien et al., 2007). Unlike in HD, where larger trinucleotide expansions cause a distinct parkinsonian phenotype, the relationship between clinical features and size of the trinucleotide repeat expansion at this point remains uncertain (Walker et al., 2003a). However, similar to other trinucleotide disorders, the size of the repeat expansions correlates inversely with the age at onset (Margolis et al., 2004). Acanthocytosis can be seen in approximately 10% of cases, confusing the diagnosis with that of other neuroacanthocytosis syndromes (Walker et al., 2003b).

The trinucleotide repeat disorder DRPLA is much more common in Japanese populations, although it has occasionally been reported in other ethnic groups (Wardle et al., 2009).

FEATURES OF MEDICAL HISTORY

Age at Onset

Infancy/Childhood Onset

Sydenham chorea may present acutely in childhood following streptococcal group A infection (Chapter 17). However, a more insidious onset, particularly in the setting of other neurological abnormalities, favors a diagnosis of AR inheritance of a metabolic disorder (Chapters 8, 13). There are a number of disorders in which a variety of movement disorders may be present. These are typically part of a constellation of neurological abnormalities which may vary with the age at presentation. Dystonia appears to be more common than chorea for the disorders with early onset, possibly due to the coexistence of rigidity or spasticity due to pyramidal tract involvement. AR inheritance of mutations of critical enzymes is the etiology. The diagnosis is made by assaying blood and urine for organic and amino acids, by enzyme assays in lymphocytes, or by genetic testing, as indicated.

Another common etiology of movement disorders in the pediatric population is cerebral palsy. Spastic di- or quadriplegia, due to pre- or perinatal ischemia or periventricular hemorrhage, may evolve to a hyperkinetic disorder in later years. The history of the disorder should be diagnostic. While dystonia is more commonly seen, chorea can also occur and in some cases can be quite violent. This can be precipitated in particular by metabolic stress such as infection and may require general anesthesia or neurosurgical intervention.

Adult Onset

Onset of neurological disease during adulthood is typical for the AD disorders. The age at onset of the trinucleotide repeat disorders varies inversely with the size of the trinucleotide repeat expansion. Most cases present in adulthood, often after the reproductive years; however, young-onset forms are not uncommon, particularly with paternal inheritance.

It is being increasingly recognized that AR disorders can present during adulthood, usually in atypical forms, for example, when the causative mutations result in only partial enzyme deficiency, such as with PKAN (Chapter 8) and AT (Verhagen et al., 2009). In other AR disorders, the cause of the late presentation is not so well understood, for example, in chorea-acanthocytosis (ChAc) (Chapter 6), although it is suspected that initial, subtle psychiatric signs of basal ganglia dysfunction may be present during adolescence. Aceruloplasminemia (Chapter 10) also presents later in life, most likely as symptoms emerge once a critical amount of iron has accumulated in the target organs.

McLeod syndrome (Chapter 7) is an X-linked disorder which characteristically presents in middle-aged men (Danek et al., 2001; Jung et al., 2001), although it may be detected at a younger age if blood typing is performed or serological tests demonstrate elevated levels of creatine kinase or liver enzymes. Occasionally, carrier females have been symptomatic, presumably due to X-chromosome inactivation (Hardie et al., 1991; Jung et al., 2001; Ueyama et al., 2000).

Late Adult Onset

Elderly patients who develop chorea should be thoroughly evaluated for a neoplastic syndrome or for an autoimmune disorder, especially if female (Chapter 18). In the absence of these, HD should be considered a possible diagnosis. Late onset is often associated with CAG repeats in the borderline range, where penetrance is reduced; but instability and expansion with vertical transmission are likely, raising genetic counseling issues. If HD has been excluded, other genetic etiologies may be considered, including HDL2, which can present at later ages with lower pathological repeat sizes (Rodrigues et al., 2008). The entity of "senile chorea" is obsolete as these cases are now recognized as most probably being due to late onset of genetic disorders.

Disease Progression

Acute Onset

As with all neurological disorders, details of disease progression are strongly suggestive of the nature of the diagnosis. Sudden onset of chorea which does not progress indicates a vascular event, either ischemic or hemorrhagic (Chapter 16).

Sudden onset of chorea related to medical illness suggests a causal relationship such as a metabolic (Chapter 15), postinfectious, or autoimmune (Chapter 18) etiology. However, the pediatric inherited metabolic disorders may be unmasked by stresses such as fever, illness, and trauma (Chapter 13), confounding the diagnosis.

A common type of sudden-onset chorea in childhood is Sydenham chorea, seen following a streptococcal throat infection (Chapter 17). Cases usually resolve after a few weeks, but symptoms may be debilitating.

Subacute Onset

Development of chorea over days to weeks may suggest a metabolic process (Chapter 15), such as nonketotic hyperglycemia in a non-insulin-dependent diabetic patient, although these patients can present quite acutely. Other metabolic disorders which present with this time frame include a range of electrolyte disturbances such as hyper- (Sparacio et al., 1976) and hyponatremia (Piccolo et al., 2003; Tang et al., 1981), hyper- (Matsis et al., 1989) and hypocalcemia (Howdle et al., 1979; Topakian et al., 2006), or hypomagnesemia.

Endocrine abnormalities related to thyroid or parathyroid disease may cause chorea (Chapter 15), specifically hyperthyroidism (Fidler et al., 1971; Fischbeck and Layzer, 1979; Lucantoni et al., 1994). Hypo- and hyperparathyroidism have also been associated with chorea, which may be paroxysmal, likely due to disturbances of calcium (Hattori and Yorifuji, 2000; Soffer et al., 1977).

A subacute presentation may be seen with prion diseases, specifically new variant Creutzfeldt-Jakob disease, related to bovine spongiform encephalopathy (Bowen et al., 2000; McKee and Talbot, 2003) (Chapter 11), or with slowly growing mass lesions (Chapter 16).

A similar time course can be seen with paraneoplastic syndromes (Albin et al., 1988; Batchelor et al., 1998; Dorban et al., 2004; Kujawa et al., 2001; Tani et al., 2000; Vernino et al., 2002) (Chapter 18) and has been reported with a variety of tumors, including renal, small cell lung, breast, and Hodgkin and non-Hodgkin lymphoma. The causative autoantibodies include anti-CRMP-5/CV2 (Muehlschlegel et al., 2005; Vernino et al., 2002), anti-Hu (Dorban et al., 2004), anti-Yo (Krolak-Salmon et al., 2006), anti-NMDA receptor, and others.

Chronic Progressive Course

A slow disease course, progressing over a number of years, particularly when accompanied by cognitive or psychiatric findings, is likely to indicate a neurodegenerative process, for example, due to HD (Chapter 3), the AD inherited ataxias (Chapter 12), a neuroacanthocytosis syndrome (Chapters 6, 7), or a neurodegeneration with iron accumulation syndrome (Chapters 8–10).

Chronic Stable Chorea

Choreiform movements which develop gradually but do not progress can sometimes be attributed to use of a medication, either as a direct side effect or as a tardive syndrome (Chapter 14). Benign hereditary chorea (Chapter 4) should also be considered, particularly if there is childhood onset and an AD family history. This condition is due to mutations of thyroid transcription factor 1 (*TITF-1*) (Breedveld et al., 2002; Devos et al., 2006; Mahajnah et al., 2007; Willemsen et al., 2005), also known as *NKX2.1*, although it may be genetically heterogeneous (Bauer et al., 2006). The chorea may respond to L-dopa (Asmus et al., 2005).

A similar, relatively stable, temporal presentation may also be due to auto-immune processes, as in lupus (Font et al., 1998; Watanabe and Onda, 2004), Sjögren syndrome (Venegas et al., 2005), and antiphospholipid antibody syndrome (Chapter 18).

Episodic Chorea

The paroxysmal hyperkinetic disorders are more typically dystonic in nature, and thus, they have been classified with the genetic dystonias, although chorea can be a component (Chapter 19). The diagnosis of these disorders was previously based upon their phenomenology and precipitating factors, but this is being replaced by molecular identification. Many appear to be due to mutations of ion channels and to respond to anticonvulsants. More rarely, episodic chorea may be psychogenic in etiology (Chapter 21).

Paroxysmal nonkinesigenic dyskinesia (paroxysmal dystonic choreoathetosis, DYT8) is due to a mutation of the myofibrillogenesis regulator gene located at 2q33 (Friedman et al., 2008; Rainier et al., 2004), which may be involved in detoxifying alcohol and caffeine (Lee et al., 2004). Episodes of dystonia and/or chorea typically occur at rest and may be precipitated by alcohol, caffeine, stress, extremes of temperature, fatigue, or fasting. Episodes are much less frequent than those of paroxysmal kinesigenic dyskinesia, and only a few may occur in a month; but they tend to be more long-lasting and severe.

Paroxysmal choreoathetosis with spasticity (DYT9) has been localized to 1p.21-p13.3 (Auburger et al., 1996). Episodes in these patients were precipitated by exercise, stress, alcohol consumption, and sleep deprivation and consisted of dystonia, choreoatherosis, and dysarthria. Spasticity also occurs and can persist between attacks.

Paroxysmal kinesigenic dyskinesia (PKD; paroxysmal kinesigenic dystonia, DYT10) of childhood onset may be familial or sporadic and is characterized by very frequent, brief episodes of limb dystonia following movement. Episodes often resolve with age. Treatment with anticonvulsants is usually beneficial (Chatterjee et al., 2002; Huang et al., 2005; Picard et al., 1998; Tsao, 2004), suggesting a channelopathy. Other cases are associated with features such as seizures (Cuenca-Leon et al., 2002; Thiriaux et al., 2002) and have been termed "benign infantile convulsions and paroxysmal choreoathetosis" (Szepetowski et al., 1997).

Paroxysmal exertional dyskinesia (DYT18) is an intermediate form with involuntary movements developing following more prolonged exertion than PKD, which can last from minutes to hours. This syndrome is one of several neurological conditions, including seizures, due to mutations of the glucose transporter GLUT1 (Suls et al., 2008; Weber et al., 2008).

Patients with episodic ataxia 1 may sometimes manifest choreoathetosis during ataxic episodes (Gancher and Nutt, 1986). More typical features are dysarthria and persistent myokymia (Litt et al., 1994; Lubbers et al., 1995). Treatment with acetazolamide can be helpful.

Medical History

The medical history may be informative in the patient with chorea. In pediatric cases nonneurological features can be very helpful in indicating a specific inherited metabolic disorder (Chapter 13).

Patients with endocrine disorders, especially diabetic patients with nonketotic hyperglycemia (Chapter 15), and autoimmune disorders (Chapter 18) may develop chorea, in some cases as the presenting symptom. Patients with aceruloplasminemia typically have diabetes mellitus due to deposition of iron in the pancreas (Chapter 10). One-third of patients with Friedreich ataxia also develop diabetes, which is thought to be due to mitochondrial dysfunction (Chapter 12).

Women of childbearing age should be evaluated for pregnancy (*chorea gravidarum*) or may develop chorea related to estrogen-/progesterone-containing medications (Caviness and Muenter, 1991; Miranda et al., 2004; Nausieda et al., 1979; Suchowersky and Muthipeedika, 2005). Hormone replacement therapy may similarly be responsible, possibly due to sensitization of dopamine receptors by estrogens. However, contradictorily, suppression of estrogen with luteinizing hormone–releasing hormone may also result in chorea (Gironell et al., 2008).

The gene identified as causing benign hereditary chorea has been reported as part of a multisystem disorder due to a mutation of the gene *TITF-1* (Breedveld et al., 2002; Devos et al., 2006; Mahajnah et al., 2007; Willemsen et al., 2005), which causes congenital hypothyroidism, hypotonia, and pulmonary problems (Doyle et al., 2004; Ferrara et al., 2008; Glik et al., 2008; Krude et al., 2002) (Chapter 4). Correction of the hypothyroidism did not prevent development of the other features, including the chorea, suggesting that these were primary effects of the mutation rather than secondary to the hypothyroidism. Differences in the mutations in these two disorders may account for the varying severity.

Polycythemia vera may be a cause of chorea (Cohen et al., 1989; Nazabal et al., 2000), although it is unclear whether this is due to the presence of autoantibodies or to hyperviscosity resulting in basal ganglia ischemia.

Celiac disease has been associated with a number of neurological complications, most likely due to an autoimmune mechanism. Chorea may occasionally respond to a gluten-free diet (Pereira et al., 2004).

Patients with hepatic disease and chorea should be evaluated for the only treatable genetic movement disorder, Wilson disease. Chorea may occasionally be seen

(Machado et al., 2006) but is not commonly reported as a presenting symptom. More typically, there is an asymmetric, coarse flapping tremor present at rest, with posture holding or with action. Dystonia, parkinsonism, and ataxia can be seen. A thorough evaluation is required, including ophthalmological slit-lamp examination. It is unusual for patients to present with neurological disease in the absence of hepatic findings. Ceruloplasmin levels are typically decreased but may be deceptively raised as it is an acute-phase reactant. Twenty-four-hour copper excretion is elevated. Rarely, Kayser-Fleischer rings may be absent in late-onset disease (Ross et al., 1985). If ceruloplasmin and 24-hour copper excretion are normal, hepatosplenomegaly in a patient with chorea suggests a neuroacantho-cytosis syndrome, either ChAc (Rampoldi et al., 2002; Walker et al., 2006a) (Chapter 6) or McLeod syndrome (Rampoldi et al., 2002) (Chapter 7). Liver disease due to a variety of etiologies may also cause acquired hepatocerebral degeneration, likely due to manganese deposition in the basal ganglia, which may be seen in brain MRI.

A condition of poorly-defined etiology known as "post-pump chorea" may occur in children after undergoing open-heart surgery or cardiopulmonary bypass. This may be due to microemboli or a hyperviscosity syndrome and appears to reduce in incidence with improvements in technology and experience (Menache et al., 2002) (Chapter 13).

Cardiac disease, specifically cardiomyopathy, is frequently found in Friedreich ataxia (Chapter 12). Similar findings, along with arrhythmias, are seen in McLeod syndrome (Chapter 7).

In children with acute onset of chorea, evaluation for a recent upper respiratory tract infection by streptococcus group A, in consideration of Sydenham chorea (Chapter 17), is essential. However, much more rarely, striatal necrosis may occur as a complication of measles encephalitis (Cambonie et al., 2000) or following undefined febrile illness (Yamamoto et al., 1997). A similar picture can be seen after *Mycoplasma pneumoniae* infection (Zambrino et al., 2000), with a mixture of chorea and dystonia, hyperreflexia, and encephalopathy. Chorea has also been reported in the setting of encephalopathy due to parvoviral infection (Fong and de Sousa, 2006) and following herpes simplex encephalitis (Kullnat and Morse, 2008).

Abnormal susceptibility to infection and a predilection to develop cancers is seen in AT (Chapter 12). The gene for chronic granulomatous disease is adjacent to the gene for McLeod syndrome on the X chromosome. With improved therapies for the chronic, recurrent infections to which these boys are susceptible, it is likely that some of them with large X-chromosome deletions could later develop McLeod syndrome.

A variety of movement disorders including chorea have been associated with human immunodeficiency viral (HIV) infection (Tse et al., 2004). Sometimes these are due to a mass lesion, such as lymphoma or abscess (Chapter 16), whereas in other cases they may be a direct result of HIV encephalopathy (Passarin et al., 2005; Sporer et al., 2005).

Chorea has been reported following correction of hyponatremia causing central pontine myelinolysis (Tison et al., 1991).

Medical findings suggestive of cancer, such as weight loss, lymphadenopathy, chronic cough, and change in bowel habit, may be indicative of a paraneoplastic syndrome (Chapter 18), although the absence of these does not rule out this diagnosis as tumor growth may be suppressed by the autoantibodies which are responsible for the paraneoplastic syndromes.

Medication and Drug Use

A number of medications may cause chorea (Chapter 14), either as a direct, and often predictable, function of their action, as seen following L-dopa in Parkinson disease, or as a side effect.

The effects of specific medications may suggest a relationship to the pathophysiology of chorea in other conditions, as information from animal models of L-dopa-induced dyskinesias may be used to further our understanding of mechanisms in other hyperkinetic disorders. The etiology of L-dopa-induced dyskinesias in Parkinson disease, namely, an increase in dopaminergic stimulation within the putamen, can be inferred from the relationship to dosing with dopaminergic medications. However, to date, alterations have been observed in a large number of parameters related to different neurotransmitters involved in striatal functioning, and agents with a variety of mechanisms of actions have been reported to reduce dyskinesias in animal models (Blandini, 2003; Brotchie et al., 2005; Monville et al., 2005; Papa and Chase, 1996).

Tardive dyskinesia (TD) is more accurately described as "chorea" and appears after an interval of 3 months following the initiation of a dopamine-blocking medication (Chapter 14). In addition to the classic neuroleptics, TD has been reported with the atypical antipsychotics, including risperidone (Harrison and Goa, 2004) and olanzapine (Bella and Piccoli, 2003; Bressan et al., 2004). The newer agents quetiapine, clozapine, aripiprazole, and ziprasidone may occasionally cause TD. Other dopaminergic antagonists, such as compazine and metoclopramide, may also be responsible.

The timing of the emergence of the symptoms and the fact that TD often does not resolve (and may even worsen) with discontinuation of the medication make it hard to confirm or refute the association of other medications with this disorder, but selective serotonin reuptake inhibitors (SSRIs), lithium, and anticonvulsant medications have also been implicated.

Chorea may be seen as a direct side effect of other medications, including gabapentin (Lai et al., 2008; Twardowschy et al., 2008; Zesiewicz et al., 2008), lamotrigine (Miller and Levsky, 2008), and lithium (Stemper et al., 2003).

Stimulants in particular, including those used therapeutically (Weiner et al., 1978) as well as those used recreationally, such as amphetamine, cocaine, and specifically "crack" cocaine, may result in chorea ("crack-dancing"). The mechanism of action of these agents, namely the release of dopamine, is probably the explanation for the appearance of the movement disorder. Usually the timing and the resolution of the movements with discontinuation of the offending agent make the diagnosis and treatment straightforward.

ASSOCIATED NEUROLOGICAL FEATURES

Distribution of Chorea

Chorea typically looks identical regardless of the etiology. The exceptions to this are when the facial and lingual muscles are markedly involved or when there is asymmetric involvement of the limbs.

Facial muscles alone are most commonly affected in neuroleptic-induced TD. Prominent orofacial and lingual involvement can be seen in ChAc and PKAN. In ChAc the tongue movements are dystonic and specifically induced by eating (Chapter 6).

Structural lesions are a common cause of unilateral chorea in adults, often due to a focal lesion involving the basal ganglia (Chapter 16). Another cause may be non-ketotic hyperglycemia, which is typically unilateral, for unknown reasons (Chapter 15).

Peripheral Neuropathy

Hyporeflexia and peripheral sensory changes suggestive of a peripheral neuropathic process are characteristic of the two core neuroacanthocytosis syndromes, ChAc (Rampoldi et al., 2002; Walker et al., 2006a,b) and McLeod syndrome. The other disorders in which peripheral neuropathy may be present in addition to chorea are some of the inherited ataxias, both AR (Friedreich ataxia [Hanna et al., 1998; Spacey et al., 2004; Zhu et al., 2002], AOA1 [Le Ber et al., 2003b; Shahwan et al., 2006], and AOA2 [Moreira et al., 2004]) and AD (SCA 1, 2 and 3 [Geschwind et al., 1997; Namekawa et al., 2001]) (Chapter 12).

Hyperreflexia

Hyperreflexia is seen in neurodegenerative disorders in which the cortex is also affected, for example, HD, HDL2, and the SCAs. Reflex asymmetry may serve to localize a focal lesion.

Ataxia

Ataxia and abnormal eye movements also suggest the inherited ataxias, which may be both AD and AR in inheritance (Chapter 12). Ataxia and hyperreflexia suggest SCA17 (Schneider et al., 2006; Stevanin et al., 2003; Zuhlke et al., 2003; Zuhlke and Burk, 2007) and DRPLA. However, the phenotype may be remarkably variable, both within and between families, and ataxia may be absent.

Cognitive and Psychiatric Symptoms

Neurodegenerative causes of chorea are frequently associated with personality changes, subcortical dementia, and frank psychiatric disease (Chapter 20). This may be due to degenerative processes affecting the frontal cortex but also to involvement of the caudate nucleus in cortical–subcortical loops. These findings are being increasingly recognized as harbingers of frank neurological disease and can often be detected even when subtle by detailed neuropsychological testing.

The use of neuroleptics for psychiatric symptoms preceding the appearance of a movement disorder may mask the diagnosis as neurological signs and symptoms may be erroneously attributed to the medication. Psychiatrists should be attuned to any atypical features of either psychiatric or neurological presentations.

Ophthalmological Findings

Abnormal eye movements are found in chorea of a variety of etiologies, including HD and ChAc, with intrusions of square-wave jerks. Impaired smooth pursuit and saccadic gaze, or ophthalmoplegia, may suggest a cerebellar disorder (Chapter 12).

Pigmentary retinopathy is indicative of PKAN and is an invariable feature of typical (young-onset) disease (Chapter 8). The characteristic telangiectactic blood vessels seen in the conjunctivae of the eye may be helpful in making the diagnosis of AT but may be absent in atypical, late-onset disease (Verhagen et al., 2009) (Chapter 12).

Other local ophthalmological findings may indicate autoimmune disease (Chapter 18).

Seizures

Seizures are seen in approximately 50% of patients with a neuroacanthocytosis syndrome (Chapters 6, 7). These can predate the appearance of the movement disorder by several years. Seizures can also be present in young-onset HD, although these patients tend to have an akinetic-rigid phenotype rather than chorea. Younger-onset patients with DRPLA tend to present with seizures, although in these cases chorea is less prominent than ataxia (Wardle et al., 2009). Older-onset patients with chorea may develop seizures later in the disease course.

Myoclonus

Myoclonus is a frequent finding in prion diseases (Chapter 11) and in DRPLA affecting younger patients.

DIAGNOSTIC TESTS

Neuroimaging

Patients with chorea should always undergo neuroimaging, ideally brain MRI, preferably with contrast to exclude the presence of a space-occupying lesion (Table 1–2). Vascular etiologies may include stroke, vasculitides, moya-moya disease, cavernous angioma, and arteriovenous malformation (Chapter 16). Rarely, movement disorders, including chorea, may be seen in multiple sclerosis (Roos et al., 1991).

Atrophy of the head of the caudate nucleus is seen in the basal ganglia neuro-degenerative disorders and is usually interpreted as being consistent with a diagnosis of HD, although this finding is not specific to this genetic cause.

The basal ganglia, and particularly the globus pallidus, are vulnerable to mineral deposition, probably due to high metabolic demands. The neuroradiological finding of calcium deposition in the brain, known as Fahr disease, may cause a variety of movement disorders, including chorea, dystonia, and parkinsonism, in addition to ataxia, cognitive impairment, and behavioral changes. The movement disorder may be due to the structural lesion caused by calcium deposition in the putamen (Chapter 16) but could also be attributable to metabolic effects upon neurotransmission (Chapter 15). The term "Fahr disease" is nonspecific and describes a number of different disorders, including those of calcium and mitochondrial metabolism. In one family, with idiopathic basal ganglia calcification (IBGC), linkage was demonstrated to 14q (IBGC1) (Geschwind et al., 1999), although the gene has not yet been identified. In several other families with AD inheritance, linkage to this locus was excluded (Brodaty et al., 2002; Oliveira et al., 2004; Wszolek et al., 2006). In other families the pattern of inheritance and additional clinical features suggest mitochondrial inheritance (Reske-Nielsen et al., 1988; Younes-Mhenni et al., 2002).

Abnormal brain iron accumulation is seen in a number of disorders due to a variety of different genetic mutations, known collectively as "neurodegeneration with brain iron accumulation" (NBIA). This term includes AD-inherited neuroferritin-opathy (Crompton et al., 2004; Mir et al., 2004; Wills et al., 2002) (Chapter 9), PKAN (Hartig et al., 2006; Hayflick et al., 2003) (Chapter 8), aceruloplasminemia (Miyajima, 2003; Xu et al., 2004) (Chapter 10), and mutations of *PLA2G6* (Gregory et al., 2008; Morgan et al., 2006; Mubaidin et al., 2003) (Chapter 8). The signature MRI finding in all these disorders, due to iron deposition in the basal ganglia, is the "eye-of-the-tiger," although there may be some variation in the different disorders (McNeill et al., 2008).

Infantile bilateral striatal necrosis, with onset in infancy of chorea and or dystonia, may be inherited in an AR manner (Basel-Vanagaite et al., 2004) but also appears to be due to mitochondrial mutations (De Meirleir et al., 1995). The diagnostic findings are of bilateral lesions in the striatum.

Although it is usually accepted that chorea originates in a disruption of basal ganglia pathways, cases of reversible chorea associated with herniated cervical discs have been reported (Tan et al., 2002).

Serological Tests

The presence of anti-streptolysin O antibodies supports the diagnosis of Sydenham chorea, as does the presence of anti-DNase B (Chapter 17).

Various autoantibodies can be tested for to support the diagnosis of autoimmune diseases such as systemic lupus erythematosis, antiphospholipid antibody syndrome, and Sjögren syndrome which can be associated with chorea (Chapter 18).

If indicated, serum and cerebrospinal fluid can be tested for the presence of autoantibodies due to neoplasm (Chapter 18). If these are found or if there is a high degree of suspicion for a neoplasm, patients should undergo computed tomographic (CT) scanning of the thorax, abdomen, and pelvis. Sometimes, for example, with ovarian teratomas, neoplasms are detected only following exploratory surgery.

The finding of elevated levels of serum liver enzymes raises the suspicion of Wilson disease, although chorea is a rare finding (Machado et al., 2006). If ceruloplasmin and 24-hour copper excretion are normal, abnormal liver enzymes in a patient with chorea suggest a neuroacanthocytosis syndrome, either ChAc (Rampoldi et al., 2002; Walker et al., 2006a,b) (Chapter 6) or McLeod syndrome (Rampoldi et al., 2002) (Chapter 7).

Elevated creatine kinase is typical of either of the neuroacanthocytosis syndromes due to myopathy. This may be high (often into the thousands), and frank myopathy is common, especially in McLeod syndrome (Danek et al., 2001; Hewer et al., 2007; Kawakami et al., 1999). This may occasionally result in rhabdomyolysis (Jung and Brandner, 2002).

In addition to Wilson disease, markedly reduced ceruloplasmin may be found in aceruloplasminemia (Chapter 10). It is also helpful to check ferritin levels as they can be reduced in neuroferritinopathy (Chapter 9).

Serum alpha-fetoprotein (AFP) levels may be elevated in AT (Chapter 12) and help to distinguish this disorder from other childhood-onset ataxias. However, atypical forms have recently been reported; thus, this may be a useful screening test for adults with unusual movement disorders (Verhagen et al., 2009).

Hypoalbuminemia (Shimazaki et al., 2002) and elevated cholesterol (Le Ber et al., 2003b) can be seen in AOA1 (Chapter 12). Findings of elevated cholesterol, creatine kinase, and AFP support the diagnosis, although AFP levels are typically lower than those seen in AT (Le Ber et al., 2004; Moreira et al., 2004).

Peripheral Blood Smear

"Acanthocytosis" refers to the finding of contracted thorny erythrocytes on peripheral blood smear. The term "neuroacanthocytosis" encompasses a group of disorders which is genetically and phenotypically heterogeneous (Walker et al., 2006a) and may be used to refer to disorders of lipoproteins and consequent vitamin E deficiency, including AR abetalipoproteinemia (Bassen-Kornzweig disease) and AD hypobetalipoproteinemia (Brin, 1993). Movement disorders are not seen in these disorders, but patients develop a peripheral neuropathy and ataxia. Acanthocytosis can also occasionally be seen in a number of other metabolic conditions, including nutritional deficiency and hepatic, renal, and thyroid disease.

The presence of acanthocytes suggests, but is not necessary for the diagnosis of, the core neuroacanthocytosis syndromes, namely, AR ChAc (Chapter 6) or X-linked recessive McLeod syndrome (Chapter 7). However, acanthocytes can be found in approximately 10% of cases of PKAN (Hayflick et al., 2003) (Chapter 8) and HDL2 (Walker et al., 2003b) (Chapter 5), which can confound the diagnosis.

The presence of acanthocytosis may vary over time (Klempir et al., 2008; Sorrentino et al., 1999) for reasons which are not understood and may not be detected even with repeated testing, despite utilization of a sensitive protocol (Storch et al., 2005). In this circumstance the serum enzymes mentioned earlier may be more informative.

Erythrocyte Phenotyping

Erythrocyte antigen phenotyping should be performed if the diagnosis of McLeod syndrome is suspected (Chapter 7). "McLeod phenotype" refers to the specific profile of the red blood cell (RBC) Kell and Kx antigens which is associated with the clinical syndrome (Allen et al., 1961). Twenty-six antigens are expressed on the RBC membrane, and Kell is the third most important of these after blood groups ABO and rhesus. Mutations of the *XK* gene result in absent or dysfunctional XK protein and absent or markedly reduced expression of the Kx antigen on the RBC membrane. As the XK protein is linked to the Kell protein via a disulfide bond, Kell antigen expression is also affected (Russo et al., 1998). Patients thus have absent Kx and reduced Kell antigen expression. Testing for these antigens requires a panel of anti-Kx and anti-Kell antibodies and is usually performed at regional blood banks, which should be asked explicitly to exclude McLeod phenotype.

The clinical importance of this antigen profile is that transfusion with heterologous blood, with normal expression of Kx and Kell antigens, may result in production of anti-Kell antibodies, which may cause massive hemolysis with any subsequent heterologous transfusions.

Electroencephalography

Electroencephalography may be informative in identifying disorders in which myoclonus and seizures co-occur with chorea. These include prion diseases, DRPLA, and the core neuroacanthocytosis syndromes.

CONCLUSION

The clinical syndrome of chorea appears to be a final common pathway for disruptions of basal ganglia function due to a wide variety of etiologies. While some of these are destructive, others merely interfere with normal neurotransmission with an identical effect upon neurological functioning (Chapter 2). The list of potential investigations of the patient with chorea continues to grow as more genetic etiologies are discovered and as the range of phenotypes for identified genetic disorders continues to expand. Increased awareness is essential for correct diagnosis and is indicated for appropriate genetic counseling. With advances in molecular medicine, we anticipate that treatment for the disorders which are of genetic etiology will eventually be more than merely symptomatic.

REFERENCES

Albin RL, Bromberg MB, Penney JB, et al. (1988) Chorea and dystonia: a remote effect of carcinoma. Mov Disord 3:162–169.

Allen FH, Krabbe SM, Corcoran PA (1961) A new phenotype (McLeod) in the Kell blood-group system. Vox Sang 6:555–560.

Asmus F, Horber V, Pohlenz J, et al. (2005) A novel TITF-1 mutation causes benign hereditary chorea with response to levodopa. Neurology 64:1952–1954.

Auburger G, Ratzlaff T, Lunkes A, et al. (1996) A gene for autosomal dominant paroxysmal choreoathetosis/spasticity (CSE) maps to the vicinity of a potassium channel gene cluster on chromosome 1p, probably within 2 cM between D1S443 and D1S197. Genomics 31:90–94.

Bardien S, Abrahams F, Soodyall H, et al. (2007) A South African mixed ancestry family with Huntington disease-like 2: clinical and genetic features. Mov Disord 22:2083–2089.

Basel-Vanagaite L, Straussberg R, Ovadia H, et al. (2004) Infantile bilateral striatal necrosis maps to chromosome 19q. Neurology 62:87–90.

Batchelor TT, Platten M, Palmer-Toy DE, et al. (1998) Chorea as a paraneoplastic complication of Hodgkin's disease. J.Neurooncol. 36:185–190.

Bauer I, Gencik M, Laccone F, et al. (2002) Trinucleotide repeat expansions in the junctophilin-3 gene are not found in Caucasian patients with a Huntington's disease-like phenotype. Ann Neurol 51:662.

Bauer P, Kreuz FR, Burk K, et al. (2006) Mutations in TITF1 are not relevant to sporadic and familial chorea of unknown cause. Mov Disord 21:1734–1737.

Bella VL, Piccoli F (2003) Olanzepine-induced tardive dyskinesia. Br J Psychiatry 182: 81–82.

Blandini F (2003) Adenosine receptors and L-DOPA-induced dyskinesia in Parkinson's disease: potential targets for a new therapeutic approach. Exp Neurol 184:556–560.

Bowen J, Mitchell T, Pearce R, et al. (2000) Chorea in new variant Creutzfeldt-Jacob disease. Mov Disord 15:1284–1285.

Breedveld GJ, van Dongen JW, Danesino C, et al. (2002) Mutations in *TITF-1* are associated with benign hereditary chorea. Hum Mol Genet 11:971–979.

Bressan RA, Jones HM, Pilowsky LS (2004) Atypical antipsychotic drugs and tardive dyskinesia: relevance of D2 receptor affinity. J Psychopharmacol 18:124–127.

Brin MF (1993) Acanthocytosis. In: Vinken PJ, Bruyn GW, Klawans HL (eds.) Handbook of Clinical Neurology: Systemic Diseases, Part I. Elsevier, Amsterdam, pp 271–299.

Brodaty H, Mitchell P, Luscombe G, et al. (2002) Familial idiopathic basal ganglia calcification (Fahr's disease) without neurological, cognitive and psychiatric symptoms is not linked to the IBGC1 locus on chromosome 14q. Hum Genet 110:8–14.

Brotchie JM, Lee J, Venderova K (2005) Levodopa-induced dyskinesia in Parkinson's disease. J Neural Transm 112:359–391.

Burke JR, Wingfield MS, Lewis KE, et al. (1994) The Haw River syndrome: dentatorubropallidoluysian atrophy (DRPLA) in an African-American family. Nat Genet 7: 521–524.

Caer M, Viala K, Levy R, et al. (2005) Adult-onset chorea and mitochondrial cytopathy. Mov Disord 20:490–492.

Cambonie G, Houdon L, Rivier F, et al. (2000) Infantile bilateral striatal necrosis following measles. Brain Dev 22:221–223.

Caviness JN, Muenter MD (1991) An unusual cause of recurrent chorea. Mov Disord 6: 355–357.

Chatterjee A, Louis ED, Frucht S (2002) Levetiracetam in the treatment of paroxysmal kinesiogenic choreoathetosis. Mov Disord 17:614–615.

Cohen AM, Gelvan A, Yarmolovsky A, et al. (1989) Chorea in polycythemia vera: a rare presentation of hyperviscosity. Blut 58:47–48.

Crimi M, Galbiati S, Moroni I, et al. (2003) A missense mutation in the mitochondrial *ND5* gene associated with a Leigh-MELAS overlap syndrome. Neurology 60:1857–1861.

Crompton DE, Chinnery PF, Bates D, et al. (2004) Spectrum of movement disorders in neuroferritinopathy. Mov Disord 20:95–99.

Cuenca-Leon E, Cormand B, Thomson T, et al. (2002) Paroxysmal kinesigenic dyskinesia and generalized seizures: clinical and genetic analysis in a Spanish pedigree. Neuropediatrics 33:288–293.

Danek A, Rubio JP, Rampoldi L, et al. (2001) McLeod neuroacanthocytosis: genotype and phenotype. Ann Neurol 50:755–764.

Debray FG, Lambert M, Gagne R, et al. (2008) Pyruvate dehydrogenase deficiency presenting as intermittent isolated acute ataxia. Neuropediatrics 39:20–23.

De Meirleir L, Seneca S, Lissens W, et al. (1995) Bilateral striatal necrosis with a novel point mutation in the mitochondrial *ATPase 6* gene. Pediatr Neurol 13:242–246.

Devos D, Vuillaume I, De Becdelievre A, et al. (2006) New syndromic form of benign hereditary chorea is associated with a deletion of *TITF-1* and *PAX-9* contiguous genes. Mov Disord 21:2237–2240.

Dorban S, Gille M, Kessler R, et al. (2004) Chorea-athetosis in the anti-Hu syndrome [in French]. Rev Neurol (Paris) 160:126–129.

Doyle DA, Gonzalez I, Thomas B, et al. (2004) Autosomal dominant transmission of congenital hypothyroidism, neonatal respiratory distress, and ataxia caused by a mutation of NKX2-1. J Pediatr 145:190–193.

Evidente VG, Advincula J, Esteban R, et al. (2002) Phenomenology of "lubag" or X-linked dystonia-parkinsonism. Mov Disord 17:1271–1277.

Evidente VG, Nolte D, Niemann S, et al. (2004) Phenotypic and molecular analyses of X-linked dystonia-parkinsonism ("lubag") in women. Arch Neurol 61:1956–1959.

Ferrara AM, De Michele G, Salvatore E, et al. (2008) A novel NKX2.1 mutation in a family with hypothyroidism and benign hereditary chorea. Thyroid 18:1005–1009.

Fidler SM, O'Rourke RA, Buchsbaum HW (1971) Choreoathetosis as a manifestation of thyrotoxicosis. Neurology 21:55–57.

Fischbeck KH, Layzer RB (1979) Paroxysmal choreoathetosis associated with thyrotoxicosis. Ann Neurol 6:453–454.

Fong CY, de Sousa C (2006) Childhood chorea-encephalopathy associated with human parvovirus B19 infection. Dev Med Child Neurol 48:526–528.

Font J, Cervera R, Espinosa G, et al. (1998) Systemic lupus erythematosus (SLE) in childhood: analysis of clinical and immunological findings in 34 patients and comparison with SLE characteristics in adults. Ann Rheum Dis 57:456–459.

Friedman A, Zakrzewska-Pniewska B, Domitrz I, et al. (2008) Paroxysmal non-kinesigenic dyskinesia caused by the mutation of MR-1 in a large Polish kindred. Eur Neurol 61: 39–41.

Friedman JR, Thiele EA, Wang D, et al. (2006) Atypical GLUT1 deficiency with prominent movement disorder responsive to ketogenic diet. Mov Disord 21:241–245.

Gancher ST, Nutt JG (1986) Autosomal dominant episodic ataxia: a heterogeneous syndrome. Mov Disord 1:239–253.

Gascon GG, Ozand PT, Brismar J (1994) Movement disorders in childhood organic acidurias. Clinical, neuroimaging, and biochemical correlations. Brain Dev 16(Suppl):94–103.

Geschwind DH, Loginov M, Stern JM (1999) Identification of a locus on chromosome 14q for idiopathic basal ganglia calcification (Fahr disease). Am J Hum Genet 65:764–772.

Geschwind DH, Perlman S, Figueroa CP, et al. (1997) The prevalence and wide clinical spectrum of the spinocerebellar ataxia type 2 trinucleotide repeat in patients with autosomal dominant cerebellar ataxia. Am J Hum Genet 60:842–850.

Gironell A, de Molina RM, Sancho G, et al. (2008) Chorea induced by a luteinizing hormone-releasing hormone analog. J Neurol 255:1264–1265.

Glik A, Vuillaume I, Devos D, et al. (2008) Psychosis, short stature in benign hereditary chorea: a novel thyroid transcription factor-1 mutation. Mov Disord 23:1744–1747.

Goldenberg PC, Steiner RD, Merkens LS, et al. (2003) Remarkable improvement in adult Leigh syndrome with partial cytochrome c oxidase deficiency. Neurology 60: 865–868.

Gregory A, Westaway SK, Holm IE, et al. (2008) Neurodegeneration associated with genetic defects in phospholipase A_2. Neurology 71:1402–1409.

Hanna MG, Davis MB, Sweeney MG, et al. (1998) Generalized chorea in two patients harboring the Friedreich's ataxia gene trinucleotide repeat expansion. Mov Disord 13: 339–340.

Hardie RJ, Pullon HW, Harding AE, et al. (1991) Neuroacanthocytosis. A clinical, haematological and pathological study of 19 cases. Brain 114:13–49.

Harrison TS, Goa KL (2004) Long-acting risperidone: a review of its use in schizophrenia. CNS Drugs 18:113–132.

Hartig MB, Hortnagel K, Garavaglia B, et al. (2006) Genotypic and phenotypic spectrum of PANK2 mutations in patients with neurodegeneration with brain iron accumulation. Ann Neurol 59:248–256.

Hattori H, Yorifuji T (2000) Infantile convulsions and paroxysmal kinesigenic choreoathetosis in a patient with idiopathic hypoparathyroidism. Brain Dev 22:449–450.

Hayflick SJ, Westaway SK, Levinson B, et al. (2003) Genetic, clinical, and radiographic delineation of Hallervorden-Spatz syndrome. N Engl J Med 348:33–40.

Hewer E, Danek A, Schoser BG, et al. (2007) McLeod myopathy revisited—more neurogenic and less benign. Brain 130:3285–3296.

Holmes SE, O'Hearn E, Rosenblatt A, et al. (2001) A repeat expansion in the gene encoding junctophilin-3 is associated with Huntington disease-like 2. Nat Genet 29: 377–378.

Howdle PD, Bone I, Losowsky MS (1979) Hypocalcaemic chorea secondary to malabsorption. Postgrad Med J 55:560–563.

Huang YG, Chen YC, Du F, et al. (2005) Topiramate therapy for paroxysmal kinesigenic choreoathetosis. Mov Disord 20:75–77.

Josephs KA, Van Gerpen MW, Van Gerpen JA (2003) Adult onset Niemann-Pick disease type C presenting with psychosis. J Neurol Neurosurg Psychiatry 74:528–529.

Jung HH, Brandner S (2002) Malignant McLeod myopathy. Muscle Nerve 26:424–427.

Jung HH, Hergersberg M, Kneifel S, et al. (2001) McLeod syndrome: a novel mutation, predominant psychiatric manifestations, and distinct striatal imaging findings. Ann Neurol 49:384–392.

Kambouris M, Bohlega S, Al Tahan A, et al. (2000) Localization of the gene for a novel autosomal recessive neurodegenerative Huntington-like disorder to 4p15.3. Am J Hum Genet 66:445–452.

Kawakami T, Takiyama Y, Sakoe K, et al. (1999) A case of McLeod syndrome with unusually severe myopathy. J Neurol Sci 166:36–39.

Klempir J, Roth J, Zarubova K, et al. (2008) The McLeod syndrome without acanthocytes. Parkinsonism Relat Disord 14:364–366.

Krolak-Salmon P, Androdias G, Meyronet D, et al. (2006) Slow evolution of cerebellar degeneration and chorea in a man with anti-Yo antibodies. Eur J Neurol 13:307–308.

Krude H, Schutz B, Biebermann H, et al. (2002) Choreoathetosis, hypothyroidism, and pulmonary alterations due to human NKX2-1 haploinsufficiency. J Clin Invest 109:475–480.

Kujawa KA, Niemi VR, Tomasi MA, et al. (2001) Ballistic-choreic movements as the presenting feature of renal cancer. Arch Neurol 58:1133–1135.

Kullnat MW, Morse RP (2008) Choreoathetosis after herpes simplex encephalitis with basal ganglia involvement on MRI. Pediatrics 121:e1003–e1007.

Lai MH, Wang TY, Chang CC, et al. (2008) Hemichorea associated with gabapentin therapy with hypoperfusion in contralateral basal ganglion—a case of a paraplegic patient with neuropathic pain. J Clin Pharm Ther 33:83–86.

Le Ber I, Bouslam N, Rivaud-Pechoux S, et al. (2004) Frequency and phenotypic spectrum of ataxia with oculomotor apraxia 2: a clinical and genetic study in 18 patients. Brain 127:759–767.

Le Ber I, Camuzat A, Castelnovo G, et al. (2003a) Prevalence of dentatorubral-pallidoluysian atrophy in a large series of white patients with cerebellar ataxia. Arch Neurol 60: 1097–1099.

Le Ber I, Moreira MC, Rivaud-Pechoux S, et al. (2003b) Cerebellar ataxia with oculomotor apraxia type 1: clinical and genetic studies. Brain 126:2761–2772.

Lee HY, Xu Y, Huang Y, et al. (2004) The gene for paroxysmal non-kinesigenic dyskinesia encodes an enzyme in a stress response pathway. Hum Mol Genet 13:3161–3170.

Lee LV, Pascasio FM, Fuentes FD, et al. (1976) Torsion dystonia in Panay, Philippines. Adv Neurol 14:137–151.

Litt M, Kramer P, Browne D, et al. (1994) A gene for episodic ataxia/myokymia maps to chromosome 12p13. Am J Hum Genet 55:702–709.

Lubbers WJ, Brunt ER, Scheffer H, et al. (1995) Hereditary myokymia and paroxysmal ataxia linked to chromosome 12 is responsive to acetazolamide. J Neurol Neurosurg Psychiatry 59:400–405.

Lucantoni C, Grottoli S, Moretti A (1994) Chorea due to hyperthyroidism in old age. A case report. Acta Neurol 16:129–133.

Machado A, Fen CH, Mitiko DM, et al. (2006) Neurological manifestations in Wilson's disease: report of 119 cases. Mov Disord 21:2192–2196.

Mahajnah M, Inbar D, Steinmetz A, et al. (2007) Benign hereditary chorea: clinical, neuroimaging, and genetic findings. J Child Neurol 22:1231–1234.

Margolis RL, Holmes SE, Rosenblatt A, et al. (2004) Huntington's disease-like 2 (HDL2) in North America and Japan. Ann Neurol 56:670–674.

Margolis RL, O'Hearn E, Rosenblatt A, et al. (2001) A disorder similar to Huntington's disease is associated with a novel CAG repeat expansion. Ann Neurol 50:373–380.

Martins S, Matama T, Guimaraes L, et al. (2003) Portuguese families with dentatorubro-pallidoluysian atrophy (DRPLA) share a common haplotype of Asian origin. Eur J Hum Genet 11:808–811.

Matsis PP, Fisher RA, Tasman-Jones C (1989) Acute lithium toxicity—chorea, hypercalcemia and hyperamylasemia. Aust N Z J Med 19:718–720.

McKee D, Talbot P (2003) Chorea as a presenting feature of variant Creutzfeldt-Jakob disease. Mov Disord 18:837–838.

McNeill A, Birchall D, Hayflick SJ, et al. (2008) T2* and FSE MRI distinguishes four subtypes of neurodegeneration with brain iron accumulation. Neurology 70:1614–1619.

Mellick G, Price L, Boyle R (2004) Late-onset presentation of pyruvate dehydrogenase deficiency. Mov Disord 19:727–729.

Menache CC, du Plessis AJ, Wessel DL, et al. (2002) Current incidence of acute neurologic complications after open-heart operations in children. Ann Thorac Surg 73:1752–1758.

Miller MA, Levsky ME (2008) Choreiform dyskinesia following isolated lamotrigine overdose. J Child Neurol 23:243.

Mir P, Edwards MJ, Curtis AR, et al. (2004) Adult-onset generalized dystonia due to a mutation in the neuroferritinopathy gene. Mov Disord 20:243–245.

Miranda M, Cardoso F, Giovannoni G, et al. (2004) Oral contraceptive induced chorea: another condition associated with anti-basal ganglia antibodies. J Neurol Neurosurg Psychiatry 75:327–328.

Miyajima H (2003) Aceruloplasminemia, an iron metabolic disorder. Neuropathology 23:345–350.

Monville C, Torres EM, Dunnett SB (2005) Validation of the l-dopa-induced dyskinesia in the 6-OHDA model and evaluation of the effects of selective dopamine receptor agonists and antagonists. Brain Res Bull 68:16–23.

Moore RC, Xiang F, Monaghan J, et al. (2001) Huntington disease phenocopy is a familial prion disease. Am J Hum Genet 69:1385–1388.

Moreira MC, Klur S, Watanabe M, et al. (2004) Senataxin, the ortholog of a yeast RNA helicase, is mutant in ataxia-ocular apraxia 2. Nat Genet 36:225–227.

Morgan NV, Westaway SK, Morton JE, et al. (2006) PLA2G6, encoding a phospholipase A$_2$, is mutated in neurodegenerative disorders with high brain iron. Nat Genet 38: 752–754.

Morimoto N, Nagano I, Deguchi K, et al. (2004) Leber hereditary optic neuropathy with chorea and dementia resembling Huntington disease. Neurology 63:2451–2452.

Mubaidin A, Roberts E, Hampshire D, et al. (2003) Karak syndrome: a novel degenerative disorder of the basal ganglia and cerebellum. J Med Genet 40:543–546.

Muehlschlegel S, Okun MS, Foote KD, et al. (2005) Paraneoplastic chorea with leukoencephalopathy presenting with obsessive–compulsive and behavioral disorder. Mov Disord 20:1523–1527.

Namekawa M, Takiyama Y, Ando Y, et al. (2001) Choreiform movements in spinocerebellar ataxia type 1. J Neurol Sci 187:103–106.

Nausieda PA, Koller WC, Weiner WJ, et al. (1979) Chorea induced by oral contraceptives. Neurology 29:1605–1609.

Nazabal ER, Lopez JM, Perez PA, et al. (2000) Chorea disclosing deterioration of polycythaemia vera. Postgrad Med J 76:658–659.

Nolte D, Niemann S, Muller U (2003) Specific sequence changes in multiple transcript system DYT3 are associated with X-linked dystonia parkinsonism. Proc Natl Acad Sci USA 100:10347–10352.

Oates CE, Bosch EP, Hart MN (1986) Movement disorders associated with chronic GM$_2$ gangliosidosis. Case report and review of the literature. Eur Neurol 25:154–159.

Ojwang PJ, Pegoraro RJ, Deppe WM, et al. (2001) Biochemical and molecular diagnosis of glutaric aciduria type 1 in a black South African male child: case report. East Afr Med J 78:682–685.

Oliveira JR, Spiteri E, Sobrido MJ, et al. (2004) Genetic heterogeneity in familial idiopathic basal ganglia calcification (Fahr disease). Neurology 63:2165–2167.

Papa SM, Chase TN (1996) Levodopa-induced dyskinesias improved by a glutamate antagonist in parkinsonian monkeys [see comments]. Ann Neurol 39:574–578.

Passarin MG, Alessandrini F, Nicolini GG, et al. (2005) Reversible choreoathetosis as the early onset of HIV-encephalopathy. Neurol Sci 26:55–56.

Pereira AC, Edwards MJ, Buttery PC, et al. (2004) Choreic syndrome and coeliac disease: a hitherto unrecognised association. Mov Disord 19:478–482.

Picard F, Tassin J, Vidailhet M, et al. (1998) Autosomal dominant paroxysmal kinesigenic choreoathetosis: a clinical and genetic study of two families. J Neurol Neurosurg Psychiatry 65:955–956.

Piccolo I, Defanti CA, Soliveri P, et al. (2003) Cause and course in a series of patients with sporadic chorea. J Neurol 250:429–435.

Rainier S, Thomas D, Tokarz D, et al. (2004) Myofibrillogenesis regulator 1 gene mutations cause paroxysmal dystonic choreoathetosis. Arch Neurol 61:1025–1029.

Rampoldi L, Danek A, Monaco AP (2002) Clinical features and molecular bases of neuroacanthocytosis. J Mol Med 80:475–491.

Reske-Nielsen E, Jensen PK, Hein-Sorensen O, et al. (1988) Calcification of the central nervous system in a new hereditary neurological syndrome. Acta Neuropathol (Berl) 75:590–596.

Richfield EK, Vonsattel JP, Macdonald ME, et al. (2002) Selective loss of striatal preprotachykinin neurons in a phenocopy of Huntington's disease. Mov Disord 17:327–332.

Rodrigues GG, Walker RH, Brice A, et al. (2008) Huntington's disease-like 2 in Brazil-Report of 4 patients. Mov Disord 23:2244–2247.

Roos RA, Wintzen AR, Vielvoye G, et al. (1991) Paroxysmal kinesigenic choreoathetosis as presenting symptom of multiple sclerosis. J Neurol Neurosurg Psychiatry 54:657–658.

Ross ME, Jacobson IM, Dienstag JL, et al. (1985) Late-onset Wilson's disease with neurological involvement in the absence of Kayser-Fleischer rings. Ann Neurol 17: 411–413.

Rottnek M, Riggio S, Byne W, et al. (2008) Schizophrenia in a patient with spinocerebellar ataxia 2: coincidence of two disorders or a neurodegenerative disease presenting with psychosis? Am J Psychiatry 165:964–967.

Russo D, Redman C, Lee S (1998) Association of XK and Kell blood group proteins. J Biol Chem 273:13950–13956.

Santos C, Wanderley H, Vedolin L, et al. (2008) Huntington disease-like 2: the first patient with apparent European ancestry. Clin Genet 73:480–485.

Schneider SA, van de Warrenburg BP, Hughes TD, et al. (2006) Phenotypic homogeneity of the Huntington disease-like presentation in a SCA17 family. Neurology 67: 1701–1703.

Sethi KD, Ray R, Roesel RA, et al. (1989) Adult-onset chorea and dementia with propionic acidemia. Neurology 39:1343–1345.

Shahwan A, Byrd PJ, Taylor AM, et al. (2006) Atypical presentation of ataxia-oculomotor apraxia type 1. Dev Med Child Neurol 48:529–532.

Shimazaki H, Takiyama Y, Sakoe K, et al. (2002) Early-onset ataxia with ocular motor apraxia and hypoalbuminemia: the aprataxin gene mutations. Neurology 59:590–595.

Shulman LM, Lang AE, Jankovic J, et al. (1995) Case 1, 1995: psychosis, dementia, chorea, ataxia, and supranuclear gaze dysfunction. Mov Disord 10:257–262.

Soffer D, Licht A, Yaar I, et al. (1977) Paroxysmal choreoathetosis as a presenting symptom in idiopathic hypoparathyroidism. J Neurol Neurosurg Psychiatry 40:692–694.

Sorrentino G, De Renzo A, Miniello S, et al. (1999) Late appearance of acanthocytes during the course of chorea-acanthocytosis. J Neurol Sci 163:175–178.

Spacey SD, Szczygielski BI, Young SP, et al. (2004) Malaysian siblings with Friedreich ataxia and chorea: a novel deletion in the frataxin gene. Can J Neurol Sci 31:383–386.

Sparacio RR, Anziska B, Schutta HS (1976) Hypernatremia and chorea. A report of two cases. Neurology 26:46–50.

Sporer B, Linke R, Seelos K, et al. (2005) HIV-induced chorea: evidence for basal ganglia dysregulation by SPECT. J Neurol 252:356–358.

Stemper B, Thurauf N, Neundorfer B, et al. (2003) Choreoathetosis related to lithium intoxication. Eur J Neurol 10:743–744.

Stevanin G, Camuzat A, Holmes SE, et al. (2002) CAG/CTG repeat expansions at the Huntington's disease-like 2 locus are rare in Huntington's disease patients. Neurology 58:965–967.

Stevanin G, Fujigasaki H, Lebre AS, et al. (2003) Huntington's disease-like phenotype due to trinucleotide repeat expansions in the *TBP* and *JPH3* genes. Brain 126:1599–1603.

Storch A, Kornhass M, Schwarz J (2005) Testing for acanthocytosis—a prospective reader-blinded study in movement disorder patients. J Neurol 252:84–90.

Suchowersky O, Muthipeedika J (2005) A case of late-onset chorea. Nat Clin Pract Neurol 1:113–116.

Suls A, Dedeken P, Goffin K, et al. (2008) Paroxysmal exercise-induced dyskinesia and epilepsy is due to mutations in SLC2A1, encoding the glucose transporter GLUT1. Brain 131:1831–1844.

Surtees RA, Matthews EE, Leonard JV (1992) Neurologic outcome of propionic acidemia. Pediatr Neurol 8:333–337.

Symmans WA, Shepherd CS, Marsh WL, et al. (1979) Hereditary acanthocytosis associated with the McLeod phenotype of the Kell blood group system. Br J Haematol 42:575–583.

Szepetowski P, Rochette J, Berquin P, et al. (1997) Familial infantile convulsions and paroxysmal choreoathetosis: a new neurological syndrome linked to the pericentromeric region of human chromosome 16. Am J Hum Genet 61:889–898.

Tan EK, Lo YL, Chan LL, et al. (2002) Cervical disc prolapse with cord compression presenting with choreoathetosis and dystonia. Neurology 58:661–662.

Tang WY, Gill DS, Chuan PS (1981) Chorea, a manifestation of hyponatraemia? Singapore Med J 22:92–93.

Tani T, Piao Y, Mori S, et al. (2000) Chorea resulting from paraneoplastic striatal encephalitis. J Neurol Neurosurg Psychiatry 69:512–515.

Thiriaux A, de St Martin A, Vercueil L, et al. (2002) Co-occurrence of infantile epileptic seizures and childhood paroxysmal choreoathetosis in one family: clinical, EEG, and SPECT characterization of episodic events. Mov Disord 17:98–104.

Tison FX, Ferrer X, Julien J (1991) Delayed onset movement disorders as a complication of central pontine myelinolysis. Mov Disord 6:171–173.

Topakian R, Stieglbauer K, Rotaru J, et al. (2006) Hypocalcemic choreoathetosis and tetany after bisphosphonate treatment. Mov Disord 21:2026–2027.

Toyoshima Y, Yamada M, Onodera O, et al. (2004) SCA17 homozygote showing Huntington's disease-like phenotype. Ann Neurol 55:281–286.

Tsao CY (2004) Effective treatment with oxcarbazepine in paroxysmal kinesigenic choreoathetosis. J Child Neurol 19:300–301.

Tse W, Cersosimo MG, Gracies JM, et al. (2004) Movement disorders and AIDS: a review. Parkinsonism Relat Disord 10:323–334.

Twardowschy CA, Teive HA, Fernandes AF, et al. (2008) Chorea due to gabapentin monotherapy in a not encephalopatic patient. Arq Neuropsiquiatr 66:107.

Ueyama H, Kumamoto T, Nagao S, et al. (2000) A novel mutation of the McLeod syndrome gene in a Japanese family. J Neurol Sci 176:151–154.

Venegas FP, Sinning M, Miranda M (2005) Primary Sjogren's syndrome presenting as a generalized chorea. Parkinsonism Relat Disord 11:193–194.

Verhagen MMM, Abdo WF, Willemsen MAAP, et al. (2009) Clinical spectrum of ataxia-telangiectasia in adulthood. Neurology 73:430–437.

Vernino S, Tuite P, Adler CH, et al. (2002) Paraneoplastic chorea associated with CRMP-5 neuronal antibody and lung carcinoma. Ann Neurol 51:625–630.

Voll R, Hoffmann GF, Lipinski CG, et al. (1993) Glutaric acidemia/glutaric aciduria I as differential chorea minor diagnosis [in German]. Klin Padiatr 205:124–126.

Walker RH, Danek A, Dobson-Stone C, et al. (2006a) Developments in neuroacanthocytosis: expanding the spectrum of choreatic syndromes. Mov Disord 21:1794–1905.

Walker RH, Jankovic J, O'Hearn E, et al. (2003a) Phenotypic features of Huntington disease-like 2. Mov Disord 18:1527–1530.

Walker RH, Liu Q, Ichiba M, et al. (2006b) Self-mutilation in chorea-acanthocytosis—manifestation of movement disorder or psychopathology? Mov Disord 21:2268–2269.

Walker RH, Rasmussen A, Rudnicki D, et al. (2003b) Huntington's disease-like 2 can present as chorea-acanthocytosis. Neurology 61:1002–1004.

Wardle M, Majounie E, Williams NM, et al. (2008) Dentatorubral pallidoluysian atrophy in South Wales. J Neurol Neurosurg Psychiatry 79:804–807.

Wardle M, Morris HR, Robertson NP (2009) Clinical and genetic characteristics of non-Asian dentatorubral-pallidoluysian atrophy: a systematic review. Mov Disord 24: 1636–1640.

Watanabe T, Onda H (2004) Hemichorea with antiphospholipid antibodies in a patient with lupus nephritis. Pediatr Nephrol 19:451–453.

Waters CH, Takahashi H, Wilhelmsen KC, et al. (1993) Phenotypic expression of X-linked dystonia-parkinsonism (lubag) in two women. Neurology 43:1555–1558.

Weber YG, Storch A, Wuttke TV, et al. (2008) GLUT1 mutations are a cause of paroxysmal exertion-induced dyskinesias and induce hemolytic anemia by a cation leak. J Clin Invest 118:2157–2168.

Weiner WJ, Nausieda PA, Klawans HL (1978) Methylphenidate-induced chorea: case report and pharmacologic implications. Neurology 28:1041–1044.

Willemsen MA, Breedveld GJ, Wouda S, et al. (2005) Brain–thyroid–lung syndrome: a patient with a severe multi-system disorder due to a de novo mutation in the thyroid transcription factor 1 gene. Eur J Pediatr 164:28–30.

Wills AJ, Sawle GV, Guilbert PR, et al. (2002) Palatal tremor and cognitive decline in neuroferritinopathy. J Neurol Neurosurg Psychiatry 73:91–92.

Wszolek ZK, Baba Y, Mackenzie IR, et al. (2006) Autosomal dominant dystonia-plus with cerebral calcifications. Neurology 67:620–625.

Xiang F, Almqvist EW, Huq M, et al. (1998) A Huntington disease-like neurodegenerative disorder maps to chromosome 20p. Am J Hum Genet 63:1431–1438.

Xu X, Pin S, Gathinji M, et al. (2004) Aceruloplasminemia: an inherited neurodegenerative disease with impairment of iron homeostasis. Ann N Y Acad Sci 1012:299–305.

Yamamoto K, Chiba HO, Ishitobi M, et al. (1997) Acute encephalopathy with bilateral striatal necrosis: favourable response to corticosteroid therapy. Eur J Paediatr Neurol 1:41–45.

Younes-Mhenni S, Thobois S, Streichenberger N, et al. (2002) Mitochondrial encephalo-myopathy, lactic acidosis and stroke-like episodes (Melas) associated with a Fahr disease and cerebellar calcifications [in French]. Rev Med Interne 23:1027–1029.

Zambrino CA, Zorzi G, Lanzi G, et al. (2000) Bilateral striatal necrosis associated with *Mycoplasma pneumoniae* infection in an adolescent: clinical and neuroradiologic follow up. Mov Disord 15:1023–1026.

Zesiewicz TA, Shimberg WR, Hauser RA, et al. (2008) Chorea as a side effect of gabapentin (Neurontin) in a patient with complex regional pain syndrome type 1. Clin Rheumatol 27:389–390.

Zhou B, Westaway SK, Levinson B, et al. (2001) A novel pantothenate kinase gene (*PANK2*) is defective in Hallervorden-Spatz syndrome. Nat Genet 28:345–349.

Zhu D, Burke C, Leslie A, et al. (2002) Friedreich's ataxia with chorea and myoclonus caused by a compound heterozygosity for a novel deletion and the trinucleotide GAA expansion. Mov Disord 17:585–589.

Zuhlke C, Burk K (2007) Spinocerebellar ataxia type 17 is caused by mutations in the TATA-box binding protein. Cerebellum 19:1–8.

Zuhlke C, Gehlken U, Hellenbroich Y, et al. (2003) Phenotypical variability of expanded alleles in the TATA-binding protein gene. Reduced penetrance in SCA17? J Neurol 250:161–163.

2

Functional Anatomy of Chorea

Jonathan W. Mink, MD, PhD

INTRODUCTION

Chorea, and the closely related movement disorder, ballism, are associated with dysfunction of basal ganglia circuits. Like other movement disorders of basal ganglia origin, chorea is best viewed as a "circuit disorder," arising from dysfunction of a complex circuit, rather than a disorder attributable to a lesion of one specific nucleus or loss of a specific cell type (Mink, 2006). To understand how circuit dysfunction can lead to chorea, it is important to first understand the broad organization of the circuit and how it may function normally. The anatomy of basal ganglia circuits has been described at length in many prior publications (Albin et al., 1989; Alexander and Crutcher, 1990; Alexander et al., 1986; Haber, 2003; Mink, 1996). For this chapter, the anatomy will be reviewed more briefly.

BASAL GANGLIA CIRCUIT ORGANIZATION

The basal ganglia include the striatum (caudate, putamen, nucleus accumbens), the subthalamic nucleus, the globus pallidus (internal segment, external segment, ventral

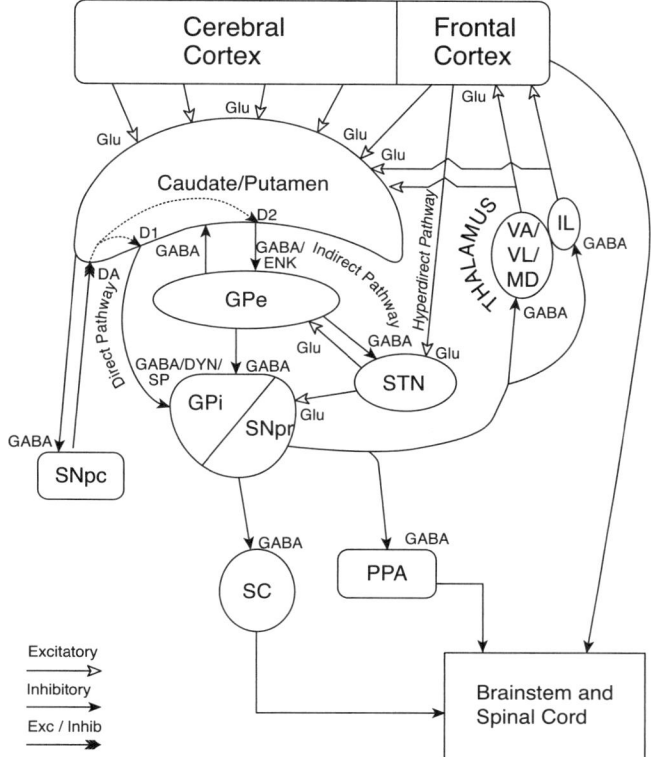

FIGURE 2–1. Simplified schematic diagram of basal ganglia–thalamocortical circuitry. Excitatory connections are indicated by *open arrows* and inhibitory connections, by *filled arrows*. The modulatory dopamine projection is indicated by a *three-headed arrow*. DA, dopamine; DYN, dynorphin; ENK, enkephalin; GABA, γ-aminobutyric acid; Glu, glutamate; GPe, globus pallidus pars externa; GPi, globus pallidus pars interna; IL, intralaminar thalamic nuclei; MD, mediodorsal nucleus; PPA, pedunculopontine area; SC, superior colliculus; SNpc, substantia nigra pars compacta; SNpr, substantia nigra pars reticulata; SP, substance P; STN, subthalamic nucleus; VA, ventral anterior nucleus; VL, ventral lateral nucleus.

pallidum), and the substantia nigra (pars compacta, pars reticulata) (Figure 2–1). The striatum and subthalamic nucleus (STN) receive the majority of inputs from outside of the basal ganglia. Most of those inputs arise from cerebral cortex, but intralaminar and ventral thalamic nuclei also provide strong inputs to the striatum. The bulk of the motor outputs from the basal ganglia arise from the globus pallidus internal segment (GPi) and substantia nigra pars reticulata (SNpr). These outputs are inhibitory to the pedunculopontine area in the brainstem and to thalamic nuclei that in turn project to the frontal lobe.

Basal Ganglia Input Nuclei

The striatum receives excitatory input from most areas of the cerebral cortex (Kemp and Powell, 1970). In addition, the ventral striatum (nucleus accumbens and rostroventral extensions of the caudate and putamen) receive inputs from the hippocampus and amygdala (Fudge et al., 2002). The cortical input to the striatum is excitatory and glutamatergic (Cherubini et al., 1988). Medium spiny striatal neurons make up 90%–95% of the striatal neuron population. They project outside of the striatum and receive a number of inputs in addition to the important cortical input, including (1) excitatory glutamatergic inputs from the thalamus; (2) cholinergic input from striatal interneurons; (3) γ-aminobutyric acid (GABA), substance P, and enkephalin input from adjacent medium spiny striatal neurons; (4) GABA input from small interneurons; (5) a large input from dopamine-containing neurons in the substantia nigra pars compacta (SNpc); and (6) a more sparse input from the serotonin-containing neurons in the dorsal and median raphe nuclei (Haber, 2003; Mink, 1996).

In recent years, there has been increasing recognition of the importance of the fast-spiking GABAergic striatal interneurons. These cells make up 2%–5% of the striatal neuron population, but they exert powerful inhibition on medium spiny neurons. Like medium spiny neurons, they receive excitatory input from the cerebral cortex. They appear to play an important role in focusing the spatial pattern of medium spiny neuron activation (Mallet et al., 2005).

The dopamine input to the striatum terminates largely on the shafts of the dendritic spines of medium spiny neurons, where it is in a position to modulate transmission from the cerebral cortex to the striatum (Bouyer et al., 1984). The action of dopamine upon striatal neurons depends on the type of dopamine receptor involved. Five types of G protein–coupled dopamine receptors have been described (D_1–D_5) (Sibley and Monsma, 1992). These have been grouped into two families (D_1 and D_2) based on their linkage to adenyl cyclase activity and response to agonists. The conventional view has been that dopamine acts at D_1 receptors to facilitate the activity of postsynaptic neurons and at D_2 receptors to inhibit postsynaptic neurons (Gerfen et al., 1990). Indeed, this is a fundamental concept for currently popular models of basal ganglia pathophysiology (Albin et al., 1989; DeLong, 1990). However, the physiological effect of dopamine on striatal neurons is more complex (Hernandez-Lopez et al., 1997; Nicola et al., 2000). Nevertheless, the basic view of dopamine being facilitatory through D_1 receptors and inhibitory through D_2 receptors is useful conceptually.

Medium spiny striatal neurons contain the inhibitory neurotransmitter GABA and colocalized peptide neurotransmitters (Penny et al., 1986). Based on the type of neurotransmitters and the predominant type of dopamine receptor they contain, the medium spiny neurons can be divided into two populations that also correspond with the type of dopamine receptor that they express. One population contains

GABA, dynorphin, and substance P and primarily expresses D_1 dopamine receptors. These neurons project to the basal ganglia output nuclei, GPi, and SNpr. The second population contains GABA and enkephalin and primarily expresses D_2 dopamine receptors. These neurons project to the external segment of the globus pallidus (GPe) (Albin et al., 1989).

The STN receives an excitatory, glutamatergic input from many areas of the frontal lobes, with especially large inputs from motor areas of the cortex (Mink, 1996). The STN also receives an inhibitory GABA input from the GPe. The output from the STN is glutamatergic and excitatory to the basal ganglia output nuclei, GPi and SNpr. The STN also sends an excitatory projection back to the GPe.

Basal Ganglia Output Nuclei

The primary basal ganglia motor output arises from the GPi and SNpr. As described above, the GPi and SNpr receive excitatory input from the STN and inhibitory input from the striatum. The pathway from the striatum to the GPi and SNpr has been called the "direct" pathway (Figure 2–1). The pathway from the frontal cortex to the STN and from the STN to the GPi and SNpr has been called the "hyperdirect" pathway (Figure 2–1). The GPi and SNpr also receive an inhibitory input from the GPe. The output from the GPi and SNpr is inhibitory and GABA-ergic. The primary output is directed to thalamic nuclei that project to the frontal lobes: the ventrolateral, ventroanterior, and mediodorsal nuclei. The thalamic targets of the GPi and SNpr project, in turn, to the frontal lobe, with the strongest output going to motor areas. Collaterals of the axons projecting to the thalamus project to an area at the junction of the midbrain and pons near the pedunculopontine nucleus (Parent, 1990). Other output neurons (20%) project to intralaminar nuclei of the thalamus, to the lateral habenula, or to the superior colliculus (Francois et al., 1988).

The basal ganglia motor output has a somatotopic organization such that the body below the neck is largely represented in the GPi and the head and eyes are largely represented in the SNpr. The separate representation of different body parts is maintained throughout the basal ganglia. Within the representation of an individual body part, it also appears that there is segregation of outputs to different motor areas of the cortex and that an individual GPi neuron sends output via the thalamus to just one area of the cortex (Hoover and Strick, 1993). Thus, GPi neurons that project via the thalamus to the motor cortex are adjacent to, but separate from, those that project to the premotor cortex or supplementary motor area. GPi neurons that project via the thalamus to the prefrontal cortex are also separate from those projecting to motor areas. The anatomic segregation of basal ganglia–thalamocortical outputs suggests functional segregation at the output level, but other anatomic evidence suggests interactions between circuits within the basal ganglia (Haber et al., 2000).

Intrinsic Nuclei

The GPe may be viewed as an intrinsic nucleus of the basal ganglia. Like the GPi and SNpr, the GPe receives an inhibitory projection from the striatum and an excitatory one from the STN. Unlike the GPi, the striatal projection to the GPe contains GABA and enkephalin but not substance P (Albin et al., 1989). The output of the GPe is quite different from the output of the GPi. The output is GABAergic and inhibitory and the majority of it projects to the STN. The connections from the striatum to the GPe, from the GPe to the STN, and from the STN to the GPi and SNpr form the "indirect" pathway (Figure 2–1). In addition, there is a monosynaptic GABAergic inhibitory output from the GPe directly to the GPi and SNpr and a GABAergic projection back to the striatum (Bolam et al., 2000). Thus, GPe neurons are in a position to provide feedback inhibition to neurons in the striatum and STN and feedforward inhibition to neurons in the GPi and SNpr.

Dopamine input to the striatum arises from the SNpc. The SNpc is made up of large dopamine-containing cells. The SNpc receives input from the striatum and frontal cortex.

BASAL GANGLIA FUNCTIONAL ORGANIZATION

Although the basal ganglia intrinsic circuitry is complex, the overall picture is of two primary pathways through the basal ganglia from the cerebral cortex with the output directed to the brainstem via the pedunculopontine area and to the cerebral cortex via the thalamus. These pathways consist of two disynaptic pathways from the cortex to the basal ganglia output (GPi and SNpr) (Figure 2–1). The two disynaptic pathways are from the cortex through (1) the striatum (the *direct pathway*) and (2) the STN (the *hyperdirect pathway*) to the basal ganglia outputs. These pathways have important anatomic and functional differences. First, the cortical input to the STN comes only from the frontal lobe, whereas the input to the striatum arises from virtually all areas of the cerebral cortex. Second, the output from the STN is excitatory, whereas the output from the striatum is inhibitory. Third, the excitatory route through the STN is faster than the inhibitory route through the striatum (Nambu et al., 2000). Finally, the STN projection to the GPi is divergent and the striatal projection is more focused (Parent and Hazrati, 1993). Thus, the two disynaptic pathways from the cerebral cortex to the basal ganglia output nuclei, GPi and SNpr, provide fast, widespread, divergent excitation through the STN and slower, focused inhibition through the striatum. This organization provides an anatomic basis for focused inhibition and surround excitation of neurons in the GPi and SNpr (Figure 2–2). Because the output of the GPi and SNpr is inhibitory, this would result in focused facilitation and surround inhibition of basal ganglia thalamocortical targets.

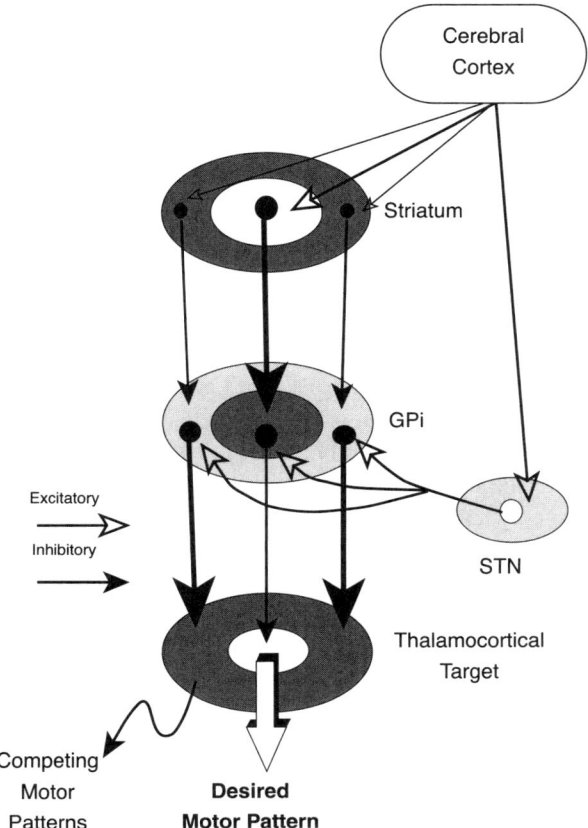

FIGURE 2–2. Schematic of normal functional organization of the basal ganglia output. Excitatory projections are indicated with *open arrows*; inhibitory projections are indicated with *filled arrows*. Relative magnitude of activity is represented by line thickness. *White areas* represent higher activity, and *shaded areas* represent lower activity. GPi, globus pallidus pars interna; STN, subthalamic nucleus. Modified from Mink (2001).

There are several multisynaptic pathways from the striatum to the GPi and SNpr involving the GPe. The most important of these is from the striatum to the GPe, from the GPe to the STN, and then from the STN to the GPi and SNpr. This is the classic indirect pathway that is in a position to modulate and focus activity mediated through the hyperdirect and direct pathways (Figure 2–1).

We have developed a scheme of normal basal ganglia motor function based on the results of anatomic, physiological, and lesion studies (Mink, 1996, 2003). In this scheme, the tonically active inhibitory output of the basal ganglia acts as a "brake" on motor pattern generators (MPGs) in the cerebral cortex (via the thalamus) and brainstem. When a movement is initiated by a particular MPG, basal ganglia output neurons projecting to competing MPGs increase their firing rate, thereby increasing inhibition and applying a "brake" on those generators. Other basal ganglia output neurons projecting to the generators involved in the desired movement decrease their discharge, thereby removing tonic inhibition and releasing the brake from the desired motor patterns. Thus, the intended movement is enabled and competing movements are prevented from interfering with the desired one.

The anatomic arrangement of the STN and striatal inputs to the GPi and SNpr form the basis for a functional center-surround organization, as shown in Figure 2–2. When a voluntary movement is initiated by cortical mechanisms, a separate signal is sent to the STN, exciting it. The STN projects in a widespread pattern and excites the GPi. The increased GPi activity causes inhibition of thalamocortical motor mechanisms. In parallel to the pathway through the STN, signals are sent from all areas of the cerebral cortex to the striatum. The cortical inputs are transformed by the striatal integrative circuitry to a focused, context-dependent output that inhibits specific neurons in the GPi. The inhibitory striatal input to the GPi is slower, but more powerful, than the excitatory STN input. The resulting focally decreased activity in the GPi selectively disinhibits the desired thalamocortical MPGs. Indirect pathways from the striatum to the GPi (striatum → GPe → GPi and striatum → GPe → STN → GPi) (Figure 2–1) result in further focusing of the output. The net result of basal ganglia activity during a voluntary movement is the inhibition ("braking") of competing motor patterns and focused facilitation (releasing the "brake") from the selected voluntary movement pattern generators. Dysfunction of these circuits can lead to impaired voluntary movements (too much braking), occurrence of involuntary movements (too little braking), or both (Mink, 1996, 2003). Specific types of involuntary movements result from specific different abnormalities in the basal ganglia circuits (Mink 2001, 2003).

NEURAL CIRCUITS IN CHOREA

Chorea is a disorder of involuntary movement that is commonly described as frequent, brief, sudden, twitch-like movements that flow from body part to body part in a chaotic manner. Although usually described as chaotic or random, chorea often resembles fragments of normal movement, and many individuals with chorea incorporate the involuntary movements into motor patterns that appear voluntary (known as "parakinesias"). Chorea exists as a spectrum of movements that can be proximal or distal, of large or small amplitude, and intermittent or nearly continuous. Chorea is seen in many different disease states, as will be described in subsequent chapters. In diseases with well-defined neuropathology, chorea is usually associated with specific abnormalities in the striatum or STN.

Experimentally, chorea can be produced by inactivation (or lesion) of the STN, disinhibition of the GPe, or administering dopaminergic agents to dopamine-depleted nonhuman primates. Study of these disease states and experimental models has led to substantial convergence of data from which the functional anatomy of chorea can be understood.

Human Chorea

Huntington Disease

Huntington disease (HD) is an autosomal dominant, neurodegenerative disease associated with trinucleotide repeat expansion that results in progressive involuntary movements and dementia (Chapter 3). The early and mid-stages of the disease in adults generally include prominent chorea. As HD progresses, parkinsonism and dystonia increase and chorea decreases. In juvenile HD, chorea is uncommon; dystonia and parkinsonism are the prominent movement disorders. The pathological hallmark of HD is a marked loss of neurons in the striatum. Medium spiny neurons are most severely affected, and within that population it is the enkephalin-containing neurons projecting to the GPe that are lost earliest in adults (Reiner et al., 1988). The substance P–containing medium spiny striatal neurons that project to the GPi and SNpr are relatively preserved until later in the disease, when rigidity typically appears. However, patients with juvenile HD or predominantly rigid-akinetic symptoms have loss of both enkephalin- and substance P–containing medium spiny neurons (Albin et al., 1990).

Consistent with the early loss of enkephalin-containing striatal neurons projecting to the GPe, it has been demonstrated that GPe discharge rates are increased and GPi discharge rates are decreased in some (Starr et al., 2008), but not all (Tang et al., 2005), patients with HD. GPi activity did not correlate in time with the presence or absence of chorea, suggesting that chorea is not caused by abnormal bursting in the GPi (Starr et al., 2008).

Subthalamic Nucleus Injury

It has long been recognized that damage to the STN by ischemic stroke or hemorrhage results in a bizarre involuntary movement that is characterized by large-amplitude, flinging (ballistic) movements of the contralateral extremities. Neuronal activity in the GPi has been shown to be decreased in a patient with hemiballism due to an STN lesion (Suarez et al., 1997). The movement abnormality is usually present immediately after the lesion and typically improves over time. The movements of hemiballism are similar to those of chorea but of larger amplitude and possibly more severity in proximal muscles. It is likely that chorea and hemiballism have similar underlying mechanisms, with the primary difference being the magnitude of the involuntary movements.

Experimental Models of Chorea

The best models of chorea involve nonhuman primates. Rodents can be induced to have involuntary movements that bear some resemblance to human chorea, but because of neuroanatomic and somatic anatomic similarities between nonhuman and human primates, nonhuman primate models have the most validity.

Striatal Lesions

The striking loss of striatal medium spiny neurons in HD has led investigators to try to produce an animal model of chorea by lesioning the striatum. However, chorea is rarely seen after experimental striatal lesions. Chorea is also uncommon after strokes affecting the striatum in humans. Certain manipulations of the striatum may produce chorea, but these appear not to be due directly to ablation of the striatal output. Crossman and colleagues found that injection of the GABA antagonist bicuculline into the ventral putamen of monkeys resulted in choreoathetosis (Crossman, 1987; Crossman et al., 1984; Jackson and Crossman, 1984). However, only sites adjacent to the GPe were effective, raising the possibility that the effect was due to spread of bicuculline into the GPe (Francois et al., 2004; Grabli et al., 2004). Chorea did not result from bicuculline injections into the caudate. Chorea can also be seen in monkeys after focal striatal lesions if they are subsequently given L-DOPA or amphetamine (Kanazawa et al., 1990). The incidence of chorea in that model correlated with dopamine depletion distal to the lesion site and likely resulted from subsequent focal hypersensitivity to dopamine. In both of the experimental models cited, the chorea could not be attributed directly to the loss of striatal neurons.

Subthalamic Nucleus Lesions

The oldest animal model of chorea involves nonhuman primates with lesions of the STN. These animals develop involuntary movements of the contralateral arm and leg that are similar to those seen in human patients with STN damage (Carpenter and Carpenter, 1951; Carpenter and Whittier, 1952; Carpenter et al., 1950; Hamada and DeLong, 1992b). The chorea or hemiballism resulting from STN lesions involves the lower extremities more than the upper extremities and can persist for days to months. Monkeys with hemichorea or hemiballism due to STN inactivation are said to be able to make normal voluntary movements (Hamada and DeLong, 1992b), but these have not been measured in detail.

After STN lesion or inactivation, there is decreased activity in the GPe and GPi. This has been shown both with 2-deoxyglucose (2-DG) autoradiography and with single-neuron recording. STN inactivation–induced hemichorea/hemiballism is associated with decreased 2-DG uptake in the GPe and GPi (Mitchell et al., 1985). There is also decreased uptake in the thalamic targets of the GPi. These results were interpreted as showing decreased excitatory input from the STN to the GPi, leading to decreased GPi inhibition of the thalamus. That interpretation is consistent with the anatomy and physiology of that pathway (see Figure 2–1). After excitotoxic lesions of the STN in monkeys, the activity of both GPe and GPi neurons was decreased during active holding of elbow position compared with prelesion activity (Hamada and DeLong, 1992a). However, these recordings were done after the hemichorea subsided, indicating that partially decreased GPi activity alone is not sufficient to produce chorea. Indeed, hemiballism due to STN ablation can be abolished by GPi lesions which reduce GPi output to zero (Carpenter et al., 1950).

Disinhibition of GPe Neurons

Injection of the GABA antagonist bicuculline into the GPe has been shown to produce reversible hemichorea (Matsumura et al., 1995). In this model, production of chorea is dependent upon the bicuculline being injected into the sensorimotor territory of the GPe (Grabli et al., 2004). Injection into other territories of the GPe produced changes in behavior but not chorea. When anatomic tracers were injected into the GPe regions in which bicuculline injection produced chorea, connection with other components of the sensorimotor basal ganglia circuits was confirmed (Francois et al., 2004). Thus, there is topographic specificity of the effect, indicating that chorea is a manifestation of dysfunction of the motor circuits in the basal ganglia.

Hemichorea produced by disinhibition of neurons in the motor territory of the GPe is associated with decreased activity of some, but not all, GPi neurons recorded at the time the chorea was present (Matsumura et al., 1995). In that study, there were tonic changes in GPi activity but no apparent bursting in correlation with the choreic movements.

A NEURAL CIRCUIT MODEL OF CHOREA

As discussed, primate models of chorea and human chorea/hemiballism have both been associated with decreased activity of GPi neurons. This would appear to be consistent with the older models of hyperkinetic movement disorders that hypothesized that GPi output was decreased in these disorders (Albin et al., 1989; DeLong, 1990). However, tonic reduction of GPi activity alone cannot explain chorea because (1) experimental lesions of the GPi do not cause chorea (Mink and Thach, 1991), (2) not all patients with chorea have decreased GPi activity (Tang et al., 2005), (3) monkeys with STN lesions have decreased GPi discharge rates even after the dyskinesia has resolved (Hamada and DeLong, 1992a), and (4) ablation of the GPi eliminates choreatic dyskinesia in Parkinson disease (Lang et al., 1997), chorea due to striatal lacunar infarction (Hashimoto et al., 2001), and hemiballismus (Suarez et al., 1997).

   If chorea is not due to tonically reduced GPi output, what is the underlying pathophysiology? It seems obvious that there is abnormal phasic, bursting neuronal activity originating somewhere in the motor system. It is not known whether the activity driving chorea originates in the basal ganglia or in thalamocortical (or brainstem) MPGs. Abnormal phasic bursting of GPi neurons has been described in some people with chorea or hemiballism. Abnormal phasic bursting of GPi neurons would intermittently and alternately disinhibit and then inhibit thalamocortical motor circuits. However, a temporal correlation between the GPi bursts and electromyographic bursts has not been demonstrated (Starr et al., 2008).

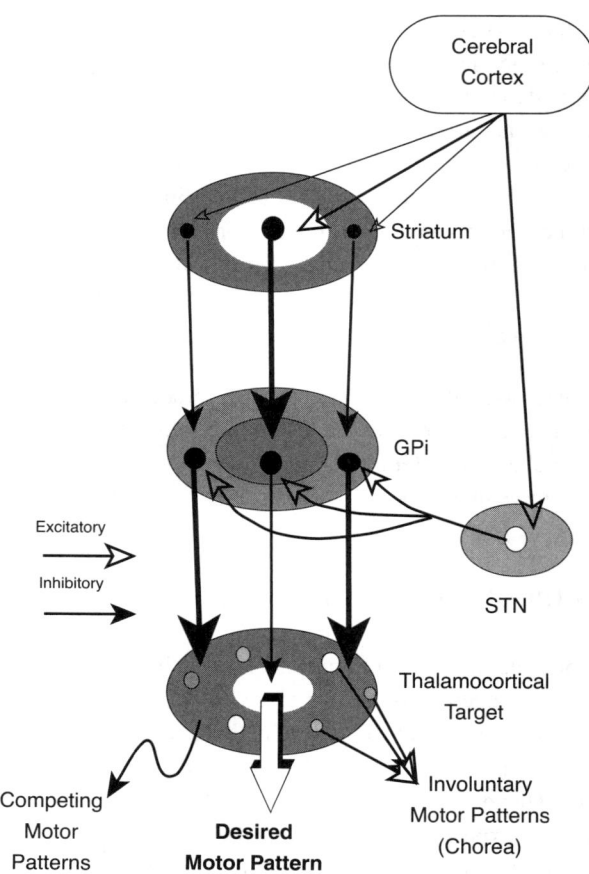

FIGURE 2–3. Schematic of abnormal basal ganglia output leading to chorea. Excitatory projections are indicated with *open arrows*; inhibitory projections are indicated with *filled arrows*. Relative magnitude of activity is represented by line thickness. *White areas* represent higher activity, and *shaded areas* represent lower activity. GPi, globus pallidus pars interna; STN, subthalamic nucleus.

Alternatively, it is possible that partial reduction of tonic GPi activity causes target neurons in the thalamus to depolarize to near threshold so that random small fluctuations in other, nonbasal ganglia inputs can cause them to fire in random bursts. In either case, cortical MPGs would be "gated in" or "gated out" in a random temporal pattern, causing the involuntary movement of chorea (Figure 2–3).

Additional work is required to determine whether abnormal phasic neuronal discharge arises from a single site within the circuit or whether it can arise from one of several sites and be propagated through the circuit. Nevertheless, it seems clear that chorea is associated with decreased inhibitory output from the basal ganglia that results in increased probability of aberrant discharge in cortical motor neurons, leading to the clinical phenomenon of chorea. Further identification of the abnormally active neurons is likely to provide important clues for future therapeutic options.

REFERENCES

Albin RL, Reiner A, Anderson KD, Penney JB, Young AB (1990) Striatal and nigral neuron subpopulations in rigid Huntington's disease: implications for the functional anatomy of chorea and rigidity-akinesia. Ann Neurol 27:357–365.

Albin RL, Young AB, Penney JB (1989) The functional anatomy of basal ganglia disorders. Trends Neurosci 12:366–375.

Alexander GE, Crutcher MD (1990) Functional architecture of basal ganglia circuits: neural substrates of parallel processing. Trends Neurosci 13:266–271.

Alexander GE, DeLong MR, Strick PL (1986) Parallel organization of functionally segregated circuits linking basal ganglia and cortex. Annu Rev Neurosci 9:357–381.

Bolam JP, Hanley JJ, Booth PA, Bevan MD (2000) Synaptic organisation of the basal ganglia. J Anat 196:527–542.

Bouyer JJ, Park DH, Joh TH, Pickel VM (1984) Chemical and structural analysis of the relation between cortical inputs and tyrosine hydroxylase-containing terminals in rat neostriatum. Brain Res 302:267–275.

Carpenter MB, Carpenter CS (1951) Analysis of somatotopic relations of the corpus Luysi in man and monkey. J Comp Neurol 95:349–370.

Carpenter MB, Whittier JB (1952) Study of methods for producing experimental lesions of the central nervous system with special reference to the stereotaxic technique. J Comp Neurol 97:73–131.

Carpenter MB, Whittier JR, Mettler FA (1950) Analysis of choreoid hyperkinesia in the rhesus monkey. Surgical and pharmacological analysis of hyperkinesia resulting from lesions in the subthalamic nucleus of Luys. J Comp Neurol 92:293–331.

Cherubini E, Herrling PL, Lanfumey L, Stanzione P (1988) Excitatory amino acids in synaptic excitation of rat striatal neurones in vitro. J Physiol 400:677–690.

Crossman AR (1987) Primate models of dyskinesia: the experimental approach to the study of basal ganglia–related involuntary movement disorders. Neuroscience 21:1–40.

Crossman AR, Sambrook MA, Jackson A (1984) Experimental hemichorea/hemiballismus in the monkey. Studies on the intracerebral site of action in a drug-induced dyskinesia. Brain 107:579–596.

DeLong MR (1990) Primate models of movement disorders of basal ganglia origin. Trends Neurosci 13:281–285.

Francois C, Grabli D, McCairn K, Jan C, Karachi C, Hirsch E-C, Feger J, Tremblay L (2004) Behavioural disorders induced by external globus pallidus dysfunction in primates II. Anatomical study. Brain 127:2055–2070.

Francois C, Percheron G, Yelnik J, Tande D (1988) A topographic study of the course of nigral axons and of the distribution of pallidal axonal endings in the centre median–parafascicular complex of macaques. Brain Res 473:181–186.

Fudge J, Kunishio K, Walsh C, Richard D, Haber S (2002) Amygdaloid projections to ventromedial striatal subterritories in the primate. Neuroscience 110:257–275.

Gerfen CR, Engber TM, Mahan LC, Susel Z, Chase TN, Monsma FJ, Sibley DR (1990) D_1 and D_2 dopamine receptor–regulated gene expression of striatonigral and striatopallidal neurons. Science 250:1429–1432.

Grabli D, McCairn K, Hirsch EC, Agid Y, Feger J, Francois C, Tremblay L (2004) Behavioural disorders induced by external globus pallidus dysfunction in primates: I. Behavioural study. Brain 127:2039–2054.

Haber SN (2003) The primate basal ganglia: parallel and integrative networks. J Chem Neuroanat 26:317–330.

Haber SN, Fudge JL, McFarland NR (2000) Striatonigrostriatal pathways in primates form an ascending spiral from the shell to the dorsolateral striatum. J Neurosci 20: 2369–2382.

Hamada I, DeLong MR (1992a) Excitotoxic acid lesions of the primate subthalamic nucleus result in reduced pallidal neuronal activity during active holding. J Neurophysiol 68:1859–1866.

Hamada I, DeLong MR (1992b) Excitotoxic acid lesions of the primate subthalamic nucleus result in transient dyskinesias of the contralateral limbs. J Neurophysiol 68:1850–1858.

Hashimoto T, Morita H, Tada T, Maruyama T, Yamada Y, Ikeda S (2001) Neuronal activity in the globus pallidus in chorea caused by striatal lacunar infarction. Ann Neurol 50:528–531.

Hernandez-Lopez S, Bargas J, Surmeier DJ, Reyes A, Galarraga E (1997) D_1 receptor activation enhances evoked discharge in neostriatal medium spiny neurons by modulating an L-type Ca^{2+} conductance. J Neurosci 17:3334–3342.

Hoover JE, Strick PL (1993) Multiple output channels in the basal ganglia. Science 259:819–821.

Jackson A, Crossman AR (1984) Experimental choreoathetosis produced by injection of a gamma-aminobutyric acid antagonist into the lentiform nucleus in the monkey. Neurosci Lett 46:41–45.

Kanazawa I, Kimura M, Murata M, Tanaka Y, Cho F (1990) Choreic movements in the macaque monkey induced by kainic acid lesions of the striatum combined with L-DOPA. Brain 113:509–535.

Kemp JM, Powell TPS (1970) The corticostriate projection in the monkey. Brain 93: 525–546.

Lang AE, Lozano AM, Montgomery E, Duff J, Tasker R, Hutchinson W (1997) Posteroventral medial pallidotomy in advanced Parkinson's disease. N Engl J Med 337: 1036–1042.

Mallet N, Le Moine C, Charpier S, Gonon F (2005) Feedforward inhibition of projection neurons by fast-spiking GABA interneurons in the rat striatum *in vivo*. J Neurosci 25:3857–3869.

Matsumura M, Tremblay L, Richard H, Filion M (1995) Activity of pallidal neurons in the monkey during dyskinesia induced by injection of bicuculline in the external pallidum. Neuroscience 65:59–70.

Mink J (2003) The basal ganglia and involuntary movements: impaired inhibition of competing motor patterns. Arch Neurol 60:1365–1368.

Mink JW (2006) Abnormal circuit function in dystonia. Neurology 66:959.

Mink JW (2001) Basal ganglia dysfunction in Tourette's syndrome: a new hypothesis. Pediatr Neurol 25:190–198.

Mink JW (1996) The basal ganglia: focused selection and inhibition of competing motor programs. Prog Neurobiol 50:381–425.

Mink JW, Thach WT (1991) Basal ganglia motor control. III. Pallidal ablation: normal reaction time, muscle cocontraction, and slow movement. J Neurophysiol 65:330–351.

Mitchell IJ, Sambrook MA, Crossman AR (1985) Subcortical changes in the regional uptake of [^{3}H]-2-deoxyglucose in the brain of the monkey during experimental choreiform dyskinesia elicited by injection of a gamma-aminobutyric acid antagonist into the subthalamic nucleus. Brain 108:405–422.

Nambu A, Tokuno H, Hamada I, Kita H, Imanishi M, Akazawa T, Ikeuchi Y, Hasegawa N (2000) Excitatory cortical inputs to pallidal neurons via the subthalamic nucleus in the monkey. J Neurophysiol 84:289–300.

Nicola S, Surmeier J, Malenka R (2000) Dopaminergic modulation of neuronal excitability in the striatum and nucleus accumbens. Annu Rev Neurosci 23:185–215.

Parent A (1990) Extrinsic connections of the basal ganglia. Trends Neurosci 13:254–258.

Parent A, Hazrati L-N (1993) Anatomical aspects of information processing in primate basal ganglia. Trends Neurosci 16:111–116.

Penny GR, Afsharpour S, Kitai ST (1986) The glutamate decarboxylase-, leucine enkephalin-, methionine enkephalin- and substance P-immunoreactive neurons in the neostriatum of the rat and cat: evidence for partial population overlap. Neuroscience 17:1011–1045.

Reiner A, Albin RL, Anderson KD, D'Amato CJ, Penney JB, Young AB (1988) Differential loss of striatal projection neurons in Huntington disease. Proc Natl Acad Sci USA 85:5733–5737.

Sibley DR, Monsma FJ (1992) Molecular biology of dopamine receptors. Trends Pharm Sci 13:61–69.

Starr PA, Kang GA, Heath S, Shimamoto S, Turner RS (2008) Pallidal neuronal discharge in Huntington's disease: support for selective loss of striatal cells originating the indirect pathway. Exp Neurol 211:227–233.

Suarez JI, Metman LV, Reich SG, Dougherty PM, Hallett M, Lenz FA (1997) Pallidotomy for hemiballismus: efficacy and characteristics of neuronal activity. Ann Neurol 42:807–811.

Tang JK, Moro E, Lozano AM, Lang AE, Hutchison WD, Mahant N, Dostrovsky JO (2005) Firing rates of pallidal neurons are similar in Huntington's and Parkinson's disease patients. Exp Brain Res 166:230–236.

3

Huntington Disease

Rebecca M. Gilbert, MD, PhD and Steven Frucht, MD

INTRODUCTION

Huntington disease (HD) is the most common form of heritable chorea. It is transmitted in an autosomal dominant fashion and is caused by a CAG expansion in exon 1 of the *IT15* or huntingtin gene. This in turn leads to a longer than normal polyglutamine stretch in the huntingtin protein product. The CAG repeat number is correlated to age at onset but not to disease severity or specific symptomatology. The polyglutamine tract is thought to have a toxic gain of function, primarily on the medium spiny neurons of the striatum, although as the disease progresses, neurodegeneration becomes more widespread. HD is characterized by cognitive decline, psychiatric disturbances, and a wide array of movement disorders, the most well-known and characteristic of which is chorea. A genetic test is widely available for symptomatic patients. It is also available to the presymptomatic children and grandchildren of HD patients, which is fraught with ethical challenges. The testing must be accompanied by genetic counseling because it can have devastating implications for the entire family. Treatments are currently only symptomatic in nature, and in the U.S. only one, tetrabenazine, has been approved for use by the Food and Drug Administration (FDA). A number of neuroprotective agents for use in the presymptomatic population are under active investigation.

OVERVIEW

HD is by far the most common form of heritable chorea, accounting for approximately 93%–99% of such cases (Andrew et al., 1994). Its hereditary nature has been recognized since the initial description in 1872, but the disease-causing mutation was elusive for decades. Finally, by studying a large HD cohort in the Lake Maracaibo region of Venezuela, the genetic abnormality was localized to chromosome 4p16.3 in 1983 (Gusella et al., 1983) and successfully cloned in 1993 (Huntington Disease Collaborative Research Group, 1993). The protein product of the gene was named "huntingtin," a 348 kDa protein without known homology to other proteins. The specific mutation in the gene, a CAG expansion in exon 1, is consistent across families and translates into a polyglutamine stretch within the protein product. When the disease-causing mutation was discovered, HD joined a group of eight other polyglutamine neurodegenerative diseases, including spinocerebellar ataxia types 1, 2, 3, 6, 7, and 17, dentatorubral-pallidoluysian atrophy (DRPLA), and spinobulbar muscular atrophy. Alteration of the huntingtin protein leads to the HD phenotype, which includes motor impairment, cognitive decline, and psychiatric disturbance.

EPIDEMIOLOGY

Although the most common form of heritable chorea, HD is still relatively rare, with a prevalence among Western European populations of approximately 2–9 per 100,000. Rates among Africans and Asians are typically 10 times lower (Conneally, 1984). Among the Venezuelan cohort described (Okun and Thommi, 2004), rates are 52 per 100,000. In this population, a founder effect among a native people with limited opportunities for genetic variability lead to much higher rates of HD— along with a unique chance to study this condition.

GENETICS

Soon after the discovery of the huntingtin gene, it was observed that the number of CAG repeats determines whether an individual develops HD (Duyao et al., 1993). Over time and with the analysis of multiple families, ranges of CAG repeat numbers and their correlation to disease status have been determined. Chromosomes with 26 or fewer repeats do not lead to disease. Chromosomes with 40 or more repeats are 100% penetrant, with repeats above 50 generally causing juvenile-onset cases. Chromosomes with 36–39 repeats have reduced penetrance and are thought to be fully penetrant if the individual lives long enough. It is generally considered that chromosomes with 27–35 repeats do not lead to disease but may be meiotically unstable, causing disease in the subsequent generation (Potter et al., 2004). The instability is more profound during spermatogenesis than during oogenesis, and it is therefore males with intermediate-length CAG repeat numbers who tend to produce offspring who manifest disease (Snell et al., 1993). In such cases, HD patients will not have a family history of the disease. Patients with seemingly *de novo* HD mutations (CAG repeat lengths of greater than 40) and no family history of disease have been studied. For each of these patients, non-diseased family members were discovered who harbored repeat lengths of 34–38. This suggests that expansion of the unstable chromosomal region occurred, thereby producing disease in a subsequent generation (Myers et al., 1993). There have also been published reports of intergenerational CAG repeat number contraction (Nahhas et al., 2009). Although a repeat number of 27–35 is not classically considered to be disease-causing, case reports of HD due to 29 repeats (Kenney et al., 2007) as well as 34 repeats (Andrich et al., 2008) have been described.

AGE AT ONSET

Age at onset of HD ranges from infancy to over 80, with a median of approximately 40 years. What was once described as "senile chorea" may turn out to be HD if genetic testing is pursued. Ten percent of HD is juvenile in onset, defined as onset before 20 years of age.

Repeat length inversely correlates with age at onset—the more repeats, the earlier the disease becomes manifest (Andrew et al., 1993; Duyao et al., 1993). Table 3–1 shows the median age at onset (the age by which 50% of individuals will have developed disease) for any given CAG repeat size as determined by Brinkman et al. (1997). Although this information is useful for risk assessment in a population, it cannot be used to accurately predict the age at onset of any particular individual. Although studies differ slightly, CAG repeat length tends to account for approximately half of the variability in age at onset. More recently, a mathematical model was created to determine the probability of a particular repeat length causing disease over a range of ages (Langbehn et al., 2004). The meiotic instability and tendency for the CAG repeat number to expand with generations cause a phenomenon known as "anticipation," in which the age at onset decreases with subsequent generations. As described, this phenomenon tends to occur when the mutation is being passed down via the individual's father.

The rare patients who are homozygous for the HD gene have been studied. Age at onset is not lower in this population, although disease severity does increase (Squitieri et al., 2003). Less variation in age of onset for a given repeat length

TABLE 3–1. Correlation of CAG Repeat Size to Age at Onset of HD

CAG REPEAT SIZE	MEDIAN AGE AT ONSET (YEARS)	95% CONFIDENCE INTERVAL
39	66	59–72
40	59	56–61
41	54	52–56
42	49	48–50
43	44	42–45
44	42	40–43
45	37	36–39
46	36	35–37
47	33	31–35
48	32	30–34
49	28	25–32
50	27	24–30

Source: Brinkman et al. (1997).

occurs between siblings than non-related individuals, suggesting the existence of other genetic modifiers to age of disease onset.

CLINICAL FEATURES

Although chorea is the hallmark motor feature of HD, dystonia, parkinsonism, eye movement abnormalities, ataxia, tics, and myoclonus commonly occur (Video 3-1). Traditionally, the onset of HD has been defined as the appearance of motor symptoms, but it has become apparent that psychiatric disturbances often predate the motor symptoms, sometimes by decades (Biglan and Shoulson, 2007). These difficulties not only may occur first but often are more functionally impairing than the motor features. Dementia usually follows onset of motor difficulties, although mild cognitive changes detectable on neuropsychiatric testing can be present before motor difficulties are evident. This is not necessarily the case in juvenile HD, where cognitive decline is often the presenting sign (Gonzalez-Alegre and Afifi, 2006). There have been case reports in which dementia has preceded motor or psychiatric features in adult-onset HD (Cooper et al., 2006).

The United Huntington's Disease Rating Scale (UHDRS) was developed to quantify impairment and follow patients as the disease progresses. It assesses motor function, cognitive function, behavioral abnormalities, and functional capacity (Huntington Study Group, 1996).

PRESENTATION

The traditional teaching has been that adult-onset HD manifests first with chorea, whereas juvenile HD, defined as age at onset less than 20, manifests with rigidity and parkinsonism. In a study of 29 juvenile HD patients, however, 66% of patients presented with severe psychiatric and cognitive difficulties in the absence of motor findings, thereby leading to some significant delays in diagnosis. As the disease progressed, motor difficulties developed, including dystonia, parkinsonism, myoclonic tremor, and chorea (Ribai, 2007). Seizures can also be present in juvenile HD.

HD that starts in adulthood can also initially manifest with cognitive or psychiatric changes, as described. The first motor signs, however, are typically eye movement abnormalities, specifically difficulty in initiating saccades as well as slowness of rapid alternating movements, found on neurological exam (Penney et al., 1990). Brief extraneous movements, which may be interpreted as "fidgetiness" by a casual observer, can sometimes be appreciated in the early stages of disease as well.

The Prospective Huntington at Risk Observational Study (PHAROS) is a large study currently in progress, under the auspices of the Huntington Study Group. It monitors individuals at risk for HD who do not have knowledge of their gene status, with the goal of identifying the very first clinical signs of disease emergence. One thousand and one individuals were recruited, and the cohort's characteristics along with the study's methodologies have been presented (Huntington Study Group PHAROS Investigators, 2006).

A parallel study, known as the Predict-HD study, is also currently under way by the Huntington Study Group and has a slightly different goal from that of PHAROS. Predict-HD was designed to monitor known presymptomatic mutation carriers and follow their neurological, cognitive, and psychiatric changes with time. The ultimate goal is to understand the natural history of HD in order to define markers and clinical end points in a trial of a putative neuroprotective agent. The initial publication presented the clinical characteristics of the 505 individuals recruited. Performance on cognitive tasks, scores on scales of psychiatric distress, and striatal volume on magnetic resonance imaging (MRI) were significantly correlated to diagnostic confidence level as determined on the UHDRS (Paulsen et al., 2006).

Predict-HD results have been very intriguing so far. One interesting finding is that presymptomatic carriers have decreased ability to discern negative emotions such as anger, fear, sadness, and disgust as represented on the human face. This change is evident prior to decreased striatal volume, implying that another set of neurons may be responsible for this early feature (Johnson et al., 2007).

DISEASE PROGRESSION

Motor Features

As time progresses, motor symptoms evolve and typically become more aggressive. The full-blown syndrome of chorea, dystonia, eye movement abnormalities, ataxia, tics, and myoclonus develops insidiously. Parkinsonism, which is evident with rigorous testing, may not be appreciable on routine testing, once it manifests along with chorea. Patients develop progressive difficulty walking, maintaining balance, and performing motor skills with their hands. Weight loss is a pervasive feature as the disease progresses, occurring despite healthy appetites. It has yet to be determined if weight loss is due solely to increased movement, although there is evidence to suggest that this is the case (Pratley et al., 2000). More recently, neurodegeneration in the hypothalamus is being studied as the cause for the intractable weight loss, as well as other related issues such as sleep disturbance (Politis et al., 2008).

In the more advanced stages of the disease, patients become akinetic and rigid. Death typically occurs 15–30 years from onset of symptoms. In juvenile HD, death typically occurs 5–20 years after onset.

Neuropsychiatric Features

Neuropsychiatric features that can become prominent include irritability and agitation, personality change, depression, apathy, impulsivity, obsessions and compulsions, mania, suicidality, and psychosis (Van Duijn et al., 2007) (see also Chapter 20). Various studies estimate the prevalence of neuropsychiatric problems in HD to be 30%–70%. Some neuropsychiatric features, such as obsessive–compulsive behavior, may affect up to 50% of HD patients. The authors hypothesized that this particular feature is consistent with other basal ganglia disorders (Anderson et al., 2001). Criminal behavior can occur, likely linked directly to impulsivity, irritability, and personality change.

Cognitive Impairment

Cognitive decline is characterized first by poor cognitive speed and multitasking abilities. This is typically followed by memory loss, visual spatial deficits, decreased attention, and impaired concentration. Toward the end of life, dementia advances to the point that self-care is impossible. These changes are nearly universal among HD patients, although there are individuals with chorea developing later in life who do not show signs of dementia before death from other causes.

Even though repeat length is correlated to disease status and age at onset, it is more difficult to correlate it to specific symptomatology or to disease severity. A case report of monozygotic twins, each carrying the same number of repeats but with different disease courses, highlights this. One of the twins showed a much more profound dementia than the other (Gomez-Esteban et al., 2007). There remains a debate in the literature, however, as to whether repeat length correlates with cognitive decline.

SPECIFIC CHARACTERISTICS OF CHOREA

Motor impersistence of tongue protrusion is a very characteristic feature of HD, which can also be thought of as negative chorea (Fahn and Jankovic, 2007). As with other forms of chorea, the individual often attempts to incorporate the choreic movements into his or her voluntary movements. As mentioned, the movement disorders characteristic of HD are varied and include eye movement abnormalities, dystonia, ataxia, and parkinsonism. These may help to distinguish HD from other forms of chorea.

DIAGNOSTIC TESTS: LABORATORY AND NEUROIMAGING FINDINGS

Currently, DNA testing has largely supplanted neuroimaging in verifying a suspected diagnosis. Prior to this, caudate atrophy was used as a confirmatory sign on MRI. Atrophy of the putamen also occurs, possibly to an even more significant degree than atrophy of the caudate. The extent of striatal atrophy correlates with CAG repeat length (Rosas et al., 2001).

Since genetic testing has become available, research into neuroimaging studies has focused on understanding the pathophysiology of HD and not on confirming diagnosis or determining carrier status. However, an imaging study that could be performed serially over time to track degeneration in a presymptomatic patient would be very valuable in clinical trials of neuroprotective agents. Voxel-based morphometry and tensor-based morphometry were investigated in normal controls and presymptomatic carriers. Atrophy of various deep gray structures increased despite the lack of clinical deterioration in mutation carriers (Kipps et al., 2005).

The standard of care for a patient manifesting signs and symptoms consistent with HD is to perform genetic testing. The test involves polymerase chain reaction

(PCR) with specific primers performed on the patient's serum sample, followed by Southern blotting of the PCR results. Specific issues that relate to the nature of the huntingtin protein make replication of the test across clinical labs difficult. For example, within huntingtin there is a CCG repeat region of 7–12 repeats which is adjacent to the CAG stretch. If primers for PCR are not carefully crafted, the CCG repeat may be amplified as well, leading to false-positive results. Extremely precise quantification of the PCR product must be determined as this can make the difference between a positive and a negative result. In addition, in the rare situation in which one PCR product size is produced, there needs to be confirmation testing to ensure that this in fact represents a homozygous situation and not a lab error (Nance et al., 1998).

The test is now readily available to symptomatic patients and accessible to asymptomatic family members who want to determine their disease status. Preimplantation genetic testing can be performed for individuals who harbor the HD mutation and want to take action in preventing the mutation from being passed on to their offspring. *In vitro* fertilization is performed, and the embryos that are created are tested for the mutation. Only healthy embryos are implanted. Preimplantation genetic testing can also be performed for at-risk individuals who do not want to know whether they carry the mutation but want to ensure that their offspring are not affected. This scenario requires very thoughtful involvement of the geneticist, obstetrician, and neurologist to make certain that the individual remains unaware of his or her disease status.

Presymptomatic diagnostic testing for a devastating and fatal disease that cannot be cured is fraught with challenges (see also Chapter 20). Long-term outcome data from both carriers and noncarriers who underwent testing show rates of depression in noncarriers that were higher than those in the general population, although rates were higher still among carriers (Gargiulo et al., 2009). This emphasizes the need for genetic counseling and psychiatric support to all those who undergo testing and suggests that even receiving reassuring news about one's HD mutation status is a difficult process. Although the genetic test is now widely available, only a small percentage of at-risk individuals take advantage of this testing. One study calculated this number to be 18% (Harper et al., 2000). Prenatal testing was used even more infrequently.

PATHOPHYSIOLOGY (STRUCTURAL/BASAL GANGLIA LEVEL)

It has been known for over a century that HD is characterized by selective atrophy of the caudate nucleus and putamen. The GABAergic medium spiny neurons of the striatum, the most common type of neuron in the striatum, are most susceptible to damage and are selectively affected in early stages (Graveland et al., 1985).

There are two populations of these neurons, those that harbor D_2 receptors, contain enkephalin, and are part of the indirect basal ganglia pathway and those that harbor D_1 receptors, contain substance P, and are part of the direct basal ganglia pathway. In adult-onset HD the D_2 dopamine receptor/enkephalin-containing neurons degenerate first. Their loss interferes with proper functioning of the indirect pathway from the striatum via the globus pallidus externa, to the subthalamic nucleus, and the globus pallidus interna, which projects to the thalamus and back to the cortex (see also Chapter 2). According to the classic model of basal

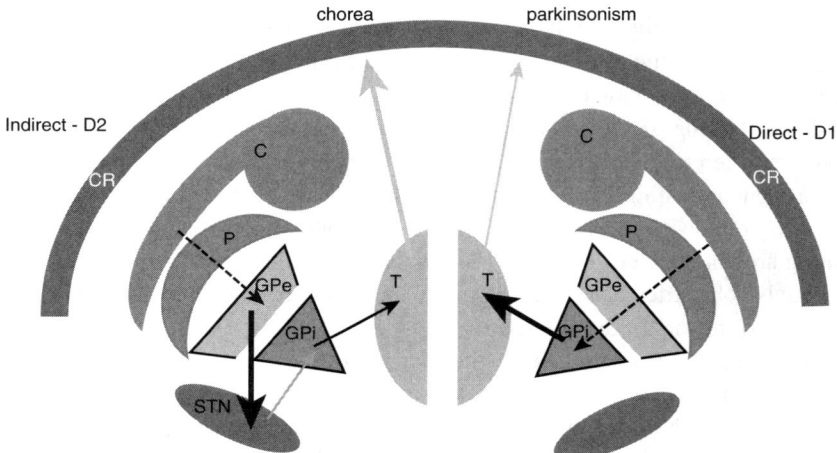

FIGURE 3–1. Basal ganglia pathophysiology in HD. *Left side of the diagram* Early on in Huntington disease(HD), the first neurons to degenerate are the GABAergic medium spiny neurons that bear D_2 dopamine receptors. When these neurons are destroyed, inhibition of the GPe is lifted. Activity of the GABAergic projection from the GPe to the STN is therefore increased. Increased inhibition of the STN causes a reduction in the excitatory output from the STN to the GPi. Decreased excitation of the GPi results in a reduction in the inhibitory output from the GPi to the thalamus. Decreased inhibition of the thalamus results in an increase of the excitatory output from the thalamus to the cortex. This increased excitation is thought to be responsible for chorea. *Right side of the diagram* As HD progresses, the D_1 receptor–bearing neurons also degenerate. When these neurons are destroyed, inhibition of the GPi is lifted. The GABAergic projection from the GPi to the thalamus is therefore increased. Increased inhibition of the thalamus results in a decrease in the excitatory output from the thalamus to the cortex. This decreased excitation is thought to be responsible for parkinsonism. In juvenile parkinsonism, the D_1 receptor–bearing neurons are affected first, leading to a parkinsonian phenotype early on. C, caudate; P, putamen; GPe, globus pallidus externa; GPi, globus pallidus interna; STN, subthalamic nucleus; T, thalamus; CR, cortex; D1, D_1 dopamine receptor–containing neurons; D2, D_2 dopamine receptor–containing neurons. *Black arrows* are GABAergic and inhibitory. *Gray arrows* are glutamatergic and excitatory. *Dashed arrows* represent degenerated neurons in the disease state.

ganglia function, the eventual outcome is the release of inhibition of the thalamus and increased excitation from the thalamus to the cortex, resulting in chorea. D_1 dopamine receptor/substance P–containing neurons appear to become susceptible at a later stage (Sapp et al., 1995). These neurons are part of the direct pathway which projects from the striatum to the globus pallidus interna. Degeneration of D_1 dopamine receptor containing neurons results in increased inhibition of the thalamus, which leads to parkinsonism (Figure 3–1).

Cases of HD that have rigidity-akinesia as the primary feature, as seen in juvenile HD, show simultaneous loss of both D_1 and D_2 striatal neurons (Albin et al., 1990).

It has recently been shown via pathological and imaging studies that, in addition to the early effects on the caudate nucleus and putamen, there is selective thinning of the cortical ribbon, with the posterior cortex affected first (Rosas et al., 2002). Although loss of the medium spiny neurons in the striatum is most prominent, there is also loss of the large striatal interneurons. As the disease progresses, there is more generalized neurodegeneration, including of the globus pallidus, subthalamic nucleus, substantia nigra, cerebellum, and thalamus (Borrell-Pages et al., 2006).

PATHOPHYSIOLOGY (CELLULAR LEVEL)

The function of wild-type huntingtin has still not been elucidated. Although the CAG repeat is responsible for pathogenesis, it may not be a crucial feature of wild-type huntingtin's role. Studies have localized huntingtin to virtually every subcellular structure, shown interactions between huntingtin and many intracellular proteins, and suggested multiple roles that huntingtin may play (Imarisio et al., 2008). Huntingtin has been implicated in antiapoptotic activity (Gervais et al., 2002), transcriptional regulation of brain-derived neurotrophic factor (BDNF) (Zuccato et al., 2001, 2003), microtubule-assisted transport (Caviston et al., 2007), and synaptic transmission (Smith et al., 2005), among other functions.

The role of mutant huntingtin is also not fully defined. The role of mutant huntingtin is also not fully defined. HD may be caused not only by a loss of function of the wild type protein, but by an additional toxic gain of function of the mutant protein. In mouse models, expressing CAG repeat expansions either in the context of the huntingtin gene or within the body of an unrelated protein causes neurodegeneration (Ordway et al., 1997).

It is known that mutant huntingtin forms inclusion bodies in the nucleus, cytoplasm, and synaptic terminals of cortical and striatal neurons (DiFiglia et al., 1997). Of note, such inclusion bodies are characteristic of all the CAG repeat diseases. In HD, the inclusions contain the ubiquitinated amino terminus of the mutant huntingtin protein, which can be cleaved from the full-length protein by a variety of proteases (Kim et al., 2001). Data exist that supports both the claim that the aggregates are responsible for neurodegeneration as well as the claim that they are neuroprotective. For example, transgenic mice expressing exon 1 of the mutant huntingtin protein develop intranuclear inclusions as neurological symptoms become evident, suggesting that the intranuclear inclusions are linked to pathogenesis (Davies et al., 1997). Other evidence, however, has suggested that the inclusions may not be pathogenic. Transgenic mice expressing exon 1 of the mutant huntingtin protein were crossed with tissue transglutaminase knockout mice, resulting in partial rescue of the disease phenotype but an increase in intranuclear inclusions (Mastroberardino et al., 2002).

Intense research into the pathophysiology of mutant huntingtin has produced evidence for the disruption of diverse cellular systems including mitochondrial function (Browne, 2008), proteasomal activity (Finkbeiner and Mitra, 2008), apoptosis (Pattison et al., 2006), protein–protein interactions (Bhattacharyya et al., 2008), endocytosis (Chen and Brodsky, 2005), transcription (Kazantsev and Hersch, 2007), intracellular trafficking (Del Toro et al., 2009), and glutamate regulation (Fan and Raymond, 2007). How significant a role each of these pathways plays and whether these effects exist in a cascade or act in parallel to cause neurodegeneration is still being worked out.

It has been well established that HD brains have impaired oxidative phosphorylation that takes place within the mitochondria. Inhibition of this process leads to free radical buildup and subsequent toxicity. What remains to be elucidated, however, is if the mechanism for mitochondrial dysregulation is mediated by a physical interaction between mutant huntingtin and the outer mitochondrial membrane or via transcriptional regulation of proteins responsible for mitochondrial function (Browne, 2008). Another line of evidence suggests that mutant huntingtin disrupts the ubiquitin–proteasomal system, leading to decreased degradation of toxic products. It has been suggested that the long polyglutamine stretch within mutant huntingtin physically clogs the proteasomal system, hindering further degradation of other proteins. Other data suggest that mutant huntingtin exerts its effects on the proteasome via transcriptional regulation of necessary proteins. Regardless, when the proteasome is dysfunctional, the cell undergoes apoptosis.

Another potential pathogenic mechanism is that the excessive tract of glutamines weakens the interaction between huntingtin and huntingtin-associated protein (HAP1). HAP1 normally interacts with kinesin, the molecular motor for anterograde transport (McGuire et al., 2006). When HAP1 cannot bind huntingtin, it loses its ability to bind kinesin, leading to disruption of cellular processes. Mutant huntingtin has also been implicated in directly enhancing apoptosis via a number of potential mechanisms. One theory implicates huntingtin's interaction with huntingtin-interacting protein (HIP1). Mutant huntingtin no longer binds HIP1 adequately, freeing it to form a proapoptotic complex which includes caspase-8 (Gervais et al., 2002).

Polyglutamine stretches can be found in the activation domain of a number of transcription factors, leading to the hypothesis that proteins of unknown function with polyglutamine repeats may also play a role in transcription. Mutant proteins with too many glutamines may therefore act to disrupt normal transcription (Perutz et al., 1994). The transcription of BDNF, among other proteins, has been shown to be altered by mutant huntingtin. Decreased levels of BDNF result in decreased neuronal cell survival. Huntingtin has also been shown to regulate transcription of cyclic adenosine monophosphate response element binding protein (CREB) binding protein (CBP), which acts as a transcriptional activator (Jiang et al., 2006). Mutant huntingtin binds CBP, thus sequestering it from participating in the transcription of cell survival signals.

Mutant huntingtin has also been implicated in the disruption of normal glutamate activity in the cell. Glutamate transporter-1 (GLT-1) transcription is regulated by huntingtin, and mutant huntingtin causes transcription of too little of GLT-1, leading to increased levels of extracellular glutamate and its resulting toxicity (Behrens et al., 2002). Another theory is that the accumulation of mutant huntingtin aggregates in the synaptic terminal, thereby interfering directly with glutamate uptake.

The field of HD biology has been substantially advanced by the introduction of numerous mouse models. These are useful both in the study of HD pathogenesis as well as in preclinical trials of potential neuroprotective or therapeutic agents. Transgenic mice, the most common of which is the R6/2 line, are created by randomly inserting either a fragment or the full-length human mutant huntingtin gene into the mouse genome. Alternatively, knock-in mice are created by replacing a portion of the mouse huntingtin gene with a portion of the human mutant huntingtin gene. This allows expression of the gene to be regulated by its natural promoter and is considered the more genetically accurate approach (Ramaswamy et al., 2007). Although more genetically accurate, the phenotype of the knock-in mice is generally quite subtle but worsens in mouse lines with CAG repeat lengths of 140 and higher. Because of the subtle phenotype, these mice are less useful for preclinical trials.

TREATMENTS

There are currently no disease-modifying therapies for HD. Symptomatic treatments are available only for the motor and behavioral features of the disease. Antipsychotics can offer some relief from chorea. Olanzapine was tested in a small open-label trial and shown to lead to improvement in Huntington chorea (Bonelli et al., 2002). Tetrabenazine (TBZ), first introduced in the 1950s, acts as a vesicular monoamine transporter-2 (VMAT-2) inhibitor. VMAT normally transports norepinephrine, serotonin, and dopamine into presynaptic vesicles.

When the transporter is inhibited, the neurotransmitters are degraded by mono-amine oxidase (MAO), thereby leading to dopamine depletion. A 2006 trial con-ducted by the Huntington Study Group demonstrated significant benefit upon chorea as well as clinical global improvement in patients taking TBZ compared to placebo. There were, however, five study withdrawals in the TBZ group (as opposed to one in the control group) and five serious adverse events, including one suicide (as opposed to none in the control group) (Huntington Study Group, 2006). Recently, the FDA approved TBZ for use in HD-related chorea in the U.S. It is also used off-label for other hyperkinetic disorders such as non-HD chorea, hemiballismus, tardive syndromes, and tics. Depression is a serious side effect of TBZ and limits its use in predisposed individuals. A very small study comparing TBZ with aripiprazole, showed similar improvements in UHDRS scores, although aripiprazole caused less sedation and was better tolerated. There was a nonsignifi-cant improvement of depression in the aripiprazole group (Brusa et al., 2009).

Selective serotonin reuptake inhibitors (SSRIs) are often prescribed for depression and the obsessive–compulsive features of HD (Chapter 20). Cognitive dysfunction has proven difficult to tackle. Two acetylcholinesterase inhibitors were tested in small patient groups in open-label, randomized, controlled studies. Treatment with rivastigmine resulted in some mild improvement in cognitive functioning (De Tommaso et al., 2004), while treatment with donepezil showed no improvement (Cubo et al., 2006). A Cochrane review analyzed all trials aimed at alleviating HD symptoms. The study concluded that good-quality data existed to support the use of TBZ alone (Mestre et al., 2009).

As more is learned about huntingtin and its function in the healthy and mutated states, rational consideration of potential neuroprotective agents becomes possible (Wagner et al., 2008). Free radical scavengers such as coenzyme Q_{10} and creatine may reverse mitochondrial damage inflicted by mutant huntingtin. Glutamate release inhibitors and glutamate receptor blockers may decrease glutamate toxic-ity, which is enhanced by mutant huntingtin. Protease inhibitors, such as minocy-cline, may be able to halt the cleavage of the N terminus of huntingtin, the portion of the mutant protein that forms aggregates. Transglutaminase is known to polym-erize mutant huntingtin, and inhibitors of this enzyme may therefore stop hunting-tin aggregation. Since huntingtin has been implicated in dysregulated gene transcription, histone deacetylase inhibitors have been tried as a mechanism to restore normal transcription. Instillation of trophic factors and fetal transplants are also under investigation. Treatments using interfering RNA aim to reduce transcription of mutant huntingtin. Caspase inhibitors may reduce abnormal activation that spirals cells into apoptosis. Autophagy is a cellular process by which protein complexes and organelles are degraded (Sarkar and Rubinsztein, 2008), as are mutant disease-causing protein aggregates. Enhancement of autophagy may therefore serve to reduce disease burden. Figure 3–2 (adapted from Fahn and Jankovic, 2007) summarizes some of the various strategies that

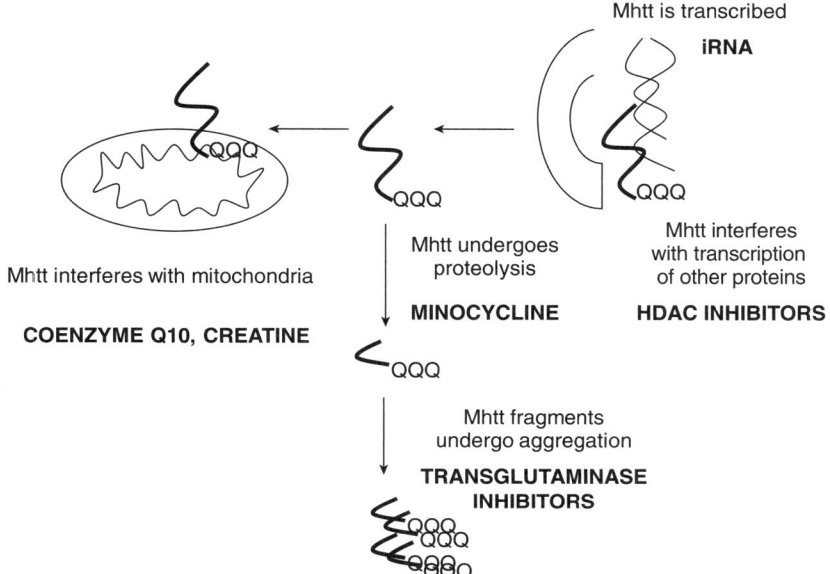

FIGURE 3–2. Potential therapeutic mechanisms to counteract the effects of mutant huntingtin. The cellular activities of mutant huntingtin are written in lower case letters; potential therapies that counteract these activities are written in capital letters. Mhtt, mutant huntingtin; QQQ, polyglutamine tract; iRNA, interfering RNA; HDAC, histone deacetylase. Adapted from Fahn and Jankovic (2007) with permission.

have been investigated or are under investigation today. Unfortunately, results so far have not yielded a successful treatment, but efforts continue valiantly to help stop the so far inevitable progression of this destructive disease.

REFERENCES

Albin RL, Reiner A, Anderson KD, Penney JB, Young AB (1990) Striatal and nigral neuron subpopulations in rigid Huntington's disease: implications for the functional anatomy of chorea and rigidity-akinesia. Ann Neurol 4:357–365.

Anderson KE, Louis ED, Stern Y, Marder KS (2001) Cognitive correlates of obsessive and compulsive symptoms in Huntington's disease. Am J Psychiatry 158(5):799–801.

Andrew SE, Goldberg YP, Kremer B, et al. (1993) The relationship between trinucleotide (CAG) repeat length and clinical features of Huntington's disease. Nat Genetics 4(4): 398–403.

Andrew SE, Goldberg YP, Kremer B, et al. (1994) Huntington disease without CAG expansion: phenocopies or errors in assignment? Am J Hum Genet 54(5):852–863.

Andrich J, Arning L, Wieczorek S, Kraus PH, Gold R, Saft C (2008) Huntington's disease as caused by 34 CAG repeats. Mov Disord 23(6):879–881.

Bhattacharyya NP, Banerjee M, Majumder P (2008) Huntington's disease: roles of huntingtin-interacting protein (HIP-1) and its molecular partner HIPPI in the regulation of apoptosis and transcription. FEBS J 275(17):4271–4279.

Behrens PF, Franz P, Woodman B, Lindenberg KS, Landwehrmeyer GB (2002) Impaired glutamate transport and glutamate–glutamine cycling: downstream effects of the Huntington mutation. Brain 125(Pt 8):1908–1922.

Biglan K, Shoulson I (2007) Juvenile-onset huntington disease: a matter of perspective. Arch Neurol 64(6):783–784.

Bonelli RM, Mahnert FA, Niederwieser G (2002) Olanzapine for Huntington's disease: an open label study. Clin Neuropharmacol 25(5):263–265.

Borrell-Pages M, Zala D, Humbert S, Saudou F (2006) Huntington's disease: from huntingtin function and dysfunction to therapeutic strategies. Cell Mol Life Sci 63(22): 2642–2660.

Brinkman RR, Mezei MM, Theilmann J, Almqvist E, Hayden MR (1997) The likelihood of being affected with Huntington disease by a particular age, for a specific CAG size. Am J Hum Genet 60(5):1202–1210.

Browne SE (2008) Mitochondria and Huntington's disease pathogenesis: insight from genetic and chemical models. Ann N Y Acad Sci 1147:358–382.

Brusa L, Orlacchio A, Moschella V, Iani C, Bernardi G, Mercuri NB (2009) Treatment of the symptoms of Huntington's disease: preliminary results comparing aripiprazole and tetrabenazine. Mov Disord 24(1):126–129.

Caviston JP, Ross JL, Antony SM, Tokito M, Holzbaur EL (2007) Huntingtin facilitates dynein/dynactin-mediated vesicle transport. Proc Natl Acad Sci USA 104(24):10045–10050.

Chen CY, Brodsky FM (2005) Huntingtin-interacting protein (Hip-1) and Hip-1 related protein (Hip1R) bind the conserved sequence of clathrin light chains and thereby influence clathrin assembly *in vitro* and actin distribution *in vivo*. J Biol Chem 280(7): 6109–6117.

Conneally PM (1984) Huntington disease: genetics and epidemiology. Am J Hum Genet 36(3):506–526.

Cooper DB, Ales G, Lange C, Clement P (2006) Atypical onset of symptoms in Huntington disease: severe cognitive decline preceding chorea or other motor manifestations. Cogn Behav Neurol 19(4):222–224.

Cubo E, Shannon KM, Tracy D, Jaglin JA, Bernard BA, Wuu J, Leurgans SE (2006) Effect of donepezil on motor and cognitive function in Huntington disease. Neurology 67(7):1268–1271.

Davies SW, Turmaine M, Cozens BA, et al. (1997) Formation of neuronal intranuclear inclusions underlies the neurological dysfunction in mice transgenic for the HD mutation. Cell 90(3):537–548.

De Tommaso M, Specchio N, Sciruicchio V, Difruscolo O, Specchio LM (2004) Effects of rivastigmine on motor and cognitive impairment in Huntington's disease. Mov Disord 19(12):1516–1518.

Del Toro D, Alberch J, Lazaro-Dieguez F, Martin-Ibanez R, Xifro X, Egea G, Canals JM (2009) Mutant huntingtin impairs post-Golgi trafficking to lysosomes by delocalizing optineurin/Rab8 complex from the Golgi apparatus. Mol Biol Cell 20(5):1478–1492.

DiFiglia M, Sapp E, Chase KO, Davies SW, Bates GP, Vonsattel JP, Aronin N (1997) Aggregation of huntingtin in neuronal intranuclear inclusions and dystrophic neurites in brain. Science 277(5334):1990–1993.

Duyao M, Ambrose C, Myers R, et al. (1993) Trinucleotide repeat length instability and age of onset of Huntington's disease. Nat Genet 4(4):387–392.

Fahn S, Jankovic J (2007) Principles and Practice of Movement Disorders. Elsevier, Philadelphia, pp 369–392.

Fan MM, Raymond LA (2007) *N*-Methyl-D-aspartate (NMDA) receptor function and excitotoxicity in Huntington's disease. Prog Neurobiol 81(5–6):272–293.

Finkbeiner S, Mitra S (2008) The ubiquitin–proteasome pathway in Huntington's disease. Sci World J 8:421–433.

Gargiulo M, Lejeune S, Tanguy ML, et al. (2009) Long-term outcome of presymptomatic testing in Huntington disease. Eur J Hum Genet 17(2):165–171.

Gervais FG, Singaraja R, Xanthoudakis S, et al. (2002) Recruitment and activation of caspase-8 by the Huntingtin-interacting protein Hip-1 and a novel partner Hippi. Nat Cell Biol 4(2):95–105.

Gomez-Esteban JC, Lezcano E, Zarranz JJ, Velasco F, Garamendi I, Perez T, Tijero B (2007) Monozygotic twins suffering from Huntington's disease show different cognitive and behavioral symptoms. Eur Neurol 57(1):26–30.

Gonzalez-Alegre P, Afifi AK (2006) Clinical characteristics of childhood-onset (juvenile) Huntington disease: report of 12 patients and review of the literature. J Child Neurol 21(3):223–229.

Graveland GA, Williams RS, DiFiglia M (1985) Evidence for degenerative and regenerative changes in neostriatal spiny neurons in Huntington's disease. Science 227(4688): 770–773.

Gusella JF, Wexler NS, Conneally PM, et al. (1983) A polymorphic DNA marker genetically linked to Huntington's disease. Nature 306(5940):234–238.

Harper PS, Lim C, Craufurd D (2000) Ten years of presymptomatic testing for Huntington's disease: the experience of the UK Huntington's Disease Prediction Consortium. J Med Genet 37(8):567–571.

Huntington's Disease Collaborative Research Group (1993) A novel gene containing a trinucleotide repeat that is expanded and unstable on Huntington's disease chromosomes. Cell 72(6):971–983.

Huntington Study Group (1996) Unified Huntington's Disease Rating Scale: reliability and consistency. Mov Disord 11(2):136–142.

Huntington Study Group (2006) Tetrabenazine as antichorea therapy in Huntington disease: a randomized controlled trial. Neurology 66(3):366–372.

Huntington Study Group PHAROS Investigators (2006) At risk for Huntington disease: the PHAROS (Prospective Huntington at Risk Observational Study) cohort enrolled. Arch Neurol 63(7):991–996.

Imarisio S, Carmichael J, Korolchuk V, et al. (2008) Huntington's disease: from pathology and genetics to potential therapies. Biochem J 412(2):191–209.

Jiang H, Poirier MA, Liang Y, et al. (2006) Depletion of CBP is directly linked with cellular toxicity caused by mutant huntingtin. Neurobiol Dis 23(3):543–551.

Johnson SA, Stout JC, Solomon AC, et al. (2007) Beyond disgust: impaired recognition of negative emotions prior to diagnosis of Huntington's disease. Brain 130(Pt 7):1732–1744.

Kazantsev AG, Hersch SM (2007) Drug targeting of dysregulated transcription in Huntington's disease. Prog Neurobiol 83(4):249–259.

Kenney C, Powell S, Jankovic J (2007) Autopsy proven Huntington's disease with 29 trinucleotide repeats. Mov Disorder 22(1):127–130.

Kim YJ, Yi Y, Sapp E, et al. (2001) Caspase-3 cleaved N-terminal fragments of wild type and mutant huntingtin are present in normal and Huntington's disease brains, associate with membranes and undergo calpain-dependent proteolysis. Proc Natl Acad Sci USA 98(22):12784–12789.

Kipps CM, Duggins AJ, Mahant N, Gomes L, Ashburner J, McCusker EA (2005) Progression of structural neuropathology in preclinical Huntington's disease: a tensor based morphometry study. J Neurol Neurosurg Psychiatry 76(5):650–655.

Langbehn DR, Brinkman RR, Falush D, Paulsen JS, Hayden MR; International Huntington's Disease Collaborative Group (2004) A new model for prediction of the age of onset and penetrance for Huntington's disease based on CAG length. Clin Genet 65(4): 267–277.

Mastroberardino PG, Iannicola C, Nardacci R, et al. (2002) Tissue tranglutaminase ablation reduced neuronal death and prolongs survival in a mouse model of Huntington's disease. Cell Death Differ 9(9):873–880.

McGuire JR, Rong J, Li SH, Li XJ (2006) Interaction of Huntingtin-associated protein-1 with kinesin light chain: implications in intracellular trafficking in neurons. J Biol Chem 281(6):3552–3559.

Mestre T, Ferreira J, Coelho MM, Rosa M, Sampaio C (2009) Therapeutic interventions for symptomatic treatment in Huntington's disease. Cochrane Database Syst Rev 3: CD006456.

Myers RH, MacDonald ME, Koroshetz WJ, et al. (1993) De novo expansion of a $(CAG)_n$ repeat in sporadic Huntington's disease. Nat Genet 5(2):168–173.

Nahhas F, Garbern J, Feely S, Feldman GL (2009) An intergenerational contraction of a fully penetrant Huntington disease allele to a reduced penetrance allele: interpretation of results and significance of risk assessment and genetic counseling. Am J Med Genet A 149A(4):732–736.

Nance M, Seltzer W, Ashizawa T, et al. (1998) ACMG/ASHG statement. Laboratory guidelines for Huntington disease genetic testing. The American College of Medical Genetics/American Society of Human Genetics Huntington Disease Genetic Testing Working Group. Am J Hum Genet 62(5):1243–1247.

Norremolle A, Budtz-Jorgensen E, Fenger K, Nielsen JE, Sorensen SA, Hasholt L (2009) 4p16.3 haplotype modifying age at onset of Huntington disease. Clin Genet 75(3): 244–250.

Okun MS, Thommi N (2004) Americo Negrette (1924–2003): diagnosing Huntington disease in Venezuela. Neurology 63(2):340–343.

Ordway JM, Tallaksen-Greene S, Gutekunst CA, et al. (1997) Ectopically expressed CAG repeats cause intranuclear inclusions and a progressive late onset neurological phenotype in the mouse. Cell 91(6):753–763.

Pattison LR, Kotter MR, Fraga D, Bonelli RM (2006) Apoptotic cascades as possible targets for inhibiting cell death in Huntington's disease. J Neurol 253(9):1137–1142.

Paulsen JS, Hayden M, Stout JC, et al. (2006) Preparing for preventive clinical trials: the Predict-HD study. Arch Neurol 63(6):883–890.

Penney JB Jr, Young AB, Shoulson I, et al. (1990) Huntington's disease in Venezuela: 7 years of follow-up on symptomatic and asymptomatic individuals. Mov Disorder 5(2):93–99.

Perutz MF, Johnson T, Suzuki M, Finch JT (1994) Glutamine repeats as polar zippers: their possible role in inherited neurodegenerative diseases. Proc Natl Acad Sci USA 91(12):5355–5358.

Politis M, Pavese N, Tai YF, Tabrizi SJ, Barker RA, Piccini P (2008) Hypothalamic involvement in Huntington's disease: an in vivo PET study. Brain 131(Pt 11):2860–2869.

Potter NT, Spector EB, Prior TW (2004) Technical standard and guidelines for Huntington disease testing. Genet Med 6(1):61–65.

Pratley RE, Salbe AD, Ravussin E, Caviness JN (2000) Higher sedentary energy expenditure in patients with Huntington's disease. Ann Neurol 47(1):64–70.

Ramaswamy S, McBride JL, Kordower JH (2007) Animal models of Huntington's disease. ILAR J 48(4):356–373.

Ribai P, Nguyen K, Hahn-Barma V, et al. (2007) Psychiatric and cognitive difficulties as indicators of juvenile huntington disease onset in 29 patients. Arch Neurol 64(6): 813–819.

Rosas HD, Goodman J, Chen YI, et al. (2001) Striatal volume loss in HD as measured by MRI and the influence of CAG repeat. Neurology 57(6):1025–1028.

Rosas HD, Liu AK, Hersch S, et al. (2002) Regional and progressive thinning of the cortical ribbon in Huntington's disease. Neurology 58(5):695–701.

Sapp E, Ge P, Aizawa H, et al. (1995) Evidence for a preferential loss of enkephalin immunoreactivity in the external globus pallidus in low grade Huntington's disease using high resolution image analysis. Neuroscience 64(2):397–404.

Sarkar S, Rubinsztein DC (2008) Huntington's disease: degradation of mutant huntingtin by autophagy. FEBS J 275(17):4263–4270.

Smith R, Brundin P, Li JY (2005) Synaptic dysfunction in Huntington's disease: a new perspective. Cell Mol Life Sci 62(17):1901–1912.

Snell RG, MacMillan JC, Cheadle JP, et al. (1993) Relationship between trinucleotide repeat expansion and phenotypic variation in Huntington's disease. Nat Genet 4(4): 393–397.

Squitieri F, Gellera C, Cannella M, et al. (2003) Homozygosity for CAG mutation in Huntington disease is associated with a more severe clinical course. Brain 126(Pt 4):946–955.

Van Duijn E, Kingma EM, van der Mast RC (2007) Psychopathology in verified Huntington's disease gene carriers. J Neuropsychiatry Clin Neurosci 19(4):441–448.

Wagner T, Menalled L, Goumeniouk AD, Brunner D, Leavitt BR (2008) Huntington disease. In: McArthur R, Bursini F (eds.) Animal and Translational Models for CNS Drug Discovery, vol 2. Elsevier, New York, pp 207–274.

Zuccato C, Ciammola A, Rigamonti D et al. (2001) Loss of huntingtin-mediated BDNF gene transcription in Huntington's disease. Science 293(5529):493–498.

Zuccato C, Tartari M, Crotti A, et al. (2003) Huntingtin interacts with REST/NRSF to modulate the transcription of NRSE-controlled neuronal genes. Nat Genet 35(1): 76–83.

4

Benign Hereditary Chorea

Octavian R. Adam, MD and Joseph Jankovic, MD

INTRODUCTION

Benign hereditary chorea (BHC) is a familial, childhood-onset disorder mani-fested primarily by chorea. This developmental disorder represents only one facet of a larger phenotype associated with mutations in the thyroid transcription factor gene (*TITF-1*) on chromosome 14q13.1–q21.1.

BHC was initially identified in the late 1960s as a new entity, distinct from other more common causes of chorea such as Huntington disease (HD) and Sydenham chorea. However, the lack of confirmatory tests and stringent clinical criteria led to a multitude of reports of poorly characterized families that blurred the BHC phenotype. As a consequence, its existence as a distinct entity started to be questioned, until the causative gene was found in 2002. Since then, our under-standing of the pathogenic mechanisms and clinical presentation of BHC has expanded, BHC becoming integrated into the larger concept of brain–lung–thyroid (BLT) disease associated with *TITF-1* mutations.

HISTORY

BHC was first described by Haerer and colleagues in 1967 in an African American family from rural Mississippi. Their report was based on the examination of two teenage brothers, an evaluation of 32 family members spanning over four generations, and collection of information from five generations. A total of 14 family members were found to exhibit "variable abnormal movements that were quick and unpredictable, not writhing and usually not violent." These movements, with onset in early childhood, were categorized as chorea, of minimal to moderate intensity, occurring mainly in the arms and hands and, in one-third of those affected, also in the facial muscles, tongue, and lower extremities. The movements were nondisabling and nonprogressive; and besides "milkmaid's grip," "hung-up" reflexes, and a general appearance of restlessness, the neurological and physical examinations were normal. One of the affected individuals scored 66 on the Wechsler Intelligence Scale, the score attributed to the "patient's educational and socioeconomic background," a sample of the immediate community averaging 80 points on the same scale. Based on their pedigree, the authors concluded that the transmission followed an autosomal dominant pattern. The nomenclature of this new condition, "hereditary nonprogressive chorea of early onset," was used to reflect its defining characteristics.

The same year, two other families sharing a very similar phenotype of nonprogressive, mild–moderate chorea affecting mainly the upper extremities and hands were identified in New Haven (Pincus and Chutorian, 1967). The physical and neurological examinations were normal with the exception of action ("intention") tremor, thus named "familial benign chorea with intention tremor." The original nomenclature reflected core clinical characteristics that made this new entity unique; early-onset chorea of a nonprogressive, benign course, dominantly transmitted, with variable penetrance, in the absence of other neurological abnormalities with the exception of action tremor, in the context of normal motor and cognitive development.

At that time, the differential diagnosis of childhood-onset chorea and the diagnostic accuracy were limited by the lack of confirmatory genetic tests (Table 4–1). BHC was identified as a new entity, causing hereditary, nonprogressive, benign, early-onset chorea, distinct from other conditions, such as HD, which carried a poorer prognosis and entailed specific genetic counseling, or transitory nonhereditary Sydenham chorea. Between 1967 and 2002, when the causative gene was identified, there have been a multitude of families reported with BHC (Table 4–2), originating in the United States, France, Germany, Japan, the United Kingdom, Italy, and Chile. Even though the core features of BHC (early onset, nonprogressive course, dominant transmission) were largely respected, these reports expanded the phenotype markedly, with additional clinical features including motor developmental delay, below-average intelligence or cognitive delay, tremor, dystonia, ataxia or dysmetria, myoclonus, weakness and amyotrophy, pyramidal signs, tics, epilepsy, dysmorphic features, psychiatric pathology, congenital deafness, apraxia, and other abnormalities (Table 4–2).

However, the lack of genetic tests raised uncertainty about the diagnosis and about the relevance of the additional features for the BHC phenotype. This made

TABLE 4–I. Differential Diagnosis of Chorea in 1967

DISEASE	INFORMATIVE CLINICAL FEATURES
Sydenham chorea	History of rheumatic fever, noninherited, self-limiting, onset later in childhood, abnormal physical examination (carditis, etc.), laboratory inflammatory testing, antistreptolysin O antibody titer
Huntington chorea	Juvenile form; rigidity, seizures, progressive, onset later in childhood, "mental deterioration"
Idiopathic hypoparathyroidism	
Familial paroxysmal choreoathetosis (paroxysmal kinesigenic dyskinesia)	Nonprogressive paroxysmal hyperkinetic movement disorder (choreoathetosis) lasting seconds to minutes, normal examination between attacks
Lesch-Nyhan syndrome	Self-mutilation, hyperuricemia, mental retardation, abnormal uric acid metabolism
Paramyoclonus multiplex	Progressive course; intellectual deterioration; massive jerks of trunk, head, and neck; characteristic electroencephalographic abnormalities
Other causes	Perinatal brain injury (cerebral palsy), encephalitis, brain tumor, drugs (dopamine receptor blockers)

Sources: Haerer et al. (1967), Pincus and Chutorian (1967).

it difficult to establish specific clinical diagnostic criteria or to accurately determine the prevalence, estimated at 1 in 500,000 (Harper, 1978). With advances in diagnostic and genetic testing, new hyperkinetic movement disorders were identified, such as myoclonus-dystonia or hereditary essential myoclonus, and the differential diagnosis and treatment of these conditions have become more refined (Jankovic, 2009).

BHC: AN ENTITY OR A SYNDROME?

The variability of the BHC clinical presentation provided a stimulus for a follow-up study of all the published cases since 1967 in an effort to better define the phenotypes and establish diagnoses (Schrag et al., 2000). Of the total of 42 families/case reports of BHC published between 1967 and 2000, the Queen Square investigators were able to obtain a follow-up on 11 families, with direct examination of three families, a review of videos in two families, and a follow-up

TABLE 4–2. BHC Families Reported Before 2002, Including Associated Features, References, and Follow-Up

REFERENCE	FAMILY	NUMBER AFFECTED	INHERITANCE	ONSET	MOTOR DELAY	COGNITIVE DELAY	CHOREA	COURSE	ASSOCIATED FEATURES	REFERENCES F/U INCLUDING FOLLOW-UP
Sleigh and Lindenbaum, 1981	1	3	AD	Infancy	Y	N	+	S	None	No F/U
	1 (2nd)	3	AD	Childhood	Y	Mildly retarded	+	S	Intention tremor, dysarthria, wobbly gait, tight pen grip	No F/U
Sleigh and Lindenbaum, 1981; Quarrell et al., 1988	1 (3rd)	2	AD	Childhood	Y	?	+/−	S	Fine action tremor, drooling, dysmetric reach	Not BHC,[a] dystonia +/− chorea, eye movement abnormalities (Schrag et al., 2000)
Quinn et al., 1988 Klein et al., 1996	1	2	AR	Childhood	N	N	+	P	Subsequently dystonia, ataxia, oculomotor apraxia, no telangiectasias	Not BHC,[a] ataxia without telangiectasia with translocation (7;14) (Klein et al., 1996)

(continued)

TABLE 4-2. (continued)

REFERENCE	FAMILY	NUMBER AFFECTED	INHERITANCE	ONSET	MOTOR DELAY	COGNITIVE DELAY	CHOREA	COURSE	ASSOCIATED FEATURES	F/U INCLUDING REFERENCES
Robinson and Thornett, 1985; Quarrell et al., 1988	1	2	AD	Infancy	Y	N	+	S	Transitory improvement of chorea with steroids	Not BHC,[a] predominantly dystonia +/- myoclonus or chorea (Schrag et al., 2000)
Garcia Ruiz et al., 1994	1	4	AD	Early onset	?	N	+	S	No	Not BHC,[b] multifocal myoclonus/ myoclonic dystonia, no chorea (Schrag et al., 2000)
Yapijakis et al., 1995	1	7	AD	2–14 years	N	N	+/–	S	Spasmodic torticollis, segmental dystonia, dysarthria, hand tremor, hyporeflexia, "spastic dysphonia"	Not BHC,[b] tics or myoclonus, without chorea (Schrag et al., 2000); no linkage to chromosome 14 (Breedveld et al., 2002a)

Reference									Clinical features	Notes
Quarrell et al., 1988; Macmillan et al., 1993a, b	1	4	AD	?	?	N	+	P	Dysarthria, limb and gait ataxia, muscle wasting	Not BHC,[c] genetically confirmed HD (CAG expansion 38–45)
Refsum and Sjaastad, 1972; Sjaastad et al., 1983	1	1	AD	Childhood	?	N	+	S	Anxiety, phobic traits, myoclonus, intention tremor	Not BHC,[c] myoclonic dystonia (no genetic testing)
Schady and Meara, 1988; Quinn, 1993	1	2	AD	Childhood	N	N	+	P	Dysarthria, torticollis, axial dystonia, shoulder girdle wasting/weakness, lower extremity hyperreflexia with extensor plantar reflexes	Not BHC,[c] hereditary idiopathic dystonia (Quinn, 1993)
Behan and Bone, 1977	1	3	AD	Childhood	N	N	+	P (after head trauma at 18)	Involuntary grunting noises	Not BHC,[c] chorea resolved in proband at 21-year F/U but had grunts, grimacing, and blepharospasm (Schrag et al., 2000)
Deonna and Voumard, 1979	1	3	AD	Early onset	Mild	Low average/N	+	I/S	Muscle weakness, hypotonia	No progression[d] (Schrag et al., 2000)

(continued)

TABLE 4–2. (continued)

REFERENCE	FAMILY	NUMBER AFFECTED	INHERITANCE	ONSET	MOTOR DELAY	COGNITIVE DELAY	CHOREA	COURSE	ASSOCIATED FEATURES	REFERENCES F/U INCLUDING
Harper, 1978; Quarrell et al., 1988	1	2	AD	Infancy	Y	N	+	S	"Behavioral disturbances"	Deletion G908 (Table 4–4) (Breedveld et al., 2002b)
	2	3	AD	Early childhood	Mild	Border-line/N	+	S/I	One member had "epileptic fits" since childhood and gait impairment, requiring "two sticks" to ambulate, with previous toe amputation to "aid walking"	No progression,[d] one member had slowly progressive paraparesis and pes cavus (Schrag et al., 2000)

Haerer et al., 1967	1	14	AD	Early childhood	N	N	+	S/I	None	No F/U
Pincus and Chutorian, 1967	1	2	AD	Late childhood	N	N	+	S	Intention tremor	No F/U
	2	1	AD	Early childhood	N	N	+	S	Intention tremor	No F/U
Nutting et al., 1969	1	2	AR	Childhood	N	N	+	S	None	No F/U
Chun et al., 1973	1	4	AD	Infancy, early childhood	N	N	+	S	Excessive drooling, severe dysarthria, wide-based gait with impaired tandem, recurrent spontaneous abortions in one member, dysmetria in another member, paroxysmal exacerbations with excessive sweating	No F/U
	2	2	AD	Early childhood	Y	N	+	S	Dysarthria, wide-based gait, poor tandem, unusual features in one (clinodactyly, mild hypospadias, hypertrophic pyloric stenosis, mild metatarsus adductus deformity)	No F/U

(continued)

TABLE 4–2. (continued)

REFERENCE	FAMILY	NUMBER AFFECTED	INHERITANCE	ONSET	MOTOR DELAY	COGNITIVE DELAY	CHOREA	COURSE	ASSOCIATED FEATURES	REFERENCES F/U INCLUDING
	3	4	AR?	Childhood	?	Borderline MR	+	S	Dysarthria, hypertrophied neck musculature, elbow hyperextensibility	No F/U
Sadjadpour and Amato, 1973	1	5	AD	Childhood	?	Lower limit of average	+	I	"Slowness," "clumsiness"; family history of mental illnesses	No F/U
Bird et al, 1976; Fernandez et al., 2001a	1	5	AD	2–5 years	N	N	+	S/I	Sudden extension neck spasms and late onset (60s), moderate memory loss, intention tremor, "sucking in and out of the lower lip," behavioral problems in two, Duane syndrome in one	Linkage confirmed to chromosome 14q (Fernandez et al., 2001a.)

Reference			Inheritance	Onset			+	S/I	Clinical features	Follow-up
Bird and Hall, 1978; Fernandez et al., 2001b	1	9	AD	Early childhood, adolescence	?	?	+	S/I	One instance each of suicide, psychosis, idiopathic epilepsy, optic nerve glioma in affected individuals; perioral and periorbital myokymia; paroxysmal dyskinesia spells	Not BHC, negative linkage to chromosome 14, diagnosis changed to familial dyskinesia with facial myokymia (Fernandez et al., 2001b)
Burns et al., 1976	1	16	AD, with bilineal transmission (propositi thought to be homozygotes)	?	N	N	+	S	Delayed speech, mild hypospadias in one; another had increased tone and expressionless face	No F/U
Damasio et al., 1977	1	2	AR? Or AD with incomplete penetrance	Childhood	N	N	+	S	Congenital deafness	No F/U
Hermier and Beaupere, 1978	1	1	AD	Childhood	?	?	+	S	Situs inversus	No F/U
Foerster and Foerster, 1978	1	2	AD	Childhood	?	Low average intelligence	+	S	Rest and intention tremor	No F/U

(continued)

TABLE 4–2. (continued)

REFERENCE	FAMILY	NUMBER AFFECTED	INHERITANCE	ONSET	MOTOR DELAY	COGNITIVE DELAY	CHOREA	COURSE	ASSOCIATED FEATURES	REFERENCES F/U INCLUDING
Rice and Terrence, 1979	1	1	AD	Childhood	N	N	+	S	Eye tic, head-nodding tremor, normal head CT, father had lifetime "nonrhythmic" head-nodding tremor since adolescence; brother had transitory chorea and confirmed rheumatic fever	No F/U
Fisher et al., 1979; Breedveld et al., 2002a	1	13	AD	<1 year	+	+/–	+	P/S	Chorea affecting predominantly lower extremities, extensor plantar reflexes, normal head CT, improved with propranolol in proband	Linkage to chromosome 14 (Breedveld et al., 2002a)

Reference			Inheritance	Onset					Clinical features	Follow-up
Ito et al., 1982	1	4	AD	Childhood	?	N	+	S	Paroxysmal choreoathetosis-like movements in proband, "occasionally manifested" choreiform movements in another	No F/U
Landrieu et al., 1984	1	4	X-linked recessive or AD with reduced penetrance	Childhood	+/−	+/−	+	S	Generalized epilepsy in proband, chorea responded to pimozide in two members	No F/U
Leli et al., 1984	1	18	AD	Infancy	+	+	+	P in childhood, S/I in adulthood	None reported	Linkage to chromosome 14 (Breedveld et al., 2002a) (see Table 4–4)
Zambrino et al., 1984	1	2	AR?	Childhood	?	+	+	S/I	Epilepsy, ataxia-telangiectasia, action myoclonus, increased HVA in CSF	No F/U
Stapert et al., 1985	1	4	AD	Childhood	Y	N	+	I	"Poor mimicry," "stereotyped facial grimacing," proximal and axial chorea	No F/U

(continued)

TABLE 4–2. (continued)

REFERENCE	FAMILY	NUMBER AFFECTED	INHERITANCE	ONSET	MOTOR DELAY	COGNITIVE DELAY	CHOREA	COURSE	ASSOCIATED FEATURES	F/U INCLUDING REFERENCES
	2	3	AD	Childhood	Y	N?	+	I	Slight intention tremor, head tremor; in one, chorea improved in adulthood to be only "occasionally" present	No F/U
Suchowersky et al., 1986	1	1	AD	Adulthood	N	N	+	P		No F/U
	2	2	AD	Childhood	Y	Y, but normal IQ testing	+	P	Mild dysarthria, facial apraxia; NL CT, abnormal caudate FDG-PET	No F/U
Kuwert et al., 1990	1	2	AD	Infancy, childhood	Y secondary to orthopedic complications	Low average IQ in proband/ NL in second	+	S	History of poliomyelitis, bilateral hip dislocation in proband; normal FDG-PET	No F/U

Loosmore and Wood, 1988	1	AD	Childhood	N	N	+	S	Psychiatric history (anxiety, depression, personality disorder, substance dependence); abnormal movements since age 3, considered tics; speech impairment; movement responsive to alcohol (multiple family members) and lorazepam (proband)	No F/U
Hageman et al., 1996	24	AD	2–6 years	N	N	+	S/P/I	Delayed speech, mild dysarthria, one with gait impairment without chorea; NL MRI, HD IT15-	Linkage to chromosome 14 not confirmed (Breedveld et al., 2002a)
Friederich, 1996	1	AD	Infancy	Y	N	+	S	Attention-deficit disorder, significant dysarthria, improvement in chorea with methylphenidate	No F/U

(continued)

TABLE 4–2. (continued)

REFERENCE	FAMILY	NUMBER AFFECTED	INHERITANCE	ONSET	MOTOR DELAY	COGNITIVE DELAY	CHOREA	COURSE	ASSOCIATED FEATURES	F/U INCLUDING REFERENCES
de Vries et al., 2000	1	9	AD	Infancy, early childhood	Y	Y	+/−	S/I	Ataxic gait, pyramidal signs, leg weakness; one individual with psychosis, intention tremor, dysarthria	Base transposition identified in *TITF-1* (Table 4)

[a] Patients examined by the Queen Square group.
[b] Video reviewed by the Queen Square group.
[c] Diagnosis revisited by the Queen Square group.
[d] Diagnosis unchanged.

AD, autosomal dominant; AR, autosomal recessive; CT, computed tomography; CSF, cerebrospinal fluid; FDG-PET, fluorodeoxyglucose positron emission tomography; F/U, follow-up; HD, Huntington disease; HVA, homovanillic acid; I, improved; MR, mental retardation; MRI, magnetic resonance imaging; N, no; NL, normal; No, number of examined affected individuals; P, progressive; S, stable; Y, yes; −, absent; +, present; +/−, present in some, but not all, affected individuals.

provided by the original authors in six families. In nine of these families the diagnosis of BHC was revised to atypical ataxia-telangiectasia (Quinn et al., 1988; Klein et al., 1996), genetically confirmed HD (Quarrell et al., 1988; MacMillan et al., 1993a, b), dystonia (Sleigh and Lindenbaum, 1981; Robinson and Thornett, 1985; Schady and Meara, 1988), myoclonic dystonia (Refsum and Sjaastad, 1972; Garcia Ruiz et al., 1994), and tics or myoclonus (Yapijakis et al., 1995). In one case, chorea resolved (Behan and Bone, 1977); and in two other cases, the diagnosis of BHC remained unchanged but the clinical presentation included additional abnormalities (Harper, 1978; Deonna and Voumard, 1979). In the remaining 31 families, obtaining follow-up was not possible: A total of 10 families were lost to follow-up, and there was no response by the original authors to the Queen Square group's inquiry in 21 families. However, in all these cases, the presence of atypical features led the Queen Square group to challenge the diagnosis of BHC (Table 4–2).

In their report, the Queen Square group also described an additional seven new families, in which the diagnosis of BHC had been contemplated at least once by any of the authors (Table 4–3). The videos were reevaluated blindly twice by all three authors separately, first to establish the presence of specific movement disorders and second to determine the most likely diagnosis. Consensus was achieved in four of the families; the diagnosis of BHC was changed in three families to hereditary essential myoclonus with dramatic response to alcohol, dystonic syndrome, and myoclonic dystonia; however, in one family, the diagnosis remained possible BHC or multifocal myoclonus. In the other three families, however, a consensus could not be reached. The interrater agreement regarding the presence of a specific movement disorder varied between 61% (myoclonus) and 100% (tics). The difficulty of accurately differentiating between chorea, myoclonus, and fast dystonic jerks, even by experienced movement disorder specialists, explains, at least partially, the inaccuracy of diagnosing BHC purely based on phenomenology, in the absence of a confirmatory test (Jankovic, 2009).

THE GENETICS OF BHC

Based on their pedigree, Haerer et al. (1967) suggested that the transmission of BHC followed an autosomal dominant pattern, with variable penetrance, considering that one obligatory carrier (the mother of six affected offspring and the daughter of one affected individual) remained asymptomatic. Subsequent studies established a nearly complete penetrance in males and 75% penetrance in females (Harper, 1978). Other modes of transmission have been reported, including autosomal recessive (Nutting et al., 1969; Chun et al., 1973; Damasio et al., 1977; Zambrino et al., 1984; Quinn et al., 1988) and X-linked recessive (Landrieu et al., 1984). However, the incomplete penetrance, the difficulties identifying

TABLE 4–3. New BHC Families Reported by the Queen Square Group (Schrag et al., 2000)

FAMILY/PATIENT [a]	AGE (YEARS)	SEX	ONSET (YEARS)	DURATION (YEARS)	F/U (YEARS)	INHERITANCE	DELAYED MOTOR DEVELOPMENT	COGNITION	OUTCOME	ETOH	AGREEMENT/DIAGNOSIS
2	35	F	2	33	20	AD (RP)	–	N	S	+++	Not BHC/hereditary essential myoclonus
6/1	45	M	3	42	14	AR	?	LA	P	0	Not BHC/dystonic syndrome
6/2	29	F	3	26	14		?				
8/1	36	M	7	29	7	AD	–	N	P	–	Not BHC/myoclonic dystonia, treated with valproic acid and clonazepam
8/2	50	F	Childhood					N	P		
8/3	38	F	Childhood				+	N	P	–	
9/1	15	F	1	14	5	AR	+	N	I		No agreement/possible BHC, myoclonic dystonia, chorea+dystonia
9/2	13	M	1	12	5		+	N	I		

10/1	34	F	2	32	4	AD	+	LA	I	+	No agreement/possible BHC, myoclonic dystonia, dystonic syndrome
10/2	6	M	1	5	4		+	LA	P		
10/3	10	M	Childhood				+	LA	I		
11/1	11	F	2.5	8.5	6	AD	+	N	I	+	No agreement/possible BHC, myoclonic dystonia, possible BHC; treated with benzhexol
11/2	34	F	2.5	31.5	6		+	N	I	+	
12/1	35	F	1	34	0	AD	+	N	P	0	Chorea or multifocal myoclonus, consensus of possible BHC or multifocal myoclonus
12/2	58	F	1	57	0		+	N	I		
12/3	15	F	6 weeks	15	0		+	N	?		

[a] Numbered according to the original paper.

AD, autosomal dominant; AR, autosomal recessive; ETOH, response to alcohol; F, female; F/U, follow-up; I, improved; LA, low average; M, male; N, normal; P, progressive; RP reduced penetrance; S, stable; −, absent; +, present; +++, robust.

mildly affected individuals, and the lack of a confirmatory test made the reports unreliable.

After identification of *IT15* as the gene responsible for HD in 1993, some patients diagnosed clinically with BHC underwent testing, showing CAG repeats within the normal range—14–16 CAG repeats (Garcia Ruiz et al., 1994), 20–23 CAG repeats (Yapijakis et al., 1995), and 17–22 CAG repeats (Hageman et al., 1996)—suggesting that the two conditions, although phenotypically alike, were not allelic. However, one family previously diagnosed with BHC (Quarrell et al., 1988) was found to have expanded CAG repeats of 39 and 45, confirming the diagnosis of HD in the two affected offspring (MacMillan et al., 1993a,b). This finding further confirms the overlap in phenotype between the two conditions and the difficulties diagnosing BHC based purely on clinical grounds.

The first breakthrough in the understanding of BHC genetics consisted of discovering linkage to a locus on chromosome 14q12-22 in a large Dutch kindred of 33 individuals spanning over four generations (de Vries et al., 2000), which included several potential genes, such as glia maturation factor-β, GTP cyclohydrolase 1, and survival of motor neurons (*SMN*)–interacting protein 1 (*SIP1*). All affected individuals had mild symptoms with onset of chorea in childhood and followed a relatively static course. Chorea involved predominantly the hands, feet, and head and improved in adolescence. The presence of atypical features (ataxic gait and pyramidal signs) in addition to more severe chorea in the youngest generation raised the suspicion of anticipation. One affected family member, not available for direct examination, also apparently suffered from psychosis. Other clinical features are summarized in Table 4–2.

The critical region on chromosome 14 was subsequently narrowed with the genetic analysis of a previously reported kindred (Bird et al., 1976) (Table 4–2). *SIP1* was excluded as a potential causative gene for BHC (Fernandez et al., 2001a). According to their pedigree, the authors concluded that there was no variable penetrance, even though there was some degree of variability in the expressivity in terms of severity and no suggestion of anticipation. The clinical presentation included typical features of BHC consisting of nonprogressive chorea with onset at 2–5 years of age, with few atypical features of unclear significance (Table 4–2). Both families with linkage to chromosome 14 presented some degree of action tremor, validating this symptom as part of the BHC phenotype, as originally described by Pincus and Chutorian (1967). The linkage to the same region on chromosome 14 was identified in two other BHC families previously reported in the United States (Fisher et al., 1979; Leli et al; 1984; Breedveld et al., 2002a). Alternate linkage to chromosome 8q21.3-23.3 was identified in a Japanese family with nonprogressive chorea of adult onset (average 54.3 years), hence named "benign hereditary chorea type 2," after excluding other causes of autosomal dominant chorea (HD, HD-like [HDL] 1 and 2, dentatorubral-pallidoluysian atrophy [DRPLA], spinocerebellar ataxia [SCA] 17, BHC) (Shimohata et al., 2007).

However, the onset in adulthood sets this condition apart as a distinct entity, probably not related to BHC.

In 2002, additional and more detailed analysis of the critical region on chromosome 14 in one small Italian family, previously diagnosed with BHC (Guala et al., 2001), revealed a 1.2 Mb genomic deletion resulting in complete loss of the thyroid transcription factor gene (*TITF-1*), also known as *TTF*, *Nkx2.1*, and *T/ebp*, suggesting that chorea in this family was caused by haploinsufficiency of the TITF-1 protein (Breedveld et al., 2002b). After determining the intron–exon boundaries of *TITF-1*, the Dutch authors sequenced the coding region in patients from three other previously reported BHC families (Harper, 1978; Leli et al., 1984; Mussell et al., 1995; de Vries et al., 2000), revealing base transversion in two families and base deletion in one (Table 4–4).

TITF-1 AND ITS FUNCTION IN THE DEVELOPING BRAIN

TITF-1 is a member of the *NK2* family of homeodomain-containing transcription factors. It is involved in the tissue-specific expression of several thyroid- and lung-specific genes and, thus, in their organogenesis (Guazzi et al., 1990). In addition, *TITF-1* is expressed in restricted areas of the developing mouse forebrain (Lazzaro et al., 1991). Its transcripts can be observed in the hypothalamic primordium at one-somite age (Shimamura et al., 1995). By 11-somite stage, *TITF-1* expression is evident in the rostrobasal telencephalon, a region that generates, among other structures, the medial ganglionic eminence (MGE). The MGE is a proliferative zone that gives rise to pallidal components of the basal ganglia. The lateral ganglionic eminence (LGE), which generates the striatum, is a distinct structure that initially lacks *TITF-1* expression. A subset of precursor cells expressing *TITF-1* migrates from the MGE to the developing striatum and the developing cortical plate. In the homozygous *TITF-1* mutant telencephalon, even though an MGE-like structure forms, it does not produce its normal derivatives (globus pallidus) and cells fail to migrate from the pallidum into the striatum (cholinergic neurons) and into the cortex (GABAergic neurons) (Sussel et al., 1999). Immunohistochemical staining of striatal tissue from a BHC-affected *post mortem* brain (Kleiner-Fisman et al., 2003) showed evidence of loss of most of the *TITF-1*-mediated striatal interneurons compared to matched control brains, supporting the role of *TITF-1* in the migration of striatal neurons in the developing human brain (Kleiner-Fisman et al., 2005).

Nuclear staining by immunohistochemistry for *TITF-1* was visible only in the human lung and thyroid gland and in the rat lung and hypothalamus, but staining was negative in the adult human and rat pallidum (Krude et al., 2002). *TITF-1* continues to be expressed postnatally in several areas of the rat brain, regulating several target genes, thus being involved in the circadian rhythm (Son et al., 2009),

TABLE 4–4. BHC Families Reported After 2002, Including Associated Features, References, and Genotype

REFERENCE	FAMILY/NO[a]	INHERITANCE	ONSET OF CHOREA	MOTOR DELAY	COGNITIVE DELAY	CHOREA	COURSE
de Vries et al., 2000; Breedveld et al., 2002a,b	1/31	AD	Infancy, early childhood	Delayed walking (13/31)	4/31	+	S/I
Leli et al., 1984; Mussell et al., 1995; Breedveld et al., 2002b	1/36	AD	4–8 years	Delayed walking (34/36)	3/13	+	I
Harper, 1978; Breedveld et al., 2002b	2/2	AD	Infancy	Y	N	+	S
Guala et al., 2001, 2008; Breedveld et al., 2002b	1/2	AD	Childhood	?	?	+	S
Kleiner-Fisman et al., 2003	1/5	AD	6 months–2 years	Delayed walking	N	+	S
Asmus et al., 2005	1/4	AD	2 years	Marked	N/A	+	I

ASSOCIATED FEATURES			COMMENTS	GENE[b]
Neurological	Lung	Thyroid		
Gait difficulty (7/31), pyramidal signs (paraparesis with extensor plantar reflexes) (2/31)	—	—	Mutation absent in individual with ataxic diplegia	Transversion C727A, R243S
CH, gait difficulty (26/36), pyramidal signs (extensor plantar reflex) (7/36), slow saccades (20/36)	—	—		Transversion G713T, W238L
"Behavioral distur- bances"	—	—		Deletion G908, G303fsx77
—	—	Occasional increase in TSH (2/2)	Oligodontia (caused by loss of function of PAX9)	Deletion of a 1.2 Mb region with complete loss of function of 5 genes, including TITF-1 and PAX9
N/A	—	—	Negative pathology	−2A→T substitution in the invariant AG splice acceptor site of intron 2, 1155fsx2
Hypotonia, atrophy, CH, response to L-dopa but dose-dependent dyskinesias	Respiratory insuffi- ciency at birth	CH	Hyperextendable knee joints, one died of leukemia	G523T, E175X

(continued)

TABLE 4–4. (continued)

REFERENCE	FAMILY/NO[a]	INHERITANCE	ONSET OF CHOREA	MOTOR DELAY	COGNITIVE DELAY	CHOREA	COURSE
Devriendt et al., 1998; Kleiner-Fisman and Lang, 2007	1/1	N/A	15 hours	Y	Y	+	N/A
Iwatani et al., 2000	1/1	N/A	Neonatal period	Y	Severe	–	S
Pohlenz et al., 2002	1/1	N/A	Neonate	Y	N/A	+	N/A
Krude et al., 2002	1/1	N/A	Neonate	?	?	+++	?
	1/1	N/A	Neonate	?	?	+++	?
	1/1	N/A	Neonate	?	?	+++	?
	1/1	N/A	Neonate	?	?	+++	?
	1/1	N/A	Neonate	?	?	-	?

ASSOCIATED FEATURES			COMMENTS	GENE[b]
Hypotonia, truncal ataxia	Respiratory insufficiency	Hypothyroidism	Normal imaging	Deletion 14q13-21 (TITF-1, PAX9), absence of protein
Pyramidal signs, hearing loss	Respiratory insufficiency	Hypothyroidism	Hyperbilirubinemia, microcephaly, hypertelorism, small mandible, high arched palate, hypertrichosis, simian crease, contractures of lower leg joints	Deletion 14q12-13.3 including TITF-1 and PAX9, absence of protein
Dyskinesia, hypotonia	Respiratory distress	CH		255insG frameshift with a nonsense, abnormally long protein, G86fsx322
—	Severe respiratory distress with frequent severe pulmonary infections	Thyroid gland hypoplasia	MRI: cystic mass craniodorsal to pituitary gland	Deletion 14q11.2q13.3 including TITF-1, absence of protein
—	Moderate respiratory distress with frequent severe pulmonary infections	Thyroid gland hypoplasia	MRI: small pallidum without visible division into lateral and medial parts, cystic mass craniodorsal to pituitary gland	G2626T, missense; V235F
—	Few mild pulmonary infections	Mild thyroid dysfunction		2595insGG, nonsense; I224fsx3
—		Thyroid gland hypoplasia		C2519A, nonsense; S199X
Severe hypotonia	Severe pulmonary distress	Agenesis of thyroid gland		C1302A, nonsense

(continued)

TABLE 4–4. (continued)

REFERENCE	FAMILY/NO[a]	INHERITANCE	ONSET OF CHOREA	MOTOR DELAY	COGNITIVE DELAY	CHOREA	COURSE
Doyle et al., 2004	1/4	AD	Neonate	Y	Y	+	S
Willemsen et al., 2005	1/1	N/A	Child-hood	Y	Y	+	S
do Carmo Costa et al., 2005	1/2	AD	10 months	Y	Y	+	S
Devos et al., 2006	1/3	AD	2 years	Y	?	+	S/I
Moya et al., 2006	1/3	AD	15 months	Y	Y	+/–	S
Mahajnah et al., 2007	1/5	AD	Before 5 years	N	N	+	S
Asmus et al., 2007	1/2	AD	Infancy	Y	N	+	S
Nagasaki et al., 2008	1	N/A	Child-hood	Y	N	+	I

ASSOCIATED FEATURES			COMMENTS	GENE[b]
Ataxia, dysarthria	Respiratory distress at birth	CH	Normal MRI studies	2A→T substitution in invariant AG splice acceptor site of intron 2, 1155fsx2
Severe hypotonia	Respiratory distress during 2nd week of life	Primary hypothyroidism	MRI: NL, large cell lung carcinoma	859-860insC, frameshift mutation; Q287fsx121
Mild lower extremity spasticity	—	—	Congenital strabismus, stuttering, pes cavus, MRI: scattered T2 hyperintense foci	745T replacement G249 for premature stop codon Q249X
–	Infant respiratory distress	Hypothyroidism, slight hypoparathyroidism	Hypodontia, interstitial pneumonopathy responsive to steroids, diarrhea associated with malabsorbtion syndrome	0.9 Mb deletion including *TITF-1*, *PAX-9*, *NKX2.8*, and *SLC25A21*; absence of protein
–	—	CH	MRI: NL	825delC nonsense mutation
Ataxia, gait impairment	—	—	MRI: NL; SPECT: decreased uptake in striatum and thalamus	978-1056 del, S330fsx24
Response of chorea to alcohol, cervical dystonia, axial and limb dystonia	—	—	SPECT: NL	376-2A>C
–	Recurrent lower respiratory tract infections during infancy	CH	MRI: NL	10 bp deletion and 3 bp insertion C.470_479 delinsGCG, frameshift mutation p.p157fsx196

(continued)

TABLE 4–4. (continued)

REFERENCE	FAMILY/NO[a]	INHERITANCE	ONSET OF CHOREA	MOTOR DELAY	COGNITIVE DELAY	CHOREA	COURSE
Ferrara et al., 2008	1/3	AD	7 years	Y	Y	+	S
Provenzano et al., 2008	1/3	AD	Before 15 months	Y (mild)	N	+	?
Glik et al., 2008	1/3	AD	Infancy	N	N	+	S
Maquet et al., 2009	1/1	N/A	Neonate	N/A	N/A	−	Death from respiratory failure
Carré et al., 2009	1/1	N/A	1 year	Y	Y (severe)	+	S
	1 (1/2 monozygotic twin)	N/A	5 years	Y	Y	+	?

ASSOCIATED FEATURES			COMMENTS	GENE[b]
–	Infant respiratory distress	CH		C609A; S145X
Dysarthria, subtle oculomotor apraxia, dystonic posture of arms	—	—	MRI: NL	C532T R178X
Myoclonic jerks of out-stretched hands, bilateral upper extremity intention tremor, foot dystonia	Lung carcinoma (one)	Hypothy-roidism	Short stature, webbed neck, psychosis (one), Ashkenazi Jewish ancestry	C650A S217X
–	Acute respiratory failure at birth	Hypothy-roidism		transversion ATC>TTC, missense mutation Ile207Phe
Hypotonia, ataxia, saccadic eye move-ments	Infant respiratory distress syndrome, chronic respiratory infections	CH	MRI: agenesis of corpus callosum	Del14q13, absence of protein
Hypotonia	Infant respiratory distress syndrome, chronic respiratory infections	CH athyreosis	MRI: NL	376-2A>G splice mutation (same as Doyle et al., 2004)

(continued)

TABLE 4-4. (continued)

REFERENCE	FAMILY/NO[a]	INHERITANCE	ONSET OF CHOREA	MOTOR DELAY	COGNITIVE DELAY	CHOREA	COURSE
	1 (2/2 mono-zygotic twin)	N/A	—	N	N	–	S
	1	N/A	2.5 years	Y	Y	+	S
	1	N/A	1.5 years	Y	Y	+	?
	1	N/A	2 years	Y	Y	+	?

[a] Number of family/individuals examined.
[b] Genetic mutation/protein product effect.
AD, autosomal dominant; CH, congenital hypothyroidism; I, improved;
MRI, magnetic resonance imaging; N, no; N/A, not applicable; NL, normal; S, stable;
SPECT, single-photon emission computed tomography; TSH, thyroid-stimulating hormone; Y, yes.

the central activation of puberty (Lee et al., 2001), the synthesis and secretion of pituitary hormones (Kim et al., 2002), the regulation of body fluid homeostasis (Son et al., 2003), feeding behavior (Kim et al., 2006), and cerebrospinal fluid formation (Kim et al., 2007). However, even though *TITF-1* has been shown to be involved in the development of both the rat and human brain and to retain some function in the adult rat brain, there is no evidence that *TITF-1* is expressed or plays any function in the adult human brain.

THE NEW PHENOTYPE

Prior to establishing a relationship between the *TITF-1* gene and BHC, very low levels of *TITF-1* expression were thought to cause congenital hypothyroidism (CH) (Acebron et al., 1995). However, initial efforts to solidify the connection between *TITF-1* and CH yielded negative results, no mutations being identified in 85 patients randomly selected from neonatal hypothyroidism screening programs (Perna et al., 1997; Lapi et al., 1997; Hishinuma et al., 1998). Subsequently, heterozygous deletions of chromosome 14, which included (but not exclusively)

	ASSOCIATED FEATURES		COMMENTS	GENE[b]
–	Infant respiratory distress syndrome	CH thyroid hemi-agenesis	MRI: NL	376-2A>G splice mutation (same as Doyle et al., 2004)
Hypotonia	Repeated episodes of bronchitis	Thyroid hypoplasia, hypothy-roidism	MRI: NL	C>G L176V
Hypotonia	—	CH	MRI: NL	C>T P202L
Hypotonia	—	CH	MRI: NL	A>C Q210P

the *TITF-1* gene, were found to be associated with thyroid and lung dysfunctions, midline abnormalities, and movement disorders (Devriendt et al., 1998; Iwatani et al., 2000). In 2002, the evidence linking mutations in *TITF-1* to CH came from a larger European study, in which one deletion and four mutations were identified in five of 150 children with CH (Krude et al., 2002). In addition, the authors observed choreoathetosis, neonatal respiratory distress, and frequent respiratory infections. However, it was unclear whether the neurological and respiratory complications were the direct consequence of *TITF-1* mutations or caused by hypothyroidism. Coincidentally, the same year, mutations in the same gene, *TITF-1*, were identified in individuals presenting with a typical BHC phenotype (Breedveld et al., 2002b). The first report of autosomal dominant transmission of CH caused by mutation in the *TITF-1* gene resulted from the study of a family in which three generations were affected (Doyle et al., 2004). In addition to CH, the affected family members presented with various degrees of respiratory dysfunction, developmental delay, chorea, and ataxia. The fact that neurological abnormalities have been reported in affected offspring of affected mothers under treatment with thyroid hormone–replacement therapy during pregnancy (Doyle et al., 2004) and the evidence that *TITF-1* is involved in the development of the basal ganglia support the theory that the neurological abnormalities are the result of abnormal embryogenesis of the nervous system caused by *TITF-1* mutations rather than inadequate thyroid hormone exposure.

The term "brain–lung–thyroid" (BLT) syndrome was introduced by Willemsen et al. (2005) to reflect the triple organ involvement associated with mutations in the *TITF-1* gene. However, the degree and severity of involvement of the three organs vary, with 50% of patients presenting with the complete triad of BLT disease, 30% with brain and thyroid involvement, and 13% with isolated chorea corresponding to BHC (Carré et al., 2009). Lung disease occurs in 54% of patients. The "lung" phenotype ranges from severe infant respiratory distress syndrome, potentially lethal, to recurrent pulmonary infections, acute respiratory distress syndrome (Iwatani et al., 2000), and chronic interstitial lung disease (Devos et al., 2006). Respiratory complications are a significant cause of mortality, 16% being fatal (Carré et al., 2009). The significance of metastatic lung carcinoma at autopsy in one case remains unknown (Willemsen et al., 2005), even though *TITF-1* has been proposed as a new lineage-specific oncogene amplified in lung cancer (Kwei et al., 2008). The thyroid dysfunction, present in 87% of patients with *TITF-1* mutations, varies between mild functional abnormalities (mild thyroid-stimulating hormone elevations) to severe developmental defects (thyroid gland agenesis) (Carré et al., 2009). Some patients without CH at birth developed hypothyroidism in adulthood, supporting the continuous role of *TITF-1* not only in the development but also in the function of the thyroid gland postnatally.

Neurological complications occur in 93% of patients with *TITF-1* mutation. Generalized and nonprogressive chorea is a predominant feature and develops at a median age of 2. Hypotonia and developmental delay may precede the movement disorder. Other neurological complications that may be present include gait difficulties, pyramidal signs, abnormal saccades, ataxia, dysarthria, dystonia, and upper extremity action tremor (Table 4–4). Cognitive delay was also described. Dysmorphic midline features, previously described in heterozygous deletions of chromosome 14, which included the *TITF-1* gene, were most likely the result of deletions of other genes localized in the vicinity, such as *PAX9* (Guala et al., 2008).

Correlations between the various clinical presentations and specific genotypes remain elusive. For example, in the same family with an identical mutation the phenotype varies between mild chorea or mild and transitory hypothyroidism during gestation to severe chorea accompanied by CH (Moya et al., 2006). Whether the theory of haploinsufficiency explains entirely the mechanism and the spectrum of disorders caused by mutations in the *TITF-1* gene or whether the mutant protein exerts a dominant negative effect remains to be established (Moya et al., 2006). Nevertheless, the type, size, location, and effect on the protein domain localization may all represent determinant factors ultimately responsible for the phenotype variability. Also, considering intrafamilial phenotypic variability caused by identical mutations (do Carmo Costa et al., 2005; Carré et al., 2009), environmental and other factors (modifier genes, hormonal factors) cannot be excluded, making the genotype/phenotype correlation very complex.

Aside from the original reports of BHC (Haerer et al., 1967; Pincus and Chutorian, 1967), the value of the majority of the "old" BHC reports published before 2002 remains questionable. Linkage to chromosome 14 was confirmed only in two (Bird et al., 1976; Fisher et al., 1979) of five "old" BHC families that were subsequently tested (Bird et al., 1976; Bird and Hall, 1978; Fisher et al., 1979; Yapijakis et al., 1995; Hageman et al., 1996). *TITF-1* mutations were found only in four previously reported families (Leli et al., 1984; Harper, 1978; de Vries et al., 2000; Guala et al., 2001). Interestingly, respiratory dysfunction was not reported in any of the "old" cases, and thyroid dysfunction was present only in two, later confirmed to carry *TITF-1* mutations (Leli et al., 1984; Guala et al., 2001). Also, spastic diplegia without chorea, described in one individual from a BHC family (de Vries et al., 2000), was subsequently excluded as part of the phenotype as this individual lacked the *TITF-1* mutation identified in the rest of the affected family members 2 years later (Breedveld et al., 2002b). This very important observation demonstrates the difficulties and potential errors of interpreting atypical features described as part of BHC in families reported before the genetic test became available.

BHC can share a similar phenotype with epsilon sarcoglycan mutations associated with the myoclonus-dystonia syndrome (Asmus et al., 2007), including the presence of dystonia, favorable response to alcohol, and involuntary "slower jerks" not easily classified clinically as either chorea or myoclonus (Glik et al., 2008). Key features that help distinguish myoclonus-dystonia from BHC include the presence of lightning-like myoclonic jerks, often precipitated or aggravated by complex tasks, and the absence of continuous chorea in myoclonus-dystonia (Asmus et al., 2007).

IMAGING STUDIES AND PATHOLOGICAL FINDINGS

Before the genetic testing became available, autopsy studies (Stapert et al., 1985) and traditional brain imaging (Rice and Terrence, 1979; Fisher et al., 1979, Hageman et al., 1996) were considered to be normal in BHC. Functional brain imaging yielded conflicting results, cerebral glucose metabolism by fluorodeoxyglucose positron emission tomographic (FDG-PET) studies were reported as normal (Kuwert et al., 1990) or abnormal but nonspecific (Suchowersky et al., 1986). Brain magnetic resonance imaging as well as functional imaging consisting of FDG-PET are usually normal in genetically confirmed BHC (Kleiner-Fisman et al., 2003). Imaging studies performed in BLT syndrome revealed cerebral atrophy, ventricle dilation, and a cyst of the cavum septum pellucidum

(Iwatani et al., 2000). Neuroimaging findings in two other BLT patients consisted of reduced size of the pallidum with a cystic mass located craniodorsally of the pituitary gland (Krude et al., 2002). Other family case reports showed evidence of scattered T2 hyperintense foci in the vermis and in both pallida and moderate cerebral and cerebellar atrophy (do Carmo Costa et al., 2005). Single-photon emission computed tomography (SPECT) performed in three children of a BHC kindred showed markedly decreased uptake in the striatum and thalamus in two (Mahajnah et al., 2007).

Autopsy of a BHC patient with a point mutation in the *TITF-1* gene who died of leukemia showed only mild frontal-parietal-temporal atrophy on gross examination and nonspecific astrocytosis and hyperplasia without noticeable neuronal loss in the globus pallidus, thalamus, hippocampus, and periaqueductal gray matter on microscopy. There were no specific pathological findings (Kleiner-Fisman et al., 2003). The thyroid and neural tissues were normal at autopsy of a 40-day-old infant with a *TITF-1* mutation who died of severe respiratory failure (Maquet et al., 2009). Evidence for the role of *TITF-1* in lung development is supported by autopsy findings in the same infant, with low alveolar counts, simplification of the pulmonary architecture with impaired pulmonary branching, and morphology suggestive of surfactant deficiency (Maquet et al., 2009).

TREATMENT

In contrast to the usual treatment of hyperkinetic movement disorders with anti-dopaminergic drugs (Jankovic, 2009), levodopa was found to ameliorate chorea and gait in a patient with BHC within 6 weeks of initiating treatment, complicated later by dose-dependent dyskinesia (Asmus et al., 2005). Chorea also was reported to improve with methylphenidate in two BHC patients (Friederich, 1996; Devos et al., 2006). In one case report, there was improvement with steroids (Robinson and Thornett, 1985); however, the diagnosis was subsequently questioned by the Queen Square group given the predominance of dystonia (Schrag et al., 2000). No curative treatment has been reported to date.

CONCLUSIONS

Our understanding of BHC has come a long way since the original report in 1967. After its original description, the variability in the clinical presentation led to legitimate questions regarding the existence of BHC as a distinct entity. However, the discovery of the causative gene provided insights into the pathogenic mechanisms of this neurodevelopmental disorder, integrating BHC into the larger phenotype of BLT associated with mutations in the *TITF-1* gene. The availability of genetic testing will allow future studies to refine the phenotype associated with *TITF-1* mutations.

REFERENCES

Acebron A, Blanc P, Rossi DL, Lamas L, Santisteban P (1995) Congenital human thyroglobulin defect due to low expression of the thyroid-specific transcription factor *TTF-1*. J Clin Invest 96:781–785.

Asmus F, Devlin A, Munz M, Zimprich A, Gasser T, Chinnery PF (2007) Clinical differentiation of genetically proven benign hereditary chorea and myoclonus-dystonia. Mov Disord 22:2104–2109.

Asmus F, Horber V, Pohlenz J, Schwabe D, Zimprich A, Munz M, Schöning M, Gasser T (2005) A novel *TITF-1* mutation causes benign hereditary chorea with response to levodopa. Neurology 64:1952–1954.

Behan P, Bone I (1977) Hereditary chorea without dementia. J Neurol Neurosurg Psychiatry 40:687–691.

Bird TD, Hall JG (1978) Additional information on familial essential (benign) chorea [letter]. Clin Genet 14:271–272.

Bird TD, Carlson CB, Hall JG (1976) Familial essential ("benign") chorea. J Med Genet 13:357–362.

Breedveld GJ, Percy AK, MacDonald ME, de Vries BB, Yapijakis C, Dure LS, Ippel EF, Sandkuijl LA, Heutink P, Arts WF (2002a) Clinical and genetic heterogeneity in benign hereditary chorea. Neurology 59:579–584.

Breedveld GJ, van Dongen JW, Danesino C, Guala A, Percy AK, Dure LS, Harper P, Lazarou LP, van der Linde H, Joosse M, Grüters A, MacDonald ME, de Vries BB, Arts WF, Oostra BA, Krude H, Heutink P (2002b) Mutations in *TITF-1* are associated with benign hereditary chorea. Hum Mol Genet 11:971–979.

Burns J, Neuhäuser G, Tomasi L (1976) Benign hereditary non-progressive chorea of early onset. Clinical genetics of the syndrome and report of a new family. Neuropadiatrie 7:431–438.

Carré A, Szinnai G, Castanet M, Sura-Trueba S, Tron E, Broutin-L'Hermite I, Barat P, Goizet C, Lacombe D, Moutard ML, Raybaud C, Raynaud-Ravni C, Romana S, Ythier H, Léger J, Polak M (2009) Five new *TTF1/NKX2.1* mutations in brain–lung–thyroid syndrome: rescue by *PAX8* synergism in one case. Hum Mol Genet 18: 2266–2276.

Chun R, Daly R, Mansheim BJ Jr, Wolcott G (1973) Benign familial chorea with onset in childhood. JAMA 1973;225:1603–1607.

Damasio H, Antunes L, Damasio AR (1977) Familial nonprogressive involuntary movements of childhood. Ann Neurol 1:602–603.

Deonna T, Voumard C (1979) Benign hereditary (dominant) chorea of early onset. Helv Paediatr Acta 34:77–83.

Devos D, Vuillaume I, de Becdelievre A, de Martinville B, Dhaenens CM, Cuvellier JC, Cuisset JM, Vallée L, Lemaitre MP, Bourteel H, Hachulla E, Wallaert B, Destée A, Defebvre L, Sablonnière B (2006) New syndromic form of benign hereditary chorea is associated with a deletion of *TITF-1* and *PAX-9* contiguous genes. Mov Disord 21:2237–2240.

Devriendt K, Vanhole C, Matthijs G, de Zegher F (1998) Deletion of thyroid transcription factor-1 gene in an infant with neonatal thyroid dysfunction and respiratory failure. N Engl J Med 338:1317–1318.

de Vries BB, Arts WF, Breedveld GJ, Hoogeboom JJ, Niermeijer MF, Heutink P (2000) Benign hereditary chorea of early onset maps to chromosome 14q. Am J Hum Genet 66:136–142.

do Carmo Costa M, Costa C, Silva AP, Evangelista P, Santos L, Ferro A, Sequeiros J, Maciel P (2005) Nonsense mutation in *TITF1* in a Portuguese family with benign hereditary chorea. Neurogenetics 6:209–215.

Doyle DA, Gonzalez I, Thomas B, Scavina M (2004) Autosomal dominant transmission of congenital hypothyroidism, neonatal respiratory distress, and ataxia caused by a mutation of *NKX2-1*. J Pediatr 145:190–193.

Fernandez M, Raskind W, Matsushita M, Wolff J, Lipe H, Bird T (2001a) Hereditary benign chorea: clinical and genetic features of a distinct disease. Neurology 57:106–110.

Fernandez M, Raskind W, Wolff J, Matsushita M, Yuen E, Graf W, Lipe H, Bird T (2001b) Familial dyskinesia and facial myokymia (FDFM): a novel movement disorder. Ann Neurol 49:486–492.

Ferrara AM, De Michele G, Salvatore E, Di Maio L, Zampella E, Capuano S, Del Prete G, Rossi G, Fenzi G, Filla A, Macchia PE (2008) A novel *NKX2.1* mutation in a family with hypothyroidism and benign hereditary chorea. Thyroid 18:1005–1009.

Fisher M, Sargent J, Drachman D (1979) Familial inverted choreoathetosis. Neurology 29:1627–1631.

Foerster K, Foerster G (1978) Benign, hereditary, non-progressive chorea—an important differential diagnosis. Nervenarzt 49:724–725.

Friederich RL (1996) Benign hereditary chorea improved on stimulant therapy. Pediatr Neurol 14:326–327.

Garcia Ruiz P, Benitez J, Garcia de Yebenes J (1994) Benign familial chorea is not genetically related to Huntington's disease. Neurology 44(Suppl 2):A397.

Glik A, Vuillaume I, Devos D, Inzelberg R (2008) Psychosis, short stature in benign hereditary chorea: a novel thyroid transcription factor-1 mutation. Mov Disord 23: 1744–1747.

Guala A, Falco V, Breedveld G, De Filippi P, Danesino C (2008) Deletion of *PAX9* and oligodontia: a third family and review of the literature. Int J Paediatr Dent 18:441–445.

Guala A, Nocita G, Di Maria E, Mandich P, Provera S, Cerruti Mainardi P, Pastore G (2001) Benign hereditary chorea: a rare cause of disability. Riv Ital Pediatr 27(Suppl): 150–152.

Guazzi S, Price M, De Felice M, Damante G, Mattei MG, Di Lauro R (1990) Thyroid nuclear factor 1 (*TTF-1*) contains a homeodomain and displays a novel DNA binding specificity. EMBO J 9:3631–3639.

Haerer A, Currier R, Jackson J (1967) Hereditary nonprogressive chorea of early onset. N Engl J Med 276:1220–1224.

Hageman G, Ippel PF, van Hout MS, Rozeboom AR (1996) A Dutch family with benign hereditary chorea of early onset: differentiation from Huntington's disease. Clin Neurol Neurosurg 98:165–170.

Harper PS (1978) Benign hereditary chorea. Clinical and genetic aspects. Clin Genet 13: 85–95.

Hermier M, Beaupere A (1978) Familial nonprogressive chorea; a propos of 1 case. Pediatrie 33:347–353.

Hishinuma A, Kuribayashi T, Kanno Y, Onigata K, Nagashima K, Ieiri T (1998) Sequence analysis of thyroid transcription factor-1 gene reveals absence of mutations in patients with thyroid dysgenesis but presence of polymorphisms in the 5' flanking region and intron. Endocr J 45:563–567.

Ito T, Suzuki H, Yamada M, Metoki K, Iinuma K, Ito H (1982) Familial nonprogressive chorea: report of four cases in a family. No To Shinkei 34:775–780.

Iwatani N, Mabe H, Devriendt K, Kodama M, Miike T (2000) Deletion of *NKX2.1* gene encoding thyroid transcription factor-1 in two siblings with hypothyroidism and respiratory failure. J Pediatr 137:272–276.

Jankovic J (2009) Treatment of hyperkinetic movement disorders. Lancet Neurol 8: 844–856.

Kim JG, Nam-Goong IS, Yun CH, Jeong JK, Kim ES, Park JJ, Lee YC, Kim YI, Lee BJ (2006) *TTF-1*, a homeodomain-containing transcription factor, regulates feeding behavior in the rat hypothalamus. Biochem Biophys Res Commun 349:969–975.

Kim JG, Son YJ, Yun CH, Kim YI, Nam-Goong IS, Park JH, Park SK, Ojeda SR, D'Elia AV, Damante G, Lee BJ (2007) Thyroid transcription factor-1 facilitates cerebrospinal fluid formation by regulating aquaporin-1 synthesis in the brain. J Biol Chem 282: 14923–14931.

Kim MS, Hur MK, Son YJ, Park JI, Chun SY, D'Elia AV, Damante G, Cho S, Kim K, Lee BJ (2002) Regulation of pituitary adenylate cyclase–activating polypeptide gene transcription by *TTF-1*, a homeodomain-containing transcription factor. J Biol Chem 277:36863–36871.

Klein C, Wenning GK, Quinn NP, Marsden CD (1996) Ataxia without telangiectasia masquerading as benign hereditary chorea. Mov Disord 11:217-220.

Kleiner-Fisman G, Lang AE (2007) Benign hereditary chorea revisited: a journey to understanding. Mov Disord 22:2297–2305.

Kleiner-Fisman G, Calingasan NY, Putt M, Chen J, Beal MF, Lang AE (2005) Alterations of striatal neurons in benign hereditary chorea. Mov Disord 20:1353–1357.

Kleiner-Fisman G, Rogaeva E, Halliday W, Houle S, Kawarai T, Sato C, Medeiros H, St George-Hyslop PH, Lang AE (2003) Benign hereditary chorea: clinical, genetic, and pathological findings. Ann Neurol 54:244–247.

Krude H, Schütz B, Biebermann H, von Moers A, Schnabel D, Neitzel H, Tönnies H, Weise D, Lafferty A, Schwarz S, DeFelice M, von Deimling A, van Landeghem F, DiLauro R, Grüters A (2002) Choreoathetosis, hypothyroidism, and pulmonary alterations due to human *NKX2-1* haploinsufficiency. J Clin Invest 109:475–480.

Kuwert T, Lange HW, Langen KJ, Herzog H, Hefter H, Aulich A, Feinendegen LE (1990) Normal striatal glucose consumption in two patients with benign hereditary chorea as measured by positron emission tomography. J Neurol 237:80–84.

Kwei KA, Kim YH, Girard L, Kao J, Pacyna-Gengelbach M, Salari K, Lee J, Choi YL, Sato M, Wang P, Hernandez-Boussard T, Gazdar AF, Petersen I, Minna JD, Pollack JR (2008) Genomic profiling identifies *TITF1* as a lineage-specific oncogene amplified in lung cancer. Oncogene 27:3635–3640.

Landrieu P, Benchet ML, Tardieu M, Lapresle J (1984) Choree familiale, non progressive, liee au sexe. Rev Neurol (Paris) 140:432–433.

Lapi P, Macchia PE, Chiovato L, Biffali E, Moschini L, Larizza D, Baserga M, Pinchera A, Fenzi G, Di Lauro R (1997) Mutations in the gene encoding thyroid transcription factor-1 (*TTF-1*) are not a frequent cause of congenital hypothyroidism (CH) with thyroid dysgenesis. Thyroid 7:383–387.

Lazzaro D, Price M, de Felice M, Di Lauro R (1991) The transcription factor *TTF-1* is expressed at the onset of thyroid and lung morphogenesis and in restricted regions of the foetal brain. Development 113:1093–1104.

Lee BJ, Cho GJ, Norgren RB Jr, Junier MP, Hill DF, Tapia V, Costa ME, Ojeda SR (2001) *TTF-1*, a homeodomain gene required for diencephalic morphogenesis, is postnatally expressed in the neuroendocrine brain in a developmentally regulated and cell-specific fashion. Mol Cell Neurosci 17:107–126.

Leli DA, Furlow TW Jr, Falgout JC (1984) Benign familial chorea: an association with intellectual impairment. J Neurol Neurosurg Psychiatry 47:471–474.

Loosmore SJ, Wood K (1988) Benign hereditary chorea. A case report. Br J Psychiatry 152:131–134.

MacMillan JC, Morrison PJ, Nevin NC, Shaw DJ, Harper PS, Quarrell OW, Snell RG (1993a) Identification of an expanded CAG repeat in the Huntington's disease gene (*IT15*) in a family reported to have benign hereditary chorea. J Med Genet 30: 1012–1013.

MacMillan JC, Snell RG, Tyler A, Houlihan GD, Fenton I, Cheadle JP, Lazarou LP, Shaw DJ, Harper PS (1993b) Molecular analysis and clinical correlations of the Huntington's disease mutation. Lancet 342:954–958.

Mahajnah M, Inbar D, Steinmetz A, Heutink P, Breedveld GJ, Straussberg R (2007) Benign hereditary chorea: clinical, neuroimaging, and genetic findings. J Child Neurol 22: 1231–1234.

Maquet E, Costagliola S, Parma J, Christophe-Hobertus C, Oligny LL, Fournet JC, Robitaille Y, Vuissoz JM, Payot A, Laberge S, Vassart G, Van Vliet G, Deladoëy J (2009) Lethal respiratory failure and mild primary hypothyroidism in a term girl with a de novo heterozygous mutation in the *TITF1/NKX2.1* gene. J Clin Endocrinol Metab 94:197–203.

Moya CM, Perez de Nanclares G, Castaño L, Potau N, Bilbao JR, Carrascosa A, Bargadá M, Coya R, Martul P, Vicens-Calvet E, Santisteban P (2006) Functional study of a novel single deletion in the *TITF1/NKX2.1* homeobox gene that produces congenital hypothyroidism and benign chorea but not pulmonary distress. J Clin Endocrinol Metab 91:1832–1841.

Mussell GM, Dure LS, Percy AK (1995) Benign familial chorea: clinical characterization of an Alabama pedigree. Neurology 45:A184.

Nagasaki K, Narumi S, Asami T, Kikuchi T, Hasegawa T, Uchiyama M (2008) Mutation of a gene for thyroid transcription factor-1 (*TITF1*) in a patient with clinical features of resistance to thyrotropin. Endocr J 55:875–878.

Nutting P, Cole B, Schimke R (1969) Benign, recessively inherited choreo-athetosis of early onset. J Med Genet 6:408–410.

Perna MG, Civitareale D, De Filippis V, Sacco M, Cisternino C, Tassi V (1997) Absence of mutations in the gene encoding thyroid transcription factor-1 (*TTF-1*) in patients with thyroid dysgenesis. Thyroid 7:377–781.

Pincus JH, Chutorian A (1967) Familial benign chorea with intention tremor: a clinical entity. J Pediatr 70:724–729.

Pohlenz J, Dumitrescu A, Zundel D, Martiné U, Schönberger W, Koo E, Weiss RE, Cohen RN, Kimura S, Refetoff S (2002) Partial deficiency of thyroid transcription factor 1 produces predominantly neurological defects in humans and mice. J Clin Invest 109:469–473.

Provenzano C, Veneziano L, Appleton R, Frontali M, Civitareale D (2008) Functional characterization of a novel mutation in *TITF-1* in a patient with benign hereditary chorea. J Neurol Sci 264:56–62.

Quarrell OW, Youngman S, Sarfarazi M, Harper PS (1988) Absence of close linkage between benign hereditary chorea and the locus D4S10 (probe G8). J Med Genet 25:191–194.

Quinn N (1993) Benign hereditary chorea or hereditary idiopathic dystonia [letter]? Mov Disord 8:401–402.

Quinn NP, Rothwell JC, Thompson PD, Marsden CD (1988) Hereditary myoclonic dystonia, hereditary torsion dystonia and hereditary essential myoclonus: an area of confusion. Adv Neurol 50:391–401.

Refsum S, Sjaastad O (1972) Hereditary non-progressive involuntary movements with early onset and intention tremors, without dementia. Acta Neurol Scand 51(Suppl): 489–491.

Rice E, Terrence C (1979) Computerized tomography in hereditary nonprogressive chorea. Arch Neurol 36:249–250.

Robinson R, Thornett C (1985) Benign hereditary chorea—response to steroids. Dev Med Child Neurol 27:814–816.

Sadjadpour K, Amato RS (1973) Hereditary nonprogressive chorea of early onset—a new entity? Adv Neurol 1:79–91.

Schady W, Meara R (1988) Hereditary progressive chorea without dementia. J Neurol Neurosurg Psychiatry 51:295–297.

Schrag A, Quinn NP, Bhatia KP, Marsden CD (2000) Benign hereditary chorea—entity or syndrome? Mov Disord 15:280–288.

Shimamura K, Hartigan DJ, Martinez S, Puelles L, Rubenstein JL (1995) Longitudinal organization of the anterior neural plate and neural tube. Development 121:3923–3933.

Shimohata T, Hara K, Sanpei K, Nunomura J, Maeda T, Kawachi I, Kanazawa M, Kasuga K, Miyashita A, Kuwano R, Hirota K, Tsuji S, Onodera O, Nishizawa M, Honma Y (2007) Novel locus for benign hereditary chorea with adult onset maps to chromosome 8q21.3 q23.3. Brain 130:2302–2309.

Sjaastad O, Sulq I, Refsum S (1983) Benign familial myoclonus-like movements, partly of early onset. J Neural Transm 19(Suppl):291–303.

Sleigh G, Lindenbaum RH (1981) Benign (non-paroxysmal) familial chorea. Paediatric perspectives. Arch Dis Child 56:616–621.

Son YJ, Hur MK, Ryu BJ, Park SK, Damante G, D'Elia AV, Costa ME, Ojeda SR, Lee BJ (2003) TTF-1, a homeodomain-containing transcription factor, participates in the control of body fluid homeostasis by regulating angiotensinogen gene transcription in the rat subfornical organ. J Biol Chem 278:27043–27052.

Son YJ, Yun CH, Kim JG, Park JW, Kim JH, Kang SG, Lee BJ (2009) Expression and role of TTF-1 in the rat suprachiasmatic nucleus. Biochem Biophys Res Commun 380: 559–563.

Stapert JL, Busard BL, Gabreëls FJ, Renier WO, Colon EJ, Verhey FH (1985) Benign (nonparoxysmal) familial chorea of early onset: an electroneurophysiological examination of two families. Brain Dev 7:38–42.

Suchowersky O, Hayden MR, Martin WR, Stoessl AJ, Hildebrand AM, Pate BD (1986) Cerebral metabolism of glucose in benign hereditary chorea. Mov Disord 1: 33-44.

Sussel L, Marin O, Kimura S, Rubenstein JL (1999) Loss of Nkx2.1 homeobox gene function results in a ventral to dorsal molecular respecification within the basal telencephalon: evidence for a transformation of the pallidum into the striatum. Development 126: 3359–3370.

Willemsen MA, Breedveld GJ, Wouda S, Otten BJ, Yntema JL, Lammens M, de Vries BB (2005) Brain–thyroid–lung syndrome: a patient with a severe multi-system disorder due to a de novo mutation in the thyroid transcription factor 1 gene. Eur J Pediatr 164:28–30.

Yapijakis C, Kapaki E, Zournas C, Rentzos M, Loukopoulos D, Papageorgiou C (1995) Exclusion mapping of the benign hereditary chorea gene from the Huntington's disease locus: report of a family. Clin Genet 47:133–138.

Zambrino CA, La Buonora I, Lanzi G, Burgio FR (1984) Corea benigna familiare: a proposito di due casi. G Neuropsichiatr Eta Evol 4:81–87.

5

Huntington Disease-Like 2

Dobrila D. Rudnicki, PhD and Russell L. Margolis, MD

INTRODUCTION

Huntington disease (HD) is caused by an expansion of a CAG repeat in the huntingtin (*HTT*) gene that is translated into a polyglutamine tract. The gene is located on chromosome 4p (Huntington's Disease Collaborative Research Group, 1993). Clinically, HD is characterized by progressive movement, emotional and cognitive abnormalities, with death occurring 15–20 years after disease onset. The disease usually begins between the ages of 35 and 50 (Harper, 1996). Neuropathological characteristics of HD include atrophy of the caudate and putamen, with a dorsal to ventral gradient of loss of medium spiny projection neurons and gliosis, as well as atrophy of the cerebral cortex and other regions (Vonsattel et al., 1985; Hedreen et al., 1991). The pathology of HD, like other diseases caused by expanded CAG tracts encoding polyglutamine, is also characterized by the presence of protein aggregates containing the protein with an expanded polyglutamine tract and a growing list of coaggregating proteins. The protein aggregates are found in neurons of multiple brain regions, including striatal and cortical neurons and their processes (DiFiglia et al., 1997; Ross, 1997; Sapp et al., 1997; Li et al., 1999). About 1% of individuals with a clinical phenotype closely resembling HD do not have the HD mutation (Margolis et al., 2004). So far, several HD-like syndromes and their corresponding genes have been described, including spinocerebellar ataxia type 17 (SCA17) (Chapter 12) caused by a repeat expansion in TATA-binding protein and three Huntington disease-like (HDL) syndromes: a prion protein mutation in the form of octapeptide repeat insertion in *PRNP* leading to HDL1 (Moore et al., 2001) (Chapter 11); HDL2, caused by a mutation in the junctophilin-3 gene (Holmes et al., 2001); and an unknown recessive mutation resulting in a syndrome designated HDL3 (Schneider et al., 2007). SCA17 has been reported as HDL4. Numerous other disorders may resemble HD.

HDL2 was first described by our group as a novel trinucleotide repeat expansion disease with clinical and neuroimaging features nearly indistinguishable from those of HD (Margolis et al., 2001; Holmes et al., 2001). The causative mutation of HDL2 is a CTG/CAG repeat expansion that on the sense strand, in the CTG orientation, falls within a variably spliced exon of junctophilin-3 (*JPH3*) and is located on chromosome 16q24.3 (Holmes et al., 2001). Our initial analyses suggest that the disease pathogenesis is complex and may involve transcripts and their protein products encoded from both the sense and antisense strands at the HDL2 locus.

CLINICAL AND PATHOLOGICAL ASPECTS OF HDL2

Epidemiology and Clinical Features

In the normal population the HDL2 repeat length ranges from six to 28 triplets, whereas affected individuals have 40–59 triplets. As in HD, the repeat length is inversely correlated with age at disease onset. Our colleagues and we have so far identified more than 30 HDL2 pedigrees. The disease predominantly affects people of African ancestry. A person with HDL2 and an apparent Middle-Eastern background (Wild et al., 2008) and another affected individual with European ancestry but the African HDL2 haplotype (Santos et al., 2008) have been recently described. In the United States, HDL2 accounts for about 1% of all cases referred for HD testing that test negative for the HD mutation, with considerably higher rates in African Americans with an autosomal dominant HD-like phenotype. The frequency is even higher among Black South Africans: 26% of all Black patients with clinical HD in Johannesburg have HDL2 (Margolis et al., 2004).

There are two main clinical presentations of HDL2. One form of the disorder, described in the index family, begins with weight loss and diminished coordination before age 40. The disease progresses to include rigidity, dysarthria, hyperreflexia, bradykinesia, and tremor. Psychiatric symptoms, dystonia, and mild chorea are frequently present. About 10–15 years after onset, HDL2 patients exhibit profound dementia and die 5–10 years thereafter. This form has a tendency to correlate with longer repeat expansions and resembles juvenile-onset or the Westphal variant of HD (Margolis et al., 2001; Walker et al., 2003). The second form of HDL2 is associated with a late onset, pronounced chorea, and less prominent dystonia, bradykinesia, tremor, and rigidity.

HDL2 Neuropathology

Five studies describing HDL2 neuropathology have been reported (Greenstein et al., 2007; Margolis et al., 2001; Walker et al., 2002a,b; Rudnicki et al., 2008). Magnetic resonance imaging (MRI) scans of HDL2 patients were indistinguishable from scans of HD patients with a similar disease duration, showing pronounced striatal atrophy, prominent cortical atrophy, and little or no atrophy of the cerebellum or brainstem (Margolis et al., 2001). MRI scans of HDL2 patients reported by Bardien and colleagues (2007) showed features atypical of HD, including cerebral atrophy with normal caudate nuclei and extensive white matter changes.

Microscopic examinations of eight HDL2 brains suggested that HDL2 neuropathology is similar, though not identical, to HD. In the first study describing a patient from the index family (Margolis et al., 2001), marked neuronal loss with relative sparing of large neurons and more prominent neuropil vacuolation of caudate compared to putamen was observed. Both the globus pallidus and substantia nigra showed neurodegeneration, though to a lesser extent than in the striatum. Similar, but not identical, features were observed in an unrelated individual with severe atrophy of the striatum and much less atrophy of the globus pallidus (Walker et al., 2002a,b). In this case substantial neuronal loss was observed in the striatum, while other brain regions, including the substantia nigra, amygdala, and locus ceruleus, exhibited milder neuronal loss. Extensive degeneration of the caudate nucleus and putamen was described in two additional cases (Greenstein et al., 2007). In the first case, mild atrophy of the accumbens, mild neurodegeneration of the locus ceruleus, and loss of large neurons in isolated regions of the parietal and occipital cortex were observed. In the second case, significant cortical changes in the occipital lobes were observed, especially in the primary visual cortex. Both cases had mildly affected substantia nigra and unaffected cerebellum and brainstem.

We have recently described in more detail five HDL2 brains for which gross and microscopic examinations were consistent with HD. The five brains showed atrophy that ranged from mild to severe. The atrophy was predominantly cerebral, with sparing of the brainstem and cerebellum; and the majority of brains showed marked atrophy of the striatum comparable to HD Vonsattel grade 3–4 (Rudnicki et al., 2008). Microscopically, all of the HDL2 brains showed degeneration of the striatum characterized by marked loss of neurons and astrocytic gliosis of the putamen and caudate, with a dorsal to ventral gradient and relative sparing of the nucleus accumbens. The globus pallidus showed slightly milder degenerative changes than the striatum. In one case, marked loss of cortical neurons and gliosis were present and most severe in the visual cortex. The same brain has shown moderate neuritic senile plaques and abundant neurofibrillary tangles (NFTs) in the entorhinal cortex. In the remainder of the cases, the hippocampus, entorhinal cortex, and amygdala were normal. No significant histological changes were present in white matter, basal forebrain, thalamus, or subthalamic nucleus. The substantia nigra showed minimal pigment incontinence but was free of Lewy bodies and NFTs. Other brain regions, including the locus ceruleus, tegmentum and basis pontis, medulla, and cerebellum, were normal.

The hallmark of HDL2 pathology is the presence of protein aggregates in affected brain regions. The HDL2 aggregates are similar to aggregates found in HD and other polyglutamine repeat disorders. They are detectable with antibodies thought to be specific for proteins with expanded polyglutamine tracts 1C2 (Trottier et al., 1995) and 3B5H10 (Peters-Libeu et al., 2005). As in the polyglutamine disorders, the aggregates also stain with anti-ubiquitin antibodies (Walker et al., 2002a,b; Greenstein et al., 2007; Rudnicki et al., 2008). We have compared the distribution of protein aggregates in five HD and five HDL2 brains and have observed a similar distribution and frequency with some notable exceptions. Two HDL2 cases with shorter repeat expansions did not have aggregates in the striatum. While in every HD case aggregates were found in the pons and/or medulla, no aggregates in these regions were found in any HDL2 case. There was no difference in the extent of gliosis in the pons and medulla between HD and HDL2 (Rudnicki et al., 2008). We observed similar ultrastructure of HD and HDL2 aggregates, as well as evidence for autophagy and early stages of apoptosis in both diseases (Rudnicki et al., 2008).

In addition to protein aggregates, HDL2 brains contain small foci that are detectable with a CAG riboprobe (Figure 5–1) and other probes specific to RNA of the exons and introns from the sense strand of *JPH3* (Rudnicki et al., 2008). These foci are very similar to the RNA foci found in myotonic dystrophy 1 (also known as dystrophia myotonica, DM1), the first disorder in which disease pathogenesis was discovered to arise, at least in part, to toxicity from a transcript (RNA) containing a long CUG repeat (Ranum and Cooper, 2006). The only other known neurodegenerative disorder characterized by both intranuclear protein aggregates and RNA foci is SCA8 (Moseley et al., 2006), suggesting that in SCA8 and HDL2 mechanisms involving both toxic RNA and toxic proteins may coexist.

Neuroacanthocytosis and HDL2

Some individuals with HDL2 have acanthocytes. This was reported by Walker et al. (2003) in a study that first demonstrated acanthocytes in three individuals belonging to a family that was later shown to have HDL2. Red blood cells from three members of a Mexican HDL2 family, two members from the HDL2 index pedigree (Margolis et al., 2001) and one member from an additional HDL2 family, were then examined for the presence of acanthocytosis; only one individual (from the Mexican family) had acanthocytes, suggesting that acanthocytosis is a variable feature of HDL2 but that the formation of red blood cell membranes may

Anti-ubiquitin	CAG riborpobe	Hoechst	Merge

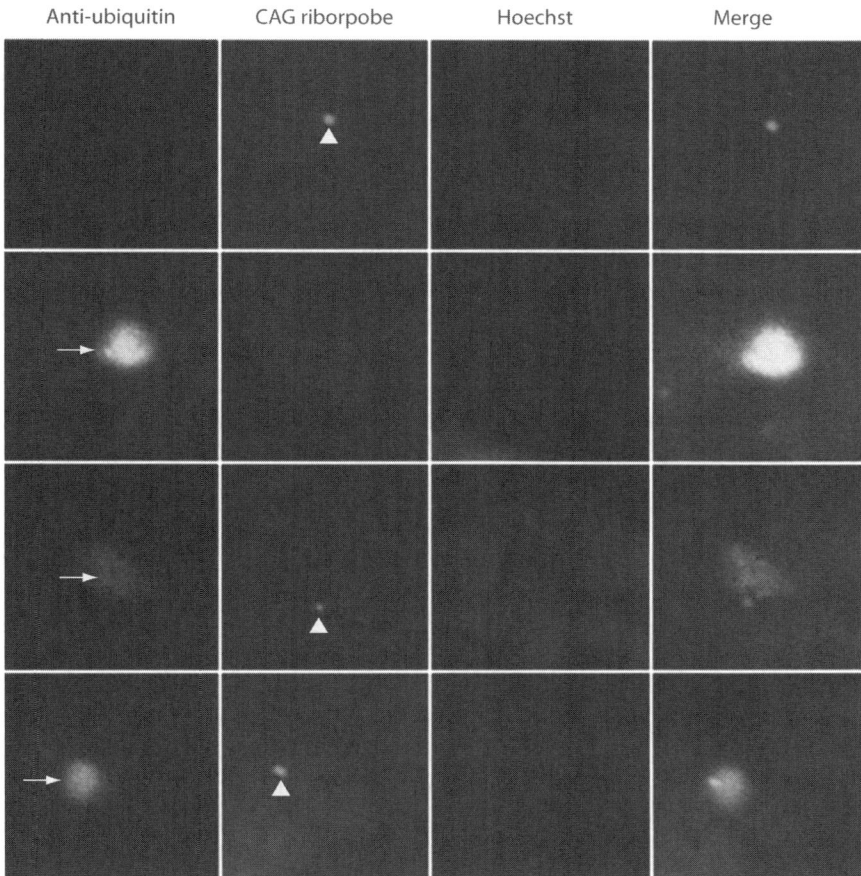

FIGURE 5–1. Ubiquitin-positive protein aggregates and small foci detectable by CAG riboprobes are pathological hallmarks of HDL2. Neurons in HDL2-affected brain regions usually contain either aggregates (*arrow*) or up to 13 RNA foci (*arrowheads*). Both aggregates and RNA foci are detected in only a fraction of neurons. Unlike in HD, where protein aggregates are found in both neurons and neuropil, in HDL2 aggregates and foci are primarily intranuclear.

provide valuable insight into the pathogenesis of HDL2, and, concomitantly, HDL2 may inform studies of the neuroacanthocytic disorders.

HDL2: GENE, MUTATION, AND PROTEIN

The gene that contains the HDL2 mutation is junctophilin-3 (*JPH3*, mouse orthologue *Jp3*). The variant of the gene that encodes the full-length protein has five exons. A sixth exon, termed "exon 2A," contains the repeat and is not part of this transcript. Other cryptic exons may exist. We have so far detected at least four *JPH3* splice variants that include exon 2A, and hence the repeat, along with exon 1. The variants differ from each other in the use of different splice acceptor sites, resulting in different reading frames and transcripts of slightly different lengths. In one variant, the repeat is in-frame to encode polyalanine, in two variants the repeat is in-frame to encode polyleucine, and in one variant the repeat is in the 3′-untranslated region. Both the full-length *JPH3* transcript and exon 2A–containing transcripts are expressed in multiple brain regions, with testis the only peripheral tissue that shows significant levels of expression. The five-exon transcript, which excludes exon 2A, is far more common than the splice variants, at least in normal tissue. Of the splice variants, the one in which the repeat encodes polyalanine appears to be the most common. Surprisingly, and unlike in HD or other repeat expansion diseases, it is difficult to detect the RNA transcript carrying an expanded repeat in the HDL2 brain; the transcript with the expansion is evident only on Southern blots, and then it appears as a smear running unexpectedly slowly (unpublished data).

Four members of the junctophilin gene family have been described (Takeshima et al., 2000; Nishi et al., 2000, 2003). *JPH1* is expressed in skeletal muscle, *JPH2* is expressed in cardiac and skeletal muscle, and *JPH3* and *JPH4* (Nishi et al., 2003) are expressed primarily in brain and to a much lesser extent in testes. The members of the junctophilin protein family have eight repeated N-terminal units of 14 amino acids, known as MORN (membrane orientation and recognition nexus) motifs, that serve to anchor the protein to the plasma membrane. The C terminus of the proteins contains an endoplasmic/sarcoplasmic reticulum transmembrane insertion domain. This structure, immunohistochemical analyses, and analysis of a *Jp1* knockout mouse model (Ito et al., 2001) have suggested that the junctophilin proteins serve to link plasma membrane voltage sensors with intracellular ion channels, including ryanodine and inositol 1,4,5-trisphosphate receptor–linked Ca^{2+} channels. The recent discovery of mutations in *JPH2* that appear to cause some cases of hypertrophic cardiomyopathy provides strong support for this hypothesis (Landstrom et al., 2007).

POSSIBLE MECHANISMS OF HDL2 PATHOGENESIS

RNA Toxic Gain of Function

One possible explanation for the extreme difficulty in detecting *JPH3* transcripts containing the expanded repeat and the clear correlation between repeat length and the age at disease onset is that the JPH3 transcript containing the mutation is toxic, similar to the toxicity of RNA observed in DM1. DM1 is caused by a CTG repeat expansion in the 3′-untranslated region of the gene *DMPK*. Prominent features include muscle weakness, myotonia, cataracts, and cardiac and endocrine abnormalities (Ashizawa, 1998; Ranum and Day, 2004); but developmental and degenerative brain abnormalities may also be present (Chang et al., 1998; Meola et al., 2003; Kassubek et al., 2003; Antonini et al., 2004). While the pathogenesis of DM1 is complicated, there is strong evidence that *DMPK* transcripts containing the expanded CUG repeat have toxic properties and substantially contribute to disease pathogenesis. RNA foci containing the mutant transcript have been detected in the nuclei of fibroblasts, muscle cells, and neurons of DM1 patients (Taneja et al., 1995; Davis et al., 1997). Expression of transcripts containing a CUG expansion leads to RNA foci or cell toxicity in various cell lines and in a transgenic mouse model (Amack et al., 1999; Mankodi et al., 2000; Quintero-Mora et al., 2002; Furuya et al., 2005). Members of the muscleblind-like (MBNL) protein family co-localize to RNA foci containing CUG repeat expansions, suggesting a role for these proteins in DM1 pathogenesis (Mankodi et al., 2001; Fardaei et al., 2002).

We have hypothesized that if RNA toxicity plays a role in HDL2 pathogenesis, RNA foci should be detected in the brains of patients with HDL2, which was indeed the case (Rudnicki et al., 2007). In addition, dual-labeled fluorescence in situ hybridization with probes specific for *JPH3* exonal and intronal sequences demonstrates that the foci contain unspliced or misspliced *JPH3* transcripts (Rudnicki et al., 2007). The HDL2 foci, like the DM1 foci, contain the protein MBNL1. This raised the possibility that muscleblind-regulated splicing could be abnormal in HDL2 as it is in DM1 (Sergeant et al., 2001; Jiang et al., 2004; Leroy et al., 2006), and preliminary evidence does indeed demonstrate altered splicing of APP and MAPT in HDL2 brains (Rudnicki et al., 2007).

One possibility is that the mutant transcript detected by riboprobes is present in protein aggregates. However, in the vast majority of neurons, the RNA foci and the protein aggregates do not co-localize (Rudnicki et al., 2008). This finding raises several intriguing hypotheses. It is possible that RNA provides the nidus for protein aggregates and that, once protein has sufficiently aggregated around the original RNA foci, the RNA foci become undetectable by RNA probes. Alternatively, the protein aggregates may form as a response to RNA-induced toxicity and may or may not contribute to pathogenesis.

The detection of RNA foci in HDL2 brains raises the possibility that *JPH3* transcripts might be neurotoxic. We have developed a cell model to test this hypothesis, using both HEK293 cells, a standard epithelial line with some neuron-like properties, and HT-22 cells, a mouse hippocampal line selected for sensitivity to glutamate toxicity (Davis and Maher, 1994). Constructs were generated that contained exon 2A with either 11 or 53 CTG triplets. The three ATG codons present in this transcript were mutated to avoid protein translation (Rudnicki et al., 2007). Constructs with the long repeat but not the short repeat lead to the formation of RNA foci in both HEK293 and HT-22 cells and are toxic to these cells (Figure 5–2) (Rudnicki et al., 2007). These findings support the hypothesis that RNA toxic gain of function may play an important role in HDL2 pathogenesis.

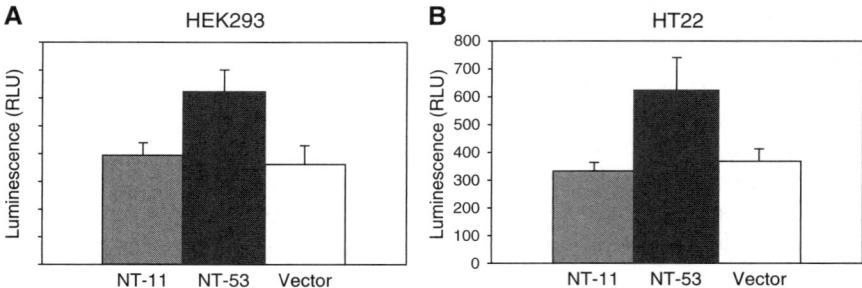

FIGURE 5–2. Cell model of RNA toxicity in HDL2. RNA transcripts corresponding to *JPH3* exon 2A with expanded, but not normal, CUG repeats are toxic to both non-neuronal HEK293 (**A**) and neuron-like HT-22 (**B**) cells. Toxicity was measured using the caspase 3/7 toxicity assay 48 hours after transfection. RLU, relative luminescence unit. From Rudnicki et al. (2007). Copyright © 2007 Wiley-Liss, Inc., a Wiley company, reprinted, with permission.

HDL2 and Gain of Function of Expanded Protein

Are *JPH3* transcripts with an expanded CUG repeat sufficient to cause neuro-degeneration, or do proteins with expanded amino tracts contribute to pathogenesis? The HDL2 repeat is much smaller than the CUG repeat in DM1, yet HDL2 is a much more devastating and rapidly progressive disease. HDL2 transcripts with CUG repeats are predominantly expressed in brain, and their regional and cell type–specific patterns and levels of expression may help to explain their high toxicity. However, it is also possible that other mechanisms contribute to HDL2 pathogenesis. At the HDL2 locus both sense (containing CTG repeats) and antisense (containing CAG repeats) strands may produce transcripts which could be translated into toxic proteins. On the sense strand the proteins would contain expanded polyleucine and polyalanine tracts. We have observed that both polyalanine- and polyleucine-expressing JPH3 isoforms readily aggregate and are quite toxic in a cell model (unpublished data). Expression of expanded polyleucine and/or polyalanine tracts in HDL2 brains could explain HDL2 brain protein aggregates as these tracts, like polyglutamine expansions, are detected by the 1C2 antibody (Dorsman et al., 2002; Sugaya et al., 2003). However, we so far have been unable to detect expanded polyalanine or polyleucine tract–containing isoforms in HDL2 brains. We therefore tentatively conclude that expanded polyalanine and polyleucine variants may still be present in HDL2 brains but at levels so low as to fall below the sensitivity of our assays and, hence, unlikely to be the primary cause of HDL2 pathogenesis.

Are protein isoforms, encoded by the antisense strand in which the repeat is in the polyglutamine orientation, present in HDL2 brains? Indeed, on the opposite strand to *JPH3*, an open reading frame exists in which the repeat is in-frame to encode polyglutamine. There are three in-frame start codons and two in-frame stop codons between the potential promoter and the polyglutamine repeat region. This region is slightly more conserved than the most conserved portion of exon 2A but less highly conserved than *JPH3* exon 1. The bioinformatic evidence for a promoter in the region is inconsistent, and the promoter activity remains to be examined experimentally. We have searched for evidence of expression of the RNA antisense to *JPH3* exon 2A using strand-specific reverse transcriptase polymerase chain reaction in HDL2 brains. We detected a transcript with the normal repeat, but not a transcript with an expanded CAG repeat. Whether this means that the repeat expansion blocks expression of the antisense transcript, destabilizes it, or in some way leads to its sequestration so that it is not extractable by normal methods of RNA isolation remains to be determined.

In parallel to a search for an antisense transcript at the HDL2 locus, we have also searched for evidence of a protein with an expanded polyglutamine tract that would be coded by this transcript in HDL2 brains. Surprisingly, 1C2 and 3B5H10 antibodies (Trottier et al., 1995; Peters-Libeu et al., 2005), thought to be specific for expanded polyglutamine tracts, detect protein aggregates in the HDL2 brain but do not detect an expanded protein on Western blots, while the antibodies stain aggregates in the HD brain and the HD protein on Western blots of protein extracted from HD brains. Why the 1C2 and 3B5H10 antibodies stain inclusions in HDL2 brains, but not on Western blots is not clear. One possible explanation is that the expanded proteins have one conformation in aggregated form and another on Western blots. It is also possible that the polyglutamine-containing protein is expressed at levels too low for detection by Western blotting but that its aggregation with other proteins, including TATA-binding protein, makes immunohistochemical detection easier. Alternatively, pathogenic polyglutamine expansion may not be necessary for the aggregation to occur so that the 1C2 and 3B5H10 antibodies may be detecting other protein epitopes with conformation similar to polyglutamine. As an example, it appears that 1C2 stains hyaline inclusions (Takahashi et al., 2000) in patients who do not have a polyglutamine disease. We conclude that, whatever the origin of the 1C2/3B5H10 staining aggregates in HDL2, it is unlikely that polyglutamine expansion can fully account for disease pathogenesis.

Antisense Transcription and HDL2

Antisense transcripts are common in the human genome, adding to its diversity and regulatory complexity (Katayama et al., 2005). As noted, an antisense transcript is expressed from the HDL2 locus, though apparently not if the repeat is expanded. The presence of this antisense transcript also links HDL2 with DM1 as an antisense transcript is located at the DM1 locus and appears to play a role in chromatin remodeling (Cho et al., 2005). In SCA8, another CAG/CTG repeat expansion disease, transcripts are expressed from both strands, with some evidence that the CAG transcript is encoded into polyglutamine and plays a potential role in disease pathogenesis (Moseley et al., 2006). In Alzheimer disease, β-secretase-1 (*BACE1*) mRNA expression is under the control of a noncoding antisense RNA that may drive Alzheimer disease–associated pathophysiology (Faghihi et al., 2008). Moreover, in the neurodegenerative disorder fragile X–associated tremor and ataxia syndrome, caused by a modest CGG expansion in the *FMR1* gene at the fragile X locus, the quantity of transcripts antisense to the *FMR1* gene is modulated by repeat length and may have a role in disease pathogenesis (Ladd et al., 2007). Given these examples, it is possible that the antisense transcripts at the HDL2 locus play a regulatory role; we have recently found evidence for such an effect at the HD locus (unpublished data), and we suspect that antisense regulation of sense expression and toxicity may be common in the repeat expansion disorders.

HDL2 and Loss of *JPH3* Function

Loss of JPH3 expression as a consequence of repeat expansion may also contribute to HDL2 pathogenesis. Indeed, total *JPH3* transcript and protein appears to be reduced in HDL2 brain (unpublished data), and knockout mice missing one or both copies of JP3 have subtle behavioral abnormalities, with no evidence of gross neuropathological changes (Nishi et al., 2002). We conclude from this mild phenotype that loss of *JPH3* expression, while potentially contributing to HDL2 pathogenesis, is unlikely to offer a full explanation.

CONCLUSION

Our preliminary data support a role of sense RNA in HDL2 pathogenesis, although it appears that HDL2 probably involves multiple pathogenic pathways, including toxicity of expanded amino acid tracts encoded from the sense (polyalanine, polyleucine) and/or antisense (polyglutamine) strands and subtle toxic effects of loss of JPH3 expression (Figure 5–3). The unexpected and intriguing complexity of HDL2 and its great clinical and pathological similarity to HD and other repeat expansion disorders suggest that RNA toxicity and bidirectional transcription may contribute to the pathogenesis of these other disorders.

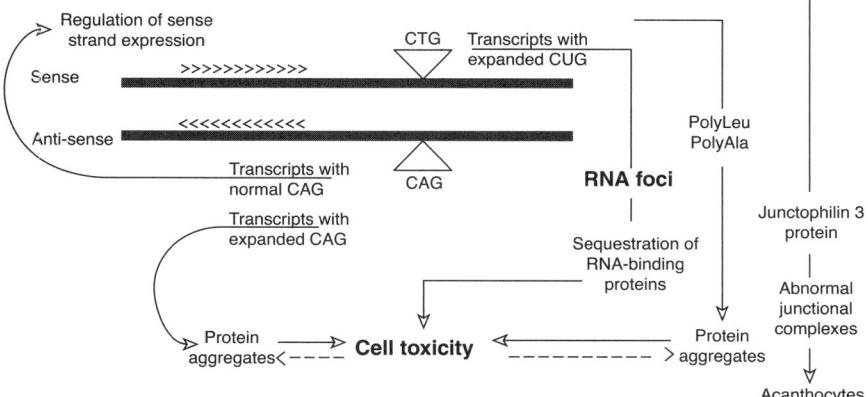

FIGURE 5–3. HDL2 pathogenesis is multimodal. In the model, RNA toxicity resulting from the expression of sense transcripts with expanded CUG repeats is central to pathogenesis. Toxicity of sense strand–encoded polyalanine- and polyleucine-containing JPH3 variants, as well as toxicity of an antisense strand–encoded polyglutamine variant, may contribute to the disease. While some evidence exists for the role of loss of junctophilin 3 function, the role of antisense transcription in HDL2 pathogenesis is so far insufficiently explored.

ACKNOWLEDGMENTS

The authors thank Christopher A. Ross, Ana Seixas, and Daniel W. Chung for valuable discussions; Ms. Chengxiu Zhiang for technical assistance; and the individuals with HDL2 and their families for their cooperation. This work was funded by the Hereditary Disease Foundation, and NIH grants NS38054, NS016375, and NS061099.

REFERENCES

Amack JD, Paguio AP, Mahadevan MS (1999) *Cis* and *trans* effects of the myotonic dystrophy (DM) mutation in a cell culture model. Hum Mol Genet 8(11):1975–1984.

Antonini G, Mainero C, Romano A, Giubilei F, Ceschin V, Gragnani F, Morino S, Fiorelli M, Soscia F, Di Pasquale A, Caramia F (2004) Cerebral atrophy in myotonic dystrophy: a voxel based morphometric study. J Neurol Neurosurg Psychiatry 75(11): 1611–1613.

Ashizawa T (1998) Myotonic dystrophy as a brain disorder. Arch Neurol 55(3): 291–293.

Bardien S, Abrahams F, Soodyall H, van der Merwe L, Greenberg J, Brink T, Carr J (2007) A South African mixed ancestry family with Huntington disease-like 2: clinical and genetic features. Mov Disord 22:2083–2089.

Chang L, Ernst T, Osborn D, Seltzer W, Leonido-Yee M, Poland RE (1998) Proton spectroscopy in myotonic dystrophy: correlations with CTG repeats. Arch Neurol 55(3):305–311.

Cho DH, Thienes CP, Mahoney SE, Analau E, Filippova GN, Tapscott SJ (2005) Antisense transcription and heterochromatin at the DM1 CTG repeats are constrained by CTCF. Mol Cell 20(3):483–489.

Davis BM, McCurrach ME, Taneja KL, Singer RH, Housman DE (1997) Expansion of a CUG trinucleotide repeat in the 3' untranslated region of myotonic dystrophy protein kinase transcripts results in nuclear retention of transcripts. Proc Natl Acad Sci USA 94(14):7388–7393.

Davis JB, Maher P (1994) Protein kinase C activation inhibits glutamate-induced cytotoxicity in a neuronal cell line. Brain Res 652(1):169–173.

DiFiglia M, Sapp E, Chase KO, Davies SW, Bates GP, Vonsattel JP, Aronin N (1997) Aggregation of huntingtin in neuronal intranuclear inclusions and dystrophic neurites in brain. Science 277(5334):1990–1903.

Dorsman JC, Pepers B, Langenberg D, Kerkdijk H, Ijszenga M, den Dunnen JT, Roos RA, van Ommen GJ (2002) Strong aggregation and increased toxicity of polyleucine over polyglutamine stretches in mammalian cells. Hum Mol Genet 11(13): 1487–1496.

Faghihi MA, Modarresi F, Khalil AM, Wood DE, Sahagan BG, Morgan TE, Finch CE, St Laurent G 3rd, Kenny PJ, Wahlestedt C (2008) Expression of a noncoding RNA is elevated in Alzheimer's disease and drives rapid feed-forward regulation of beta-secretase. Nat Med 14(7):723–730.

Fardaei M, Rogers MT, Thorpe HM, Larkin K, Hamshere MG, Harper PS, Brook JD (2002) Three proteins, MBNL, MBLL and MBXL, co-localize *in vivo* with nuclear foci of expanded-repeat transcripts in DM1 and DM2 cells. Hum Mol Genet 11(7): 805–814.

Furuya H, Shinnoh N, Ohyagi Y, Ikezoe K, Kikuchi H, Osoegawa M, Fukumaki Y, Nakabeppu Y, Hayashi T, Kira J (2005) Some flavonoids and DHEA-S prevent the *cis*-effect of expanded CTG repeats in a stable PC12 cell transformant. Biochem Pharmacol 69(3):503–516.

Greenstein PE, Vonsattel JP, Margolis RL, Joseph JT (2007) Huntington's disease like-2 neuropathology. Mov Disord 22(10):1416–1423.

Harper PS (1996) New genes for old diseases: the molecular basis of myotonic dystrophy and Huntington's disease. The Lumleian Lecture 1995. J R Coll Physicians Lond 30(3):221–231.

Hedreen JC, Peyser CE, Folstein SE, Ross CA (1991) Neuronal loss in layers V and VI of cerebral cortex in Huntington's disease. Neurosci Lett 133(2):257–261.

Holmes SE, Hearn EO, Ross CA, Margolis RL (2001a) SCA12: an unusual mutation leads to an unusual spinocerebellar ataxia. Brain Res Bull 56(3–4):397–403.

Holmes SE, O'Hearn E, Rosenblatt A, Callahan C, Hwang HS, Ingersoll-Ashworth RG, Fleisher A, Stevanin G, Brice A, Potter NT, Ross CA, Margolis RL (2001b) A repeat expansion in the gene encoding junctophilin-3 is associated with Huntington disease-like 2. Nat Genet 29(4):377–378.

Huntington's Disease Collaborative Research Group (1993) A novel gene containing a trinucleotide repeat that is expanded and unstable on Huntington's disease chromosomes. Cell 72(6):971–983.

Ito K, Komazaki S, Sasamoto K, Yoshida M, Nishi M, Kitamura K, Takeshima H (2001) Deficiency of triad junction and contraction in mutant skeletal muscle lacking junctophilin type 1. J Cell Biol 154(5):1059–1067.

Jiang H, Mankodi A, Swanson MS, Moxley RT, Thornton CA (2004) Myotonic dystrophy type 1 is associated with nuclear foci of mutant RNA, sequestration of muscleblind proteins and deregulated alternative splicing in neurons. Hum Mol Genet 13(24): 3079–3088.

Kassubek J, Juengling FD, Hoffmann S, Rosenbohm A, Kurt A, Jurkat-Rott K, Steinbach P, Wolf M, Ludolph AC, Lehmann-Horn F, Lerche H, Weber YG (2003) Quantification of brain atrophy in patients with myotonic dystrophy and proximal myotonic myopathy: a controlled 3-dimensional magnetic resonance imaging study. Neurosci Lett 348(2): 73–76.

Katayama S, Tomaru Y, Kasukawa T, Waki K, Nakanishi M, Nakamura M, Nishida H, Yap CC, Suzuki M, Kawai J, Suzuki H, Carninci P, Hayashizaki Y, Wells C, Frith M, Ravasi T, Pang KC, Hallinan J, Mattick J, Hume DA, Lipovich L, Batalov S, Engstrom PG, Mizuno Y, Faghihi MA, Sandelin A, Chalk AM, Mottagui-Tabar S, Liang Z, Lenhard B, Wahlestedt C (2005) Antisense transcription in the mammalian transcriptome. Science 309(5740):1564–1566.

Ladd PD, Smith LE, Rabaia NA, Moore JM, Georges SA, Hansen RS, Hagerman RJ, Tassone F, Tapscott SJ, Filippova GN (2007) An antisense transcript spanning the CGG repeat region of FMR1 is upregulated in premutation carriers but silenced in full mutation individuals. Hum Mol Genet 16(24):3174–3187.

Landstrom AP, Weisleder N, Batalden KB, Bos JM, Tester DJ, Ommen SR, Wehrens XH, Claycomb WC, Ko JK, Hwang M, Pan Z, Ma J, Ackerman MJ (2007) Mutations in JPH2-encoded junctophilin-2 associated with hypertrophic cardiomyopathy in humans. J Mol Cell Cardiol 42(6):1026–1035.

Leroy O, Dhaenens CM, Schraen-Maschke S, Belarbi K, Delacourte A, Andreadis A, Sablonniere B, Buee L, Sergeant N, Caillet-Boudin ML (2006) ETR-3 represses Tau exons 2/3 inclusion, a splicing event abnormally enhanced in myotonic dystrophy type I. J Neurosci Res 84(4):852–859.

Li H, Li SH, Cheng AL, Mangiarini L, Bates GP, Li XJ (1999) Ultrastructural localization and progressive formation of neuropil aggregates in Huntington's disease transgenic mice. Hum Mol Genet 8(7):1227–1236.

Mankodi A, Logigian E, Callahan L, McClain C, White R, Henderson D, Krym M, Thornton CA (2000) Myotonic dystrophy in transgenic mice expressing an expanded CUG repeat. Science 289(5485):1769–1773.

Mankodi A, Urbinati CR, Yuan QP, Moxley RT, Sansone V, Krym M, Henderson D, Schalling M, Swanson MS, Thornton CA (2001) Muscleblind localizes to nuclear foci of aberrant RNA in myotonic dystrophy types 1 and 2. Hum Mol Genet 10(19): 2165–2170.

Margolis RL, Holmes SE, Rosenblatt A, Gourley L, O'Hearn E, Ross CA, Seltzer WK, Walker RH, Ashizawa T, Rasmussen A, Hayden M, Almqvist EW, Harris J, Fahn S, MacDonald ME, Mysore J, Shimohata T, Tsuji S, Potter N, Nakaso K, Adachi Y, Nakashima K, Bird T, Krause A, Greenstein P (2004) Huntington's disease-like 2 (HDL2) in North America and Japan. Ann Neurol 56(5):670–674.

Margolis RL, O'Hearn E, Rosenblatt A, Willour V, Holmes SE, Franz ML, Callahan C, Hwang HS, Troncoso JC, Ross CA (2001) A disorder similar to Huntington's disease is associated with a novel CAG repeat expansion. Ann Neurol 50(3):373–380.

Meola G, Sansone V, Perani D, Scarone S, Cappa S, Dragoni C, Cattaneo E, Cotelli M, Gobbo C, Fazio F, Siciliano G, Mancuso M, Vitelli E, Zhang S, Krahe R, Moxley RT (2003) Executive dysfunction and avoidant personality trait in myotonic dystrophy type 1 (DM-1) and in proximal myotonic myopathy (PROMM/DM-2). Neuromuscul Disord 13(10):813–821.

Moore RC, Xiang F, Monaghan J, Han D, Zhang Z, Edstrom L, Anvret M, Prusiner SB (2001) Huntington disease phenocopy is a familial prion disease. Am J Hum Genet 69(6):1385–1388.

Moseley ML, Zu T, Ikeda Y, Gao W, Mosemiller AK, Daughters RS, Chen G, Weatherspoon MR, Clark HB, Ebner TJ, Day JW, Ranum LP (2006) Bidirectional expression of CUG and CAG expansion transcripts and intranuclear polyglutamine inclusions in spinocerebellar ataxia type 8. Nat Genet 38(7):758–769.

Nishi M, Hashimoto K, Kuriyama K, Komazaki S, Kano M, Shibata S, Takeshima H (2002) Motor discoordination in mutant mice lacking junctophilin type 3. Biochem Biophys Res Commun 292(2):318–324.

Nishi M, Mizushima A, Nakagawara K, Takeshima H (2000) Characterization of human junctophilin subtype genes. Biochem Biophys Res Commun 273(3):920–927.

Nishi M, Sakagami H, Komazaki S, Kondo H, Takeshima H (2003) Coexpression of junctophilin type 3 and type 4 in brain. Brain Res Mol Brain Res 118(1–2):102–110.

Peters-Libeu C, Newhouse Y, Krishnan P, Cheung K, Brooks E, Weisgraber K, Finkbeiner S (2005) Crystallization and diffraction properties of the Fab fragment of 3B5H10, an antibody specific for disease-causing polyglutamine stretches. Acta Crystallogr F Struct Biol Cryst Commun 61(Pt 12):1065–1068.

Quintero-Mora ML, Depardon F, Waring J, Korneluk Robert G, Cisneros B (2002) Expanded CTG repeats inhibit neuronal differentiation of the PC12 cell line. Biochem Biophys Res Commun 295(2):289–294.

Ranum LP, Cooper TA (2006) RNA-mediated neuromuscular disorders. Annu Rev Neurosci 29:259–277.

Ranum LP, Day JW (2004) Myotonic dystrophy: RNA pathogenesis comes into focus. Am J Hum Genet 74(5):793–804.

Ross CA (1997) Intranuclear neuronal inclusions: a common pathogenic mechanism for glutamine-repeat neurodegenerative diseases? Neuron 19(6):1147–1150.

Rudnicki DD, Holmes SE, Lin MW, Thornton CA, Ross CA, Margolis RL (2007) Huntington's disease-like 2 is associated with CUG repeat-containing RNA foci. Ann Neurol 61(3):272–282.

Rudnicki DD, Pletnikova O, Vonsattel JP, Ross CA, Margolis RL (2008) A comparison of Huntington disease and Huntington disease-like 2 neuropathology. J Neuropathol Exp Neurol 67(4):366–374.

Santos C, Wanderley H, Vedolin L, Pena SD, Jardim L, Sequeiros J (2008) Huntington disease-like 2: the first patient with apparent European ancestry. Clin Genet 73(5): 480–485.

Sapp E, Schwarz C, Chase K, Bhide PG, Young AB, Penney J, Vonsattel JP, Aronin N, DiFiglia M (1997) Huntingtin localization in brains of normal and Huntington's disease patients. Ann Neurol 42(4):604–612.

Schneider SA, Walker RH, Bhatia KP (2007) The Huntington's disease-like syndromes: what to consider in patients with a negative Huntington's disease gene test. Nat Clin Pract Neurol 3(9):517–525.

Sergeant N, Sablonniere B, Schraen-Maschke S, Ghestem A, Maurage CA, Wattez A, Vermersch P, Delacourte A (2001) Dysregulation of human brain microtubule-associated tau mRNA maturation in myotonic dystrophy type 1. Hum Mol Genet 10(19): 2143–2155.

Sugaya K, Matsubara S, Miyamoto K, Kawata A, Hayashi H (2003) An aggregate-prone conformational epitope in trinucleotide repeat diseases. Neuroreport 14(18): 2331–2335.

Takahashi J, Fukuda T, Tanaka J, Minamitani M, Fujigasaki H, Uchihara T (2000) Neuronal intranuclear hyaline inclusion disease with polyglutamine-immunoreactive inclusions. Acta Neuropathol (Berl) 99(5):589–594.

Takeshima H, Komazaki S, Nishi M, Iino M, Kangawa K (2000) Junctophilins: a novel family of junctional membrane complex proteins. Mol Cell 6(1):11–22.

Taneja KL, McCurrach M, Schalling M, Housman D, Singer RH (1995) Foci of trinucle-otide repeat transcripts in nuclei of myotonic dystrophy cells and tissues. J Cell Biol 128(6):995–1002.

Trottier Y, Lutz Y, Stevanin G, et al. (1995) Polyglutamine expansion as a pathological epitope in Huntington's disease and four dominant cerebellar ataxias. Nature 378(6555):403–406.

Vonsattel JP, Myers RH, Stevens TJ, Ferrante RJ, Bird ED, Richardson EP Jr (1985) Neuropathological classification of Huntington's disease. J Neuropathol Exp Neurol 44(6):559–577.

Walker RH, Brin MF, Sandu D, Good PF, Shashidharan P (2002a) TorsinA immunoreactiv-ity in brains of patients with DYT1 and non-DYT1 dystonia. Neurology 58(1): 120–124.

Walker RH, Jankovic J, O'Hearn E, Margolis RL (2003) Phenotypic features of Hunting-ton's disease-like 2. Mov Disord 18(12):1527–1530.

Walker RH, Morgello S, Davidoff-Feldman B, Melnick A, Walsh MJ, Shashidharan P, Brin MF (2002b) Autosomal dominant chorea-acanthocytosis with polyglutamine-containing neuronal inclusions. Neurology 58(7):1031–1037.

Wild EJ, Mudanohwo EE, Sweeney MG, Schneider SA, Beck J, Bhatia KP, Rossor MN, Davis MB, Tabrizi SJ (2008) Huntington's disease phenocopies are clinically and genetically heterogeneous. Mov Disord 23(5):716–720.

6

Chorea-Acanthocytosis

Benedikt Bader, MD; Adrian Danek, MD;
and Ruth H. Walker, MB, ChB, PhD

INTRODUCTION

Understanding of the disorder now known as chorea-acanthocytosis (ChAc) (OMIM 200150) has undergone significant evolution since the 1960s, when it was first described and termed "Levine-Critchley syndrome." Subsequent reports used variable terms such as "amyotrophic chorea with acanthocytosis" (Kito et al., 1980) and "amyotrophic choreo-acanthocytosis" (Serra et al., 1986). The remarkably numerous Japanese observations from the 1980s (Hirose, 2008) have favored the term "chorea-acanthocytosis" (Toyokura et al., 1982). This designation is now internationally accepted for the disease resulting from mutations of the *VPS13A* gene (initially called *CHAC*) on chromosome 9q (Rampoldi et al., 2001; Ueno et al., 2001) and absence of the chorein protein (Dobson-Stone et al., 2004). This is despite the fact that acanthocytes may not be detected in every single case and are no longer a prerequisite for diagnosing ChAc and that chorea is not a consistent feature.

The term "neuroacanthocytosis" (NA) has been, and continues to be, widely used, resulting in diagnostic confusion both with phenotypically similar disorders and with entities such as the abetalipoproteinemia of Bassen and Kornzweig, which features neuropathy and ataxia. Further analysis of the 19 NA cases reported in the once seminal reference of Hardie and colleagues (1991) demonstrated that at least one-third were not affected by ChAc (Gandhi et al., 2008). ChAc was diagnosed only in nine cases (families H and B corresponding to *CHAC* families 01 and 09 [Rampoldi et al., 2001] and three further cases were analyzed individually for *VPS13A* mutations [Dobson-Stone et al., 2002]). Six cases (L family) carried a McLeod mutation (Ho et al., 1996), and one patient was clearly distinct because of his retinitis pigmentosa and pallidal degeneration (Orrell et al., 1995), most likely due to pantothenate kinase–associated neurodegeneration (PKAN).

Reports that lack sufficient diagnostic evidence for ChAc, on the basis of either molecular methods or circumstantial evidence from pedigree or clinical findings, are of questionable use for the present review, even if they are recent. Some cases reported in the premolecular era underwent subsequent genetic analysis and were reported at a later date, but in others the precise diagnosis has not been confirmed. In order not to discard a wealth of potentially useful information regarding this very rare disorder, we include here cases where ChAc is the likely diagnosis. In the absence of confirmatory testing, this can be inferred in many cases from the involvement of females, the age of onset, and the prominence of orofacial and lingual movements.

EPIDEMIOLOGY

The number of patients currently identified worldwide is estimated to be in the hundreds, but this disorder is likely to be substantially underdiagnosed. From our own experience with the internationally open free diagnostic service (chorein Western blot, see later section "Diagnostic Tests"), we estimate its prevalence at 1 in 10 million. The higher figure for Japan (Hirose, 2008; Iwata et al., 1984; Kuroiwa et al., 1984; Sato et al., 1984; Yamamoto et al., 1982) is striking and could indicate the effect of a founder gene. The absence of reports mainly from Africa and the former Soviet Union might be due to their inaccessibility or to insufficient diagnostic resources. ChAc was first recognized in the 1960s in two kindreds from North America (Critchley et al., 1967; Levine et al., 1968), but subsequent reports have come from practically all ethnic backgrounds (Bharucha and Bharucha, 1989; Gross et al., 1985; Kutcher et al., 1999; Nielsen and Temlett, 1997; Ong et al., 1989; Rodrigues et al., 2008; Walker et al., 2006b).

GENETICS

ChAc is inherited in an autosomal recessive manner. Carrier testing requires the knowledge of the specific mutation in the family. Prenatal testing is currently not feasible. To date, more than 90 mutations of the *VPS13A* gene (formerly known as *CHAC*) have been found (Dobson-Stone et al., 2002, 2004; Ichiba et al., 2007;

Ishida et al., 2009; Miki et al., 2010; Rampoldi et al., 2001; Ueno et al., 2001; Velayos-Baeza et al., 2008). Mutations affect 43 of the 73 exons as well as several introns, without any significant hot spot, and lead to absent or markedly reduced levels of chorein protein. The majority of the mutations detected in exons consist of small deletions or insertions (49%) leading to frameshift of the open reading frame of *VPS13A* and to premature termination codons. Nonsense mutations (32%) and gross deletions (10%) were also found frequently, followed by missense mutations (8%) and mutations affecting splice sites of exons (2%).

Presently available data are insufficient for conclusions about genotype–phenotype correlation in ChAc (Danek et al., 2005), although it is tempting to speculate that certain mutations may confer a higher risk of epilepsy (Al-Asmi et al., 2005). An instructive example, however, of phenotypic variability of the same genotype is provided by a pair of siblings in their 30s (Aasly et al., 1999). The sister initially presented with orofacial dyskinesia and ataxia of stance and gait and became wheelchair-dependent and mute, while her brother suffered from epilepsy and developed only a minor movement disorder.

Consanguinity of patients' parents has been noted in a number of reports (Sorrentino et al., 1999), but many cases are sporadic. In the French-Canadian group, pseudodominant inheritance was attributed to consanguinity (Dobson-Stone et al., 2005).

CLINICAL FEATURES

The mean age of onset is about 30 years, although ChAc can develop as early as the first or as late as the seventh decade. The typical appearance is of dysarthria, orofacial hyperkinesias, and choreic leg movements. However, there can be considerable phenotypic variation, especially in the early stages. ChAc runs a chronic progressive course and may lead to major disability within a few years. Some patients become bedridden or wheelchair-dependent by their third decade (Aasly et al., 1999; Alonso et al., 1989). Life expectancy is reduced, and several instances of death during epileptic seizures are on record. Ages at death have ranged between 28–61 years.

As the hyperkinetic orofacial state progresses to mutism, there is a gradual development of the choreatic and dystonic syndrome into parkinsonism in the majority of patients. There may be increased muscle tone, rest tremor, impaired postural reflexes, bradykinesia, facial masking, and micrographia. The pyramidal tracts do not seem to be involved, and the plantar reflexes are usually flexor. Abnormalities of eye movements consist of square-wave jerks, impaired saccades, and smooth pursuit (Gradstein et al., 2005).

Illustrative case reports are provided in the appendix and Video 6–1 (Chorea-acanthocytosis). These patients were examined by Adrian Danek in 2000–2001 at the Cognitive Neuroscience Section, Medical Neurology Branch, National Institute of Neurologic Disorders and Stroke, National Institutes of Health (Bethesda, MD, USA) and subsequently reported in detail (Danek et al., 2004).

Gait

Stance and gait are severely impaired due to a combination of chorea and limb dystonia (Aasly et al., 1999; Burbaud et al., 2002a; Malandrini et al., 1993; Wihl et al., 2001), and this impairment can be characterized as "rubber man appearance" (Thomas and Jankovic, 2006). There may be flinging arm and leg movements, shoulder shrugs, and pelvic thrusts (Burbaud et al., 2002a). Violent trunk spasms cause sudden flexion and extension movements (Burbaud et al., 2002a), with head dropping and head banging, resulting in local bruising, hair loss, and the risk of more serious injuries to the head and neck. Falls may result from impaired postural reflexes (Wihl et al., 2001), sudden buckling of the knees (Hiersemenzel et al., 1996), and equinovarus foot deformity, the latter related to dystonia as well as distal limb muscle atrophy.

Orofacial and Tongue Protrusion Dystonia

Characteristic of ChAc are the involuntary movements that affect the face, mouth, tongue, pharynx, and larynx, which are a major cause of morbidity. Involuntary vocalizations (vocal tics) are present in about two-thirds of patients and may consist of clicking, gasping, sighing, whistling, blowing, sucking, and grunting noises as well as perseveration of word elements, phrases, and continuous humming. There may be habitual teeth grinding (bruxism) and spitting as well as involuntary belching (Hiersemenzel et al., 1996; Wihl et al., 2001). Tongue and lip biting can lead to severe mutilation (Aasly et al., 1999), which patients typically try to avoid by keeping objects such as a handkerchief or cotton swabs between their jaws (Malandrini et al., 1993). These probably function both as a mechanical obstacle and as a sensory trick to reduce dystonia. Bruxism may cause severe dental damage, and local infections can be life-threatening.

Swallowing is often severely impaired and may necessitate tube feeding to avoid malnutrition. The main cause of dysphagia is the action dystonia of the tongue that, once in contact with solid food, forcefully pushes it out of the mouth (tongue protrusion and feeding dystonia) (Aasly et al., 1999; Bader et al., 2009). This feature was noted in the seminal publication by Critchley et al. (1968. p. 134): "When he ate, his tongue would involuntarily push food out on to his plate." Only a few conditions are associated with tongue protrusion dystonia (Schneider et al., 2006) and are not specifically precipitated by eating, as seen in ChAc. Tongue dystonia is usually milder during other tasks such as talking, swallowing saliva, and drinking. Patients may develop a technique of swallowing with their heads tipped back and facing the ceiling (authors' personal observation), to allow passage of the food bolus by gravity. Although no fatalities have yet been recorded, this maneuver certainly carries a high risk of aspiration. Feeding dystonia may occasionally be absent.

Dysarthria is very common, and slurred speech may be a presenting symptom (Alonso et al., 1989). In the course of the disease, communication may be limited to grunting or whispering and patients become mute and require computer-based speech aids (Aasly et al., 1999, and case 4).

Neuropsychiatric Features

Changes in personality and behavior along with psychopathological abnormalities occur in about two-thirds of patients (Chapter 20). Patients may be apathetic and depressed and show bradyphrenia but can also be hyperactive, irritable, distractable, and emotionally unstable. They may behave in an immature or disinhibited manner, including sexual disinhibition. Obsessive–compulsive behaviors are common and may be a presenting symptom (Walterfang et al., 2008). Loss of insight, self-neglect, anxiety, and paranoia are observed. Aggression against others as well as autoaggression (Walker et al., 2006b) occur. Both suicidal ideation and suicidal actions are part of the disease spectrum (Alonso et al., 1989; Hiersemenzel et al., 1996; Malandrini et al., 1993; Sorrentino et al., 1999).

Progressive cognitive deterioration is typical. Memory and executive functions, such as the ability to sustain concentration over time, to plan, and to change behavior to reach a particular goal, seem particularly affected. These findings, as well as the psychopathology described, resemble the frontal lobe syndrome (Danek et al., 2004).

Cognitive and neuropsychiatric findings in ChAc were previously mainly interpreted on the basis of striatal involvement (Henkel et al., 2006; Danek et al., 2004), but recent stereological data also suggest considerable cortical neuronal loss (Arzberger et al., 2005). Deficits of learning and memory (Danek et al., 2004) point to hippocampal structures as additional targets of dysfunction.

Origination of seizures in the temporal lobe also suggests involvement of this region (Al-Asmi et al., 2005; Scheid et al., 2009).

Other Symptoms

Epilepsy, usually described as generalized seizures (probably secondarily generalized originating in the mesial temporal lobe), is observed in almost half of patients and can be the initial disease manifestation (Aasly et al., 1999; Kazis et al., 1995; Scheid et al., 2009; Schwartz et al., 1992). Seizures also may relate to the reduced life expectancy in ChAc. Interictal electroencephalography shows temporal or independent bitemporal abnormalities (Vance et al., 1987) and temporal seizure onset (Al-Asmi et al., 2005; Andermann et al., 2005, Scheid et al., 2010). Polysomnography has been reported for a few cases (Ghorayeb et al., 2009).

Neuropathic and myopathic involvement of the disease is responsible for ankle areflexia in almost all patients and for muscle atrophy and weakness in at least half. Vibration sensation may be reduced. The presence of myopathy is obvious from the elevation of muscle creatine kinase (CK), and correspondingly, there are central nuclei and atrophic fibers on biopsy. Most changes on biopsy, however, support the predominance of neurogenic atrophy, with variation in muscle fiber diameters and occurrence of small angulated fibers (Alonso et al., 1989; Limos et al., 1982).

Autonomic dysfunction, manifesting as a postganglionic sympathetic dysfunction, has been reported (Kihara et al., 2002) and may explain sudden death in ChAc.

In three cases an association of ChAc with cardiomyopathy has been reported: one case of the dilated type (Kageyama et al., 2000), one with asymmetric left ventricular nonobstructive hypertrophy (Lossos et al., 2005), and one not further characterized (Shizuka et al., 1997). The relationship of this observation to ChAc remains to be clarified, but in contrast to McLeod syndrome is atypical (Danek et al., 2001).

A presumed connection with hypothalamic and other endocrine abnormalities (Terao et al., 1995) also needs confirmation. Splenomegaly and hepatomegaly are occasionally noted and can be attributed to erythrocyte dysfunction and hemolysis. The abnormal acanthocytic shape of the erythrocytes does not have any other apparent hematological consequences apart from a mild hemolytic anemia with reduced levels of hemoglobin and haptoglobin. Low glycohemoglobin A_{1c}, as observed in one patient, was interpreted on the basis of reduced erythrocyte half-life, not abnormal glucose metabolism (Ogawa et al., 1993).

The basic defect of the acanthocytic membrane has not yet been uncovered, in spite of a variety of physicochemical studies on red cells (Asano et al., 1985; Copeland et al., 1982; Oshima et al., 1985; Sakai et al., 1991; Terada et al., 1999; Ueno et al., 1982).

In a few possible cases of ChAc, diverse autoantibodies of unknown significance have been described (Bosman et al., 1994; Hirayama et al., 1997; Kay et al., 1990; Lagreze et al., 1988). Cerebrospinal fluid studies, if reported, have been normal.

DIAGNOSTICS

Laboratory Findings

Acanthocytes are found in the blood of ChAc patients in highly variable proportions, usually 5%–50%; and their presence should not be regarded as a criterion for diagnosis. The percentage of acanthocytes is not correlated with disease severity, and the relationship to neurodegeneration and to absence of chorein has not been identified. For unknown reasons, acanthocytosis can be absent (Bayreuther et al., 2010; Malandrini et al., 1993) or may be detected only late in the course of the disease (Sorrentino et al., 1999).

A standard procedure for the determination of acanthocytosis has been established: After diluting a fresh blood sample 1:1 with 0.9% saline and 10 U/mL heparin and incubation for at least 30 minutes, fixation is performed with Karnofsky solution and the slide is examined under Nomarski optics.

Blood was drawn into 10 ml plastic syringes and immediately mixed with 5 ml of isotonic sodium chloride solution containing 10 units of heparin per ml. gently shaken and incubated at room temperature for 30 to 120 min. For wet unfixed blood preparations a bubble-free monolayer of blood cells was mounted between a glass object slide and a glass cover slip. All blood preparations were investigated on photomicrographs using a phase-contrast microscope (Axiophot125; Zeiss, Germany) at a magnification of 1000× (oil immersion). (Storch et al., 2005, p. 85)

Serum chemistry shows chronic elevation of muscle CK levels in the great majority of patients. CK appears to be a much more useful laboratory test than the unreliable testing for acanthocytes. Lactate dehydrogenase, aspartate aminotransferase, and alanine aminotransferase may also be elevated.

Neuroimaging

Structural neuroimaging (computed tomography [CT] and magnetic resonance imaging [MRI]) discloses atrophy of the caudate nuclei with dilatation of the anterior horns and is often reported as being consistent with a diagnosis of Huntington disease (HD). There may be slight generalized cortical atrophy. The extent of basal ganglia atrophy is best appreciated on sections in the frontal plane. MRI may show a T2-weighted signal increase in the caudate and putamen.

Imaging of brain metabolism with fluorodeoxyglucose positron emission tomography (FDG-PET) or hexamethylpropylene-amine oxime single-photon emission CT (HMPAO-SPECT) shows reduced tracer accumulation in the caudate nucleus and putamen (Brin, 1993; Hosokawa et al., 1987) and occasionally in the thalamus and in cortical, mainly frontal, regions (Brooks et al., 1991; Delecluse et al., 1991).

Imaging studies of dopaminergic transmission reveal reduced presynaptic dopamine storage capacity in the posterior putamen and loss of postsynaptic D_2 receptor binding (Brooks et al., 1991).

Electrophysiology

Electrophysiological tests demonstrate a mainly sensory axonopathy with normal nerve conduction velocities and reduced sensory action potentials (Aasly et al., 1999; Vance et al., 1987). Peripheral nerve biopsies correspondingly show loss of myelinated fibers, particularly those of larger diameter. Unmyelinated fibers may also be affected, and signs of regeneration are observed (Alonso et al., 1989; Ferrer et al., 1990; Malandrini et al., 1993; Sorrentino et al., 1999).

Frank myopathy is suggested both clinically, with distally pronounced muscle wasting, and on CT scanning of leg muscles, which reveals a selective pattern of fatty change. This is in contrast to McLeod syndrome, in which findings tend to be symmetrical (Ishikawa et al., 2000). However, neurogenic changes are more commonly detected on electromyography.

Diagnostic Tests

Genetic sequencing of the *VPS13A* gene with proof of mutation is the diagnostic gold standard (Dobson-Stone et al., 2002). The diagnosis of the disease is clear if one homozygous or two heterozygous mutations are found on both alleles of the gene. This test has recently become commercially available (see www.mgz-muenchen.de). Genetic analysis is difficult due to the large size of the *VPS13A* gene and the fact that mutations are distributed among all introns and exons. In a few patients, a mutation is found only on one allele. This is likely due to technical issues, for example, methodology which does not detect large deletions, rather than to dominant transmission, which remains controversial (Bader et al., 2009; Ishida et al., 2009; Saiki et al., 2003).

Detection of the protein product of *VPS13A* (chorein) is a simpler and cheaper test than genetic analysis. Absent or markedly reduced chorein from blood samples (erythrocyte membrane preparations) is suggestive of ChAc (Dobson-Stone et al., 2004). The chorein Western blot is available free of charge (see www.naadvocacy.org or www.euro-hd.net/html/na/submodule).

Chronically increased CK values of more than 500 U/l are seen in two-thirds of ChAc patients and, in addition to elevated liver enzymes, may be more useful in indicating the diagnosis than the presence of acanthocytes.

THERAPY

Physical Therapy, Medical Aids, and Appliances

There is as yet no curative treatment for ChAc. Mechanical protective devices are advisable in the case of teeth grinding and head banging. In addition to reducing the jaw closure dystonia, bite guards have been reported to reduce obsessive–compulsive symptoms, suggesting a common pathophysiology (Fontenelle and Leite, 2008). Splints can be tried for foot drop. Often, mealtime assistance and feeding are necessary to prevent aspiration (Aasly et al., 1999). Patients usually profit from swallowing and speech therapy and, with progression to mutism, should be equipped with computer-based speech systems (Aasly et al., 1999; McIntosh, 2008).

Drug Treatment

Drug treatment is based on conventional, symptomatic approaches. Common antiepileptic regimes should be used and usually result in good seizure control; however, carbamazepine and lamotrigine have been reported to worsen the involuntary movements (Andermann et al., 2005). As in HD, psychiatric issues should be addressed with antidepressant or antipsychotic drugs, as indicated, because these symptoms can result in significant morbidity and mortality.

Dopamine antagonists/depletors such as sulpiride, tiapride, and tetrabenazine can be used for symptomatic treatment of chorea or tics (Jankovic, 2001). Patients report that dopamine antagonists show an effect on especially orofacial dyskinesias and improve swallowing and feeding. Patients should be carefully monitored for development of parkinsonism, in particular with tetrabenazine, which can also cause depression.

The atypical dopamine antagonist clozapine was at least temporarily effective in a single observation (Wihl et al., 2001). Levetiracetam may alleviate trunk dyskinesia (Lin et al., 2006) and control seizures at the same time. An effect of verapamil on the movement disorder has not been substantiated (Brenes et al., 1990).

The combination of masseter muscle and tongue protrusion dystonia appears to be the cause of the very common mutilations of the tongue, lips, and cheeks and may result in significant weight loss and lethal infection (Lossos et al., 2005). Botulinum toxin injections into the masseter muscle may be helpful to decrease the jaw dystonia that interferes with feeding. Injections into the submental muscle complex (genioglossus and hyoglossus muscles) or into the tongue itself have been tried in specialized centers (Kasravi and Jog, 2009; McIntosh, 2008; Schneider et al., 2006). These can lead to reductions in bruxism, tongue protrusion, and feeding dystonia but carry a significant risk of worsening dysphagia, and increasing the risk of aspiration and asphyxia. Since the equinovarus deformity has a dystonic component, local injections of botulinum toxin have been used. Although anecdotally in use in a number of ChAc patients, a more systematic assessment of botulinum effects is desired.

Systematic collection of therapeutic experience is still lacking in ChAc. To achieve the goal of standardized case assessment, we have set out to document observations on ChAc and other NA syndromes in a Web-based databank within the European Huntington's Disease Network (www.euro-hd.net/html/na/submodule).

Neurosurgical Treatment

Neurosurgical approaches have been employed with mixed outcomes. Staged bilateral posteroventral pallidotomy reportedly improved feeding in one patient (Fujimoto et al., 1997). For an alternative ablative procedure, unilateral ventral lateral thalamic coagulation, the outcome was not reported (Cavalli et al., 1995).

Bilateral thalamic stimulation very successfully reduced incapacitating trunk spasms, reestablished ambulation, and improved feeding (Burbaud et al., 2002a,b). Stimulation of the internal globus pallidus (GPi) was judged effective in two recent studies (Guehl et al., 2007; Ruiz et al., 2009) and rapidly improved both dystonia and chorea. While chorea responded faster than dystonia, no benefit was noted in dysarthria (Ruiz et al., 2009). Another study of GPi stimulation found better responses of both dystonia and chorea at lower frequencies (40–50 Hz) (Gupta et al., 2008). Although other reports are less favorable (Wihl et al., 2001) and long-term experience is not available, deep brain stimulation can be discussed as a therapeutic option in patients not responsive to medication.

DIFFERENTIAL DIAGNOSIS

Because of the protean manifestations of ChAc (Walker et al., 2006a, 2007), there is a wide range of differential diagnoses among the general categories of parkinsonian and choreatic syndromes (including tardive dyskinesias), epilepsies, myopathies (Felker et al., 2000, Scheid et al., 2009), and the laboratory problem of "hyperCKemia" (Reijneveld et al., 2001; Fernandez et al., 2006; Walker et al., 2007b).

The spectrum of symptoms in ChAc patients significantly overlaps with that of McLeod syndrome (Danek et al., 2001; Jung et al., 2007; Rampoldi et al., 2002; Walker et al., 2007a) (Chapter 7). The distinctive feature of the latter is an absence or marked reduction of the red blood cell Kx and Kell antigens. Thus, specific immunohematological studies are necessary to differentiate the two disorders. Genetic analysis of the *XK* gene confirms the diagnosis of McLeod syndrome. Older reports have certainly mistaken some cases for ChAc. This diagnostic error was proven for one report (Faillace et al., 1982; Marsh et al., 1983) and is not unlikely for others (Aminoff, 1972; Lupo et al., 1987; Cavalli et al., 1995).

Abetalipoproteinemia (ABL, Bassen-Kornzweig disease) and hypobetalipoproteinemia (HBL) share acanthocytosis with ChAc and McLeod syndrome. Cerebellar dysarthria, neuropathy, and areflexia are also features; but these disorders are distinguished by the hallmark of pigmentary retinopathy. ABL and HBL are caused by mutations affecting the microsomal triglyceride transfer protein (ABL, autosomal recessive) and apolipoprotein B (HBL, clinical manifestations in the homozygous as well the heterozygous states), respectively. These cause vitamin E deficiency due to impaired lipid absorption from the gastrointestinal tract. The neurological presentation is of a progressive spinocerebellar degeneration; a sensorimotor, demyelinating, as well as axonal peripheral neuropathy with hyporeflexia, diminished vibration, and position sense; ataxia of gait; dysmetria; and dysarthria, rarely with pyramidal tract signs and cranial nerve involvement.

Even if damage to the basal ganglia can be demonstrated in patients with vitamin E deficiency, there are no overt clinical signs or symptoms (Dexter et al., 1994).

Patients with a movement disorder due to basal ganglia dysfunction and pigmentary retinopathy should also be examined for PKAN (Hayflick et al., 2003; Zhou et al., 2001) (Chapter 8). Some of these cases may have acanthocytosis and myopathy (Malandrini et al., 1995, 1996). HARPP syndrome (hypoprebetalipoproteinemia, acanthocytosis, retinitis pigmentosa, and pallidal degeneration [Higgins et al., 1992; Orrell et al., 1995]) is also allelic with PKAN (Ching et al., 2002).

Tourette syndrome is often misdiagnosed during the initial stages of ChAc (Hiersemenzel et al., 1996; Saiki et al., 2004). The picture of motor and vocal tics, obsessive–compulsive behavior, and impaired impulse control (Jankovic, 2001) can be very similar to parts of the ChAc spectrum. In contrast to Tourette syndrome, coprolalia is not common in ChAc. The latter will eventually develop the additional features of neuromyopathy, seizures, dysphagia, and orolingual dystonia.

Self-mutilation and head banging in ChAc are shared with Lesch-Nyhan syndrome, an X-linked condition caused by dysfunction of hypoxanthine guanine phosphoribosyltransferase. It is characterized by slight elevation in the blood of uric acid, yet high levels of renal excretion, that causes urinary stone formation and gouty arthropathy (Visser et al., 2000; Jinnah, 2009).

Wilson disease is another multisystem disease with various movement abnormalities due to basal ganglia involvement. It results from abnormal copper metabolism and may lead to severe, often lethal, disease of the liver. Copper deposition is the likely cause of the Kayser-Fleischer ring at the periphery of the cornea, which may be detected in about two-thirds of patients. Serum ceruloplasmin typically is low and urinary copper excretion high, yet no single feature appears reliable on its own. Although usually not considered beyond 30 years, Wilson disease may present in older age groups and, as one of the few treatable disorders in this class, should be considered in any patient with unusual liver, neurological, or psychiatric abnormalities (Gow et al., 2000; Wild et al., 2007).

In the past, particularly before the molecular diagnosis of HD was possible, the diagnosis of ChAc may have been missed because of its close resemblance to HD (Harper, 1996) (Chapter 3). ChAc is an important differential diagnosis for those presumed HD cases where the *IT15* gene has not disclosed the diagnostic increase in CAG repeat number (Rosenblatt et al., 1998). Some older reports of presumed HD in association with additional degenerative features such as muscle atrophy or motor neuron disease may well have represented ChAc cases (Frank and Vuia, 1973). Examination of blood smears may not be helpful, as mentioned; and acanthocytes might be found in patients with a molecular diagnosis of HD, for example, in the setting of malnutrition. In addition to the almost identical choreic movement disorder and indistinguishable imaging findings, there are similar changes in personality and behavior in HD and ChAc (Kutcher et al., 1999).

Clinically, the disorders can be distinguished by the presence of severe orolingual dystonia, which seems to be unique for ChAc (Bader et al., 2010), and seizures, which are seen only in juvenile-onset (Westphal variant) HD. Hyporeflexia and CK elevation are not typical of HD (Sakai et al., 1981). If available, a family history of autosomal dominant transmission supports the diagnosis of HD.

Genetic advances have defined a series of new entities, such as dentatorubral-pallidoluysian atrophy (DRPLA) (Chapter 12), that may mimic HD as phenocopies (Curtis et al., 2001; de Vries et al., 2000; Fernandez et al., 2001; Kambouris et al., 2000; Margolis et al., 2001; Quinn and Schrag, 1998; Ross et al., 1997; Schneider et al., 2007; Xiang et al., 1998) and should therefore also be considered in the differential diagnosis of ChAc.

PATHOPHYSIOLOGY

Cellular Level

Full-length chorein is an abundant protein in the central nervous system and was found to be absent in brain tissue of ChAc patients (Bader et al., 2007). Two alternative splicing variants of *VPS13A* are known: variant 1A (exons 1-68 and 70-73; 317 kDa) and 1B (exons 1-69; 309 kDa) (Velayos-Baeza et al., 2008). In brain tissue of healthy humans, two chorein fragments of 160 kDa and 94 kDa probably reflect additional alternative splicing variants or posttranslational modifications (Bader et al., 2007).

In mice, chorein is highly expressed in brain, testis, kidney, spleen, and muscle (Kurano et al., 2007). In humans, chorein is found in brain, blood and at a high level in testis. Minor expression can be observed in muscle tissue. ChAc muscle tissue has not yet been examined systematically, but a single case report shows nemaline rods as a sign of myopathic muscle degeneration (Tamura et al., 2005).

In yeast, the homologous Vps13p protein has been described as being associated with membranes and forming a high–molecular weight complex (Brickner and Fuller, 1997). It was shown to be involved in the trans-Golgi network localization of transmembrane proteins. Vps13p is not required for transport of proteins between the trans-Golgi network and the prevacuolar compartment directly but is involved in transport regulation by recruiting trans-Golgi network membrane proteins into transport vesicles from the trans-Golgi network as well as the prevacuolar compartment (Brickner and Fuller, 1997).

In studies of acanthocytes from NA patients which included ChAc cases, the structure of band 3 complex in erythrocytes was altered, affecting the binding of the spectrin cytoskeleton to erythrocyte membranes. As a result, the signal transduction pathways are altered and may lead to deficiency in that process. While relatively harmless in erythrocytes, these changes might have a striking effect in neurons that depend very much on an intact intracellular trafficking system (Bosman et al., 1994; De Franceschi et al., 2004; Kay et al., 1990).

Structural Pathology

In most other neurodegenerative diseases, including HD, Parkinson disease, Alzheimer disease, prion diseases, and the spinocerebellar ataxias, pathological accumulations of proteins either appear to contribute to pathophysiology or are found as by-products of neurodegeneration. These protein aggregations have been the target of much research for clues to disease pathogenesis and, hence, prevention. In contrast, in ChAc the absence of chorein apparently results in neurodegeneration with cell loss and gliosis, without the formation of any type of protein aggregations.

On autopsy the cerebral cortex appears macroscopically unaffected (Alonso et al., 1989; Arzberger et al., 2007; Bader et al., 2007, 2008; Bird et al., 1978; Ishida et al., 2009; Rinne et al., 1994b; Vital et al., 2002). There is macroscopic atrophy bilaterally of the caudate nucleus, the putamen, and the globus pallidus, corresponding to histological loss of neurons, microglial activation, and astroglial and oligodendroglial activation. This is particularly severe in the caudate nucleus and less so in the putamen and the external and internal pallidum (Alonso et al., 1989; Arzberger et al., 2005; Vital et al., 2002).

Within the caudate nucleus and globus pallidus, antibodies against the striatal neurotransmitters methionine-enkephalin, leucine-enkephalin, and substance P show reduced reactivity (Ishida et al., 2009).

Pronounced neuronal loss in the substantia nigra is the likely correlate of parkinsonism (Rinne et al., 1994a,b). There is also extraneuronal pigment, but there are no Lewy bodies in the nigra. The locus ceruleus, inferior olives, and cerebellum appear unaffected. Loss of spinal cord anterior horn cells, a correlate of neurogenic muscle atrophy, was seen in a few autopsy cases.

It is intriguing to speculate about the possibility of a fixed developmental sequence of the clinical features of ChAc that ought to reflect the progression of neuropathological changes. It appears as if striatal dysfunction is followed by involvement of the nigrostriatal system as the hyperkinetic state is commonly followed by parkinsonism. In some reports, however, parkinsonism was noted already at initial presentation (Bostantjopoulou et al., 2000; Peppard et al., 1990).

CONCLUSIONS

Identification of the gene for ChAc has permitted the correct diagnosis of many patients and, hence, genetic counseling for their families. The causes of neurodegeneration and of acanthocytes and their relationships to mutant chorein remain obscure. We hope that advances in molecular medicine will lead to therapy, for example, by using stem cells to replace the absent chorein or to pharmacologically replace functional aspects of chorein.

As with other molecular disorders, identification of the causative gene may lead to expansions of the recognized phenotype. Phenotypes without caudate atrophy but prominent spinocerebellar degeneration (Tsai et al., 1997) may eventually be classified, as may cases with features of ChAc but no acanthocytes (Johnson et al., 1998), including the so-called Fotopulos syndrome (Fotopoulos, 1966; Grotjahn, 1934; Pageot et al., 2000). Finally, it may be of interest that the diagnosis of ChAc has been suggested for a historic case of atypical chorea ("Bu42") along with the proposal to rename ChAc as the "Vogt-Hopf syndrome" (Brin, 1993; Hopf, 1952; Lange et al., 1976; Vogt and Vogt, 1937).

ACKNOWLEDGMENTS

The chorein Western blot is funded by the Advocacy for Neuroacanthocytosis Patients (www.naadvocacy.org) and is carried out at the Zentrum für Neuropathologie und Prionforschung (Prof. Hans A. Kretzschmar, Munich, Germany). We thank Mark Hallett, Elaine Considine, Barbara Karp, Linda Nee, Gangadhar Madupu, Eric Wassermann, Laura Sheesley, Michael Tierney, Milan Makale, Saidi Mohiddin, Lameh Fananapazir, Dotti Tripodi, Lev Goldfarb, McDonald Horne, Jolynn Procter, David Stroncek, Luca Rampoldi, and Tony Monaco for collaborating with us in the study of these patients. The video teams at the National Institutes of Health and Munich University Hospital provided expert assistance. We are much indebted to our patients and their families.

APPENDIX: CASE REPORTS (see Videos)

Case 1 was first noted to exhibit echolalia, lip smacking, teeth grinding, and clicking and grunting noises at the age of 27 years. Subsequently, he showed micrographia, deterioration of gait, and chorea (including head banging and sudden trunk flexions and extensions), which subsided over the ensuing years. By the age of 34 he had developed parkinsonism with hypophonia as well as epilepsy, including prolonged status epilepticus. On examination at the age of 44, he was severely dysphonic and communicated via a keyboard-driven speech synthesizer. There was hypomimia and a dystonic grin, impaired tongue movements, reduced gag and tendon reflexes, unsteady gait, bradykinesia, muscle atrophy, and reduction of performance IQ. Further details are on record (see Tables 6–1 and 6–2). He is alive at 52 years and maintains lively communication via the Internet.

TABLE 6–1. Patients with Chorea-Acanthocytosis Due to Mutations in the *VPS13A* Gene: Mutations Are Described According to the Nomenclature Recommended by http://www.hgvs.org/mutnomen

CASE	GENDER	AGE AT EXAMINATION (YEARS)	*VPS13A* MUTATIONS (EXON/INTRON)	CASE NUMBER IN MUTATION REPORT (DOBSON-STONE ET AL., 2002)	CASE NUMBER IN OTHER PUBLICATIONS; COMMENTS
1	M	44	c.6419C>G (48), c.9190del (70)	24	Case 1 (Danek et al. 2004), case 3 (Gradstein et al. 2005), case A (Henkel et al. 2006), case (Stamey et al. 2006)
2	M	35	c.8390del (61), c.9399+2_+8del (71)	14	Case 2 (Danek et al. 2004), case B (Henkel et al. 2006)
3	F	30	c.1208_1211del (14), c.7867C>T (56)	23	Case 3 (Danek et al. 2004), case 2 (Gradstein et al. 2005)
4	M	51	c.883-1_892del (11), c.8007del (57)	22	Case 4 (Danek et al. 2004); died age 52
5	M	42	Sibling of case 4	—	Case 5 (Danek et al. 2004), case C (Henkel et al. 2006)
6	F	40	Sibling of case 4	—	Case 6 (Danek et al. 2004), case D (Henkel et al. 2006); died age 43
7	M	36	c.3283G>C (31), c.4835del (39)	21	Case 7 (Danek et al. 2004), case E (Henkel et al. 2006)
8	M	36	c.6059del (46), c.6059del (46)	37	Case 2 (Lossos et al. 2005); died age 38

TABLE 6–2. Clinical Features and Ages at Onset in Eight Patients with Chorea-Acanthocytosis

CASE	UHDRS TOTAL MOTOR SCORE	FUNCTIONAL IMPAIRMENT (ON TASKS OUT OF 25 FROM UHDRS)	DYSPHAGIA, FEEDING DYSTONIA	DYSARTHRIA	VOCAL TICS	ORAL MUTILATION	BALANCE, GAIT PROBLEM	CHOREA	TRUNK SPASMS	LIMB DYSTONIA	PARKINSONISM	NEUROPATHY, AREFLEXIA	SEIZURES	BEHAVIORAL OR COGNITIVE CHANGES
1	20	12	30	27	27	27	28	28	30	28	34	–	33	32
2	23	1	34	31	31	34	34	27	–	35	–	35	–	30
3	36	10	25	25	24	–	26	27	–	26	–	26	28	25
4	27	12	43	46	35	44	40	35	–	46	51	43	43	–
5	14	0	35	34	29	+	42	29	–	–	–	33	24	+
6	23	1	34	36	30	37	34	34	–	–	–	32	21	–
7	16	4	–	33	33	–	+	29	–	–	–	33	32	32
8	nt	nt	31	31	29	31	26	26	33	26	–	+	–	29

nt, not tested; UHDRS, Unified Huntington's Disease Rating Scale; –, absent; +, present, onset age not known.

Case 2, a 35-year-old college graduate with excellent educational records, developed slight gait difficulties at the age of 24 years. Inability to sit still from about the age of 27 years was followed by deterioration of gait, handwriting, speech, and feeding, with his tongue temporarily pushing food out of the mouth. At the age of 31 fidgety movements, occasional grunts, and anxiety were described. Shortly after, he developed alcohol and marijuana abuse. A change of manners and personality was noted, with difficulties in keeping jobs and social interactions, increasing disorderliness, and excessive consumption of food. On examination, his gait was impaired by truncal instability and foot dystonia. There was trunk and leg chorea as well as mumbling speech with almost continuous muttering of phrases such as "OK, what's next." Saccades were slowed. There was no tongue or lip biting but slight drooling. He regurgitated water during a test drink, but chewing of solids was not impaired. Froment's maneuver brought out arm rigidity. There was slight distal extremity weakness and equinovarus foot posture bilaterally. Tendon reflexes were obtained only in the brachioradialis muscles; plantar responses were flexor. He continuously handled cigarettes, was easily distracted, and behaved impulsively. Social interactions were inappropriate: He would interrupt conversations, ask intimate questions, pass gas or belch without excuse, and leave for extended cigarette breaks. Verbal learning was slightly impaired. On follow-up at the age of 39, he reported increased restlessness while sitting but not while lying down. He has started using a four-wheeled walking device because of deterioration of gait and balance with occasional falls.

Case 3, a 30-year-old female, had developed general clumsiness and uneven handwriting at age 23, followed a year later by throat clicking and teeth grinding. Dysphagia and feeding dystonia were first noted at the age of 25, along with dysarthria, memory lapses, and vocal tics. She subsequently developed tongue biting, involuntary stereotypic movements, seizures, cognitive decline, and gait difficulties. On examination, she showed frequent square-wave jerks, slow saccades, as well as dysarthria, chorea, hand and foot dystonia, ataxia, abnormal gait, and hyporeflexia. To overcome the dysphagia caused by her tongue pushing food out of the mouth, she would rapidly extend her neck and tilt her head up so that solid foods could advance by gravity. Laboratory testing was significant for acanthocytosis and slightly elevated CK (298 U/l, range 38–252). Chorein was absent from erythrocyte preparations of the patient (Dobson-Stone et al., 2004). MRI disclosed atrophy of the basal ganglia. Neuroimaging and cognitive testing details are available (for references see Table 6–1). At 38 years, she lives under the care of her parents, who report an increase in her cognitive problems. The reduction in her quality of life is mainly due to impaired mobility and dysphagia (Bader et al., 2010, case 2), problems that have essentially remained unaltered over 8 years.

Cases 4–6 were from a series of seven siblings from unrelated parents. The oldest, case 4, was diagnosed with Tourette syndrome in his mid-30s because of oral dyskinesia. Later, he developed limb chorea as well as difficulties with balance, gait, and fine motor skills. At the age of 43, he experienced a first series of focal seizures and displayed choreatic lip and mouth movements, and transient involuntary lip biting. At the age of 46, dysphagia, dysarthria, and dysphonia were observed as well as tongue dystonia, facial grimacing, and clicking oral sounds. He moved into assisted living because of increasing motor problems, stuttering, hypophonia, and dysphagia that necessitated a liquid diet and, for a while, a gastric tube because of aspiration pneumonia. His handwriting became micrographic, and he was wheelchair-dependent because of numerous falls.

On examination at the age of 51 he was mute but with excellent communication through a computer speech device. Cognitive testing showed superior memory but visuoconstructive and attentional impairment. There was generalized bradykinesia. His face was masked, with a dystonic smile; and the mouth was open and drooling. Forward/backward and up/down tongue movements were slow and limited, but lateral tongue motion was rapid. There was generalized muscle weakness and atrophy, particularly affecting the interdigital muscles and the peroneal muscles bilaterally, with equinovarus foot posture. Tendon reflexes were absent, and the plantar response was lacking. There was a stocking and glove distribution of decreased sensation to light touch, pinprick, and temperature.

Acanthocytosis was repeatedly documented. CK was 508 U/l (upper limit of normal 386) but had on previous occasions reached values up to 5,859 U/l. Haptoglobin and lactate dehydrogenase (LDH) were slightly elevated. Cardiological evaluation showed borderline systolic left ventricular function on echocardiography but did not explain the reason for external placement of a pacemaker after loss of consciousness several years ago. CT scan of the head demonstrated widening of the anterior horns of both lateral ventricles subsequent to caudate nucleus atrophy. The patient died suddenly of undetermined cause at the age of 52.

His brother, case 5, sixth of the siblings, was a 42-year-old, right-handed salesperson who had noted generalized restlessness and experienced one generalized seizure at the age of 24 years. This was followed 10 years later by seizures with focal onset (olfactory aura). Isolated auras occasionally recur in spite of chronic treatment with phenytoin and phenobarbital (520 and 100 mg).

Involuntary movements were first noted at age 29 in the orofacial region, the trunk, and the limbs. Tongue clicking or grunting, preceded by the build-up of a feeling of internal pressure which the patient could temporarily resist, were prominent. After more than 10 years, his vocal tics spontaneously ceased at age 40.

At the age of 33, echolalia, tongue dystonia, involuntary facial movement, and general areflexia were noted. He displayed some atrophy of hand and distal leg muscles as well as mild generalized chorea and gait impairment. There was reduction of sensation for pinprick, temperature, and vibration in a stocking and glove distribution corresponding to a generalized axonal sensory neuropathy on nerve conduction testing. By age 35 his speech had become increasingly slurred and he displayed involuntary shoulder shrugs. He had also developed dysphagia for solid foods.

This is presently his chief complaint along with weakness of mastication. Because of his tongue pushing out food, he had adopted the strategy of holding his chin up to facilitate the passage of solid food but had mainly resorted to a liquid diet taken with straws. Due to involuntary lip biting, he held cotton buds between his teeth. His speech was slurred, and there was drooling. Both temporalis muscles were atrophic. Distal hand muscles were atrophic; but there was no muscle weakness, the tongue included. However, vertical tongue motion was slow and restricted. There was slight generalized chorea, and parkinsonian features were not detected. Writing was poor due to involuntary movements. Except for trace patella reflexes, he was areflexic and showed diminished vibration perception. Cognitive testing suggested an acquired reduction of his IQ from the difference between the value of 111, estimated on the basis of word knowledge (National Adult Reading Test), and the Wechsler Adult Intelligence Scale-III full IQ of 87.

Acanthocytosis was present, and CK and LDH were clearly elevated. Alkaline phosphatase was slightly above normal. Aspartate aminotransferase (AST) and alanine aminotransferase (ALT) were only transiently elevated.

Case 8 died suddenly at the age of 38 years (Lossos et al., 2005) but was examined 2 years previously. He was a former Talmud student, whose parents were second cousins. He first developed difficulties walking, with occasional falls. After continuous progression over 10 years, he spent most of his time in a recumbent position but also had developed rocking trunk movements. Dexterity of his dominant left hand decreased, with objects falling from the hand and deterioration of writing. His personality and manners had changed (unexcused passing of gas and belching, unkempt attire, negligence in religious matters, defiance, indecision, repetitive eating and drinking), and he was depressed, according to his parents who took him in after his divorce.

Non-suppressible vocalizations (sucking noises) first appeared at the age of 29, and 2 years later he developed continuous mumbling, dysarthria, and drooling. He tended to place objects into his mouth to suppress an urge to clench his teeth but commonly destroyed these objects so that at present he constantly keeps several fingers of one hand in his mouth. His teeth were severely worn, and a night-guard was of no help since he destroyed it by the force of his bite. He required feeding because of severe swallowing problems, causing a weight loss of almost 30 kg, and was unable to take solid food. His tongue habitually pushed food out, and he had to throw himself back on the bed to assist the swallowing process.

On examination, he maintained his recumbent position, kept one hand in his mouth, and rarely engaged in conversation. He could not produce voluntary oral movements except for brief periods of mouth opening. These were regularly brought to an end by moans and grunts, lip smacking, jaw opening and closing, as well as slow movements of the deeply scarred tongue. According to him, some of these were truly involuntary without any preceding urge to move, whereas others followed such an urge. With the onset of the involuntary mouth movements, the patient immediately tried to stick his fingers back into his mouth. There were scars also on his left lower lip, ulcers on the inside of both cheeks, and several bite marks on the fingers of both hands.

Both feet were held in inversion and showed calluses over the lateral ankle joints. His legs were in continuous, restless motion of small amplitude. There was slight distal muscle weakness and areflexia. The sensory exam was remarkable only for slightly reduced distal vibration perception. Stance and gait were highly abnormal, with episodes of spontaneous retropulsion.

He showed imitative behavior, was easily distracted, and appeared environment-dependent as he unexpectedly took a series of sudden small steps to walk over to a table and rapidly touch food items with his forefinger. Brain MRI showed circumscribed ventricular widening due to bilateral, symmetric atrophy of the caudate nucleus and the putamen as well as slightly increased signal. There was acanthocytosis, pronounced elevation of CK and LDH, and slight elevation of AST and ALT. Echocardiography with asymmetric left ventricular hypertrophy indicated hypertrophic nonobstructive cardiomyopathy.

One year later, after onset of generalized seizures, he was admitted to an outside hospital, where neuropsychological testing showed cognitive impairment mainly in the domains of attention, memory, and executive functions.

REFERENCES

Aasly J, Skandsen T, Ro M (1999) Neuroacanthocytosis—the variability of presenting symptoms in two siblings. Acta Neurol Scand 100:322–325.

Al-Asmi A, Jansen AC, Badhwar A, et al. (2005) Familial temporal lobe epilepsy as a presenting feature of choreoacanthocytosis. Epilepsia 46:1256–1263.

Alonso ME, Teixeira F, Jimenez G, et al. (1989) Chorea-acanthocytosis: report of a family and neuropathological study of two cases. Can J Neurol Sci 16:426–431.

Aminoff MJ (1972) Acanthocytosis and neurological disease. Brain 95:749–760.

Andermann F, Jansen A, Al-Asmi A, et al. (2005) Epilepsy in neuroacanthocytosis. Mov Disord 20:1680.

Arzberger T, Heinsen H, Buresch N, et al. (2005) The neuropathology of chorea-acanthocytosis: from stereology to an immunohistochemical detection of chorein. Mov Disord 20:1679.

Asano K, Osawa Y, Yanagisawa N, et al. (1985) Erythrocyte membrane abnormalities in patients with amyotrophic chorea with acanthocythosis. Part 2. Abnormal degradation of membrane proteins. J Neurol Sci 68:161–173.

Bader B, Arzberger T, Velayos-Baeza A, et al. (2007) Detection of chorein in *post mortem* brain tissue of chorea-acanthocytosis patients and nonaffected controls by Western blot. Mov Disord 22 (Supplement):VI.

Bader B, Arzberger T, Heinsen H, et al. (2008) Neuropathology of chorea-acanthocytosis. In: Walker RH, Saiki S, Danek A (eds.) Neuroacanthocytosis Syndromes II. Springer, Heidelberg, pp 187–195.

Bader B, Velayos-Baeza A, Walker RH, et al. (2009) Dominant transmission of chorea-acanthocytosis with VPS13A mutations remains speculative. Acta Neuropathol 117:95–96.

Bader B, Walker RH, Vogel M, et al. (2010) Tongue protrusion and feeding dystonia: a hallmark of chorea-acanthocytosis. Mov Disord 25:127–129.

Bayreuther C, Borg M, Ferrero-Vacher C, Chaussenot A, Lebrun C (2010). Choreo-acanthocytose sans acanthocytes. Revue Neurologique 166:100-103.

Bharucha EP, Bharucha NE (1989) Choreo-acanthocytosis. J Neurol Sci 89:135–139.

Bird TD, Cederbaum S, Valpey RW, et al. (1978) Familial degeneration of the basal ganglia with acanthocytosis: a clinical, neuropathological, and neurochemical study. Ann Neurol 3:253–258.

Bosman GJ, Bartholomeus IG, De Grip WJ, et al. (1994) Erythrocyte anion transporter and antibrain immunoreactivity in chorea-acanthocytosis. A contribution to etiology, genetics, and diagnosis. Brain Res Bull 33:523–528.

Bostantjopoulou S, Katsarou Z, Kazis A, et al. (2000) Neuroacanthocytosis presenting as parkinsonism. Mov Disord 15:1271–1273.

Brenes LG, Sanchez MI, Antillon A (1990) Verapamil induces complete remission of the clinical and laboratory findings in a patient with chorea-acanthocytosis. Clin Res 38:93A.

Brickner JH, Fuller RS (1997) SOI1 encodes a novel, conserved protein that promotes TGN-endosomal cycling of Kex2p and other membrane proteins by modulating the function of two TGN localization signals. J Cell Biol 139:23–36.

Brin MF (1993) Acanthocytosis. In: Vinken PJ, Bruyn GW, Klawans HL (eds.) Handbook of Clinical Neurology: Systemic Diseases, Part I (Goetz CG, Tanner CM, Aminoff MJ, vol. eds.). Elsevier, Amsterdam, pp 271–299.

Brooks DJ, Ibanez V, Playford ED, et al. (1991) Presynaptic and postsynaptic striatal dopaminergic function in neuroacanthocytosis: a positron emission tomographic study. Ann Neurol 30:166–171.

Burbaud P, Rougier A, Ferrer X, et al. (2002a) Improvement of severe trunk spasms by bilateral high-frequency stimulation of the motor thalamus in a patient with chorea-acanthocytosis. Mov Disord 17:204–207.

Burbaud P, Vital A, Rougier A, et al. (2002b) Minimal tissue damage after stimulation of the motor thalamus in a case of chorea-acanthocytosis. Neurology 59:1982–1984.

Cavalli G, de Gregorio C, Nicosia S, et al. (1995) Cardiac involvement in familial amyotrophic chorea with acanthocytosis: description of two new clinical cases [in Italian]. Ann Ital Med Int 10:249–252.

Ching KHL, Westaway SK, Gitschier J, et al. (2002) HARP syndrome is allelic with pantothenate kinase–associated neurodegeneration. Neurology 58:1673–1674.

Copeland BR, Todd SA, Furlong CE (1982) High resolution two-dimensional gel electrophoresis of human erythrocyte membrane proteins. Am J Hum Genet 34:15–31.

Critchley EM, Clark DB, Wikler A (1967) An adult form of acanthocytosis. Trans Am Neurol Assoc 92:132–137.

Critchley EM, Clark DB, Wikler A (1968) Acanthocytosis and neurological disorder without betalipoproteinemia. Arch Neurol 18:134–140.

Curtis AR, Fey C, Morris CM, et al. (2001) Mutation in the gene encoding ferritin light polypeptide causes dominant adult-onset basal ganglia disease. Nat Genet 28: 350–354.

Danek A, Rubio JP, Rampoldi L, et al. (2001) McLeod neuroacanthocytosis: genotype and phenotype. Ann Neurol 50:755–764.

Danek A, Sheesley L, Tierney M, et al. (2004) Cognitive and neuropsychiatric findings in McLeod syndrome and in chorea-acanthocytosis. In: Danek A (ed.) Neuroacanthocytosis Syndromes, Springer, Dordrecht, The Netherlands, pp 95–115.

Danek A, Dobson-Stone C, Velayos-Baeza A, et al. (2005) The phenotype of chorea-acanthocytosis: a review of 106 patients with *VPS13A* mutations. Mov Disord 20:1678.

De Franceschi L, Olivieri O, Corrocher R (2004) Erythrocyte aging in neurodegenerative disorders. Cell Mol Biol (Noisy-le-Grand) 50:179–185.

de Vries BB, Arts WF, Breedveld GJ, et al. (2000) Benign hereditary chorea of early onset maps to chromosome 14q. Am J Hum Genet 66:136–142.

Delecluse F, Deleval J, Gerard JM, et al. (1991) Frontal impairment and hypoperfusion in neuroacanthocytosis. Arch Neurol 48:232–234.

Dexter DT, Brooks DJ, Harding AE, et al. (1994) Nigrostriatal function in vitamin E deficiency: clinical, experimental, and positron emission tomographic studies. Ann Neurol 35:298–303.

Dobson-Stone C, Danek A, Rampoldi L, et al. (2002) Mutational spectrum of the *CHAC* gene in patients with chorea-acanthocytosis. Eur J Hum Genet 10:773–781.

Dobson-Stone C, Velayos-Baeza A, Filippone LA, et al. (2004) Chorein detection for the diagnosis of chorea-acanthocytosis. Ann Neurol 56:299–302.

Dobson-Stone C, Velayos-Baeza A, Jansen A, et al. (2005) Identification of a *VPS13A* founder mutation in French Canadian families with chorea-acanthocytosis. Neurogenetics 6:151–158.

Faillace RT, Kingston WJ, Nanda NC, et al. (1982) Cardiomyopathy associated with the syndrome of amyotrophic chorea and acanthocytosis. Ann Intern Med 96:616–617.

Felker GM, Thompson RE, Hare JM, et al. (2000) Underlying causes and long-term survival in patients with initially unexplained cardiomyopathy. N Engl J Med 342: 1077–1084.

Fernandez C, de Paula AM, Figarella-Branger D, et al. (2006) Diagnostic evaluation of clinically normal subjects with chronic hyperCKemia. Neurology 66:1585–1587.

Fernandez M, Raskind W, Wolff J, et al. (2001) Familial dyskinesia and facial myokymia (FDFM): a novel movement disorder. Ann Neurol 49:486–492.

Ferrer X, Julien J, Vital C, et al. (1990) La choree-acanthocytose. Rev Neurol (Paris) 146:739–745.

Fontenelle LF, Leite MA (2008) Treatment-resistant self-mutilation, tics, and obsessive–compulsive disorder in neuroacanthocytosis: a mouth guard as a therapeutic approach. J Clin Psychiatry 69:1186–1187.

Fotopoulos D (1966) Huntington's chorea and chronic-progressive spinal muscular atrophy [in German]. Psychiatr Neurol Med Psychol (Leipz) 18:63–70.

Frank G, Vuia O (1973) Chorea Huntington—Amyotrophische Lateralsklerose—Spastische Spinalparalyse. Zur Kombination von Systemerkrankungen. Z Neurol 205:207–220.

Fujimoto Y, Isozaki E, Yokochi F, et al. (1997) A case of chorea-acanthocytosis successfully treated with posteroventral pallidotomy [in Japanese]. Rinsho Shinkeigaku 37: 891–894.

Gandhi S, Hardie RJ, Lees AJ (2008) An update on the Hardie neuroacanthocytosis series. In: Walker RH, Saiki S, A Danek A (eds.) Neuroacanthocytosis Syndromes II. Springer, Heidelberg, pp 43–51.

Ghorayeb I, Dolenc-Groselj L, Kobal J, et al. (2009) Sleep disorders in neuroacanthocytosis. In: Walker RH, Saiki S, Danek A (eds.) Neuroacanthocytosis Syndromes II. Springer, Heidelberg, pp 249–253.

Gow PJ, Smallwood RA, Angus PW, et al. (2000) Diagnosis of Wilson's disease: an experience over three decades. Gut 46:415–419.

Gradstein L, Danek A, Grafman J, et al. (2005) Eye movements in chorea-acanthocytosis. Invest Ophthalmol Vis Sci 46:1979–1987.

Gross KB, Skrivanek JA, Carlson KC, et al. (1985) Familial amyotrophic chorea with acanthocytosis. New clinical and laboratory investigations. Arch Neurol 42:753–756.

Grotjahn M (1934) Chronische, progressive Chorea und spinale Muskelatrophie. Zentralbl Neurol Psychiatr 73:251–253.

Guehl D, Cuny E, Tison F, et al. (2007) Deep brain pallidal stimulation for movement disorders in neuroacanthocytosis. Neurology 68:160–161.

Gupta F, Chan N, Alterman R, et al. (2008) DBS frequency screening for programming optimization in a patient with chorea-acanthocytosis. Mov Disord 23:S384.

Hardie RJ, Pullon HWH, Harding AE, et al. (1991) Neuroacanthocytosis: a clinical, haematological and pathological study of 19 cases. Brain 114:13–49.

Harper PS (1996) New genes for old diseases: the molecular basis of myotonic dystrophy and Huntington's disease. The Lumleian Lecture 1995. J R Coll Physicians Lond 30:221–231.

Hayflick SJ, Westaway SK, Levinson B, et al. (2003) Genetic, clinical, and radiographic delineation of Hallervorden-Spatz syndrome. N Engl J Med 348:33–40.

Henkel K, Danek A, Grafman J, et al. (2006) Head of the caudate nucleus is most vulnerable in chorea-acanthocytosis: a voxel-based morphometry study. Mov Disord 21: 1728–1731.

Hiersemenzel LP, Johannes S, Themann P, et al. (1996) Die Choreoakanthozytose. Ein neurologisch–hämatologisches Syndrom. Nervenarzt 67:490–495.

Higgins JJ, Patterson MC, Papadopoulos NM, et al. (1992) Hypoprebetalipoproteinemia, acanthocytosis, retinitis pigmentosa, and pallidal degeneration (HARP syndrome). Neurology 42:194–198.

Hirayama M, Hamano T, Shiratori M, et al. (1997) Chorea-acanthocytosis with polyclonal antibodies to ganglioside GM$_1$. J Neurol Sci 151:23–24.

Hirose G (2008) Neuroacanthocytosis in Japan—review of the literature and cases. In: Walker RH, Saiki S, Danek A (eds.) Neuroacanthocytosis Syndromes II. Springer, Heidelberg, pp 75–84.

Ho MF, Chalmers RM, Davis MB, et al. (1996) A novel point mutation in the McLeod syndrome gene in neuroacanthocytosis. Ann Neurol 39:672–675.

Hopf A (1952) Über eine patho-anatomische Sonderform der Chorea. J Nerv Ment Dis 116:608–618.

Hosokawa S, Ichiya Y, Kuwabara Y, et al. (1987) Positron emission tomography in cases of chorea with different underlying diseases. J Neurol Neurosurg Psychiatry 50: 1284–1287.

Ichiba M, Nakamura M, Kusumoto A, et al. (2007) Clinical and molecular genetic assessment of a chorea-acanthocytosis pedigree. J Neurol Sci 263:124–132.

Ishida C, Makifuchi T, Saiki S, et al. (2009) A neuropathological study of autosomal-dominant chorea-acanthocytosis with a mutation of VPS13A. Acta Neuropathol 117:85–94.

Ishikawa S, Tachibana N, Tabata KI, et al. (2000) Muscle CT scan findings in McLeod syndrome and chorea-acanthocytosis. Muscle Nerve 23:1113–1116.

Iwata M, Fuse S, Sakuta M, et al. (1984) Neuropathological study of chorea-acanthocytosis. Jpn J Med 23:118–122.

Jankovic J (2001) Tourette's syndrome. N Engl J Med 345:1184–1192.

Jinnah HA (2009) Lesch-Nyhan disease: from mechanism to model and back again. Dis. Model. Mech. 2:116–121.

Johnson SE, Dahl A, Sjaastad O (1998) Progressive pseudobulbar paresis, early choreiform movements, and later rigidity: appearance in two sets of dizygotic twins in the same family. Mov Disord 13:556–562.

Jung HH, Danek A, Frey BM (2007). McLeod syndrome: a neurohaematological disorder. Vox Sang 93:112–121.

Kageyama Y, Kodama Y, Tadano M, et al. (2000). A case of chorea-acanthocytosis with dilated cardiomyopathy and myopathy [in Japanese]. Rinsho Shinkeigaku 40: 816–820.

Kambouris M, Bohlega S, Al Tahan A, et al. (2000) Localization of the gene for a novel autosomal recessive neurodegenerative Huntington-like disorder to 4p15.3. Am J Hum Genet 66:445–452.

Kasravi N, Jog MS (2009) Botulinum toxin in the treatment of lingual movement disorders. Mov Disord 24:2199–2202.

Kay MMB, Goodman J, Lawrence C, et al. (1990) Membrane channel protein abnormalities and autoantibodies in neurological disease. Brain Res Bull 24:105–111.

Kazis A, Kimiskidis V, Georgiadis G, et al. (1995) Neuroacanthocytosis presenting with epilepsy. J Neurol 242:415–417.

Kihara M, Nakashima H, Taki M, et al. (2002) A case of chorea-acanthocytosis with dysautonomia; quantitative autonomic deficits using CASS. Autonom Neurosci Basic Clin 97:42–44.

Kito S, Itoga E, Hiroshige Y, Matsumoto N, Miwa S (1980) A pedigree of amyotrophic chorea with acanthocytosis. Arch Neurol 37:514–517.

Kurano Y, Nakamura M, Ichiba M, et al. (2007) *In vivo* distribution and localization of chorein. Biochem Biophys Res Commun 353:431–435.

Kuroiwa Y, Ohnishi A, Sato Y, et al. (1984) Chorea acanthocytosis: clinical pathological and biochemical aspects. Int J Neurol 18:64–74.

Kutcher JS, Kahn MJ, Andersson HC, et al. (1999) Neuroacanthocytosis masquerading as Huntington's disease: CT/MRI findings. J Neuroimaging 9:187–189.

Lagreze HL, Kornguth SE, Brooks BR, et al. (1988) Delayed immune response in chorea-amyotrophy with spherocytosis. Neurology 38:1642–1643.

Lange H, Thorner G, Hopf A, et al. (1976) Morphometric studies of the neuropathological changes in choreatic diseases. J Neurol Sci 28:401–425.

Levine IM, Estes JW, Looney JM (1968) Hereditary neurological disease with acanthocytosis. A new syndrome. Arch Neurol 19:403–409.

Limos LC, Ohnishi A, Sakai T, et al. (1982) "Myopathic" changes in chorea-acanthocytosis. Clinical and histopathological studies. J Neurol Sci 55:49–58.

Lin FC, Wei LJ, Shih PY (2006) Effect of levetiracetam on truncal tic in neuroacanthocytosis. Acta Neurol Taiwan 15:38–42.

Lossos A, Dobson-Stone C, Monaco AP, et al. (2005) Early clinical heterogeneity in choreoacanthocytosis. Arch Neurol 62:611–614.

Lupo I, Aragona F, Fierro B, et al. (1987) Choreo-acanthocytosis with myopathy. Report of a case. Acta Neurol (Napoli) 9:334–338.

Malandrini A, Bonuccelli U, Parrotta E, et al. (1995) Myopathic involvement in two cases of Hallervorden-Spatz disease. Brain Dev 17:286–290.

Malandrini A, Fabrizi GM, Bartalucci P, et al. (1996) Clinicopathological study of familial late infantile Hallervorden-Spatz disease: a particular form of neuroacanthocytosis. Childs Nerv Syst 12:155–160.

Malandrini A, Fabrizi GM, Palmeri S, et al. (1993) Choreo-acanthocytosis like phenotype without acanthocytes: clinicopathological case report. A contribution to the knowledge of the functional pathology of the caudate nucleus. Acta Neuropathol (Berl) 86: 651–658.

Margolis RL, O'Hearn E, Rosenblatt A, et al. (2001) A disorder similar to Huntington's disease is associated with a novel CAG repeat expansion. Ann Neurol 50:373–380.

Marsh WL, Schnipper EF, Johnson CL, et al. (1983) An individual with McLeod syndrome and the Kell blood group antigen K(K1). Transfusion 23:336–338.

Miki Y, Nishie M, Ichiba M, et al. (2010) Chorea-acanthocytosis with upper motor neuron degeneration and 3419_3420 delCA and 3970_3973 delAGTC VPS13A mutations. Acta Neuropathol 119:271-273.

McIntosh J (2008) Multidisciplinary neurorehabilitation in chorea-acanthocytosis; a case study. In: Walker RH, Saiki S, Danek A (eds.) Neuroacanthocytosis Syndromes II. Springer, Heidelberg, pp 271–284.

Nielsen SM, Temlett JA (1997) Neuro-acanthocytosis—a rare cause of chorea. South Afr Med J 87:897–898.

Ogawa T, Seki H, Okita N, et al. (1993) A case of chorea-acanthocytosis associated with low glycohemoglobin A1c [in Japanese]. Rinsho Shinkeigaku 33:344–346.

Ong B, Devathasan G, Chong PN (1989) Choreoacanthocytosis in a Chinese patient—a case report. Singapore Med J 30:506–508.

Orrell RW, Amrolia PJ, Heald A, et al. (1995) Acanthocytosis, retinitis pigmentosa, and pallidal degeneration: a report of three patients, including the second reported case with hypoprebetalipoproteinemia (HARP syndrome). Neurology 45:487–492.

Oshima M, Osawa Y, Asano K, et al. (1985) Erythrocyte membrane abnormalities in patients with amyotrophic chorea with acanthocytosis. Part 1. Spin labeling studies and lipid analyses. J Neurol Sci 68:147–160.

Pageot N, Vial C, Remy C, et al. (2000) Progressive chorea and amyotrophy without acanthocytes: a new case of Fotopoulos syndrome? J Neurol 247:392–394.

Peppard RF, Lu CS, Chu NS, et al. (1990) Parkinsonism with neuroacanthocytosis. Can J Neurol Sci 17:298–301.

Quinn N, Schrag A (1998) Huntington's disease and other choreas. J Neurol 245: 709–716.

Rampoldi L, Danek A, Monaco AP (2002) Clinical features and molecular bases of neuroacanthocytosis. J Mol Med 80:475–491.

Rampoldi L, Dobson-Stone C, Rubio JP, et al. (2001) A conserved sorting-associated protein is mutant in chorea-acanthocytosis. Nat Genet 28:119–120.

Reijneveld JC, Notermans NC, Linssen WH, et al. (2001) Hyper-CK-aemia revisited. Neuromuscul Disord 11:163–164.

Rinne JO, Daniel SE, Scaravilli F, et al. (1994a) Nigral degeneration in neuroacanthocytosis. Neurology 44:1629–1632.

Rinne JO, Daniel SE, Scaravilli F, et al. (1994b) The neuropathological features of neuroacanthocytosis. Mov Disord 9:297–304.

Rodrigues GR, Walker RH, Bader B, et al. (2008) Chorea-acanthocytosis: report of two Brazilian cases. Mov Disord 23:2090–2093.

Rosenblatt A, Ranen NG, Rubinsztein DC, et al. (1998) Patients with features similar to Huntington's disease, without CAG expansion in huntingtin. Neurology 51:215–220.

Ross CA, Margolis RL, Rosenblatt A, et al. (1997) Huntington disease and the related disorder, dentatorubral-pallidoluysian atrophy (DRPLA). Medicine 76:305–338.

Ruiz PJ, Ayerbe J, Bader B, et al. (2009) Deep brain stimulation in chorea acanthocytosis. Mov Disord 24:1546–1547.

Saiki S, Hirose G, Sakai K, et al. (2004) Chorea-acanthocytosis associated with Tourettism. Mov Disord 19:833–836.

Saiki S, Sakai K, Kitagawa Y, et al. (2003) Mutation in the *CHAC* gene in a family of autosomal dominant chorea-acanthocytosis. Neurology 61:1614–1616.

Sakai T, Antoku Y, Iwashita H, et al. (1991) Chorea-acanthocytosis: abnormal composition of covalently bound fatty acids of erythrocyte membrane proteins. Ann Neurol 29: 664–669.

Sakai T, Mawatari S, Iwashita H, et al. (1981) Choreoacanthocytosis. Clues to clinical diagnosis. Arch Neurol 38:335–338.

Sato Y, Ohnishi A, Tateishi J, et al. (1984) An autopsy case of chorea-acanthocytosis. Special reference to the histopathological and biochemical findings of basal ganglia [in Japanese]. No To Shinkei 36:105–111.

Scheid R, Bader B, Ott DV, et al. (2009) Development of mesial temporal lobe epilepsy in chorea-acanthocytosis. Neurology 73:1419–1422.

Schneider SA, Aggarwal A, Bhatt M, et al. (2006) Severe tongue protrusion dystonia: clinical syndromes and possible treatment. Neurology 67:940–943.

Schneider SA, Walker RH, Bhatia KP (2007) The Huntington's disease-like syndromes: what to consider in patients with a negative Huntington's disease gene test. Nat Clin Pract Neurol 3:517–525.

Schwartz MS, Monro PS, Leigh PN (1992) Epilepsy as the presenting feature of neuroacanthocytosis in siblings. J Neurol 239:261–262.

Serra S, Arena A, Xerra A, et al. (1986) Amyotrophic choreoacanthocytosis: is it really a rare disease? Ital J Neurol Sci 7:521-524.

Shizuka M, Watanabe M, Aoki M, et al. (1997) Analysis of the McLeod syndrome gene in three patients with neuroacanthocytosis. J Neurol Sci 150:133–135.

Sorrentino G, De Renzo A, Miniello S, et al. (1999) Late appearance of acanthocytes during the course of chorea-acanthocytosis. J Neurol Sci 163:175–178.

Stamey W, Fernandez HH, Rodriguez R (2006) Neuroacanthocytosis, www.medlink.com/cip.asp?uid=MLT000AE.

Storch A, Kornhass M, Schwarz J (2005) Testing for acanthocytosis—A prospective reader-blinded study in movement disorder patients. J Neurol 252:84–90.

Tamura Y, Matsui K, Yaguchi H, et al. (2005) Nemaline rods in chorea-acanthocytosis. Muscle Nerve 31:516–519.

Terada N, Fujii Y, Ueda H, et al. (1999) Ultrastructural changes of erythrocyte membrane skeletons in chorea-acanthocytosis and McLeod syndrome revealed by the quick-freezing and deep-etching method. Acta Haematol (Basel) 101:25–31.

Terao S, Sobue G, Takahashi M, et al. (1995) Disturbance of hypothalamic–pituitary hormone secretion in familial chorea-acanthocytosis [in Japanese]. No To Shinkei 47:57–61.

Thomas M, Jankovic J (2006) Neuroacanthocytosis. In: Noseworthy JH (ed.) Neurological Therapeutics: Principles and Practice, vol. 2. Informa Healthcare, Abingdon, UK, pp 2882–2889.

Toyokura Y, Kamakura K, Shimada Y (1982) Familial chorea-acanthocytosis (the Levine-Critchley syndrome)—a review of the reported cases in Japan. In: Annual Report of the Research Committee of CNS Degenerative Diseases. Ministry of Health and Welfare of Japan, Tokyo, pp 335–351.

Tsai CH, Chen RS, Chang HC, et al. (1997) Acanthocytosis and spinocerebellar degeneration: a new association? Mov Disord 12:456–459.

Ueno E, Oguchi K, Yanagisawa N (1982) Morphological abnormalities of erythrocyte membrane in the hereditary neurological disease with chorea, areflexia and acanthocytosis. J Neurol Sci 56:89–97.

Ueno S, Maruki Y, Nakamura M, et al. (2001) The gene encoding a newly discovered protein, chorein, is mutated in chorea-acanthocytosis. Nat Genet 28:121–122.

Vance JM, Pericak Vance MA, Bowman MH, et al. (1987) Chorea-acanthocytosis: a report of three new families and implications for genetic counselling. Am J Med Genet 28:403–410.

Velayos-Baeza A, Levecque C, Dobson-Stone C, et al. (2008) The function of chorein. In: Walker RH, Saiki S, Danek A (eds.) Neuroacanthocytosis Syndromes II. Springer, Heidelberg, pp 87–105.

Visser JE, Bar PR, Jinnah HA (2000) Lesch-Nyhan disease and the basal ganglia. Brain Res Brain Res Rev 32:449–475.

Vital A, Bouillot S, Burbaud P, et al. (2002) Chorea-acanthocytosis: neuropathology of brain and peripheral nerve. Clin Neuropathol 21:77–81.

Vogt C, Vogt O (1937) Sitz und Wesen der Krankheiten im Lichte der topischen Hirnforschung und des Variierens der Tiere, vol. 1. J Psychol Neurol (Leipzig, Germany) 47: 237–457.

Walker RH, Danek A, Dobson-Stone C, et al. (2006a) Developments in neuroacanthocytosis: expanding the spectrum of choreatic syndromes. Mov Disord 21:1794–1905.

Walker RH, Jung HH, Dobson-Stone C, et al. (2007a) Neurologic phenotypes associated with acanthocytosis. Neurology 68:92–98.

Walker RH, Jung HH, Danek A, (2007b) Diagnostic evaluation of clinically normal subjects with chronic hyperCKemia. Neurology 68:1086.

Walker RH, Liu Q, Ichiba M, et al. (2006b) Self-mutilation in chorea-acanthocytosis—manifestation of movement disorder or psychopathology? Mov Disord 21:2268–2269.

Walterfang M, Yucel M, Walker R, et al. (2008) Adolescent obsessive compulsive disorder heralding chorea-acanthocytosis. Mov Disord 23:422–425.

Wihl G, Volkmann J, Allert N, et al. (2001) Deep brain stimulation of the internal pallidum did not improve chorea in a patient with neuro-acanthocytosis. Mov Disord 16: 572–575.

Wild EJ, Tabrizi SJ (2007) The differential diagnosis of chorea. Pract Neurol 7:360–373.

Xiang F, Almqvist EW, Huq M, et al. (1998) A Huntington disease-like neurodegenerative disorder maps to chromosome 20p. Am J Hum Genet 63:1431–1438.

Yamamoto T, Hirose G, Shimazaki K, et al. (1982) Movement disorders of familial neuroacanthocytosis syndrome. Arch Neurol 39:298–301.

Zhou B, Westaway SK, Levinson B, et al. (2001) A novel pantothenate kinase gene (*PANK2*) is defective in Hallervorden-Spatz syndrome. Nat Genet 28:345–349.

7

McLeod Syndrome

Hans H. Jung, MD

INTRODUCTION

The X-linked McLeod neuroacanthocytosis syndrome (MLS) is a neurological disorder resembling Huntington disease (HD) with onset ranging between 25 and 60 years. It is defined by the combination of neurological and neuromuscular signs and symptoms and the presence of the McLeod phenotype of the Kell blood group system (Jung et al., 2007).

The McLeod blood group phenotype was first detected by routine screening for allogenic antibodies at Harvard University blood bank in 1960 (Allen et al., 1961). The red blood cells (RBCs) of the propositus, Hugh McLeod, showed a weak reactivity to Kell antisera. Immunohematologically, the McLeod blood group phenotype was later characterized by absent expression of Kx RBC antigen, weak expression of Kell glycoprotein RBC antigens, and X-linked inheritance (Wimer et al., 1977). Subsequently, the McLeod blood group phenotype was also observed in boys with X-linked chronic granulomatous disease as part of a contiguous gene syndrome (Francke et al., 1985). Most carriers of the McLeod blood group phenotype have RBC acanthocytosis (Figure 7–1). For reliable detection of RBC acanthocytosis, a standardized protocol with 1:1 dilution of the blood in heparinized saline and phase-contrast microscopy should be used

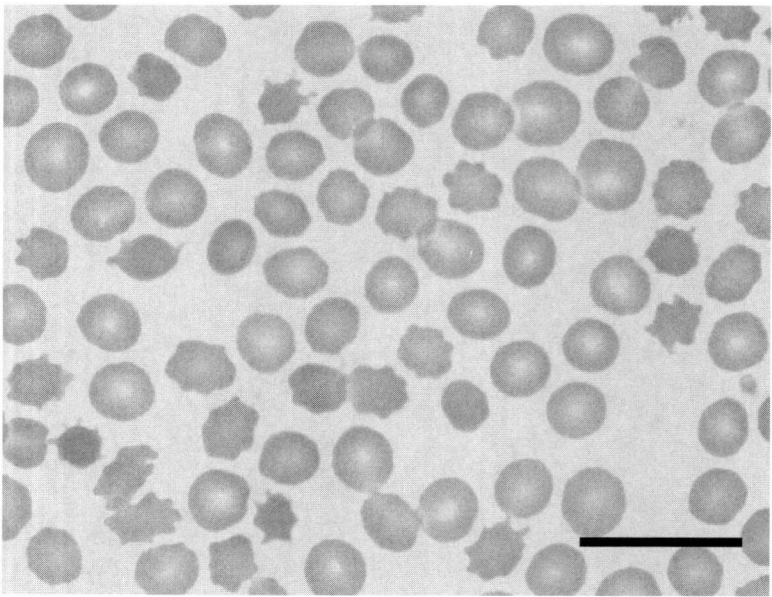

FIGURE 7–I. Acanthocytes. Peripheral blood smear showing significant acanthocytosis (May-Grünwald–Giemsa, ×100, scale bar = 25 μm).

(Storch et al., 2005). Marsh and colleagues (1981) demonstrated that male carriers of the McLeod blood group phenotype have elevated serum levels of creatine kinase (CK), reflecting muscle cell pathology. Later, it was recognized that McLeod carriers had a "neurological disorder characterized by involuntary dystonic or choreiform movements, areflexia, wasting of limb muscles, elevated CK, and congestive cardiomyopathy" (Schwartz et al., 1982). This first, short description as well as the subsequent clinical observations defined MLS as a multisystem disorder with hematological, neuromuscular, and central nervous system (CNS) involvement.

In addition to chorea, which is seen in most patients, CNS symptoms include variable psychiatric and cognitive manifestations. A subset of patients has seizures, which are mostly generalized. About half of patients develop a cardiomyopathy manifesting with atrial fibrillation, malignant arrhythmias, and dilated cardiomyopathy, which may be determinants of survival.

MLS is caused by mutations of the *XK* gene encoding the XK protein. Although the exact function of the human XK protein is not yet known, available data suggest a possible role in apoptosis regulation. Thus, MLS might be a model disorder to study the principal mechanisms that are involved not only in RBC physiology but also in neurodegeneration.

MOLECULAR BASIS

MLS is caused by mutations of the *XK* gene, which contains three exons and is located on Xp21.1. *XK* shares important homologies with the ced-8 protein of the nematode *Caenorhabditis elegans*, where it controls the timing of programmed cell death (Stanfield and Horvitz, 2000). The XK protein is predicted to have 10 trans-membrane domains and shows structural characteristics of prokaryotic and eukary-otic membrane transport proteins (Ho et al., 1994; Calenda et al., 2006; Russo et al., 2000). The XK protein carries the Kx RBC antigen and is linked to the Kell glycoprotein by a single disulfide bond (XKcys347-KellCys72) (Lee et al., 2000). Databank analysis demonstrated that the human *XK* gene belongs to a family of nine full-length human genes related to *ced-8*, as well as a series of eight Y chro-mosome–linked partial sequences (Calenda et al., 2006). Sequence comparisons confirmed that highly conserved motifs in *ced-8* and *XK* are shared with the related genes. Although several residues in these motifs were identical between ced-8 and other family members, these were not conserved in XK (Phelan et al., 2005).

The Kell protein is a 93 kDa glycoprotein encoded by the *KEL* gene on chromo-some 7q34. *KEL* contains 19 exons and shares a consensus sequence with a large family of zinc-dependent endopeptidases (Lee et al., 1999). The Kell glycoprotein is a type II RBC membrane protein with a short intracellular amino-terminal, a single transmembrane, and a large extracellular domain (Lee, 1997). It shows substantial homology with the M13 subfamily of mammalian neutral endopepti-dases, including endothelin converting enzyme-1 (ECE-1), which converts big endothelin-3 into endothelin-3, the bioactive peptide (Lee et al., 1999).

Several studies demonstrated that XK and Kell are coexpressed in erythroid tissue and most probably form a functional complex (Ho et al., 1994; Calenda et al., 2006; Russo et al., 2000; Claperon et al., 2007). In other tissues, however, the Kell and XK proteins had a differential expression pattern. In skeletal muscle, Kell and XK were not co-localized (Jung et al., 2001b). In rodent and human brain, XK was expressed in intracellular compartments of neurons, whereas Kell expression was restricted to RBCs in cerebral vessels (Claperon et al., 2007). XK, but not Kell, was significantly expressed in spinal cord, muscle, heart, small intestine, stomach, bladder, and kidney, as well as in brain, where it was predominantly expressed in neuronal cells (Lee et al., 2007). Coexpression of Kell and XK in erythroid tissues and the different expression patterns in nonerythroid tissues suggest that XK may have a comple-mentary hematological function with Kell and a separate role in other tissues.

HEMATOLOGICAL INVOLVEMENT

Most patients with MLS have subclinical non-immune-mediated, extravascular hemolysis. Hepatosplenomegaly is found in about one-third of McLeod patients and is most likely due to an MLS-associated extravascular hemolytic state (Jung et al., 2007). Boys with X-linked chronic granulomatous disease (CGD) are at risk of developing anti-Kx antibodies, which may lead to serious transfusion reactions when receiving multiple transfusions. Rarely, carriers of the McLeod phenotype without CGD may develop anti-Kx antibodies. Therefore, transfusion risks must be considered in all carriers of the McLeod phenotype due to allogenic antibody production, which occurs exclusively in male carriers of the McLeod mutation and requires previous exposure to Kx antigens as a result of homologous blood transfusion. Autologous blood banking for males with the McLeod blood-group phenotype should be considered before elective surgical procedures that may require transfusions. Female carriers of McLeod mutations are always hemizygous mutation carriers and therefore not prone to anti-Kx generation and subsequent transfusion hazards.

CNS INVOLVEMENT

CNS manifestations of MLS closely resemble HD and comprise the prototypic triad of a progressive neurodegenerative basal ganglia disease including a choreatic movement disorder, frontotemporal cognitive impairment, and psychiatric symptoms.

Chorea of MLS

Choreatic movements are the presenting sign in about 30% of MLS patients (Danek et al., 2001a, b; Jung et al., 2001a). Abnormal motor findings may be subtle, such as a slight generalized restlessness with frequent changes of posture or with tic-like movements (Danek et al., 2001a, b; Jung et al., 2001a; see Video 7–1 McLeod Syndrome). During the course of the disease, most patients develop chorea, which may be indistinguishable from that of HD (Danek et al., 2001a; Jung et al., 2001a). Additional involuntary movements include facial dyskinesia as well as involuntary vocalizations (Danek et al., 2001a, b; Jung et al., 2001a). There is a considerable inter- and intrafamilial variability with respect to the type and severity of the movement disorder (Walker et al., 2007a, b). In contrast to autosomal recessive chorea-acanthocytosis (ChAc), very few McLeod patients have habitual lip or tongue biting, dysphagia, dystonia, or parkinsonism (Danek et al., 2001a,b; Walker et al., 2007a, b).

Cognitive and Psychiatric Manifestations

Cognitive impairment is usually not a major presenting finding in MLS. During the disease course, however, about 50% of patients develop cognitive deficits with a frontotemporal pattern similar to that seen in HD (Danek et al., 2001a, 2004; Jung et al., 2001a). The severity of cognitive alterations shows a remarkable intrafamilial variability and ranges from slight memory impairment to frank dementia (Danek et al., 2004). About 20% of McLeod patients manifest with psychiatric abnormalities including personality disorder, anxiety, depression, obsessive–compulsive disorder, bipolar disorder, and schizoaffective disorder (Danek et al., 2001a; Jung et al., 2001a; Jung and Haker, 2004) (Chapter 20). A psychiatric presentation may predominate in certain families (Jung et al., 2001a) and develops in a majority of McLeod patients during the course of disease (Danek et al., 2001a; Jung et al., 2001a). The spectrum of psychiatric abnormalities is comparable to that of other neurodegenerative basal ganglia disorders such as HD (Danek et al., 2004; Ring and Serra-Mestres, 2002).

Seizures

About 20% of McLeod patients present with generalized seizures, and up to 40% experience them during the course of disease, usually with secondary generalization (Danek et al., 2001a).

Neuroradiology

Computed tomographic and magnetic resonance imaging studies demonstrate atrophy of the caudate nucleus and putamen, particularly with advanced disease (Danek et al., 2001a; Jung et al., 2001a). This atrophy shows slow progression over time (Valko et al., 2010). Exceptionally, white matter changes have been described (Nicholl et al., 2004). [18F]-Fluorodeoxyglucose (FDG)-positron emission tomography (PET) demonstrates impaired striatal glucose metabolism without evidence of cortical involvement (Figure 7–2) (Jung et al., 2001a; Oechsner et al., 2001). By contrast, magnetic resonance spectroscopy demonstrates subtle metabolic abnormalities in different extrastriatal brain regions related to the psychiatric and cognitive findings (Dydak et al., 2006).

Neuropathology

Neuropathological examination reveals marked neuronal loss and astrocytic gliosis in the caudate nucleus and putamen. In contrast, no alterations were found in the cortex, thalamus, subthalamic nucleus, brainstem, and cerebellum (Brin et al., 1993; Geser et al., 2008). Similar findings were observed in the exceptional case of a female XK mutation carrier who clinically manifested MLS (Hardie et al., 1991). Although the prominent psychiatric and cognitive manifestations in McLeod patients indicate a significant and widespread cortical, rather than purely subcortical, dysfunction, the cerebral pathological alterations were restricted to

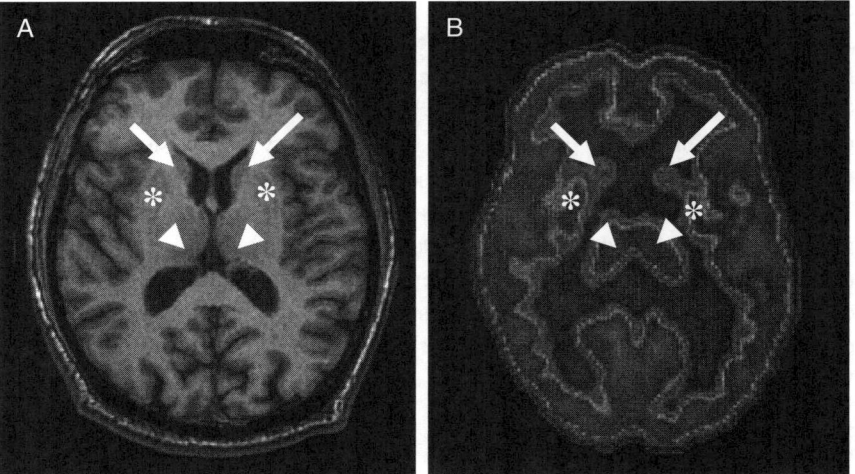

FIGURE 7–2. Neuroradiology. **A** T1-weighted cerebral MRI, performed on a 1.5-tesla MRI system (GE Medical Systems, Milwaukee, WI) using routine parameters, demonstrates only subtle atrophy of the head of the caudate nucleus (*arrow*). **B** FDG-PET (Advance PET Scanner, GE Medical Systems) demonstrates severe impairment of FDG uptake of the head of the caudate nucleus (*arrow*), which is less pronounced in the putamen (∗). FDG uptake in the thalamus (*arrowhead*) and the cerebral cortex was normal.

the striatum. Therefore, the clinical symptoms may be explained by neuronal dysfunction due to impaired basal ganglia–cortical circuits.

NEUROMUSCULAR INVOLVEMENT

Peripheral Neuropathy

All McLeod patients reported to date have reduced or absent deep tendon reflexes. About one-third of McLeod patients have reduced vibration sense in the feet, but only a minority of patients has sensory symptoms. Neurography demonstrates a sensorimotor axonal neuropathy, and electromyography may reveal myopathic as well as neurogenic changes (Danek et al., 2001a; Hewer et al., 2007).

Skeletal Muscle Involvement

Elevated serum CK levels are present in virtually all carriers of the McLeod blood group as a sign of subclinical or manifest myopathy (Danek et al., 2001a; Jung et al., 2001a, b; Swash et al., 1983; Hewer et al., 2007). CK elevation is usually below 4,000 U/l. As many as 50% of McLeod patients develop a clinically significant muscle weakness or atrophy with slow progression, and only few McLeod patients have severe weakness leading to gait difficulties. Sural and femoral nerves displayed a nonspecific sensorimotor axonal neuropathy (Hewer et al., 2007). Histological findings of skeletal muscle in McLeod patients revealed fiber type grouping, type 1 fiber predominance, type 2 fiber atrophy, increased variability in fiber size, and increased central nucleation (Jung et al., 2001b; Hewer et al., 2007). In normal skeletal muscle, XK immunohistochemistry showed a type 2 fiber–specific intracellular staining, possibly confined to the sarcoplasmic reticulum. XK staining was absent in McLeod myopathy. This finding correlated to the observed type 2 fiber atrophy and suggested that the XK protein is crucial for the maintenance of normal structure and function (Jung et al., 2001b).

Cardiomyopathy

Cardiac manifestations of MLS include congestive cardiomyopathy, dilated cardiomyopathy, atrial fibrillation, and tachyarrhythmia (Oechslin et al., 2009). Cardiac muscle at autopsy showed nonspecific focal myocyte hypertrophy, slight variation of myofiber size, and patchy interstitial fibrosis (Oechslin et al., 2009). Up to 60% of McLeod patients develop cardiac manifestations during the course of the disease (Danek et al., 2001a). Cardiac problems such as malignant arrhythmia or heart failure might be a significant cause of death (Danek et al., 2001a; Hewer et al., 2007). Due to the possibility of a curative intervention, MLS patients should be carefully monitored for cardiac disease.

MANIFESTING FEMALE HETEROZYGOTES

Manifesting female heterozygous mutation carriers have occasionally been reported (Hardie et al., 1991; Kawakami et al., 1999). In addition, reduction of striatal glucose uptake was seen in asymptomatic female heterozygotes, indicating subclinical CNS involvement (Jung et al., 2001a). The most probable reason for these findings is a skewed inactivation of the chromosome carrying the normal XK gene, as demonstrated in one heterozygote (Ho et al., 1996). Female heterozygotes with or without clinical manifestation of MLS may demonstrate a Kell blood-group mosaicism detectable by Kell antigen flow cytometry (Jung et al., 2007).

DISEASE COURSE AND THERAPY

MLS has an insidious onset, usually between 30 and 40 years of age, but rarely also as young as 20 or as late as 60 years (Danek et al., 2001a; Jung et al., 2001a). Disease progression is usually slow, and reported disease durations ranged

7–51 years. Mean age at death was 53 years, ranging 31–69 years (Danek et al., 2001a; Jung et al., 2001a; Hewer et al., 2007). Cardiovascular events, epileptic seizures, and aspiration pneumonia appear to be the major causes of death (Danek et al., 2001a, b; Jung et al., 2001a, b). At present, no disease-modifying therapy is available to alter the progression of the syndrome. Recognition of treatable MLS complications, for example, cardiac problems and seizures, is presently the most important issue. Because of possible rhabdomyolysis, serum CK levels should be carefully monitored, in particular if an excessive movement disorder or neuro-leptic medication is present (Jung and Brandner, 2002). Psychiatric problems should be treated according to their clinical presentation. Dopamine antagonists such as tiapride, clozapine, and quetiapine may be useful to ameliorate choreatic movements. And—last but not least—an extended and continuous multidisci-plinary psychosocial support should be provided for patients and their families.

CONCLUSION

Although the CNS manifestations of MLS have many similarities with HD, the neuromuscular manifestations and laboratory findings of elevated CK levels sug-gest the correct diagnosis, which is further confirmed by determination of the McLeod blood-group phenotype that is available in specialized immunohemato-logical laboratories. Possibly treatable complications such as seizures and cardio-myopathy warrant special attention in the management of MLS patients.

REFERENCES

Allen FH, Krabbe SMR, Corcoran PAl. (1961) A new phenotype (McLeod) in the Kell blood-group system. Vox Sang 6:555–560.
Brin MF, Hays A, Symmans WA et al. (1993) Neuropathology of McLeod phenotype is like choreaacanthocytosis (CA). Can J Neurol Sci 20(Suppl):S234.
Calenda G, Peng J, Redman CM et al. (2006) Identification of two new members, XPLAC and XTES, of the XK family. Gene 370:6–16.
Claperon A, Hattab C, Armand V et al. (2007) The Kell and XK proteins of the Kell blood group are not co-expressed in the central nervous system. Brain Res 1147:12–24.
Danek A, Rubio JP, Rampoldi Let al. (2001a) McLeod neuroacanthocytosis: genotype and phenotype. Ann Neurol 50:755–764.
Danek A, Sheesley L, Tierney M et al. (2004) Cognitive and neuropsychiatric findings in McLeod syndrome and in chorea-acanthocytosis. In: Danek A (ed.) Neuroacanthocy-tosis Syndromes. Springer, Dordrecht, The Netherlands, pp 95–115.
Danek A, Tison F, Rubio J et al. (2001b) The chorea of McLeod syndrome. Mov Disord 16(5):882–889.
Dydak U, Mueller S, Sandor PS et al. (2006) Cerebral metabolic alterations in McLeod syndrome. Eur Neurol 56(1):17–23.

Francke U, Ochs HD, de Martinville B et al. (1985) Minor Xp21 chromosome deletion in a male associated with expression of Duchenne muscular dystrophy, chronic granulomatous disease, retinitis pigmentosa, and McLeod syndrome. Am J Hum Genet 37(2):250–267.

Geser F, Tolnay M, Jung HH et al. (2008). The neuropathology of McLeod syndrome. In: Walker RH, Saiki S, Danek A (eds.) Neuroacanthocytosis Syndromes II. Springer, Heidelberg, pp 197–203.

Hardie RJ, Pullon HW, Harding AE et al. (1991) Neuroacanthocytosis. A clinical, haematological and pathological study of 19 cases. Brain 114(Pt 1A):13–49.

Hewer E, Danek A, Schoser BG et al. (2007) McLeod myopathy revisited: more neurogenic and less benign. Brain 130(Pt 12):3285–3296.

Ho M, Chelly J, Carter M et al. (1994) Isolation of the gene for McLeod syndrome that encodes a novel membrane transport protein. Cell 77(6):869–880.

Ho MF, Chalmers RM, Davis MB et al. (1996) A novel point mutation in the McLeod syndrome gene in neuroacanthocytosis. Ann Neurol 39(5):672–675.

Jung HH, Brandner S (2002) Malignant McLeod myopathy. Muscle Nerve 26:424–427.

Jung HH, Danek A, Frey BM (2007) McLeod syndrome: a neurohaematological disorder. Vox Sang 93(2):112–121.

Jung HH, Haker H (2004) Schizophrenia as a manifestation of X-linked McLeod-neuroacanthocytosis syndrome. J Clin Psychiatry 65(5):722–723.

Jung HH, Hergersberg M, Kneifel S et al. (2001a) McLeod syndrome: a novel mutation, predominant psychiatric manifestations, and distinct striatal imaging findings. Ann Neurol 49(3):384–392.

Jung HH, Russo D, Redman C et al. (2001b) Kell and XK immunohistochemistry in McLeod myopathy. Muscle Nerve 24(10):1346–1351.

Kawakami T, Takiyama Y, Sakoe K et al. (1999) A case of McLeod syndrome with unusually severe myopathy. J Neurol Sci 166(1):36–39.

Lee S (1997) Molecular basis of Kell blood group phenotypes. Vox Sang 73(1):1–11.

Lee S, Lin M, Mele A et al. (1999) Proteolytic processing of big endothelin-3 by the kell blood group protein. Blood 94(4):1440–1450.

Lee S, Russo D, Redman CM (2000) The Kell blood group system: Kell and XK membrane proteins. Semin Hematol 37(2):113–121.

Lee S, Sha Q, Wu X et al. (2007) Expression profiles of mouse Kell, XK, and XPLAC mRNA. J Histochem Cytochem 55(4):365–374.

Marsh WL, Marsh NJ, Moore A et al. (1981) Elevated serum creatine phosphokinase in subjects with McLeod syndrome. Vox Sang 40(6):403–411.

Nicholl DJ, Sutton I, Dotti MT et al. (2004) White matter abnormalities on MRI in neuroacanthocytosis. J Neurol Neurosurg Psychiatry 75:1200–1201.

Oechslin E, Kaup D, Jenni R, Jung HH (2009) Cardiac abnormalities in McLeod syndrome. Int J Cardiol 132:130–132.

Oechsner M, Buchert R, Beyer W, Danek A (2001) Reduction of striatal glucose metabolism in McLeod choreoacanthocytosis. J Neurol Neurosurg Psychiatry 70(4):517–520.

Phelan JK, Wong K, Jung HH, Hengartner MO (2005) Sequence analysis identifies a family of human genes related to ced-8. Presented at the 15th Biennial International *C. elegans* Conference, University of California, Los Angeles, June 25–29.

Ring HA, Serra-Mestres J (2002) Neuropsychiatry of the basal ganglia. J Neurol Neurosurg Psychiatry 72(1):12–21.

Russo D, Wu X, Redman CM, Lee S (2000) Expression of Kell blood group protein in nonerythroid tissues. Blood 96:340–346.

Schwartz SA, Marsh WL, Symmans A et al. (1982) New clinical features of McLeod syndrome. Transfusion 22:404.

Stanfield GM, Horvitz HR (2000) The *ced-8* gene controls the timing of programmed cell deaths in C. *elegans*. Mol Cell 5(3):423–433.

Storch A, Kornhass M, Schwarz J (2005) Testing for acanthocytosis: a prospective reader-blinded study in movement disorder patients. J Neurol 252(1):84–90.

Swash M, Schwartz MS, Carter ND et al. (1983) Benign X-linked myopathy with acanthocytes (McLeod syndrome). Its relationship to X-linked muscular dystrophy. Brain 106(Pt 3):717–733.

Valko PO, Hänggi J, Meyer M, Jung HH. Evolution of striatal degeneration in McLeod syndrome. Eur J Neurol 2010; 17: 612–618

Walker RH, Jung HH, Dobson-Stone C et al. (2007a) Neurologic phenotypes associated with acanthocytosis. Neurology 68(2):92–98.

Walker RH, Jung HH, Tison F et al. (2007b). Phenotypic variation among brothers with the McLeod neuroacanthocytosis syndrome. Mov Disord 22:244–248.

Wimer BM, Marsh WL, Taswell HF, Galey WR (1977) Haematological changes associated with the McLeod phenotype of the Kell blood group system. Br J Haematol 36(2): 219–224.

8

Neurodegeneration with Brain Iron Accumulation

Penelope Hogarth, MD and Susan Hayflick, MD

INTRODUCTION: NOSOLOGY

Neurodegeneration with brain iron accumulation (NBIA, formerly Hallervorden-Spatz disease) encompasses at least five different disorders, with chorea being rare in all but neuroferritinopathy (Chapter 9). Therefore, though individual patients with chorea and high brain iron have been described, this association is uncommon. A diagnostic algorithm (see Gregory et al., 2009) can be employed to help guide the evaluation, which, if chorea is prominent, will usually lead away from the disorders covered in this section.

As with many neurological disorders, NBIA nosology has evolved as newly discovered disease genes have been linked to specific phenotypes. The nosology has been further complicated by two additional factors: differing and conflicting usage of terms in the medical literature and a push to discontinue use of the eponym "Hallervorden-Spatz syndrome," requiring the creation of a new set of terms.

As the genetic bases of the various forms of NBIA have become clear, it has become evident that the earlier literature often presented cases and conclusions that cannot be translated into our current framework. It is difficult to apply the conclusions of these publications to the genetically defined disorders that we now recognize, especially for collections of cases that predate the routine use of magnetic resonance imaging (MRI), since they often represent a lumping together of entirely different disorders. Moreover, authors have used the terms "Hallervorden-Spatz syndrome" to refer to the genetic or inherited form and "Hallervorden-Spatz disease" to encompass the more heterogeneous collection of apparently nongenetic phenotypes. We now know that these distinctions are artificial.

Since Shevell (1992) brought to light the involvement of Julius Hallervorden and Hugo Spatz in Nazi programs of active euthanasia of people deemed "mentally defective," the neurology community has sought to discontinue use of this eponym. After the major gene had been mapped but before it was identified, the locus was named *NBIA1* as a first step toward dissociating the disorder from the eponym (Taylor et al., 1996). *NBIA1* was simply a placeholder until the gene (*PANK2*) was discovered. Once the gene was identified, a new descriptive term, "pantothenate kinase–associated neurodegeneration" (PKAN), was proposed (Zhou et al., 2001). "PKAN" is now the favored term, and "Hallervorden-Spatz syndrome" has fallen into disuse.

In order to acknowledge its genetic heterogeneity, we retained the term "NBIA" to encompass all of the disorders that previously had been grouped together on the basis of the common feature of high levels of brain iron. Not surprisingly, as genes have been discovered and phenotypes linked to these genes, some individuals with mutations in an NBIA gene have been found to have normal brain iron levels. Despite this, we have proposed a nosology that retains flexibility yet tries to discern the groups of patients who share a common disease pathogenesis. By continuing to lump together the group of disorders that share the feature of high brain iron levels, we hope to be able to use knowledge gleaned about one form of NBIA to advance investigations of the others.

Currently, NBIA comprises four genetically distinct disorders, in addition to the disorders found in the remaining patients who have clear evidence of high basal ganglia iron levels but who lack mutations in the known genes. These latter patients are said to have "idiopathic NBIA," and they represent a small but significant subset. Each specific form of NBIA is defined by the association of mutations in a single gene, and not surprisingly, the phenotypic spectrum of each continues to expand as new cases are discovered (Gregory et al., 2009; Thomas et al., 2004). For the clinician, the diagnostic evaluation usually veers toward NBIA when the brain MRI demonstrates the changes that typify high levels of iron. While the MRI findings may suggest a specific form of NBIA, genetic testing is recommended in order to establish a diagnosis.

CLINICAL FEATURES

The four genetic forms of NBIA are PKAN, neuroaxonal dystrophy (NAD), neuroferritinopathy (Chapter 9) and aceruloplasminemia (Chapter 10), which are caused by mutations in *PANK2*, *PLA2G6*, *FTL*, and *CP*, respectively. This chapter will focus on PKAN, NAD, and idiopathic NBIA.

Pantothenate Kinase–Associated Neurodegeneration

PKAN is an autosomal recessive disorder caused by mutations in *PANK2* (Zhou et al., 2001). The clinical spectrum of disease is broad. Age at onset spans from early childhood to adulthood. Presenting features may include a movement disorder or neuropsychiatric impairment, and the rate of disease progression may be rapid or slow. Despite these ranges, the phenotype may be divided into classic and atypical PKAN (Hayflick et al., 2003). Classic PKAN is a relatively homogeneous clinical disorder with onset around 3 years of age and typified by dystonia that progresses to require wheelchair use often by age 10 years. Pigmentary retinopathy and acanthocytosis are common features of classic PKAN. Atypical PKAN includes the remainder; onset is later in childhood or early in adulthood, presenting signs and symptoms are more diverse, and the disease usually progresses slowly to preserve ambulation into mid- or late adulthood. Although these categories are useful for prognostic purposes, the range of PKAN phenotypes in fact represents a continuum.

Classic PKAN

Chorea is *not* a common feature of the classic form of PKAN. Early-onset, rapidly progressive PKAN typically presents with dystonia as the predominant movement disorder, often manifesting early in the disease as a change in gait. The child may start tripping and falling, and a neurological exam may reveal foot intorsion or upper limb dystonia, which is generally asymmetric. As the disease progresses, involvement of the axial musculature increases, manifesting initially with dystonic facies (sometimes with widened staring eyes and a smile reminiscent of the "risus sardonicus" of Wilson disease) and later with a characteristic retrocollic or even opisthotonic posturing of the neck and trunk. Orobuccolingual dystonia may be severe, resulting in tongue and lip trauma. Upper limb involvement generally remains asymmetric; it is common for one arm to be held in a posture with the elbow and wrist flexed and the fingers flexed at the metacarpophalangeal joints with the phalanges extended or for the entire upper extremity to be extended backward at the shoulder. Dysarthria and dysphagia become more prominent over time, and corticospinal tract signs may emerge, with brisk deep tendon reflexes, upgoing toes, and spasticity superimposed on parkinsonian rigidity.

The dystonia of PKAN fluctuates throughout the day and may be exacerbated by physical activity, emotional excitement, or pain. The resulting movements could be described as "choreiform"; however, they are usually repetitive and stereotyped, rather than the more usual random movements of true chorea. One limb might intermittently flail in a stereotyped fashion, or the head might repeatedly retroflex. Also, the child with classic PKAN attempting voluntary movement with a severely dystonic upper extremity might appear choreic, but the experienced observer will recognize dystonia as the underlying movement disorder.

Atypical PKAN

In contrast to the rather homogeneous picture of classic PKAN, patients presenting in the second decade of life and beyond have a much more heterogeneous clinical picture and, thus, are designated as having "atypical" PKAN. Neurological signs and symptoms may be overt or quite subtle. As a general rule, adolescent or young adult patients with atypical PKAN present with a *hyperkinetic* movement disorder and older adult patients, with a *hypokinetic* picture of parkinsonism.

Psychiatric symptoms may precede the onset of a movement disorder in atypical PKAN. Patients may develop overt affective or even psychotic symptoms but more commonly show nonspecific impulsivity, obsessive–compulsive behaviors, a decline in school or work performance, or a change in personality. These symptoms may not be recognized as part of a larger neurological disorder until the onset of the movement disorder, which may present as dystonia, tourettism, parkinsonism, or infrequently, chorea (Carod-Artal et al., 2004; Grimes et al., 2000; Hayflick et al., 2003; Klepper et al., 2003; Nardocci et al., 1994; Pellecchia et al., 2005). The motor presentation tends to be asymmetric in the limbs, often in combination with prominent axial involvement. Although the literature prior to discovery of the *PANK2* gene suggests that chorea and choreoathetosis are common presenting symptoms (Dooling et al., 1974), our own experience with mutation-positive atypical PKAN patients reveals chorea to be a relatively uncommon finding, at least at presentation. More commonly, younger patients present with facial, neck, and truncal dystonia, with eating dystonia being a particularly interesting and characteristic feature. Other action-induced dystonias, such as writer's cramp, are also common. Older patients present with a picture of atypical parkinsonism. Asymmetric bradykinesia and rigidity may be present, but tremor, if it is present, tends to occur with action rather than at rest. Freezing of gait and disabling palilalia are common (Guimaraes and Santos, 1999). Rarely, the phenotype in older patients may be mild enough to go undetected until MRI reveals the highly specific pattern of abnormalities on T2-weighted sequences.

Neuroaxonal Dystrophy

NAD is a recessive neurodegenerative disorder caused by mutations in the *PLA2G6* gene (Morgan et al., 2006). It has been classified as a disorder of neurodegeneration with brain iron accumulation because some cases show iron accumulation on MRI and on pathological examination; however, many cases do not have this feature. Prior to the 2006 gene discovery, the disease was diagnosed based on clinical and pathological criteria; but now it is more properly defined on the basis of mutation analysis.

Previously considered a disorder of infancy, NAD is now recognized to have a more heterogeneous phenotype and thus, like PKAN, may be divided into classic and atypical disease subtypes. The clinical spectrum of disease is continuing to expand, and the nomenclature is likely to change to reflect our evolving understanding.

Classic or Infantile Neuroaxonal Dystrophy

The classic form of NAD presents in the first 3 years of life with hypotonia progressing to quadriparesis and global psychomotor regression (Carrilho et al., 2008). Although some children with infantile NAD (INAD) show signs of cerebellar ataxia, chorea is not a feature of classic NAD. The child may show signs of visual impairment, with ophthalmological exam demonstrating optic atrophy. MRI commonly shows cerebellar atrophy and, less often, T2 hypointensity of the globus pallidus, suggesting iron accumulation, the reason for the disease's inclusion as a disorder of brain iron accumulation (Gregory et al., 2008; Kurian et al., 2008). Pathological examination of tissue from conjunctiva, skin, rectum, or peripheral nerve shows dystrophic axons, which provides the basis for the descriptive name of the disease in the older literature.

Atypical Neuroaxonal Dystrophy

Like PKAN, atypical NAD presenting after the age of 3 years has a more variable phenotype and may manifest with chorea, but this is very rare: We have seen only one patient with chorea in our own database of 40+ patients with *PLA2G6* mutations, and we are not aware of any other reported cases in the literature. Karak syndrome includes chorea and mutations in *PLA2G6* (Mubaidin et al., 2003). However, as this term was applied to only a single consanguineous family, we favor instead the more inclusive term "atypical NAD." Like other disorders in which the molecular basis has only recently been defined, the phenotype of *PLA2G6*-associated disease is expected to evolve over the coming years, illustrated by the recent description of parkinsonism-dystonia associated with mutations in the gene (Paisan-Ruiz et al., 2009).

Idiopathic Neurodegeneration with Brain Iron Accumulation

As might be expected, patients presenting with evidence of basal ganglia brain iron accumulation but without mutations in the *PANK2* or *PLA2G6* gene have a widely variable phenotype as they likely represent many different diseases. Some of these patients will have chorea when their particular pattern of basal ganglia pathology disturbs the circuitry in such a way as to cause chorea; others will have dystonia, parkinsonism, tics, or athetosis; still others will have limited or no movement disorder.

DIAGNOSTIC STUDIES

The diagnosis of NBIA may be suspected from the clinical examination. More commonly, the diagnosis is suggested by the results of a brain MRI. PKAN, NAD, and idiopathic NBIA are all characterized by high levels of basal ganglia iron, though the specific nuclei involved may differ. Iron is demonstrated on MRI by its characteristic pattern of marked hypointensity on T2-weighted imaging, with isointensity of the same regions on T1 weighting (Figure 8–1).

Iron is evident on brain MRI in all cases of PKAN, though it may be less evident early in the course of disease. The MRI changes of PKAN are virtually pathognomonic, showing the "eye of the tiger" sign. This sign describes the appearance of the globus pallidus, with T2 hypointensity representing iron and a central hyperintense spot within the globus pallidus that probably represents tissue damage or edema (Sethi et al., 1988). The central bright spot surrounded by a dark rim is the specific finding in PKAN that is not found in other forms of NBIA or in other disorders (Hayflick et al., 2003). Later in the disease, iron also is high in the substantia nigra (Hayflick et al., 2006).

In NAD, basal ganglia iron levels may be high, especially later in the disease. When present, the regions of high iron levels include the globus pallidus and substantia nigra; however, the appearance on MRI is of only T2 hypointensity, with no central hyperintensity in the globus pallidus. This distinguishes the MRI from that of PKAN. In NAD, cerebellar atrophy is also a common feature.

In idiopathic NBIA, the brain MRI findings include high iron levels in the basal ganglia. Since this term still encompasses a collection of several disorders, additional findings are often present and may be disease-specific (Hayflick et al., 2006).

With high–field strength MRI scanners now in routine use in many countries, we recommend caution in the interpretation of T2 signal hypointensity as evidence of pathological iron accumulation. Several of the basal ganglia are normally iron-rich structures, and readers accustomed to 1.5T imaging may overcall iron accumulation on T2-weighted imaging performed on 3T or higher–field strength magnets. A useful point of comparison to determine if iron accumulation is pathological is the red nucleus, which is normally iron-rich but does not typically show abnormal signal intensity in PKAN, NAD, or most cases of idiopathic NBIA. Therefore, if the basal ganglia signal intensity appears equivalent to that of the red nucleus, consultation with an experienced neuroradiologist is recommended before interpreting the signal intensity of the basal ganglia as abnormal.

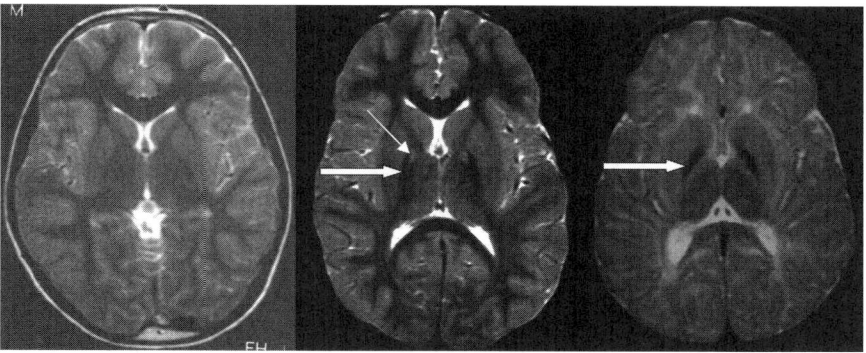

FIGURE 8–1. Patterns on T2-weighted brain magnetic resonance imaging. The image on the *left* is of a normal patient. An image of a patient with PKAN (*center*) shows hypointensity (*thick arrow*) with a central region of hyperintensity (*thin arrow*) in the medial globus pallidus ("eye of the tiger" sign). In an image of a patient with idiopathic NBIA (*right*), only a region of hypointensity (*arrow*) is seen in the medial globus pallidus.

While MRI remains an essential tool to direct diagnostic suspicions toward NBIA, genetic testing can confirm the diagnosis in most cases. Clinical genetic testing for PKAN and NAD is available through a worldwide network of referral labs. Current information about specific laboratories that offer testing can be found at the Genetests Web site (http://www.Genetests.org).

MANAGEMENT

As yet, there are no evidence-based guidelines for the management of PKAN, INAD, or idiopathic NBIA; thus, treatment recommendations are based on anecdotal evidence, case reports, and small case series, with specific options dictated by the particular clinical phenotype. Most patients require a combination of medical therapy and rehabilitation services, and some patients may benefit from surgical intervention for their movement disorder.

For the rare NBIA patient presenting with chorea, tetrabenazine may be helpful; and this drug has also been used with some success when dystonia is the primary issue. Dopamine antagonists for chorea or tics may result in parkinsonism in NBIA patients and should be used with great caution, if at all. Younger PKAN patients with dystonia frequently derive some benefit from anticholinergic drugs such as trihexyphenidyl. Children can generally tolerate higher doses of this class of compounds than older adults, who may develop dry mouth, blurred vision, constipation, urinary retention, or adverse cognitive effects before a beneficial effect is observed.

When spasticity is an issue, baclofen or tizanidine may be helpful; and intrathecal baclofen has been used with benefit in some patients (Albright et al., 1996; Kyriagis et al., 2004). Benzodiazepines are sometimes added to the drug regimen of patients with refractory spasticity and dystonia. Focal or segmental dystonia may be improved by targeted intramuscular botulinum toxin injections.

The response of NBIA patients with parkinsonism to dopaminergic drugs is unpredictable, reflecting the heterogeneous pathogenesis and phenotypic variability of these disorders. We have seen few PKAN patients tolerate or be responsive to this class of agents, but there have been no controlled studies to confirm this observation. However, we are aware of a small subset of idiopathic NBIA patients with mental retardation who show levodopa-responsive parkinsonism complicated by motor fluctuations and dyskinesias.

Despite pathological and radiological evidence of brain iron accumulation, there is no evidence of systemic iron abnormalities in NBIA. Further, it is not clear if the central nervous system iron accumulation contributes to the pathogenesis of any of these disorders or if it is simply a nonspecific "tombstone" marker (Schneider et al., 2009). Several prospective studies currently under way to assess the effects of deferiprone, a centrally active iron chelator, may shed light on this question (Forni et al., 2008).

Stereotactic lesion surgeries targeting the globus pallidus and, more recently, implantation of pallidal deep brain stimulation electrodes have been reported to be beneficial in case reports and small case series in PKAN (Castelnau et al., 2005; Justesen et al., 1999; Krause et al., 2004; Kyriagis et al., 2004; Mikati et al., 2009; Umemura et al., 2004). A recent multi center retrospective study also reported benefits, albeit more modest than previous reports, in a cohort that included PKAN and other forms of NBIA (Timmerman 2010). An international prospective study is under way to objectively assess the efficacy of deep brain stimulation in PKAN and non-PKAN forms of NBIA.

Multidisciplinary rehabilitation services with physical, occupational, speech, and nutrition therapy have an important role in the management of NBIA patients. Quality of life may be improved by maintaining mobility and communication and preventing secondary complications such as contractures, skin breakdown, nutritional deficiency, and infections.

SUMMARY

Chorea is uncommon in PKAN, INAD, and idiopathic NBIA. These disorders are typically first suspected following MRI of the brain, when high levels of basal ganglia iron become evident. Diagnosis can be confirmed for PKAN and INAD using molecular genetic testing. Management remains primarily palliative, with promise for more rational therapeutics as disease pathogenesis becomes better understood.

REFERENCES

Albright AL, Barry MJ, Fasick P, Barron W, Shultz B (1996) Continuous intrathecal baclofen infusion for symptomatic generalized dystonia. Neurosurgery 38(5):934–938, discussion 938–939.

Carod-Artal FJ, Vargas AP, Marinho PB, Fernandes-Silva TV, Portugal D (2004) Tourettism, hemiballism and juvenile parkinsonism: expanding the clinical spectrum of the neurodegeneration associated to pantothenate kinase deficiency (Hallervorden Spatz syndrome) [in French]. Rev Neurol 38(4):327–331.

Carrilho I, Santos M, Guimaraes A, Teixeira J, Chorao R, Martins M, Dias C, Gregory A, Westaway S, Nguyen T, Hayflick S, Barbot C (2008) Infantile neuroaxonal dystrophy: what's most important for the diagnosis? Eur J Paediatr Neurol 12(6):491–500.

Castelnau P, Cif L, Valente EM, Vayssiere N, Hemm S, Gannau A, Digiorgio A, Coubes P (2005) Pallidal stimulation improves pantothenate kinase–associated neurodegeneration. Ann Neurol 57(5):738–741.

Dooling EC, Schoene WC, Richardson EP Jr (1974) Hallervorden-Spatz syndrome. Arch Neurol 30(1):70–83.

Forni GL, Balocco M, Cremonesi L, Abbruzzese G, Parodi RC, Marchese R (2008) Regression of symptoms after selective iron chelation therapy in a case of neurodegeneration with brain iron accumulation. Mov Disord 23(6):904–907.

Genetests: Medical genetics information resource (database online). Copyright, University of Washington, Seattle. 1993–2009, http://www.Genetests.org (accessed September 2009).

Gregory A, Polster BJ, Hayflick SJ (2009) Clinical and genetic delineation of neurodegeneration with brain iron accumulation. J Med Genet 46(2):73–80.

Gregory A, Westaway SK, Holm IE, Kotzbauer PT, Hogarth P, Sonek S, Coryell JC, Nguyen TM, Nardocci N, Zorzi G, Rodriguez D, Desguerre I, Bertini E, Simonati A, Levinson B, Dias C, Barbot C, Carrilho I, Santos M, Malik I, Gitschier J, Hayflick SJ (2008) Neurodegeneration associated with genetic defects in phospholipase A$_2$. Neurology 71(18):1402–1409.

Grimes DA, Lang AE, Bergeron C (2000) Late adult onset chorea with typical pathology of Hallervorden-Spatz syndrome. J Neurol Neurosurg Psychiatry 69(3):392–395.

Guimaraes J, Santos JV (1999) Generalized freezing in Hallervorden-Spatz syndrome: case report. Eur J Neurol 6(4):509–513.

Hayflick SJ, Hartman M, Coryell J, Gitschier J, Rowley H (2006) Brain MRI in neurodegeneration with brain iron accumulation with and without *PANK2* mutations. Am J Neuroradiol 27(6):1230–1233.

Hayflick SJ, Westaway SK, Levinson B, Zhou B, Johnson MA, Ching KH, Gitschier J (2003) Genetic, clinical, and radiographic delineation of Hallervorden-Spatz syndrome. N Engl J Med 348(1):33–40.

Justesen CR, Penn RD, Kroin JS, Egel RT (1999) Stereotactic pallidotomy in a child with Hallervorden-Spatz disease. Case report. J Neurosurg 90(3):551–554.

Klepper J, Schaper J, Raca G, Coryell J, Das S, Hayflick SJ, Voit T (2003) Progressive dystonia in a 12-year-old boy. Eur J Paediatr Neurol 7(2):85–88.

Krause M, Fogel W, Kloss M, Rasche D, Volkmann J, Tronnier V (2004) Pallidal stimulation for dystonia. Neurosurgery 55(6):1361–1368, discussion 1368–1370.

Kurian MA, Morgan NV, MacPherson L, Foster K, Peake D, Gupta R, Philip SG, Hendriksz C, Morton JE, Kingston HM, Rosser EM, Wassmer E, Gissen P, Maher ER (2008) Phenotypic spectrum of neurodegeneration associated with mutations in the *PLA2G6* gene (PLAN). Neurology 70(18):1623–1629.

Kyriagis M, Grattan-Smith P, Scheinberg A, Teo C, Nakaji N, Waugh M (2004) Status dystonicus and Hallervorden-Spatz disease: treatment with intrathecal baclofen and pallidotomy. J Paediatr Child Health 40(5–6):322–325.

Mikati MA, Yehya A, Darwish H, Karam P, Comair Y (2009) Deep brain stimulation as a mode of treatment of early onset pantothenate kinase–associated neurodegeneration. Eur J Paediatr Neurol 13(1):61–64.

Morgan NV, Westaway SK, Morton JE, Gregory A, Gissen P, Sonek S, Cangul H, Coryell J, Canham N, Nardocci N, Zorzi G, Pasha S, Rodriguez D, Desguerre I, Mubaidin A, Bertini E, Trembath RC, Simonati A, Schanen C, Johnson CA, Levinson B, Woods CG, Wilmot B, Kramer P, Gitschier J, Maher ER, Hayflick SJ (2006) PLA2G6, encoding a phospholipase A₂, is mutated in neurodegenerative disorders with high brain iron. Nat Genet 38(7):752–754.

Mubaidin A, Roberts E, Hampshire D, Dehyyat M, Shurbaji A, Mubaidien M, Jamil A, Al-Din A, Kurdi A, Woods CG (2003) Karak syndrome: a novel degenerative disorder of the basal ganglia and cerebellum. J Med Genet 40(7):543–546.

Nardocci N, Rumi V, Combi ML, Angelini L, Mirabile D, Bruzzone MG (1994) Complex tics, stereotypies, and compulsive behavior as clinical presentation of a juvenile progressive dystonia suggestive of Hallervorden-Spatz disease [letter]. Mov Disord 9(3):369–371.

Paisan-Ruiz C, Bhatia KP, Li A, Hernandez D, Davis M, Wood NW, Hardy J, Houlden H, Singleton A, Schneider SA (2009) Characterization of PLA2G6 as a locus for dystonia-parkinsonism. Ann Neurol 65(1):19–23.

Pellecchia MT, Valente EM, Cif L, Salvi S, Albanese A, Scarano V, Bonuccelli U, Bentivoglio AR, D'Amico A, Marelli C, Di Giorgio A, Coubes P, Barone P, Dallapiccola B (2005) The diverse phenotype and genotype of pantothenate kinase–associated neurodegeneration. Neurology 64(10):1810–1812.

Schneider SA, Hardy J, Bhatia KP (2009) Iron accumulation in syndromes of neurodegeneration with brain iron accumulation 1 and 2: causative or consequential? J Neurol Neurosurg Psychiatry 80(6):589–590.

Sethi KD, Adams RJ, Loring DW, el Gammal T (1988) Hallervorden-Spatz syndrome: clinical and magnetic resonance imaging correlations. Ann Neurol 24(5):692–694.

Shevell M (1992) Racial hygiene, active euthanasia, and Julius Hallervorden. Neurology 42(11):2214–2219.

Timmermann L, Pauls KA, Wieland K, Jech R, Kurlemann G, Sharma N, Gill SS, Haenggeli CA, Hayflick SJ, Hogarth P, Leenders KL, Limousin P, Malanga CJ, Moro E, Ostrem JL, Revilla FJ, Santens P, Schnitzler A, Tisch S, Valldeoriola F, Vesper J, Volkmann J, Woitalla D, Peker S, (2010). Dystonia in neurodegeneration with brain iron accumulation: outcome of bilateral pallidal stimulation. Brain. 2010 Mar;133 (Pt 3):701–712.

Taylor TD, Litt M, Kramer P, Pandolfo M, Angelini L, Nardocci N, Davis S, Pineda M, Hattori H, Flett PJ, Cilio MR, Bertini E, Hayflick SJ (1996) Homozygosity mapping of Hallervorden-Spatz syndrome to chromosome 20p12.3-p13. Nat Genet 14(4):479–481.

Thomas M, Hayflick SJ, Jankovic J (2004) Clinical heterogeneity of neurodegeneration with brain iron accumulation (Hallervorden-Spatz syndrome) and pantothenate kinase–associated neurodegeneration. Mov Disord 19(1):36–42.

Umemura A, Jaggi JL, Dolinskas CA, Stern MB, Baltuch GH (2004) Pallidal deep brain stimulation for longstanding severe generalized dystonia in Hallervorden-Spatz syndrome. Case report. J Neurosurg 100(4):706–709.

Zhou B, Westaway SK, Levinson B, Johnson MA, Gitschier J, Hayflick SJ (2001) A novel pantothenate kinase gene (PANK2) is defective in Hallervorden-Spatz syndrome. Nat Genet 28(4):345–349.

9

Neuroferritinopathy

Alisdair McNeill, MRCP and
Patrick F. Chinnery, PhD, FRCPath, FRCP, FMedSci

INTRODUCTION

Neuroferritinopathy (MIM 606159, also labeled "hereditary ferritinopathy" and "neurodegeneration with brain iron accumulation type 2," NBIA2) was first recognized as a clinical entity distinct from Huntington disease among families in the northeast of England, transmitted as an autosomal dominant choreiform movement disorder with preserved cognition (Curtis et al., 2001). The most frequent presentation is with chorea (50%), followed by dystonia (42.5%) and parkinsonism (7.5%). Neuroferritinopathy is distinguished clinically from Huntington disease by the lack of major neuropsychiatric involvement and preserved eye movements, from spinocerebellar ataxias by less prominent cerebellar signs, and from dentatorubral-pallidoluysian atrophy by lack of seizures. The clinical diagnosis can be confirmed by brain magnetic resonance imaging (MRI), which reveals characteristic features in patients with chorea due to neuroferritinopathy. This should be followed with molecular genetic analysis. Neuroferritinopathy follows a prolonged clinical course, with patients remaining ambulant 20 years after diagnosis, which serves to further differentiate it from choreiform disorders with more aggressive clinical courses such as prion diseases.

Mutations in the ferritin light chain gene have been identified as causative, the most common being the 460insA mutation (Curtis et al., 2001). Seven different mutations are known; six insertions in exon 4 and a missense mutation in exon 3. In neuroferritinopathy, high levels of brain iron deposition are present both on MRI of the brain and on histological examination of cerebral tissue. As a result, neuroferritinopathy is considered to be a member of the NBIA group. Neuropathological studies have demonstrated neuronal loss in the cerebral cortex, cerebellum, and basal ganglia. Ferritin inclusion bodies were demonstrated within neurons and glia. Increased expression of hemeoxygenase-1, suggesting oxidative stress, and caspase-3, an apoptotic marker, was also noted. Autopsy studies have shown loss of fibers within the indirect striatopallidal pathway. This suggests that loss of inhibitory input from the putamen to the globus pallidus externus is responsible for chorea.

EPIDEMIOLOGY

Neuroferritinopathy is a rare neurogenetic disorder, which has been described in families from England (Chinnery et al., 2007), France (Devos et al., 2008), Spain (Maciel et al., 2005), North America (Mancuso et al., 2005), and Japan (Ohta et al., 2008). The largest number of neuroferritinopathy cases originates from the Cumbrian region of England, due to a founder effect in the mutation in the ferritin light chain. Neuroferritinopathy is predominantly an adult disorder, with a mean age at onset of 39 years. However, it can present as early as 13 years of age or as late as 63 years, and we have observed asymptomatic brain iron accumulation on MRIs collected in early childhood. There is no sex predominance.

CLINICAL FEATURES

The phenotype of neuroferritinopathy due to the common 460insA mutation in the ferritin light chain was defined by a cohort study of European patients (Chinnery et al., 2007). The major presentation was with a movement disorder; in 50% of cases chorea, in 42.5% focal dystonia (which affected the leg in 76% of cases and the arm in 24%), and in 7.5% parkinsonism (Chinnery et al., 2007). With disease progression, the majority developed both chorea and limb or foot dystonia. Infrequent features included ballism, writer's cramp, and blepharospasm. Oromandibular dystonia and dysarthrophonia were also seen.

Neuroferritinopathy caused by the less common *FTL* mutations has a subtly different phenotype from that of 460insA. The phenotype of the 458insA mutation is broadly similar to that of the 460insA cases. However, the 458insA family had more severe cognitive involvement and cerebellar ataxia, which was not seen in the 460insA cases (Devos et al., 2008).

A duplication of the 469–484 sequence of exon 4 (c.469_484dup16nt) was reported in a 42-year-old Japanese male with postural tremor, hypotonia, aphonia, micrographia, and abnormal gait (Ohta et al., 2008). He did not have the typical hyperkinetic features associated with neuroferritinopathy.

A 498-499insTC mutation was reported in a French-Canadian family (Vidal et al., 2004). The proband presented in her 20s with a postural hand tremor. She developed a severe cerebellar syndrome in her late 40s and 50s. She was also noted to have cog-wheel rigidity, facial chorea, and severe cognitive impairment. The marked tremor, cerebellar ataxia, and dementia differed from the 460insA phenotype.

The 646insC mutation was reported in a large French-Canadian/Dutch kindred. The proband presented at age 63 with cerebellar ataxia, pseudobulbar affect, and chorea. The proband's sister presented at age 49 with festinant gait, emotional lability, oromandibular and cervical dystonia, and mild proximal leg weakness. There was no parkinsonism or dementia in either. It is intriguing that the presentation of two individuals with identical mutations should differ so substantially, and the explanation is unclear.

The 474G>A missense mutation in exon 3 identified in a Spanish-Portuguese family was associated with gait ataxia at age 13 in the proband, followed by acute psychosis; subsequent to treatment with valproate and trazodone, the patient developed an akinetic-rigid syndrome. This improved with drug withdrawal, but the patient still had a parkinsonian syndrome with ataxia 1 year after medication withdrawal. Given that the boy's mother and brother were asymptomatic and carried the same mutation and that the motor features could be due to medication, it is not totally clear that the phenotype is actually a direct consequence of the exon 3 missense mutation.

Kubota et al. (2009) report a family with a four-nucleotide duplication in exon 4 (c.641-642GACC) which presented with chorea, dystonia, parkinsonism, and cognitive impairment in middle age. Kubota et al. (2009) propose that families with insertions at the 5' portion of exon 4 present with middle age–onset chorea and mild cognitive impairment, while those families with insertions in the 3' portion of exon 4 present with early-onset tremor and ataxia. However, given the small numbers of families reported with mutations other than 460insA, it is difficult to draw firm conclusions at this stage. Orolingual chorea and dystonia are consistent motor features across all *FTL* mutations, while cerebellar ataxia, action tremor, and overt dementia appear not to be features of the 460ins A mutation.

UNIQUE FEATURES OF CHOREA DUE TO NEUROFERRITINOPATHY

There are several clinical features which serve to differentiate neuroferritinopathy from other inherited causes of chorea. It is important to note that an isolated case of neuroferritinopathy would have to be distinguished from a case of chorea due to a sporadic cause. Here, we restrict ourselves to factors differentiating between causes of autosomal dominant chorea and refer readers to the relevant sections of this book for an approach to diagnosing sporadic chorea. The major differential diagnosis for neuroferritinopathy is Huntington disease (CAG expansion in the gene for huntingtin) (Chapter 3). However, neuroferritinopathy can be distinguished from Huntington disease by the facts that psychiatric and cognitive manifestations are relatively minor and that oculomotor disturbance does not occur in neuroferritinopathy (Wild and Tabrizi, 2007). Aceruloplasminemia, an autosomal recessive cause of NBIA due to ceruloplasmin mutations, can cause adult-onset chorea (Miyajima et al., 1995) (Chapter 10). This is frequently accompanied by diabetes and retinopathy, which are not seen in neuroferritinopathy. Moreover, brain MRI permits distinction of neuroferritinopathy and aceruloplasminemia (McNeill et al., 2008). Spinocerebellar ataxia (SCA) types 1 (CAG expansion in *ATXN1*), 3 (CAG expansion in *ATXN3*), and 17 (CAG expansion in *TBP*) can present with chorea (Wild and Tabrizi, 2007) (Chapter 12). However, the majority of cases of neuroferritinopathy have no cerebellar signs, or only minor cerebellar features, and no pyramidal tract signs, thus distinguishing chorea due to SCA from chorea due to neuroferritinopathy. Dentatorubral-pallidoluysian atrophy (DRPLA, CAG expansion in *ATN1*) can cause chorea with a dominant family history, but myoclonic seizures are often present in DRPLA and not in neuroferritinopathy (Wild and Tabrizi, 2007). The neuroacanthocytosis syndromes can cause chorea (Chapters 6, 7), which can be distinguished from neuroferritinopathy by an autosomal recessive (*VPS13A*) or X-linked (*XK* gene) family history and the absence of a peripheral neuropathy or seizures in neuroferritinopathy (Chinnery et al., 2007). Benign hereditary chorea caused by *TITF1* mutations is an autosomal dominant cause of chorea (Breedveld et al., 2002), which can be distinguished from neuroferritinopathy by the childhood onset of chorea and normal brain imaging (Chapter 4). "Senile chorea" can rarely occur with an autosomal dominant pedigree linked to 8q (Shimohata et al., 2007); normal MRI and a very benign clinical course without the development of dystonia distinguish it from neuroferritinopathy. The natural history of neuroferritinopathy, in which there is slow progression, with most patients still ambulant 20 years after onset, also serves to distinguish it from other inherited choreiform disorders, such as prion diseases (*PRNP*) (Chapter 11), with more rapid clinical courses (Chinnery et al., 2007).

INVESTIGATIONS

Routine blood tests play a minor role in the diagnosis of neuroferritinopathy. The serum ferritin is low in most males and postmenopausal females but only a quarter of premenopausal women with neuroferritinopathy (Chinnery et al., 2007). Hemoglobin and serum iron are normal. Neurophysiological tests are unremarkable

(Chinnery et al., 2007). Routine neurological investigations such as lumbar puncture may be required to differentiate a simple case of neuroferritinopathy from a case of chorea due to a sporadic cause. These tests are detailed elsewhere in this book and will not be dealt with here.

The most useful investigation in suspected neuroferritinopathy is brain MRI, which serves both to make the diagnosis and to distinguish neuroferritinopathy from other causes of chorea (McNeill et al., 2008). Using appropriate MR sequences, all symptomatic cases have abnormal imaging. Totally normal MRIs in a patient with chorea would make the diagnosis of neuroferritinopathy extremely unlikely. In early disease (460insA *FTL* mutation) there is cerebral iron deposition as evidenced by hypointensity of the red nucleus, caudate, globus pallidus, putamen, thalamus, substantia nigra, and cerebral cortex on T2-weighted scans (Figure 9–1A). With disease progression and tissue damage, areas of hyperintensity develop within the globus pallidus and caudate heads on T2-weighted scans (Figure 9–1B). This probably represents tissue edema and correlates with fluid-filled cysts found in the globus pallidus at autopsy. In two neuroferritinopathy cases an "eye of the tiger" sign was observed. In the c.469_484dup16nt case there was marked cerebellar atrophy on brain imaging (Ohta, personal communication). The most sensitive MRI sequence for detection of brain iron is gradient echo imaging (T2*), and the earliest imaging changes in presymptomatic carriers are hypointensity of the putamen and/or globus pallidus and substantia nigra (McNeill et al., 2008; Chinnery et al., 2007). The imaging features of neuroferritinopathy

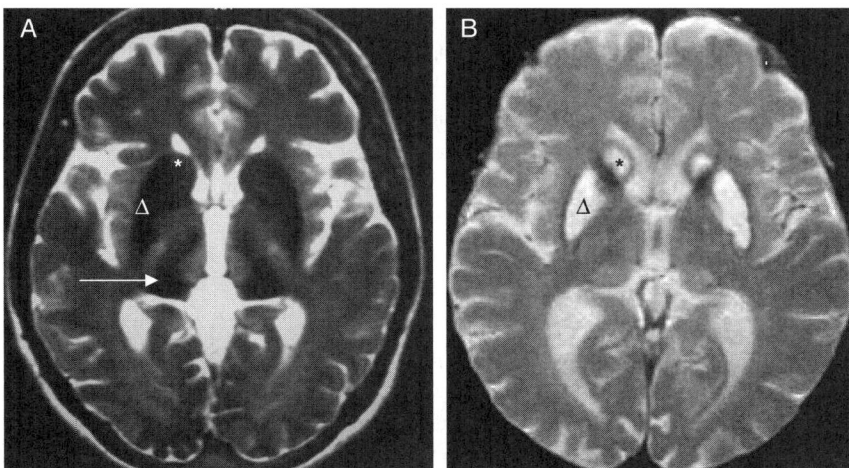

FIGURE 9–1. Magnetic resonance images of neuroferritinopathy. **A** Gradient echo (T2*) of a 60-year-old woman with neuroferritinopathy; note hypointensity of caudate nuclei (*), putamen (Δ), and thalamus (*arrow*). **B** Fast spin echo (T2) of a 65-year-old woman with neuroferritinopathy; note cavitation of caudate nuclei (*) and putamen (Δ).

are characteristic and clearly distinguish it from other causes of chorea such as Huntington disease; and while there is some overlap between MRI appearances of neuroferritinopathy and mitochondrial disease, a radiological algorithm can be used to differentiate them (McNeill et al., 2008).

The definitive diagnosis of neuroferritinopathy ultimately relies upon molecular genetic tests. To date, six of the seven identified mutations lie in exon 4 and the other in exon 3; six are insertions (460insA, 458insA, 498-499insTC, 646insC, c.469_484dup16nt, and c.641_642GACC) and one is a missense mutation (474G>A). The most frequently reported mutation is 460insA, with the remaining mutations being private to individual families. If the imaging and clinical history are highly suggestive and exon 4 sequencing is normal, then sequencing the whole of the ferritin light chain gene is sensible, although only one mutation has been identified outside exon 4.

PATHOPHYSIOLOGY: CELLULAR LEVEL

Ferritin is a hollow shell composed of a polymer of ferritin light chains (FTL) and ferritin heavy chains (FTH) (Curtis et al., 2001). FTL offers acidic residues to aid iron nucleation around the ferritin molecule, while FTH acts as a ferroxidase. The 460insA, 646insC, 498-499insTC, and 458dupA mutations all extend the carboxy terminus of FTL, disrupting the dodecahedral structure of ferritin, interfering with its ability to transport iron, and resulting in iron deposition in the brain. Analysis of fresh frozen neuroferritinopathy brains has confirmed the presence of grossly elevated nanocrystalline iron oxide (magnetite) (Hautot et al., 2007).

The neuropathology of neuroferritinopathy in a case due to the 498insTC mutation was described by Vidal et al. (2004). Grossly, there was atrophy of the cerebrum and cerebellum, with small cavities in the putamen. Microscopically, there was neuronal loss in the cerebral cortex, cerebellum, thalamus, caudate nuclei, putamen, and globus pallidus. Neuronal loss was particularly severe in the putamen. Ferritin-immunopositive inclusion bodies were seen in neurons and glia throughout the brain but most densely in the putamen. This description was confirmed by Mancuso et al. (2005), who studied the neuropathology of the 646insC mutation. Grossly, there was atrophy of the cerebrum and cerebellum, with cavitation of the putamen and softening of the globus pallidus. Microscopically, there was loss of neurons in the putamen, red nucleus, cerebellar vermis, and subthalamic nucleus. There was extensive loss of putaminal fibers in the globus pallidus externus, while the globus pallidus internus and thalamus were spared. Hyaline deposits which stained positively for iron were observed in the globus pallidus externus.

Histological studies of neuroferritinopathy due to the 646insC mutation provide evidence of neuronal oxidative stress as there are hemeoxygenase-1– and hydroxyl-nonenal-immunoreactive neurons in the putamen (Mancuso et al., 2005).

In the same patient there was evidence of mitochondrial damage, with depletion of cyclooxygenase I (COX I) and COX II neuronal immunostaining and neuronal apoptosis with caspase-3 and TUNEL-positive cells (Mancuso et al., 2005). These findings support a model of neurodegeneration whereby iron deposition leads to oxidative stress, mitochondrial damage, and neuronal apoptosis.

A mouse model of neuroferritinopathy was generated by expressing 499insTC in a transgene (Vidal et al., 2008). The transgenic mice had a reduced lifespan and abnormal posturing. Histologically, there was neuronal and glial ferritin accumulation accompanied by positive Perl's staining of the cytoplasm. Interestingly, ubiquitin and proteosome staining was observed at sites of ferritin accumulation, suggesting the involvement of this pathway in the pathogenesis of neuroferritinopathy (Vidal et al., 2008).

PATHOPHYSIOLOGY: BASAL GANGLIA

In one simplified model of the neuroanatomy of chorea, increased glutamatergic drive from the motor nuclei of the thalamus leads to excessive activation of the motor cortex and, hence, involuntary movements (Chapter 2). Increased activation of the motor nuclei of the thalamus can result from either degeneration of the inhibitory motor projections (indirect pathway) of the putamen or excessive activity of the facilitatory motor projection (direct pathway) of the putamen. There are no studies which directly address the pathophysiology of chorea in neuroferritinopathy; however, given that neuroferritinopathy is a neurodegenerative disorder, it seems most likely that chorea will result from degeneration of the indirect pathway. Evidence for this comes from MRI studies of neuroferritinopathy, which demonstrated lesions of the putamen and globus pallidus externus in one-third of cases due to the 460insA mutation (McNeill et al., 2008). Moreover, loss of afferent fibers from the putamen was observed in the lateral portion of the globus pallidus externus of a neuroferritinopathy case due to the 646insC mutation (Mancuso et al., 2005), suggesting that degeneration of the inhibitory indirect pathway might be associated with chorea in neuroferritinopathy. The foregoing discussion is highly speculative, and definitive delineation of the pathophysiology of chorea in neuroferritinopathy will require functional neuroimaging studies.

A CLINICAL APPROACH TO SUSPECTED
NEUROFERRITINOPATHY

The presentation of neuroferritinopathy overlaps significantly with common movement disorders such as idiopathic dystonia, Parkinson disease, and Huntington disease. However, given the relative rarity of neuroferritinopathy, molecular genetic testing for *FTL* mutations should be undertaken only in patients in whom certain criteria are met. The most important factors are a family history of autosomal dominant chorea with evidence of the characteristic imaging features of neuroferritinopathy on brain MRI. Imaging has revealed elevated levels of basal ganglia iron (globus pallidus) even in presymptomatic carriers, so the absence of elevated brain iron on gradient echo (T2∗) MRI makes a diagnosis of neuroferritinopathy most unlikely. An autosomal dominant family history, adult onset of chorea, and low serum ferritin are also supportive of a diagnosis of neuroferritinopathy. Investigations such as neurophysiology and examination of cerebrospinal fluid do not help in the diagnosis of neuroferritinopathy; and in the presence of a compatible clinical presentation and characteristic imaging, molecular genetic testing of *FTL* should be undertaken. It should be remembered that making a diagnosis of an autosomal dominant neurodegenerative disorder such as neuroferritinopathy has implications for the patient's family and appropriate genetic counseling should be offered.

Currently, there is no effective disease-modifying treatment for neuroferritinopathy (Chinnery et al., 2007). Symptomatic treatment of dystonia with either benzodiazepines or botulinum toxin injection is effective, and the dystonia may also respond to antipsychotics or anticholinergics. Deep brain stimulation was ineffective in one case (unpublished observations, McNeill A, Jenkinson A, Burns DJ & Chinnery PF), possibly because of difficulties placing the electrodes in severely damaged or cystic basal ganglia. It is important to note that parkinsonian syndromes in neuroferritinopathy patients do not generally respond to L-DOPA. Attempts at iron chelation or depletion do not appear clinically effective, although limited data are available. This is in contrast to aceruloplasminemia, in which iron chelation can be affective at preventing disease progression (Miyajima et al., 1995). The different response to iron chelation in neuroferritinopathy and aceruloplasminemia underscores the need for accurate clinical and molecular diagnosis. If there is any doubt as to the precise diagnosis, then the opinion of clinicians involved in NBIA research programs should be sought.

REFERENCES

Breedveld GJ, von Dongen JWF, Danesin C, et al. (2002) Mutations in *TITF-1* are associated with benignhereditarychorea. Hum Mol Genet 8:971–979.

Chinnery PF, Crompton DE, Birchall D, et al. (2007) The clinical features and natural history of neuroferritinopathy caused by the *FTL1* 460insA mutation. Brain 130:110–119.

Curtis AR, Fey C, Morris CM, et al. (2001) Mutation in the gene encoding ferritin light polypeptide causes dominant adult onsetbasal ganglia disease. Nat Genet 28:350–354.

Devos D, Tchofo J, Vuillaume I, et al. (2008) Clinical features and natural history of neuroferritinopathy caused by the 458dupA FTL mutation. Brain. doi:10.1093/brain/awn274.

Hautot D, Pankhurst QA, Morris CM, et al. (2007) Preliminary observation of elevated levels of nanocrystalline iron oxide in the basal ganglia of neuroferritinopathy patients. Biochem Biophys Acta 1772:21–25.

Kubota A, Hida A, Ichikawa Y, et al. (2009) A novel ferritin light chain gene mutation in a japanese family with neuroferritinopathy: description of clinical features and implications for genotype–phenotype correlations. Mov Disord 24:441–445.

Maciel P, Cruz VT, Constante M, et al. (2005) Neuroferritinopathy: missense mutation in FTL causing early-onset bilateral pallidal involvement. Neurology 65:603–605.

Mancuso M, Davidzon G, Kurlan RM, et al. (2005) Hereditary ferritinopathy: a novel mutation, its cellular pathology, and pathogenetic insights. J Neuropathol Exp Neurol 64:280–294.

McNeill A, Birchall D, Hayflick SJ, et al. (2008) T2* and FSE MRI distinguishes 4 subtypes of neurodegeneration with brain iron accumulation. Neurology 70:1614–1619.

Miyajima H, Ikeda S, Yamamoto K, et al. (1995) Hereditary ceruloplasmin deficiency: a clinicopathological study of a Japanese family. Ann Neurol 36:646–656.

Ohta E, Nagasaka T, Shindo K, et al. (2008) Neuroferritinopathy in a Japanese family with a duplication in the ferritin light chain gene. Neurology 70:1493–1494.

Shimohata T, Hara K, Sanpei K, et al. (2007) Novel locus for benign hereditary chorea with adult onset maps to chromosome 8q21.3–q23.3. Brain 130:2302–2309.

Vidal R, Ghetti B, Takao M, et al. (2004) Intracellular ferritin accumulation in neuronal and extra-neuronal tissues characterises a neurodegenerative disorder associated with a mutation in the ferritin light polypeptide gene. J Neuropathol Exp Neurol 63:363–380.

Vidal R, Miravalle L, Gao X, et al. (2008) Expression of a mutant form of the ferritin l ight chain gene induces neurodegeneration and iron overload in transgenic mice. J Neurosci 28:60–67.

Wild EJ, Tabrizi SJ. The differential diagnosis of chorea. Pract Neurol 2007; 7: 360–373.

10

Aceruloplasminemia

Frank Skidmore, MD

INTRODUCTION

Aceruloplasminemia is an autosomal recessive neurodegenerative disease caused by a loss-of-function mutation in the ceruloplasmin gene. The disorder is characterized by iron deposition in the brain and visceral organs. As a systemic disease, aceruloplasminemia often presents with neurological disease, asymptomatic retinal degeneration, mild anemia, and diabetes mellitus. Symptoms referable to the nervous system include movement disorders (characteristically facial grimacing and blepharospasm, chorea, dystonia, and tremor) as well as ataxia and dysarthria, corresponding to the location of iron deposition in the brain. Iron deposition characteristically occurs primarily in the caudate nucleus, putamen, and dentate nucleus of the cerebellum and to a lesser extent in other basal structures such as the thalamus, globus pallidus, red nucleus, and cerebellar Purkinje cell layers. The diagnosis of aceruloplasminemia is strongly supported by the finding of absent serum ceruloplasm and low T1- and T2-weighted signal intensity in the striatum, thalamus, and dentate nucleus of the cerebellum on magnetic resonance imaging (MRI).

Because aceruloplasminemia typically presents with a movement disorder, absent ceruloplasmin, and low serum copper, the disorder is often initially confused with the also rare but relatively more common disorder, Wilson disease. However, unlike Wilson disease, aceruloplasminemia does not result in any

178

functional abnormality in copper metabolism and urine 24-hour copper levels are normal. The additional laboratory findings of low serum iron (often combined with anemia), elevated serum ferritin, and absent plasma ceruloplasmin ferroxidase activity can suggest the diagnosis. If further evaluation is necessary, a liver biopsy can show the distinctive finding of elevated liver iron and confirm the diagnosis. Like Wilson disease, aceruloplasminemia is a treatable disorder; however, treatments are distinct from the treatments for Wilson disease, and specific diagnosis is required to appropriately manage this disorder. Congenital disorders of intestinal copper transport (Menke's disease and occipital horn syndrome) can also present with low or absent ceruloplasmin; however, these are not among the conditions in the differential diagnosis of chorea.

While aceruloplasminemia is rare, as a treatable condition it is an important consideration in the differential of chorea, particularly with respect to individuals with chorea related to apparent Wilson disease. The purpose of this chapter is to review the clinical features, diagnosis, molecular genetics and pathogenesis, and treatment of this disorder.

MOLECULAR CHARACTERISTICS AND PATHOLOGY

Ceruloplasmin is a 132-kilodalton $\alpha 2$-glycoprotein that is a member of a family of proteins known as the "multicopper oxidase family." Localized to 3q23-24, the gene consists of 19 exons that encode for a 1,046–amino acid protein (Royle et al., 1987; Daimon et al., 1995; Koschinsky et al., 1986). Synthesized in secreted form primarily by the liver, the protein is also present in the brain as a membrane-bound astrocyte protein (Klomp and Gitlin, 1996; Patel and David, 1997). Peripherally, secreted ceruloplasmin incorporates six copper molecules and plays a role in the mobilization and oxidation of ferrous iron (Fe^{2+}) from tissue stores and ferric iron (Fe^{3+}), which is carried by transferrin. Lack of ceruloplasmin peripherally prevents recycling of iron into a form readily accessible by the bone marrow for producing hemoglobin, leading to anemia.

Serum ceruloplasmin does not cross the blood–brain barrier, and glycosyl-phosphatidylinositol (GPI)–anchored, membrane-bound ceruloplasmin on the surface of astrocytes contains >95% of all brain-localized copper. Bound ceruloplasmin plays a critical role in brain iron metabolism and homeostasis (Jeong and David, 2003). Astrocytes and oligodendrocytes cooperate in the process of iron homeostasis and transport. While astrocytes through ceruloplasmin ensure that iron remains in the appropriate redox state, oligodendrocytes produce transferrin, which binds the ferric iron for transport. Brain iron is a crucial component for many physiological functions of the brain, particularly in the development of myelin; myelin in fact represents the largest endogenous sink of bound iron within the central nervous system (CNS).

In aceruloplasminemia, absence of membrane-bound ceruloplasm results in an increase in ferrous iron (Fe^{2+}) (Xu et al., 2004). While ferric iron binds to transferrin, ferrous iron may be bound to ascorbate or citrate or may be free (e.g., unbound). The presence of increased quantities of unbound, oxidizable iron in the CNS leads to an overall shift in redox balance favoring oxidation and lipid peroxidation in individuals with aceruloplasminemia (Figure 10–1) (Miyajima et al., 1996; Yoshida et al., 2000). In addition, there are mitochondrial enzyme abnormalities (Kono et al., 2000; Miyajima et al., 2002) and oxidatively modified glial fibrillary acid protein, suggestive of glial dysfunction (Kaneko et al., 2002).

On the cellular level, iron is deposited predominantly in terminal astrocytic processes in association with cerebral capillaries; astrocytic cell bodies are also noted to have excess iron (Gonzalez-Cuyar et al., 2008). Gonzalez-Cuyar et al. demonstrated iron in aceruloplasminemia as small, granular structures staining intensely for Fe^{2+}.

Macroscopically, iron deposition is present throughout the cerebral cortex, cerebellum, and brainstem; but it is pathologically most heavily concentrated in the caudate nucleus, putamen, and dentate nucleus of the cerebellum, with moderate

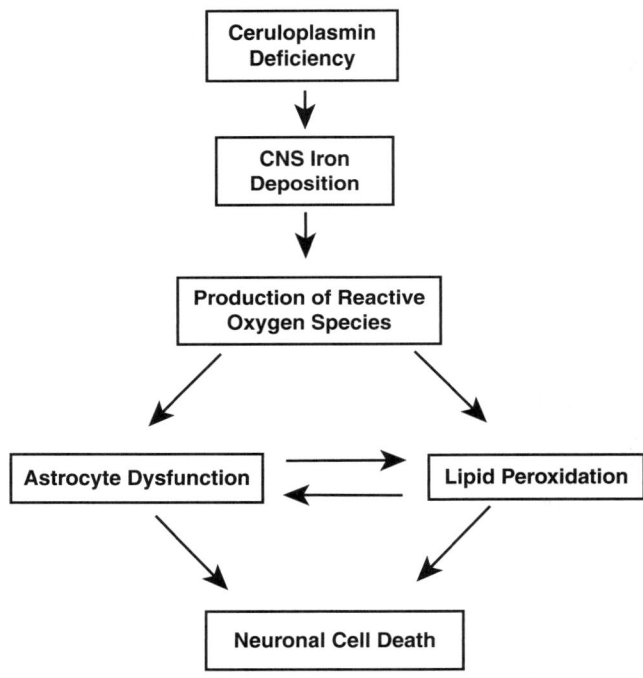

FIGURE 10–1. Diagram of processes leading to neuronal death in aceruloplasminemia.

TABLE 10–1. Pathological Localization of Iron Deposition in Aceruloplasminemia

Liver	+++
Myocardium	+++
Pancreas	+++
Thyroid	++
Kidney	++
Pituitary	++
CNS	
Caudate nucleus	+++
Putamen	+++
Dentate (cerebellum)	+++
Globus pallidus	++
Thalamus	++
Hippocampus	++
Red nucleus	++
Cerebellar Purkinje cell layer	++
Neocortex	+
Cerebellar granule cell layer	+
Substantia nigra	+

+++, severe; ++, moderate; +, mild.

staining in the globus pallidus, thalamus, and hippocampus. Peripherally, iron deposition is ubiquitous but most concentrated in the liver, myocardium, and pancreas. Table 10–1 shows the regions of greatest pathologically-defined iron deposition in aceruloplasminemia (from Gonzalez-Cuyar et al., 2008).

PREVALENCE AND GENETICS

Aceruloplasminemia is an autosomal recessive disorder. To date, approximately 40 mutations of the gene have been described. Frequency studies have been performed in Japan, and the estimated prevalence of aceruloplasminemia in this population was estimated at 1 per 2,000,000 adults (Miyajima et al., 1999), with heterozygote frequency among the general population in Japan of 0.1% (Daimon et al., 1997). Prevalence studies have not been conducted outside of Japan.

CLINICAL FEATURES AND EVALUATION

Aceruloplasminemia has characteristic systemic and CNS manifestations, although expression of the symptoms is variable from individual to individual, even within the same family. The largest case series of individuals with aceruloplasminemia was published by Miyajima et al. (2003; Miyajima, 2003). In this population of 45 Japanese individuals, while onset of systemic disease (anemia, diabetes) occurred most typically before the age of 40, 98% of neurological presentations occurred after the age of 40. Neurological symptoms included ataxia and dysarthria in 86%; hyperkinesia such as chorea, blepharospasm, or dystonia in 60%; parkinsonism (bradykinesia and rigidity) in 41%; and dementia in 25%.

Laboratory Evaluation

Clinical evaluation of an individual with suspected aceruloplasminemia starts with evaluation of serum and urine markers of copper and iron metabolism. Atypical cases with nondiagnostic laboratory or neuroimaging findings have been reported, and these cases are discussed later (see "Atypical Cases"). In a typical case of aceruloplasminemia, ceruloplasmin is absent in the serum and undetectable. This contrasts with the finding in Wilson disease, in which production of secreted ceruloplasmin is defective but can still occur. In Wilson disease, consequently, serum ceruloplasmin levels are low but often detectable (Xu et al., 2004). Serum copper is typically low in both Wilson disease and aceruloplasminemia; however, urine copper in aceruloplasminemia is normal (and would be expected to be dramatically elevated in Wilson disease).

Serum markers of iron metabolism are an important part of the evaluation of aceruloplasminemia. Individuals with aceruloplasminemia have a normocytic, normochromic anemia with low serum iron, despite having a high ferritin level suggestive of tissue iron overload. Plasma ceruloplasmin ferroxidase activity, a measure of ceruloplasmin's capacity to oxidize ferrous iron (Fe^{2+}) to ferric iron (Fe^{3+}), is absent (Kono and Miyajima, 2006). Table 10–2 shows expected copper and iron metabolism laboratory findings in aceruloplasminemia.

In a case in which differentiation from Wilson disease is difficult, a liver biopsy can clearly define the two disorders. Iron in the liver is commonly measured by determining the hepatic iron index. First, hepatic iron is determined as micromoles per gram of dry weight. The hepatic iron index is calculated by dividing hepatic iron concentration by age (in years) of the individual. Individuals with

TABLE 10–2. Expected Laboratory Findings in Hereditary Aceruloplasminemia and Wilson Disease

LABORATORY	ACERULOPLASMINEMIA	WILSON DISEASE	NORMAL
Serum ceruloplasmin	Undetectable	5–20 µg/dl[a]	20–80 mg/dl
Serum copper	<10 µg/dl	<70 µg/dl[a]	80–160 µg/dl
Serum iron	<45 µg/dl	10–180 µg/dl	10–180 µg/dl
Serum ferritin	850–4,000 ng/ml	30–200 ng/ml	30–200 ng/ml
Plasma ceruloplasmin ferroxidase activity	Undetectable	500–680 U/l	500–680 U/l

[a]Typically in a low detectable range but may not be detectable by some laboratories.

aceruloplasminemia typically show a hepatic iron index of >1.3, while normal healthy adults typically show an index of <1.1. Despite iron overload, individuals with aceruloplasminemia do not develop cirrhosis from the disorder, in contrast to Wilson disease, which typically shows chronic hepatitis or cirrhosis (Scott et al., 1978; Hoffman, 2008).

Imaging

Aceruloplasminemia is included among a clinically defined grouping of disorders with neurodegeneration with brain iron accumulation (NBIA). Known causes of NBIA include pantothenate kinase–associated neurodegeneration (Chapter 8), neuroferritinopathy (Chapter 9), infantile neuroaxonal dystrophy (Chapter 8), and aceruloplasminemia. Recent research suggests that MRI T2* and fast spin echo sequences may be used to distinguish the various genetic causes of brain iron deposition (McNeill et al., 2008). In typical cases of aceruloplasminemia, uniform iron deposition is noted in the caudate nucleus and thalamus. Unlike other causes of NBIA, cavitation is typically not seen (McNeill et al., 2008).

Molecular Genetic Testing

The ceruloplasmin gene is the only gene known to be associated with the clinical syndrome of aceruloplasminemia. Sequence analysis of the ceruloplasmin gene is at present performed on a research basis. In a series of 45 patients (Miyajima, 2003; Miyajima et al., 2003), 92% of individuals with suspected aceruloplasminemia based on clinical findings, laboratory markers, and imaging had detectable sequence abnormalities. Mutations in the disorder are spread throughout the gene, with no specific identified genetic "hot spot." In almost all cases, mutations cause defects in the ceruloplasmin gene, resulting in absence of the ceruloplasmin protein. However, a few rare cases of compound heterozygotes with normal ceruloplasm levels related to nonfunctional, secreted ceruloplasm have been described. No clinical tests are currently available.

Screening for Anemia and Diabetes

In individuals in whom there is a presumptive diagnosis of aceruloplasminemia on the basis of laboratory results, screening for these comorbid systemic problems is appropriate. A complete blood count should be performed to detect the normochromic, normocytic anemia associated with the disorder. Serum glucose, hemoglobin A_{1c}, and possibly glucose tolerance tests should also be considered to evaluate for diabetes mellitus.

Atypical Cases

Rarely, this disorder may present with atypical laboratory findings. Takeuchi et al. (2002) described an individual with typical symptoms of aceruloplasminemia but normal serum ceruloplasmin levels. Measurement of serum ceruloplasmin ferroxidase activity revealed no ferroxidase activity. The individual was found to be a compound heterozygote, with one allele encoding a nonfunctioning, secreted ceruloplasmin protein and the other allele encoding a nonfunctioning, nonsecreted ceruloplasmin protein. Another group (Kono and Miyajima, 2006) described an individual with retinal degeneration and diabetes who similarly secreted a form of ceruloplasmin with no ferroxidase activity.

Although it has not been described, a defect in the CNS-specific, GPI-anchored form of the protein might present with normal serum ceruloplasmin and ceruloplasmin ferroxidase activity and a purely CNS presentation of iron overload.

Almost all imaging studies describe the typical findings of iron overload; however, these can occasionally be absent. One recent case was reported of an individual with absent ceruloplasmin, anemia, hepatic iron overload, mood changes, chorea, and ataxia, who had no visible signs of cerebral iron overload on T2-weighted images and T2* imaging (Skidmore, 2008). In this individual, despite lack of visible iron deposition, progressive atrophy of the basal ganglia, thalamus, and cerebral cortex were noted along with the progression of symptoms. Despite the lack of visible cerebral iron, the patient had a modest response to chelation therapy, suggesting that iron might still be the etiological cause of CNS insult.

It is likely that other variants of this disorder will be described; therefore, the constellation of anemia, diabetes, and development of a movement disorder should warrant evaluation of not just ceruloplasmin levels but also the serum iron profile and serum ferroxidase activity to fully characterize the nature of the disorder and exclude aceruloplasminemia.

TREATMENT OF ACERULOPLASMINEMIA

Due to the small number of cases of this rare disorder, large, well-controlled clinical trials have not been performed and the majority of treatments have been evaluated in individual cases in an unblinded setting. Chelation with iron-chelating agents is the primary proposed treatment for aceruloplasminemia. Intravenous desferrioxamine can decrease serum ferritin concentration and liver and brain iron stores, and can prevent progression of neurological symptoms (Miyajima et al., 1997). While anemia can be exacerbated acutely with chelation therapy, in the study of Miyajima et al. (1997) the chronic effect of chelation was a slight improvement in the anemia, as well as improvement in markers of diabetes. Plasma markers of lipid peroxidation also improved. Coinfusion of fresh frozen plasma (FFP) during chelation (Yonekawa et al., 1999) has been proposed to be potentially helpful; immediately after infusion of FFP, serum iron concentration increases due to the presence of ceruloplasmin in the FFP. Treatment with desferrioxamine and FFP requires frequent intravenous infusions and can be complicated. Other, newer oral chelating agents that are able to cross the blood–brain barrier have been used in individual cases (Skidmore et al., 2008).

Oral zinc sulfate (Kuhn et al., 2007) and vitamin E have both been proposed (Fraga and Oteiza, 2002). Proposed treatments for aceruloplasminemia, along with proposed doses, are listed in Table 10–3.

TABLE 10–3. Proposed Treatments for Aceruloplasminemia

TREATMENT	DOSE	BENEFITS
Desferrioxamine	500 mg dissolved in 100 ml of isotonic saline biweekly over 6–10 weeks for 6–10 months, do not start if hemoglobin concentration is <9 and maintain hemoglobin concentration >9	Increased MRI iron signal intensity, improved anemia and diabetes, decreased plasma markers of lipid peroxidation
Fresh frozen plasma	15 ml/kg biweekly for 6–10 months	Temporary increase in serum iron, improved neurological symptoms
Zinc sulfate	50 mg/day po, increasing to 200 mg/day po	Anecdotal: prevention of iron-related neurodegeneration
Vitamin E	Not established	Anecdotal: prevention of iron-related neurodegeneration

MRI, magnetic resonance imaging; po, per os (by mouth).

CONCLUSIONS

Aceruloplasminemia is a rare, usually autosomal recessive, disorder of iron metabolism resulting in cerebral and systemic iron deposition. Laboratory markers of the disorder include absent ceruloplasmin with low serum copper but normal urine copper, and absent serum ceruloplasmin ferroxidase activity. Liver biopsy typically shows significant iron overload. Almost all individuals with the disorder have presented with visible cerebral iron deposition in the CNS localized primarily in the basal ganglia and cerebellum. Rare heterozygous presentations as well as individuals with normal ceruloplasmin levels and a single individual without visible iron overload on neuroimaging have all been described, suggesting that recognition of the full spectrum of this disorder is still developing. Proposed treatments including chelation, FFP, oral zinc, and vitamin E have been described to be helpful in individual cases.

REFERENCES

Daimon M, Yamatani K, Igarashi M, et al. (1995) Fine structure of the human ceruloplasmin gene. Biochem Biophys Res Commun 208:1028–1035.

Daimon M, Yamatani K, Tominaga M, Manaka H, Kato T, Sasaki H (1997) NIDDM with a ceruloplasmin gene mutation. Diabetes Care 20:678.

Fraga CG, Oteiza PI (2002) Iron toxicity and antioxidant nutrients. Toxicology 180(1): 123–132.

Gonzalez-Cuyar LF, Perry G, Miyajima H, Atwood CS, Riveros-Angel M, Lyons PF, Siedlak SL, Smith MA, Castellani RJ (2008) Redox active iron accumulation in aceruloplasminemia. Neuropathology 28:466–471.

Hoffman R (2008) Disorders of iron metabolism: iron deficiency and iron overload. In: Hoffman R, Furie B, Benz EJ Jr, McGlave P, Silberstein LE, Shattil SJ (eds.) Hematology: Basic Principles and Practice, 5th ed. Churchill Livingstone, New York.

Jeong SY, David S (2003) Glycosylphosphatidylinositolanchored ceruloplasmin is required for iron efflux from cells in the central nervous system. J Biol Chem 278:27144–27148.

Kaneko K, Nakamura A, Yoshida K, Kametani F, Higuchi K, Ikeda S (2002) Glial fibrillary acidic protein is greatly modified by oxidative stress in aceruloplasminemia brain. Free Radic Res 36:303–306.

Klomp LWJ, Gitlin JD (1996) Expression of the ceruloplasmin gene in the human retina and rain: implications for the pathogenic model in aceruloplasminemia. Hum Mol Genet 5:1989–1996.

Kono S, Miyajima H (2006) Molecular and pathological basis of aceruloplasmineinia. Biol Res 39:15.

Kono S, Miyajima H, Takahashi Y, et al. (2000) Defective electron transfer in complexes I and IV in patients with aceruloplasminemia. J Neurol Sci 182:57–60.

Koschinsky ML, Funk WD, van Oost BA, MacGillivray RT (1986) Complete cDNA sequence of human preceruloplasmin. Proc Natl Acad Sci USA 83:5086–5090.

Kuhn J, Bewermeyer H, Miyajima H, Takahashi Y, Kuhn KF, Hoogenraad TU (2007) Treatment of symptomatic heterozygous aceruloplasminemia with oral zinc sulphate. Brain Dev 29:450–453.

McNeill A, Birchall D, Hayflick SJ, Gregory A, Schenk JF, Zimmerman EA, Shang H, Miyajima H, Chinnery PF (2008) T2* and FSE MRI distinguishes four subtypes of neurodegeneration with brain iron accumulation. Neurology 70(18):1614–1619.

Miyajima H (2003) Aceruloplasminemia, an iron metabolic disorder. Neuropathology 23(4):345–350.

Miyajima H, Kohno S, Takahashi Y, Yonekawa O, Kanno T (1999) Estimation of the gene frequency of aceruloplasminemia in Japan. Neurology 53:617–619.

Miyajima H, Kono S, Takahashi Y, Sugimoto M (2002) Increased lipid peroxidation and mitochondrial dysfunction in aceruloplasminemic brains. Blood Cells Mol Dis 29: 433–438.

Miyajima H, Takahashi Y, Kamata T, Shimizu H, Sakai N, Gitlin JD (1997) Use of desferrioxamine in the treatment of aceruloplasminemia. Ann Neurol 41:404–407.

Miyajima H, Takahashi Y, Serizawa M, Kaneko E, Gitlin JD. (1996). Increased plasma lipid peroxidation in patients with aceruloplasminemia. Free Radic Biol Med 20(5): 757–760.

Miyajima H, Takahashi Y, Kono S (2003) Aceruloplasminemia, an inherited disorder of iron metabolism. Biometals 16(1):205–213.

Patel BN, David S (1997) A novel glycophosphatidylinositol-anchored form of ceruloplasmin is expressed by mammalian astrocytes. J Biol Chem 272:20185–20190.

Royle NJ, Irwin DM, Koschinsky ML, MacGillivray RT, Hamerton JL (1987) Human genes encoding prothrombin and ceruloplasmin map to 11p11-q12 and 3q21-24, respectively. Somat Cell Mol Genet 13:285–292.

Scott J, Gollan JL, Samourian S, Sherlock S (1978) Wilson's disease, presenting as chronic active hepatitis. Gastroenterology 74:645–651.

Skidmore FM, Drago V, Foster P, Schmalfuss IM, Heilman KM, Streiff RR. (2008). Aceruloplasminaemia with progressive atrophy without brain iron overload: treatment with oral chelation. J Neurol Neurosurg Psychiatry. 79(4):467–470.

Takeuchi Y, Yoshikawa M, Tsujino T, Kohno S, Tsukamoto N, Shiroi A, Kikuchi E, Fukui H, Miyajima H (2002) A case of aceruloplasminaemia: abnormal serum ceruloplasmin protein without ferroxidase activity. J Neurol Neurosurg Psychiatry 72: 543–545.

Xu X, Pin S, Gathinji M, Fuchs R, Harris ZL (2004) Aceruloplasminemia: an inherited neurodegenerative disease with impairment of iron homeostasis. Ann N Y Acad Sci 1012:299–305.

Yonekawa M, Okabe T, Asamoto Y, Ohta M (1999) A case of hereditary ceruloplasmin deficiency with iron deposition in the brain associated with chorea, dementia, diabetes mellitus and retinal pigmentation: administration of fresh-frozen human plasma. Eur Neurol 42:157–162.

Yoshida K, Kaneko K, Miyajima H, et al. (2000) Increased lipid peroxidation in the brains of aceruloplasminemic patients. J Neurol Sci 175:91–95.

11

Chorea in Prion Diseases

Nayana Lahiri, BSc, MBBS, MRCP;
Simon Mead, BMBChir, MBBS, PhD;
and Sarah J. Tabrizi, BSc, MBChB, FRCP, PhD

INTRODUCTION

The prion diseases, or transmissible spongiform encephalopathies, are a group of rare, progressive neurodegenerative conditions that affect both humans and other animals.

Mammalian prions ("small proteinaceous infectious particles that resist inactivation by procedures which modify nucleic acids"), were purified by Prusiner (1982) and are the causative agents of prion diseases. The protein purified by Prusiner, which he termed the "prion protein" (PrP), exists in at least two conformational states. The normal protein, PrP^C ("C" for cellular), is a cell surface protein expressed in a wide range of cell types, particularly in neuronal and immune cells. It is protease-sensitive and soluble in detergents. The pathogenic prion protein, PrP^{Sc} ("Sc" for scrapie), is a conformational isoform of PrP^C and is associated with prion disease. It is protease-resistant and insoluble in detergents. PrP^{Sc} is thought to be derived from PrP^C by an autocatalytic posttranslational process, which accounts for its infectious properties (Collinge, 2001). Human prion diseases show marked clinical phenotypic variability. A major factor in explaining this diversity is the existence of distinct prion strains. Prion strains, analogous to strains of bacteria or viruses in microbiology, are distinguished by pathological and clinical characteristics and are associated with different biochemical properties of PrP^{Sc} (Bruce, 1993).

Symptoms of prion diseases generally include cognitive impairment and a movement disorder. Prion diseases are included in the differential diagnosis of Huntington disease, particularly as the inherited forms of prion disease all have an autosomal dominant inheritance pattern. Chorea forms part of the diagnostic criteria of variant Creutzfeldt-Jakob disease (vCJD), but it has also been described in a number of patients with other human prion diseases, notably the inherited prion diseases. Consequently, prion disease should be considered in the differential diagnosis of a patient presenting with chorea. This chapter gives a general overview of the clinical features, investigations, and pathophysiology of the human prion diseases, as well as reviewing specific case reports describing patients for whom chorea was a prominent feature.

CLINICAL FEATURES

Prion diseases of humans include acquired diseases such as vCJD and kuru, iatrogenic CJD and inherited syndromes caused by mutation of the prion protein gene such as Gerstmann-Sträussler-Scheinker syndrome (GSS) and fatal familial insomnia (FFI). Some prion diseases are etiologically unexplained, termed "sporadic Creutzfeldt-Jakob disease" (sCJD) (see Table 11–1) (Rossor et al., 2009). These conditions form a spectrum of diseases with overlapping signs and symptoms.

Sporadic Prion Disease

Typically, sCJD is a rapidly progressive multifocal dementia. It remains the most common of the human prion diseases, although it is still rare, with an annual incidence of one to two cases per million, with an equal incidence in men and women (Masters et al., 1979). It generally affects those between the ages of 45 and 75 years, with peak incidence in the 60s. It has a rapid clinical course, with a median survival of 4–6 months (Pocchiari et al., 2004). Diagnostic criteria require a rapidly progressive dementia and a minimum of 2 of 4 additional symptoms of myoclonus, visual or cerebellar disturbances, pyramidal or other extrapyramidal dysfunction, and akinetic mutism (WHO, 2003) (see Table 11–2). Prodromal features occur in approximately one-third of cases and include fatigue, insomnia, depression, weight loss, headaches, general malaise, and ill-defined pain sensations.

The etiology of sCJD is unclear: It may arise from somatic mutations of *PRNP* or spontaneous conversion of PrP^{C} to PrP^{Sc}; further, some patients with sCJD may

TABLE 11–1. Classification of Human Prion Disease

ETIOLOGY	PHENOTYPE	PROPORTION OF CASES/ LOCATION
Sporadic		
Unknown: random distribution worldwide, incidence of 1–2 per million per annum	Sporadic CJD: subacute myoclonic form and range of atypical forms, multiple distinct prion strains associated with distinct clinicopathological phenotypes	~85%
Acquired		
Iatrogenic infection with human prions via medical or surgical procedures, human cadaveric–derived pituitary hormones, tissue grafts, and contaminated neurosurgical instruments	Iatrogenic CJD: typical CJD when direct CNS exposure, ataxic onset when peripheral infections	<5% (most for United States, United Kingdom, France, and Japan)
Exposure to human prions via cannibalism	Kuru	Unique to small area of Papua New Guinea: major epidemic in 1950s
Enviromental exposure (dietary) to BSE prion strain	vCJD	Total to date ~200, mainly in United Kingdom but now reported from a number of countries
Iatrogenic infection via blood transfusion from healthy donor infected with vCJD prions	Secondary vCJD	United Kingdom only to date
Inherited		
Autosomal dominantly inherited conditions with high penetrance, all forms have germline *PRNP* coding mutations	Extremely variable: over 30 mutations identified, includes familial CJD, GSS, and FFI	~10%–15%

BSE, bovine spongiform encephalopathy; CJD, Creutzfeldt-Jakob disease; vCJD, variant CJD; CNS, central nervous system; FFI, fatal familial insomnia; GSS, Gerstmann-Sträussler-Scheinker syndrome.
Source: Adapted from Rosser et al. (2009).

TABLE 11–2. Diagnostic Criteria for Sporadic CJD

Possible	• Progressive dementia and
	• EEG atypical or not known and
	• Duration <2 years and
	• At least two of the following clinical features
	  ○ Myoclonus
	  ○ Visual or cerebellar disturbance
	  ○ Pyramidal/extrapyramidal dysfunction
	  ○ Akinetic mutism

Probable (in the absence of an alternative diagnosis from routine investigation)	• Progressive dementia and
	• At least two of the following four clinical features
	  ○ Myoclonus
	  ○ Visual or cerebellar disturbance
	  ○ Pyramidal/extrapyramidal dysfunction
	  ○ Akinetic mutism and
	• A typical EEG, whatever the clinical duration of the disease, and/or
	• A positive 14-3-3 assay for CSF and
	• A clinical duration to death of <2 years

Definite CJD	• Neuropathological confirmation and/or • Confirmation of protease-resistant prion protein (immunohistochemistry or Western blot) and/or • Presence of scrapie-associated fibrils

CJD, Creutzfeldt-Jakob disease; CSF, cerebrospinal fluid; EEG, electroencephalogram.
Source: Adapted from WHO (2003).

have an unrecognized environmental source. Investigation of the prion protein gene (*PRNP)* has revealed a common PrP polymorphism at codon 129, where either methionine (Met) or valine (Val) can be encoded. Homozygosity at this point has been shown to confer genetic susceptibility to acquired and sporadic prion disease (Collinge et al., 1991; Palmer et al., 1991). Codon 129 genotype also has a key role in determining clinicopathological phenotypes, in part via an effect on selection of particular prion strains (Collinge, 1999; Collinge and Clarke, 2007).

Acquired Prion Disease

Kuru

Kuru is an acquired human prion disease affecting the Fore linguistic group in the Eastern Highlands of Papua New Guinea. Kuru predominantly affects adult women and children of both sexes. It is transmitted when the brain and internal organs of deceased relatives are consumed during cannibalistic feasts. It has been speculated that the trigger for the kuru epidemic was a member of the population with sCJD. The recycling of prions in this relatively isolated population led to a substantial epidemic that was the major cause of death among children and adult women in the region, although cannibalistic practises ended by 1960. More than 2,700 cases were reported between 1957 and 2004 (Collinge et al., 2006). The mean incubation period for development of kuru is 12 years, although incubation periods can exceed 50 years (Collinge et al., 2006).

The onset of disease ranges from age 5 to over 60. The mean clinical duration of illness is 12 months, with a range of 3 months to 3 years. The condition presents predominantly with a progressive cerebellar ataxia. Dementia is clearly a feature of the established disease (Collinge et al., 2008).

Iatrogenic CJD

Iatrogenic routes for the transmission of CJD include inadequately sterilized intracerebral electrodes, dura mater and corneal grafting, and the use of cadaveric pituitary-derived growth hormone or gonadotrophin.

The incubation for intracerebral cases is much shorter than that of peripherally acquired forms.

vCJD

A new variant of CJD was first reported in 1996 (Will et al., 1996). vCJD has been established to be caused by exposure to the prion strain which causes bovine spongiform encephalopathy (BSE) (Collinge et al., 1996). This finding raised the possibility of an epidemic of vCJD in countries that have had BSE in their cattle and occurring as a result of dietary exposure to BSE (Collinge, 1999).

The clinical presentation is very different from that of sCJD (see Table 11–3). The median age is 26 years and the median duration of illness is 13 months. Early in the course of the disease, psychiatric symptoms predominate, with behavioral change, dysphoria, irritability, anxiety, and insomnia being common. Gait disturbance and slurred speech are common early neurological features (Spencer et al., 2002), and in most patients a progressive cerebellar syndrome develops. Myoclonus and dementia occur later in the clinical course.

Inherited Prion Disease

Inherited prion diseases are responsible for 10–15% of the incidence of human prion disease, and are all accounted for by mutations in the prion protein gene (*PRNP*). More than 30 disease-causing mutations have been described (Figure 11–1), and they are inherited in an autosomal dominant fashion. These are either point mutations, leading to an amino acid substitution or premature stop codon, or alteration in the number of octapeptide repeats (OPRI). The most

TABLE 11–3. Diagnostic Criteria for Variant CJD

Criteria I	A	Progressive neuropsychiatric disorder
	B	Duration of illness <6 months
	C	Routine investigations do not suggest an alternative diagnosis
	D	No history of potential iatrogenic exposure
	E	No evidence of a familial form of CJD
Criteria II	A	Early psychiatric symptoms
	B	Persistent painful sensory symptoms
	C	Ataxia
	D	Myoclonus or chorea or dystonia
	E	Dementia
Criteria III	A	EEG does not show typical appearance of sporadic CJD (or no EEG performed)
	B	MRI brain scan shows bilateral symmetrical pulvinar high signal
Criteria IV	A	Positive tonsil biopsy

Definite: IA and neuropathological confirmation of variant CJD

Probable: I and 4/5 of II and IIIA and IIIB *or* I and IVA

Possible: I and 4/5 of II and IIIA

CJD, Creutzfeldt-Jakob disease; EEG, electroencephalogram; MRI, magnetic resonance imaging.
Source: Adapted from WHO (2003).

common worldwide *PRNP* mutations are E200K, D178N, P102L, and OPRI (for review, see Mead, 2006). Approximately 50% of hereditary cases lack a clear family history of a similar disorder. Some patients with mutations were initially misidentified as "sporadic" cases as they had no relevant family history. This might be due to reduced penetrance of the disease, misdiagnosis of affected family members, or occurrence of a new mutation.

Prior to the availability of molecular genetic diagnosis, inherited prion diseases were subclassified as GSS, FFI, or familial CJD.

GSS presents in adult life (20–60 years) with progressive limb and truncal ataxia, dysarthria, personality change, and cognitive decline. GSS typically differs from CJD by exhibiting early and prominent cerebellar ataxia, longer duration of illness, and the presence of morphologically distinct multicentric amyloid plaques in the cerebellum (Collins et al., 2001).

FFI also affects adults, with an average age at onset of 50 years. The condition is characterized by insomnia, dysautonomia, and motor deficits. Autonomic dysfunction occurs early and includes increased lacrimation, salivation, sweating, raised body temperature, and impotence in males. Ataxia, dysarthria, and dysphagia

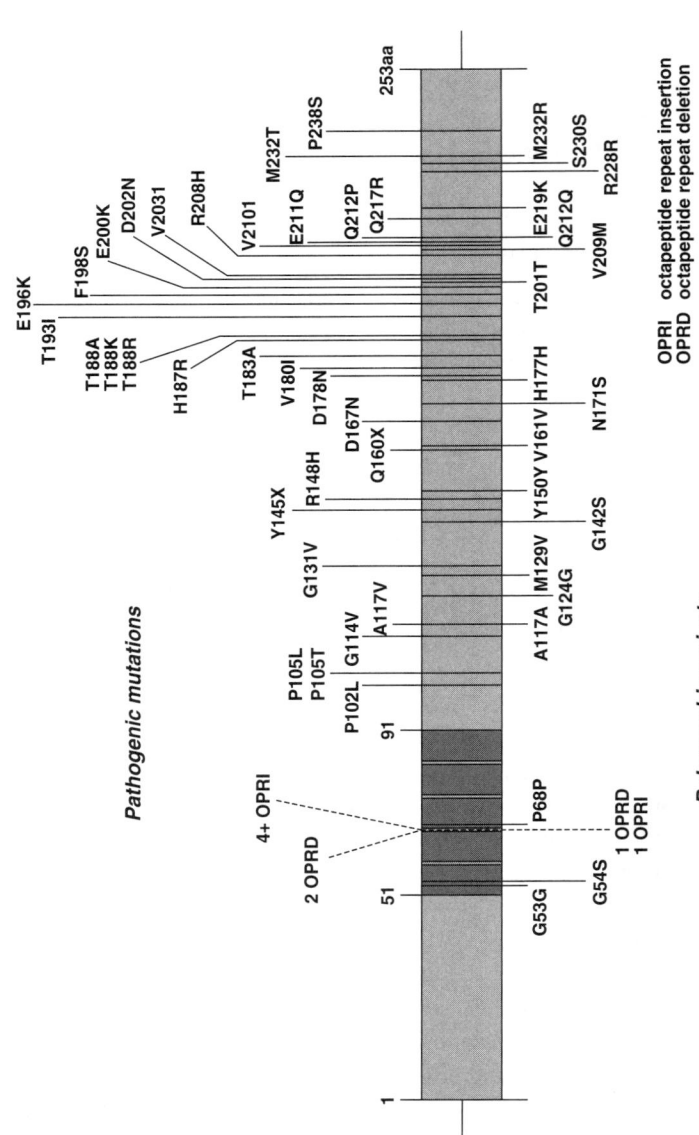

FIGURE 11–1. Definite or suspected pathogenic mutations are shown above this representation of the prion protein gene. Neutral or prion disease susceptibility/modifying polymorphisms are shown below. This figure appears courtesy of Dr John Beck.

are among the early motor signs, while cognitive functions remain relatively spared until late in the course of the illness. The clinical course runs over 7–18 months. It is mostly associated with a missense mutation at codon 178 of *PRNP* (Lugaresi et al., 1986; Montagna et al., 2003).

Familial CJD presents like sCJD. The E200K/129M mutation accounts for approximately 70% of familial CJD cases worldwide. All patients have dementia, with a large proportion showing cerebellar signs and myoclonus.

There is, however, a large overlap between these three inherited prion disease syndromes; and since the advent of genetic testing, it may be more accurate to categorize patients according to genotype. It is also clear that some of the mutations are associated with particular clinical phenotypes, while others are phenotypically heterogeneous. For example, E200K mutations typically have a clinical presentation very similar to that of sCJD (Kahana et al., 1991), whereas patients with OPRI mutations can have extremely variable phenotypes.

With OPRI mutations, both the number of repeats and the order of the repeat elements may vary (Croes et al., 2004). Clinical features are largely determined by the number of repeats. It is likely that small OPRI (i.e., 1 to 3 extra repeats) are neutral, rare polymorphisms that have been detected in sCJD cases. Patients with 4 extra repeats have a later-onset disease (average age 67 years) with a shorter duration (4 months) and generally follow a similar course to sCJD, with a rapidly progressive dementia, ataxia, myoclonus, and periodic sharp wave complexes (PSWCs) on electroencephalogram (EEG). Pathologically, changes are also consistent with those of sCJD, including spongiform degeneration, astrogliosis, and neuronal loss (Vital et al., 1998). In contrast, patients with 6 to 9 extra repeats develop the disease earlier (average 35 years). They can expect to have a longer duration of illness (8 years) characterized by a slowly progressive mental deterioration with cerebellar and extrapyramidal signs, often without PSWCs. Neuropathologically, they display PrP amyloid plaques located in the molecular layer of the cerebellum and the cerebral gray matter. These changes are similar to GSS (Vital et al., 1998).

CHOREA AND OTHER MOVEMENT DISORDERS IN PRION DISEASE

Approximately 90% of patients develop a movement disorder during the course of their illness. The most common movement disorders associated with all human prion diseases are myoclonus and ataxia. However, dystonia, tremor, hemiballismus, and atypical parkinsonian syndromes (i.e., corticobasal degeneration and supranuclear palsy) have all been described in a significant number of patients (Maltête et al., 2006). Chorea has generally been reported as a later-stage characteristic, but there are a number of reports of chorea occurring at an early stage or as an initial manifestation of human prion disease in sCJD, vCJD, and inherited prion diseases (Bowen et al., 2000; Moore et al., 2001; McKee and Talbot, 2003; Donmez et al., 2005). The prominence of chorea in prion disease is consistent with the observation that the caudate nucleus and the thalamus are the noncortical areas most commonly affected by prion lesions (Maltête et al., 2006) as these areas are implicated in the mechanisms of chorea.

sCJD

Despite the internationally accepted criteria for diagnosis (WHO, 2003), symptoms can be extremely variable and it can be difficult to distinguish sCJD from other neurodegenerative diseases on a clinical basis during the patient's lifetime. This is made more challenging by the fact that no readily available, accurate, surrogate markers for the disease exist. Clinical characterization of movement disorders in sCJD may assist in making an accurate diagnosis (Weller and Aguzzi, 2009).

A recent study carried out at the German Surveillance unit for Spongiform Encephalopathies (Edler et al., 2009) aimed to improve the clinical characterization of sCJD. They reviewed the medical records of 143 patients referred to the unit. One hundred of these were neuropathologically confirmed as having sCJD, 29 were confirmed as having Alzheimer disease, 7 had dementia with Lewy bodies, and 7 received other diagnoses. The aim of the study was to determine the value of motor disturbances in diagnosing sCJD. The most common movement disorders in the sCJD group were gait disturbances (80%), myoclonus (80%), and cerebellar ataxia (77%). Ataxia and dysmetria, along with an absence of hypokinesia, suggested a diagnosis of sCJD rather than one of Alzheimer disease or dementia with Lewy bodies. Interestingly, 9% of patients with CJD had athetosis and 11% had chorea. Unfortunately, there are no further details as to the specific characteristics of chorea in this study.

It is unusual for chorea to be a presenting or early feature of sCJD (Will and Matthews, 1984; Rabinovici et al., 2006). However, Donmez et al. (2005) described a 47-year-old woman who presented with generalized chorea, dystonic posture, and myoclonic jerks. A diagnosis of sCJD was made on the basis of clinical course, EEG findings, and the presence of 14-3-3 protein in the cerebrospinal fluid (CSF), although this was not neuropathologically confirmed *post mortem*. Alternative diagnoses at the onset of the disease were all excluded with appropriate laboratory tests. This case exemplifies the challenges of making a diagnosis of sCJD when there is atypical clinical onset.

vCJD

The early stages of vCJD are dominated by psychiatric symptoms or a combination of psychiatric and neurological symptoms. Chorea is more common in vCJD and forms part of the diagnostic criteria (see Table 11–3). In a review of the first 100 cases diagnosed as having vCJD at the National CJD Surveillance Unit (Spencer et al., 2002), chorea was a less common feature (occurring in 25–50 patients) and occurred between 6 and 11 months from the onset of the illness. A number of other movement disorders, myoclonus, and ataxia were more common and occurred earlier in the disease course.

There have also been a number of case reports of patients presenting with chorea in the early course of the disease (Bowen et al., 2000; McKee and Talbot, 2003). Bowen et al. described a 28-year-old woman who initially presented with behavioral disturbances and cognitive decline and gross chorea 4 months after the onset of the illness. Physical examination showed florid, generalized chorea with superimposed dysarthria and a predominantly axial ataxia. Diagnosis of vCJD was confirmed with a positive assay for 14-3-3 protein in the CSF and a tonsil biopsy showing the abnormal isoform of cellular prion protein.

McKee and Talbot (2003) reported the case of a 27-year-old man in whom chorea was the presenting feature of the disease and was not preceded by any psychiatric or behavioral features. On examination 2 months into the course of the illness, he had continuous choreiform movements of all four limbs and the neck. This became significantly more florid within several weeks, and he deteriorated with dementia and sensory symptoms. He died 8 months after his initial presentation, and a diagnosis of vCJD was confirmed *post mortem*.

Both of these cases highlight that vCJD should be considered in the differential diagnosis of chorea in younger patients.

Inherited Prion Diseases

"Huntington disease-like 1" (HDL1) is a historical term for an autosomal dominant, progressive, adult-onset, neurodegenerative disorder. In the initial report of this condition (Moore et al., 2001), cases had an early adult–onset (mean 29.7 years) syndrome consisting of personality change, cognitive decline, motor disturbance with chorea, dysarthria, and ataxia together with atrophy of the basal ganglia. Chorea in this pedigree was a prominent clinical feature, being present in 4 of 6 affected individuals. In the absence of a genetic diagnosis of Huntington disease, the *PRNP* gene was sequenced; and all affected family members examined were found to have an octapeptide repeat expansion of 8 extra repeats (8-OPRI). A previous report of a family with 8-OPRI was described as having prominent psychiatric features (Laplanche et al., 1999). One member of this family had "motor discharges" causing falls, but none of the other affected family members was diagnosed as having chorea. This stark contrast in clinical features between families with the same mutation highlights the phenotypic heterogeneity of inherited prion diseases and the difficulty in making comparisons between families seen in different countries and by different neurologists.

Interestingly, the first described mutation of *PRNP* was a 6-OPRI (Owen et al., 1989) in a U.K. pedigree. This pedigree has been updated and expanded over the years through contact with the National Prion Clinic (www.nationalprionclinic.org) (Collinge et al., 1992), and there now is information available from eight generations (Mead et al., 2006). Six out of 86 affected members of this family have had chorea documented as a significant feature. Myoclonus was much more frequently observed in 30 individuals.

Chorea is a less prominent feature but has been described with other *PRNP* mutations. Libyan Jews living in Israel have a high prevalence of familial CJD caused by the E200K mutations. In a study of 65 heterozygotes, only 4 had chorea as a prominent feature (Meiner et al., 1997).

INVESTIGATIONS IN HUMAN PRION DISEASES

sCJD

Routine hematological and biochemical investigations are normal. Routine CSF examination is normal; but the detection of 14-3-3 in the CSF has a high degree of sensitivity and specificity for the diagnosis of sCJD, and this may be increased by the assessment of other CSF markers, namely tau, S-100b, and neuron-specific enolase (Sanchez-Juan et al., 2006).

Magnetic resonance imaging (MRI) is now widely acknowledged to be the most sensitive investigation in the diagnosis of prion disease. The recognized features of sCJD on MRI are bilateral high signal in the caudate and putamen and in the cerebral cortex (see Figure 11–2A–C). Sensitivity of axial diffusion-weighted imaging (DWI) may be better than T2-weighted imaging or fluid attenuated inversion recovery (FLAIR) (Macfarlane et al., 2007). Cortical atrophy is a late feature, and the degree of atrophy generally correlates with disease duration.

The EEG exhibits changes ranging from nonspecific findings in sCJD, such as diffuse slowing and frontal rhythmic delta activity in the early stages, to disease-typical PSWCs in the middle and late stages. PSWCs occur in about two-thirds of patients with sCJD, with a positive predictive value of 95% (Wieser et al., 2006). Serial EEG is recommended to demonstrate this feature.

Mutation analysis of *PRNP* should be carried out to exclude pathogenic mutations even in the absence of a family history.

Brain biopsy may be considered in certain cases to exclude treatable alternative diagnoses.

vCJD

CSF analysis for 14-3-3 protein may be elevated or normal but does not help differentiate sCJD from vCJD. The pulvinar sign on MRI now forms part of the World Health Organization's diagnostic criteria for vCJD (WHO, 2003). This is bilateral symmetrical pulvinar high signal relative to the signal intensity of other

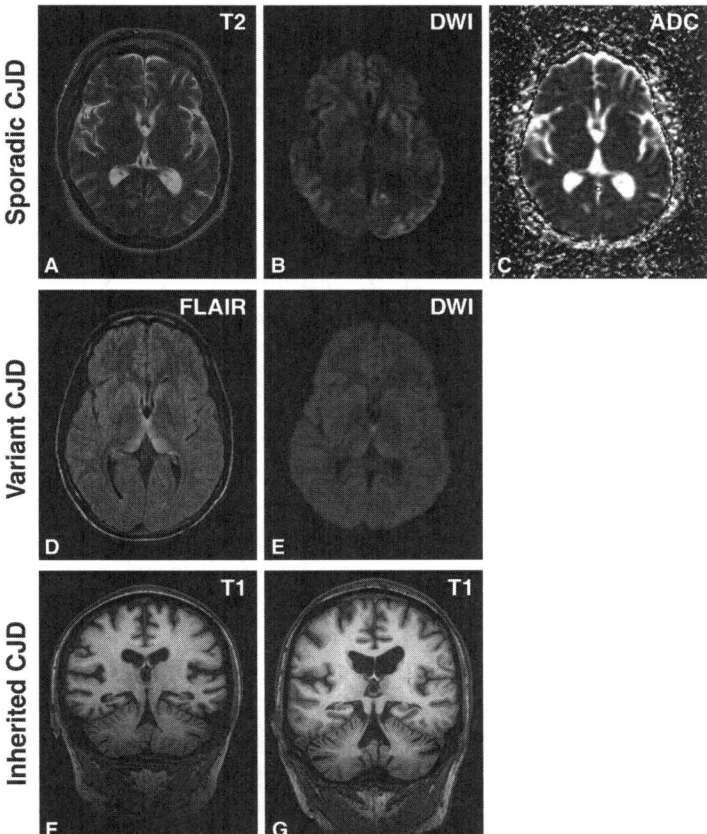

FIGURE 11–2. A–C Sporadic Creutzfeldt-Jakob disease (CJD). A Axial T2-weighted magnetic resonance imaging (MRI) shows a subtle increase in signal intensity of the left putamen anteriorly. The remainder of the basal ganglia and cortex appear normal. B Axial diffusion-weighted image (DWI) shows hyperintense signal in the heads of both caudate nuclei and in both putamina. In addition, there are gyriform areas of hyperintensity in both the insulae and the frontal temporal and occipital cortices. C A map of the apparent diffusion coefficient (ADC) shows reduced signal in the areas which appear hyperintense on the DWI (B), confirming that the diffusion of water is restricted in these regions. D, E Variant CJD. D Axial fluid attenuated inversion recovery image (FLAIR) demonstrates hyperintensity in the dorsomedial thalamic nuclei and pulvinar bilaterally ("hockey stick sign"). E DWI acquired at the same time as D also shows hyperintense signal change. It is, however, less marked than on the FLAIR images, appears more linear, and affects predominantly the dorsomedial nuclei. F, G Coronal T1-weighted images of a volumetric MRI study in two cases with inherited CJD. F 6-Octapeptide repeat insertion. MRI shows cerebellar atrophy with widening of the cerebellar fissures and supratentorial atrophy with enlarged lateral ventricles and very prominent sylvian fissures. G P102L mutation. There is marked cerebellar atrophy with pronounced enlargement of the horizontal cerebellar fissure and fourth ventricle. There is also supratentorial atrophy, mostly of the central type with ventricular enlargement. Modified from Macfarlane et al. (2007). This figure appears courtesy of Dr Harpreet Hyare.

deep gray matter nuclei and cortical gray matter using T2-weighted imaging, proton density weighted, FLAIR, and DWI sequences (Macfarlane et al., 2007) (see Figure 11–2D,E).

EEG recordings in vCJD usually show nonspecific slow-wave abnormalities, but some patients have had normal tracings, even in the later phases of the disease when clinical signs and cognitive impairment were present. PSWCs are not generally observed.

It is essential to rule out pathogenic mutations in *PRNP* as a number of inherited prion diseases present in younger patients and may clinically mimic vCJD. To date, all definite cases of vCJD have been homozygous for the codon 129 Met/Met genotype.

Tonsillar biopsy is a sensitive and specific diagnostic procedure for vCJD. Tonsillar PrP^{Sc} is present in vCJD but not in other forms of human prion disease (Hill et al., 1997).

Inherited Prion Diseases

PRNP should be analyzed in all suspected cases of CJD and will reveal a mutation in the inherited prion diseases. A missense mutation at codon 178 of *PRNP* is the most common mutation seen in FFI, whereas P102L is the most common mutation reported in GSS (Mead, 2006).

Investigations depend on the predominant presenting syndrome. For example, PSWCs on EEG occur in about 10% of patients with inherited prion disease but are much more frequent in familial CJD than in GSS or FFI (Wieser et al., 2006). EEG features consistent with a reduction in sleep time are apparent in FFI (Montagna et al., 2003).

Neuroimaging may be normal, may show nonspecific atrophy affecting the cerebral hemispheres and cerebellum, or may be more typical of sCJD in familial CJD syndromes.

PATHOLOGY OF HUMAN PRION DISEASES

There is wide variation in the neuropathology of different forms of human prion disease. PrP^{Sc} can be detected on Western blot (see Figure 11–3). There are often no recognizable abnormalities on macroscopic examination; however, microscopic examination of the central nervous system reveals characteristic histopathological changes.

sCJD

Neuropathological features of sCJD include spongiform change, neuronal loss, and astrocytosis together with positive PrP immunohistochemistry (see Figure 11–4).

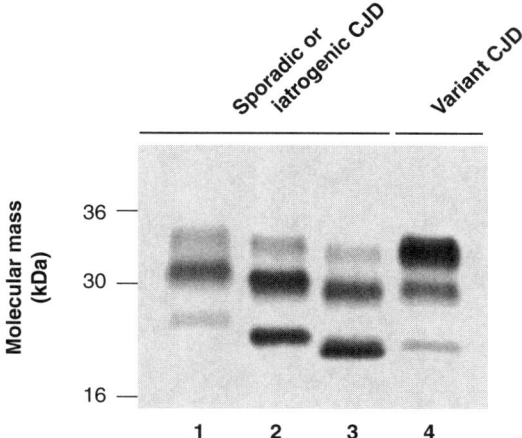

FIGURE 11–3. Western blot demonstrating the presence of PrPSc in brain and tonsil from patients with sporadic and variant Creutzfeldt-Jakob disease (CJD). The presence of PrPSc is revealed after proteinase K treatment, which digests the normal form of PrP (PrPC) but not the pathological form (PrPSc). Three common PrPSc types (1–3) in sporadic CJD can be distinguished by differing fragment sizes of the three PrP glycoforms. This figure appears courtesy of Dr Jonathan Wadsworth and Dr Susan Joiner.

PrP amyloid plaques are not usually present. PrPSc can be demonstrated by immunoblotting of brain homogenates and is diagnostic of prion disease. In the London classification system, PrPSc strain types 1–3 are seen on Western blotting (see Figure 11–3).

vCJD

There are widespread spongiform changes, gliosis, and neuronal loss, most severe in the basal ganglia and thalamus. There are also abundant PrP amyloid plaques in the cerebral and cerebellar cortex. These consist of kuru-like "florid" and multicentric plaque types. PrPSc strain type 4 (London classification) is seen, which is pathognomonic of vCJD (see Figure 11–3).

Inherited Prion Diseases

The histopathological hallmark of FFI is the loss of neurons and astrogliosis in the mediodorsal and anterior thalamic nuclei. The inferior olives show neuronal loss and gliosis in most cases. Deposition of PrPSc is scant relative to other prion diseases (Montagna et al., 2003).

The pathognomonic feature of GSS is the presence of widespread, large, multicentric amyloid plaques which are selectively immunostained by antibodies

normal cortex   Sporadic CJD

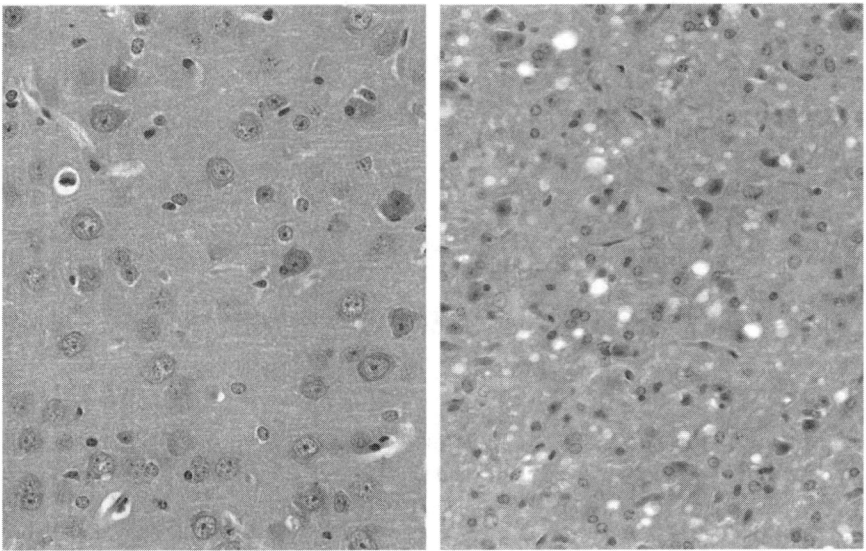

FIGURE 11–4. Cerebral cortex of normal brain (*left*) and a case of sporadic Creutzfeldt-Jakob disease (sCJD, *right*) (H&E stain). sCJD is characterized by the presence of neuronal vacuolation and degeneration, which gives the cerebral gray matter a microvacuolated or "spongiform" appearance. There is typically astrocytic gliosis and neuronal loss. This figure appears courtesy of Dr Sebastian Brandner.

to PrP. White matter degeneration, spongiform change, and gliosis may also be present (Collins et al., 2001).

Familial CJD usually gives appearances similar to those seen in sCJD.

TREATMENT OF HUMAN PRION DISEASES

As with chorea of any etiology, antichoreic medication should be used sparingly as no drug is particularly effective and adverse effects may worsen functional disability. There is a report of choreic and dystonic postures in prion disease reduced with a low dose of haloperidol (Donmez et al., 2005).

Prion diseases are invariably fatal, and the cause of neuronal death remains unclear. Improvements in early diagnostic markers and markers of disease progression are urgently required to assess putative therapies. A number of therapeutic strategies are being investigated (for review, see Mallucci and Collinge, 2005), and the development of neuroprotective agents that may slow down disease progression as well as pre- and postexposure prophylaxis are also important. The first

U.K. therapeutic drug trial, PRION-1, has recently reported on the use of quinacrine in humans (Collinge et al., 2009). No significant benefit was seen for either the primary outcome (cognitive function) or the secondary outcome (survival); however, the study highlights the feasibility of carrying out further clinical trials in human prion diseases.

CONCLUSIONS

It is important to consider all forms of prion diseases in the differential diagnosis of chorea. Chorea can be a significant feature in human prion diseases, which are extremely phenotypically heterogeneous conditions. It may be that the incidence of chorea is rather higher than reported as many phenotypic studies have been carried out retrospectively using historic case note reviews. In addition, it can sometimes be difficult to assess the presence or absence of chorea, and it may be confused with, or overlap with, other involuntary movement disorders (athetosis, ballismus, dystonia, and myoclonus) that can also be significant features of prion disease. Future studies to correlate the clinical phenotypes of the disease with imaging and CSF or blood-based biochemical markers, *PRNP* genotypes, and PrP^{Sc} strain types will be invaluable in improving the early diagnosis of prion disease.

ACKNOWLEDGMENT

We thank Mr. Ray Young for his help with producing the figures. We also thank the patients and families of the National Prion Clinic and Professor John Collinge, director of the MRC Prion Unit, for allowing us to use these figures.

REFERENCES

Bowen J, Mitchell T, Pearce R, Quinn N (2000) Chorea in new variant Creutzfeldt-Jacob disease. Mov Disord 15(6):1284–1285.
Bruce ME (1993) Scrapie strain variation and mutation. Br Med Bull 49(4):822–838.
Collinge J (1999) Variant Creutzfeldt-Jakob disease. Lancet 354(9175):317–323.
Collinge J (2001) Prion diseases of humans and animals: their causes and molecular basis. Annu Rev Neurosci 24:519–550.
Collinge J, Brown J, Hardy J, et al. (1992) Inherited prion disease with 144 base pair gene insertion. 2. Clinical and pathological features. Brain 115(Pt 3):687–710.
Collinge J, Clarke AR (2007) A general model of prion strains and their pathogenicity. Science 318(5852):930–936.

Collinge J, Gorham M, Hudson F, et al. (2009) Safety and efficacy of quinacrine in human prion disease (PRION-1 study): a patient-preference trial. Lancet Neurol 8(4):334–344.

Collinge J, Palmer MS, Dryden AJ (1991) Genetic predisposition to iatrogenic Creutzfeldt-Jakob disease. Lancet 337(8755):1441–1442.

Collinge J, Sidle KC, Meads J, Ironside J, Hill AF (1996) Molecular analysis of prion strain variation and the aetiology of "new variant" CJD. Nature 383(6602):685–690.

Collinge J, Whitfield J, McKintosh E, et al. (2006) Kuru in the 21st century—an acquired human prion disease with very long incubation periods. Lancet 367(9528):2068–2074.

Collinge J, Whitfield J, McKintosh E, et al. (2008) A clinical study of kuru patients with long incubation periods at the end of the epidemic in Papua New Guinea. Philos Trans R Soc Lond B Biol Sci 363(1510):3725–3739.

Collins S, McLean CA, Masters CL (2001) Gerstmann-Straussler-Scheinker syndrome, fatal familial insomnia, and kuru: a review of these less common human transmissible spongiform encephalopathies. J Clin Neurosci 8(5):387–397.

Croes EA, Theuns J, Houwing-Duistermaat JJ, et al. (2004) Octapeptide repeat insertions in the prion protein gene and early onset dementia. J Neurol Neurosurg Psychiatry 75(8):1166–1170.

Donmez B, Cakmur R, Men S, Oztura I, Kitis A (2005) Coexistence of movement disorders and epilepsia partialis continua as the initial signs in probable Creutzfeldt-Jakob disease. Mov Disord 20(9):1220–1223.

Edler J, Mollenhauer B, Heinemann U, et al. (2009) Movement disturbances in the differential diagnosis of Creutzfeldt-Jakob disease. Mov Disord 24(3):350–356.

Hill AF, Zeidler M, Ironside J, Collinge J (1997) Diagnosis of new variant Creutzfeldt-Jakob disease by tonsil biopsy. Lancet 349(9045):99–100.

Kahana E, Zilber N, Abraham M (1991) Do Creutzfeldt-Jakob disease patients of Jewish Libyan origin have unique clinical features? Neurology 41(9):1390–1392.

Laplanche JL, Hachimi KH, Durieux I, et al. (1999) Prominent psychiatric features and early onset in an inherited prion disease with a new insertional mutation in the prion protein gene. Brain 122(Pt 12):2375–2386.

Lugaresi E, Medori R, Montagna P, et al. (1986) Fatal familial insomnia and dysautonomia with selective degeneration of thalamic nuclei. N Engl J Med 315(16):997–1003.

Macfarlane RG, Wroe SJ, Collinge J, Yousry TA, Jager HR (2007) Neuroimaging findings in human prion disease. J Neurol Neurosurg Psychiatry 78(7):664–670.

Mallucci G, Collinge J (2005) Rational targeting for prion therapeutics. Nat Rev Neurosci 6(1):23–34.

Maltête D, Guyant-Maréchal L, Mihout B, Hannequin D (2006) Movement disorders and Creutzfeldt-Jakob disease: a review. Parkinsonism Relat Disord 12(2):65–71.

Masters CL, Harris JO, Gajdusek DC, et al. (1979) Creutzfeldt-Jakob disease: patterns of worldwide occurrence and the significance of familial and sporadic clustering. Ann Neurol 5(2):177–188.

McKee D, Talbot P (2003) Chorea as a presenting feature of variant Creutzfeldt-Jakob disease. Mov Disord 18(7):837–838.

Mead S (2006) Prion disease genetics. Eur J Hum Genet 14(3):273–281.

Mead S, Poulter M, Beck J, et al. (2006) Inherited prion disease with six octapeptide repeat insertional mutation—molecular analysis of phenotypic heterogeneity. Brain 129 (Pt 9):2297–2317.

Meiner Z, Gabizon R, Prusiner SB (1997) Familial Creutzfeldt-Jakob disease. Codon 200 prion disease in Libyan Jews. Medicine (Baltimore) 76(4):227–237.

Montagna P, Gambetti P, Cortelli P, Lugaresi E (2003) Familial and sporadic fatal insomnia. Lancet Neurol 2(3):167–176.

Moore RC, Xiang F, Monaghan J, et al. (2001) Huntington disease phenocopy is a familial prion disease. Am J Hum Genet 69(6):1385–1388.

Owen F, Poulter M, Lofthouse R, et al. (1989) Insertion in prion protein gene in familial Creutzfeldt-Jakob disease. Lancet 1(8628):51–52.

Palmer MS, Dryden AJ, Hughes JT, Collinge J (1991) Homozygous prion protein genotype predisposes to sporadic Creutzfeldt-Jakob disease. Nature 352(6333):340–342.

Pocchiari M, Puopolo M, Croes EA, et al. (2004) Predictors of survival in sporadic Creutzfeldt-Jakob disease and other human transmissible spongiform encephalopathies. Brain 127(10):2348–2359.

Prusiner SB (1982) Novel proteinaceous infectious particles cause scrapie. Science 216(4542):136–144.

Rabinovici GD, Wang PN, Levin J, et al. (2006) First symptom in sporadic Creutzfeldt-Jakob disease. Neurology 66(2):286–287.

Rossor M, Collinge J, Fox N, et al. (2009) Cognitive impairment and dementia. In: Clarke C, Howard R, Rossor M, Shorvon S (eds) Neurology: A Queen Square Textbook., Wiley-Blackwell Publishing, Oxford, pp 245–289.

Sanchez-Juan P, Green A, Ladogana A, et al. (2006) CSF tests in the differential diagnosis of Creutzfeldt-Jakob disease. Neurology 67(4):637–643.

Spencer MD, Knight RSG, Will RG (2002) First hundred cases of variant Creutzfeldt-Jakob disease: retrospective case note review of early psychiatric and neurological features. BMJ 324(7352):1479–1482.

Vital C, Gray F, Vital A, et al. (1998) Prion encephalopathy with insertion of octapeptide repeats: the number of repeats determines the type of cerebellar deposits. Neuropathol Appl Neurobiol 24(2):125–130.

Weller M, Aguzzi A (2009) Prion diseases: movement disorders reveal Creutzfeldt-Jakob disease. Nat Rev Neurol 5(4):185–186.

WHO (2003) Manual for surveillance of human transmissible spongiform encephalopathies including variant Creutzfeld-Jakob disease, www.who.int/bloodproducts/TSE-manual2003.pdf.

Wieser HG, Schindler K, Zumsteg D (2006) EEG in Creutzfeldt-Jakob disease. Clin Neurophysiol 117(5):935–951.

Will RG, Ironside JW, Zeidler M, et al. (1996) A new variant of Creutzfeldt-Jakob disease in the UK. Lancet 347(9006):921–925.

Will RG, Matthews WB (1984) A retrospective study of Creutzfeldt-Jakob disease in England and Wales 1970–1979. I: Clinical features. J Neurol Neurosurg Psychiatry 47(2):134–140.

12

Chorea in the Inherited Ataxias

Guilherme G. Riccioppo Rodrigues, MD, MSc
and Jennifer G. Goldman, MD, MS

INTRODUCTION

Chorea may be a clinical feature in the inherited ataxias. This chapter will discuss several of the autosomal recessive and autosomal dominant ataxias in which chorea may occur, including the recessively inherited Friedreich ataxia, ataxia-telangiectasia, and ataxia with oculomotor apraxia types 1 and 2 and the dominantly inherited spinocerebellar ataxias types 1–3 and 17 and dentatorubral-pallidoluysian atrophy.

AUTOSOMAL RECESSIVE ATAXIAS

Friedreich Ataxia

Friedreich ataxia (FRDA) is an autosomal recessive disorder characterized by early-onset ataxia, absent tendon reflexes in the legs, and extensor plantar responses, secondary to degeneration of the dorsal root ganglia, posterior columns of the spinal cord, and corticospinal tracts (Harding, 1981) (Table 12–1). FRDA is the most common cause of autosomal recessive inherited ataxia, with an estimated prevalence of 1/50,000 inhabitants in Europe (Filla et al., 1992); however, it seems to be very rare in Finland (Juvonen et al., 2002), sub-Saharan Africa, and southeast Asia (Labuda et al., 2000). In Caucasians, FRDA accounts for about 50% of the hereditary ataxias and 75% of those before age 25.

Genetics

In approximately 95% of cases, FRDA is caused by an unstable expansion of GAA repeats, within the first intron of the frataxin gene, on chromosome 9q13. Normal allele length varies from seven to 22 triplets, and the size of expanded

TABLE 12–1. Differential Diagnosis of Autosomal Recessive Ataxias that Cause Chorea

	FA	AT	AOA I	AOA2
Age at onset	±15 years	<5 years	±7 years	±15 years
Gait ataxia	+++	+++	+++	+++
Oculomotor apraxia	–	++	+++	+
Chorea	+/–	+++	++	+
Cognitive impairment	+	+	++	+
Neuropathy	S	SM	SM	SM
Babinski sign	+	–	–	+/–
Optic atrophy	+	–	+	–
Telangiectasia	–	+++	–	–
Cerebellar atrophy on MRI	+/–	+++	+++	+++
Cardiomyopathy	++	–	–	–
Diabetes	+	+/–	–	–
Scoliosis/pes cavus	++	+	++	++
Radiosensitivity	–	+++	–	–
Immunodeficiency	–	+++	–	–
Cancer susceptibility	–	+++	–	–
↑ AFP	–	+++	–	++
↑ Cholesterol	–	–	+++	+
↓ Albumin	–	–	+++	+
Gene	*frataxin*	*ATM*	*aprataxin*	*senataxin*

AFP, alpha-fetoprotein; AOA1/2, ataxia with oculomotor apraxia types 1 and 2; AT, ataxia-telangiectasia; FA, Friedreich ataxia; MRI, magnetic resonance imaging; S, sensory; SM, sensorimotor; –, absent; +/–, rare; +, occasionally present; ++, common; +++, very common.

alleles usually ranges from 200 to more than 900 triplets (Campuzano et al., 1996). About 4%–5% of cases are due to an association of the GAA expansion and a frataxin point mutation (Delatycki et al., 1999).

Pathophysiology

The exact mechanism underlying the decrease of frataxin levels is unknown; possibly, the GAA repeat expansion may disturb the normal DNA structure and reduce frataxin gene transcription (Bidichandani et al., 1998). Frataxin is a mito-chondrial protein (Campuzano et al., 1997) involved in iron homeostasis and con-trol of free radical production (Babcock et al., 1997; Cavadini et al., 2000; Bulteau et al., 2004). The frataxin knockout mouse model leads to embryonic lethality a few days after implantation, in some cases associated with significant morpho-logical abnormalities, without evidence of iron accumulation (Cossée et al., 2000). Conditional (tissue-specific) knockout mouse models and knock-in transgenic mice exhibit FRDA pathological features, such as progressive intramitochondrial iron accumulation, cardiac hypertrophy, and large sensory neuron dysfunction (Puccio et al. 2001; Simon et al., 2004; Al-Mahdawi et al., 2006), confirming the role of frataxin in the etiology of FRDA.

Clinical Features

Dürr et al. (1996) screened for GAA expansion in the frataxin gene in 187 patients with progressive ataxia and possible autosomal recessive inheritance. Expanded GAA repeats, ranging from 120 to 1,700, were found on both alleles of the frataxin gene in 140 (75%) patients. The presenting symptom in 133 patients was gait ataxia. Other symptoms, such as dysarthria, lower-limb areflexia, cardiomyo-pathy, loss of vibration sense, scoliosis, extensor plantar reflexes, muscle weak-ness in lower limbs, and pes cavus, occurred in >50% of patients. In their series, 34 patients had an atypical clinical presentation, including 19 patients who pre-sented with onset of symptoms after 25 years old, 13 patients who had retained tendon reflexes, and 21 patients who lacked the extensor plantar response. They found an inverse relation between the size of the GAA expansion and age at onset, presence of cardiomyopathy, and time until the patient become wheelchair-bound. Larger repeat expansions were associated with earlier age of disease onset and more severe clinical phenotype. The importance of the length of the GAA expan-sion in the age at onset and clinical variability has been confirmed by other authors (Filla et al., 1996; Monrós et al., 1997).

Among the nonneurological manifestations, hypertrophic cardiomyopathy is present in approximately 65% of patients. The electrocardiogram frequently is abnormal, mainly due to widespread T-wave inversion; however, FRDA patients are often asymptomatic, and rarely the cardiomyopathy progresses to heart failure or fatal arrhythmias. Scoliosis and pes cavus are the most common skeletal abnormalities found in FRDA patients. These are secondary to the neurological impairment and may worsen the respiratory and gait problems. Diabetes and impaired glucose tolerance occur in 30% of patients and are probably due to mitochondrial dysfunction.

Chorea

In general, reports of chorea as a clinical feature of FRDA are rare. The first cases of chorea in genetically confirmed FRDA patients were described by Hanna et al. (1998). The first case was a 21-year-old man with generalized chorea since age 19. The chorea was severe enough to disturb his gait and lead to occasional falls. He was areflexic, had flexor plantar responses and scoliosis, but did not have any cerebellar signs, cardiomyopathy, diabetes, or family history of neurological disease. Brain and spinal magnetic resonance imaging (MRI) were normal, and acanthocytes were not found in three peripheral blood films. Frataxin gene analysis revealed two expanded alleles, with 500 and 800 repeats, respectively, confirming the diagnosis of FRDA. The second case was a 13-year-old boy with mild generalized chorea, mainly in his head, neck, and shoulders. He had absent tendon reflexes, mild hypertrophic cardiomyopathy, flexor plantar responses, and dubious cerebellar signs. He did not have diabetes, and blood film examination was normal. Frataxin gene analysis demonstrated a homozygous expansion of 1,000 repeats. In this brief report of two cases, the authors propose that chorea may be part of the phenotypic variability found in FRDA; however, they do not conceive a putative pathophysiology to explain the chorea in these cases. Anatomical studies, through structural neuroimaging or pathological series, do not demonstrate significant involvement of the cortex or basal ganglia in FRDA (Lamarche et al., 1984; Klockgether et al., 1991; Wüllner et al., 1993). However, functional studies reveal some abnormalities in cortical perfusion (De Michele et al., 1998) and activation (Mantovan et al., 2006), not related to regional atrophy. FRDA patients also have impairments in visuoconstructive abilities, verbal fluency, and memory, suggesting that frataxin deficiency might have a greater impact on cerebral physiology (Mantovan et al., 2006), which could explain rare cases with supratentorial manifestations, such as chorea. In addition to these cases, two compound heterozygous FRDA patients have been reported to have chorea. Zhu et al. (2002) described a 14-year-old boy who presented with a combination of chorea and myoclonus since about age 4. Spacey et al. (2004) reported a 10-year-old boy with choreiform movements of the tongue and hands. The authors suggest that atypical phenotypes are more likely to be associated with compound heterozygosity.

Treatment

The course of FRDA is variable; however, most patients are wheelchair-bound by age 40–50. There is no curative treatment of FRDA, and the main therapy has been supportive. To date, the most promising treatment has been idebenone, a free-radical scavenger. In 1999, Rustin et al. conducted *in vitro* and *in vivo* studies on the effects of idebenone on heart homogenates and myocardial thickness in three FRDA patients. They found that idebenone protected membrane lipids against iron-induced injury and was associated with a substantial decrease in myocardial hypertrophy. The protective effects were confirmed in a mouse model experiment (Seznec et al., 2004) and in an open trial with 38 patients (Hausse et al., 2002). A long-term follow-up study (Pineda et al., 2008) corroborated the cardiac improvement and demonstrated that idebenone may stabilize cerebellar dysfunction in pediatric patients. In addition, a randomized, placebo-controlled trial suggested that high-dose idebenone may improve neurological function (Di Prospero et al., 2007).

Ataxia-Telangiectasia

Ataxia-telangiectasia (AT) is the second most common recessive disorder that causes ataxia, with a birth frequency estimated at 1/300,000 (Swift et al., 1986; Woods et al., 1990).

Genetics

AT is caused by truncating mutations in the *ATM* (ataxia-telangiectasia mutated) gene (Savitsky et al., 1995), which extends over 150 kb of genomic DNA and encodes a protein of ~350 kDa (Watters et al., 1997), ATM. In classical forms, the ATM protein is completely inactive (Gilad et al., 1996). Some residual function is associated with milder clinical phenotype (McConville et al., 1996).

Pathophysiology

ATM has an important role in DNA damage response, mainly in double strand breakage and cell cycle regulation (Beamish et al., 1996). The exact mechanism implicated in neurodegeneration in AT is unknown. Presumed mechanisms include programmed cell death in neurons with excessive damage (Lee and McKinnon, 2000) and neuronal death through increased oxidative stress (Kamsler et al., 2001). ATM knockout mice show mild motor impairment, without significant ataxia or histological evidence of cerebellar abnormalities, and several systemic findings, such as growth retardation, infertility, immunodeficiency, and cancer (Barlow et al., 1996; Xu et al., 1996; Elson et al., 1996).

Clinical Features

Clinical manifestations are first noticed by age 2, due to progressive unsteady gait and ataxia. Oculocutaneous telangiectasia typically develop between ages 3 and 5, being more visible in the bulbar conjunctiva (Figure 12–1). By age 10, patients usually need a wheelchair. Deficiency of cell-mediated and humoral immunity may lead to recurrent sinopulmonary infections (Nowak-Wegrzyn et al., 2004).

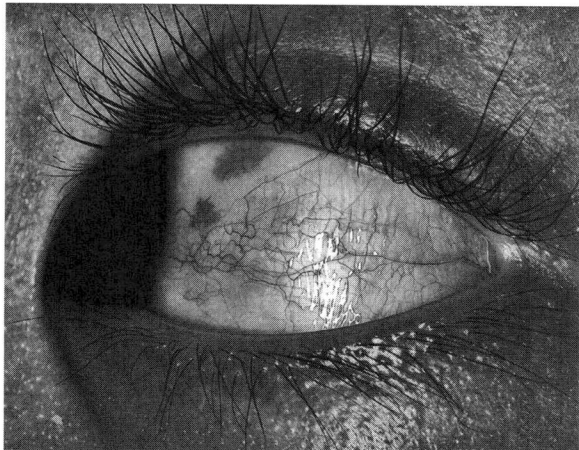

FIGURE 12–1. Ocular telangiectasia in a 5-year-old ataxia-telangiectasia patient (Courtesy of Dr. Percio Roxo Júnior, School of Medicine of Ribeirão Preto, University of São Paulo, Brazil).

Growth retardation and susceptibility to cancer, mainly lymphoid malignancies (Taylor et al., 1996), complete the classical clinical picture. Median survival is between 19 and 25 years, and most deaths are due to cancer or infectious complications (Crawford et al., 2006). In addition to ataxia, other neurological abnormalities include oculomotor apraxia (difficulty in initiating saccades without ophthalmoplegia), cognitive disturbances, peripheral neuropathy, dystonia, and choreoathetosis.

In a suspected case of AT, a high serum alpha-fetoprotein (AFP) level makes the diagnosis probable. The demonstration of increased sensitivity of lymphocytes to ionizing radiation (colony survival assay) (Sun et al., 2002) or absent expression of ATM on Western blot analysis supports the diagnosis. As there are several disease-associated mutations in the large *ATM* gene, complete gene sequencing is not obligatory in a clinical setting.

Chorea

Chorea occurs in approximately 90% of AT patients and is usually associated with other neurological symptoms. Occasionally, chorea can precede the onset of ataxia by several years, thereby suggesting alternative diagnoses such as Sydenham chorea (Chapter 17), cerebral palsy, Huntington disease (HD) (Chapter 3), and benign hereditary chorea (Chapter 4). With the availability of genetic tests, some cases previously reported to be AT with chorea were found to be an AT-like disorder (Klein et al., 2001). The pathogenesis of chorea in AT is unclear. It is probably caused by primary degeneration of basal ganglia but in some cases is associated with vascular abnormalities, as demonstrated by perfusion studies

(Koepp et al., 1994) and pathological descriptions (Agamanolis and Greenstein, 1979; Bodensteiner et al., 1980).

Treatment

To date, there is no curative therapy for AT. Treatment aims are to control infections and cancer and to minimize neurological impairment. Infections can be treated using wide-spectrum antibiotics; occasionally, intravenous immunoglobulin is used in those patients with recurrent infections. As AT patients have increased sensitivity to ionizing radiation and antitumor drugs, the treatment of malignancies must be performed with caution and on an individual basis. Chorea usually responds to neuroleptics, as often used in the treatment of other causes of chorea. Ataxia may be managed with physical, occupational, and speech therapies.

Ataxia with Oculomotor Apraxia Type 1

Ataxia with oculomotor apraxia type 1 (AOA1) is the most frequent cause of autosomal recessive ataxia in Japan and the second most frequent cause in Portugal (Moreira et al., 2001a). It was first described in 14 patients with a slowly progressive history of ataxia, choreoathetosis, and oculomotor apraxia. Initially, the authors pointed out that, although similar to AT, AOA1 did not present with systemic abnormalities such as telangiectasias, infections, or cancer susceptibility (Aicardi et al., 1988). AOA1 has been frequently associated with hypoalbuminemia and hypercholesterolemia.

Genetics

AOA1 is caused by mutations on the gene *APTX* (Date et al., 2001; Moreira et al., 2001b), which contains seven exons and is located on 9p13. To date, all missense mutations have been detected in exons 5, 6, and 7.

Pathophysiology

APTX produces a nuclear protein named aprataxin, which belongs to the histidine-triad superfamily protein and is involved in DNA single-strand break repair (Gueven et al., 2004; Sano et al., 2004). Both missense and frameshift mutations have been related to severe forms of disease (Date et al., 2001; Shimazaki et al., 2002); milder cases may have missense mutations (Criscuolo et al., 2004, 2005).

Clinical Features

Clinically, cerebellar ataxia is first noticed as unstable gait and dysarthria, usually between ages 1 and 16 (Video 12–1 Apraxia with Oculomotor Ataxia I). There is slow progression, and patients usually require assistance to walk after 7–10 years of disease (Barbot et al., 2001). The oculomotor apraxia is characterized by difficulty moving the eyes on command, without weakness of extraocular muscles.

There is excessive blinking, and patients frequently make compensatory head movements when initiating saccades. For this reason, the head reaches the target before the eyes (Figure 12–2). Pursuit is preserved in initial phases of disease; however, the oculomotor abnormality usually progresses to external ophthalmoplegia. Patients also frequently exhibit signs of axonal neuropathy, such as areflexia, distal atrophy, and weakness. Pes cavus, scoliosis, optic atrophy, mental retardation, and movement disorders including dystonia and chorea are also reported. Brain MRI findings typically reveal severe cerebellar atrophy (Barbot et al., 2001).

Chorea

In contrast to FRDA, chorea is a frequent symptom in AOA1. In some patients, chorea is more prominent than ataxia at onset (Le Ber et al., 2003), which may lead to an incorrect diagnosis. As aprataxin is expressed in the caudate nucleus (Date et al., 2001), chorea may be due to striatal dysfunction secondary to abnormal aprataxin function. Although abnormal findings were not found in the striatum on neuropathological examination (Sekijima et al., 1998), one study demonstrated caudate hypoperfusion on single-photon emission computed tomography (SPECT) (Le Ber et al., 2003). Chorea tends to decrease during the disease course, possibly related to degeneration of lower motor neurons (Shimazaki et al., 2002) or decreased striatal dopaminergic inflow, secondary to progressive nigrostriatal dysfunction (Salvatore et al., 2008).

Ataxia with Oculomotor Apraxia Type 2

Following linkage studies, patients with a clinical phenotype compatible with AOA were divided into two groups. The first, described in the previous section, is known as AOA1. The second had a mutation linked to 9q34 (Nemeth et al., 2000; Bomont et al., 2000) and was classified as AOA2. As oculomotor apraxia is not a cardinal feature of this disease, some concerns have been raised about using the term "AOA2." Although some authors suggest using the name "spinocerebellar ataxia, autosomal recessive, with axonal neuropathy-2" (Duquette et al., 2005), we will use the traditional name, "AOA2," in this section.

Genetics

AOA2 is caused by mutations in the senataxin (*SETX*) gene, which encodes a protein containing a seven-motif domain found in the superfamily 1 of helicases and shares extensive homologies with the fungal Sen1p proteins (Moreira et al., 2004). Missense mutations in the helicase domain cause disease (Fogel and Perlman, 2006). Missense mutations in *SETX* can also produce a juvenile form of amyotrophic lateral sclerosis (ALS4). Unlike AOA2, ALS4 is autosomal dominantly inherited. It has been speculated that a toxic gain of function of senataxin could lead to development of ALS4 (Chen et al., 2004).

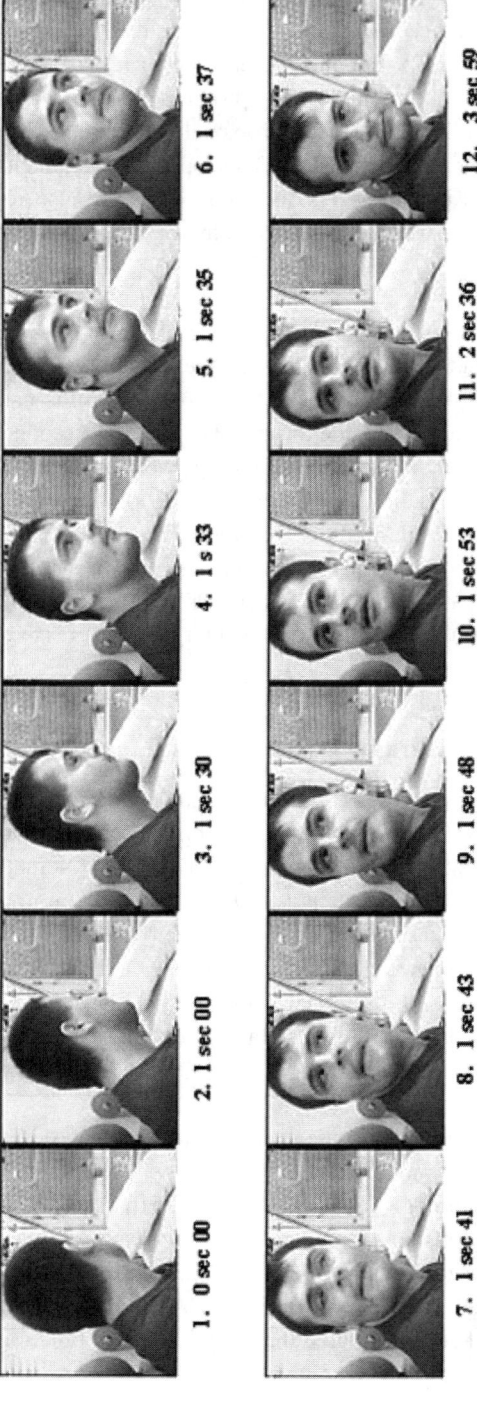

FIGURE 12–2. Eye–head dissociation, characterized by a lateral head movement that precedes the eye movement when the patient attempts to look toward a lateral target. From Le Ber et al. (2003) Cerebellar ataxia with oculomotor apraxia type 1: clinical and genetic studies. Brain 126(12): 2761–2772 © Oxford University Press, 2003. Used with permission.

Pathophysiology

Senataxin is related to RNA splicing and termination (Moreira et al., 2004) and plays a role in the response against oxidative DNA damage (Suraweera et al., 2007). Clinical and pathological studies suggest that senataxin is important to cerebellar, anterior horn, and dorsal root survival (Criscuolo et al., 2006).

Clinical Features

Symptoms in AOA2 patients typically start at around age 15, most frequently with progressive gait ataxia. Other common features include cerebellar dysarthria, saccadic ocular pursuit, and sensorimotor neuropathy. Oculomotor apraxia can be absent (Duquette et al., 2005) or found in less than half of patients (Criscuolo et al., 2006; Tazir et al., 2009). In one study of 18 AOA2 patients, oculomotor apraxia was found in 56% (Le Ber et al., 2004). Recently, Anheim et al. (2009) retrospectively analyzed 90 AOA2 patients and reported chorea in 9.5% of cases. Other movement disorders, such as head tremor and dystonia, were observed in 14% and 13.5%, respectively. Mild cognitive impairment with predominant executive dysfunction has been observed (Le Ber et al., 2004). Laboratory evaluation demonstrated increased AFP levels in all patients, if at least three measurements were performed (Le Ber et al., 2004). Brain MRI revealed cerebellar atrophy. Increased total cholesterol and low albumin levels have been found occasionally (Le Ber et al., 2004). The clinical progression of AOA2 is slower than that of AOA1. The majority of patients approaching age 25 are still able to walk alone but eventually need a wheelchair for long distances.

Chorea

Involuntary movements are not reported as frequently in AOA2 as in AT or AOA1. In a series with 18 patients identified by linkage analysis, chorea was found in 22% (Le Ber et al., 2004). In a report of 10 cases, Criscuolo et al. (2006) found chorea in one case, which disappeared with disease evolution. In a series of seven AOA2 patients, chorea was not found, and upper limb dystonia was diagnosed in one (Anheim et al., 2008). Similarly, in 19 AOA2 patients, chorea was not found, but writer's cramp was diagnosed in one (Tazir et al., 2009). As there are few cases reported to date, the pathogenesis of involuntary movements in AOA2 remains to be clarified.

AUTOSOMAL DOMINANT ATAXIAS

The spinocerebellar ataxias (SCAs) represent a heterogeneous group of autosomal dominantly inherited ataxias with varied clinical manifestations and different genetic mutations. Although primarily considered disorders of cerebellar degeneration, the SCAs are often accompanied by extracerebellar features such as

TABLE 12–2. Differential Diagnosis of Autosomal Dominant Ataxias that Cause Chorea

	SCA1	SCA2	SCA3	SCA17	DRPLA
Mean onset age	40s	30s–40s	30s–40s	30s	30s
Gait ataxia	+++	+++	+++	+++	+++
Spasticity	++	+	+++	+	+/–
Neuropathy	++	++	+++	+/–	+/–
Dementia	–	–	–	+++	+++
Psychiatric	–	–	–	+++	+++
Epilepsy	–	–	–	++	+++
Parkinsonism and dystonia	–	+++	+++	++	+
Ophthalmoplegia	+/–	+/–	+++	–	–
Slowed saccades	++	+++	++	+	+
Cerebellar atrophy on MRI	+++	+++	+++	+++	+++
Mutation	CAG	CAG	CAG	CAG	CAG
Chromosome	6p23	12q24	14q32	6q27	12p13
Gene	*Ataxin-1*	*Ataxin-2*	*Ataxin-3*	*TATA-BP*	*Atrophin-1*

DRPLA, dentatorubral-pallidoluysian atrophy; MRI, magnetic resonance imaging; SCA, spinocerebellar ataxia; –, absent; +/–, rare; +, occasionally present; ++, common; +++, very common.

basal ganglia (e.g., chorea, dystonia, parkinsonism), pyramidal, neuropathic, and cognitive changes (Table 12–2). A recent study of the frequency of non-ataxic symptoms in 526 patients with SCA1, SCA2, SCA3, and SCA6 found that chorea/dyskinesia were reported on the Inventory of Non-Ataxia Symptoms in 6.8% of SCA1 and SCA2, 10.1% of SCA3, and 1.9% of SCA6 (Schmitz-Hübsch et al., 2008) cases. Although chorea may be found in other SCAs, such as SCA2 (Geschwind et al., 1997; Rottnek et al., 2008) (Video 12–2 Spinocerebellar Ataxia 2) and SCA3 (Cancel et al., 1995; Tang et al., 2000), this section will focus on SCA types 1 and 17 as well as the dominantly inherited dentatorubral-pallidoluysian atrophy (DRPLA), in which chorea may occur.

SCA1

SCA1 is a progressive neurodegenerative disorder characterized by cerebellar ataxia, pyramidal signs, neuropathy, and occasionally chorea. SCA1 is caused by a CAG trinucleotide repeat expansion on chromosome 6p23. Prior to the discovery of specific genetic mutations responsible for the different SCA types, SCA1 was classified by Harding (1982) as one of the autosomal dominant cerebellar ataxias, type I (ADCA I); those ataxias grouped as ADCA I (e.g., SCA1, SCA2, SCA3) had signs and symptoms of cerebellar ataxia in combination with variable presentations of other neurological features, such as spasticity, hyperreflexia, parkinsonism, dystonia, neuropathy, and dementia, among others. SCA1 is one of the more common SCA types, representing about 10% of the SCAs worldwide. SCA1 is most frequent in South Africa but also common in Australia, India, Italy, and Japan; SCA1 is rare in Brazil, central Japan, and Portugal.

Genetics

The locus of SCA1 on the short arm of chromosome 6 was reported initially by Yakura et al (1974) on the basis of its linkage to the human major histocompatibility complex (HLA). This was subsequently confirmed by Jackson et al. (1977) through HLA typing and linkage analysis performed on 19 members of a kindred with an autosomal dominantly inherited SCA. A more specific gene locus was identified and found to be closely linked to D6S90 by two groups in 1991 (Zoghbi et al., 1991; Ranum et al., 1991). Using a positional cloning strategy, the *SCA1* gene was isolated in 1993, and mutations were found to be due to an unstable CAG trinucleotide repeat located within the gene coding region (Orr et al., 1993; Banfi et al., 1994). Affected alleles in SCA1 have expansions of 39–82 CAG repeats, whereas normal alleles contain 6–39 repeats. About 98% of unexpanded alleles have a CAT interruption, which may help to maintain genetic stability across generations (Chung et al., 1993). If CAT interruptions are absent, patients with intermediate or marginal numbers of CAG repeats (i.e., 39–44 repeats) may develop SCA1. Similar to other trinucleotide repeat disorders, such as HD, a greater number of CAG repeats is associated with earlier age of disease onset and greater disease severity; this phenomenon is particularly evident with paternal transmission (Chung et al., 1993; Matilla et al., 1993).

Pathophysiology

The *SCA1* (or ATXN1) gene encodes ataxin-1, a protein of about 800 amino acids, depending on the length of the expanded trinucleotide or polyglutamine tract. Ataxin-1 expression is widespread in normal brain and peripheral tissues. Although mainly localized within neuronal nuclei, ataxin-1 also may be found in the cytoplasm of Purkinje cells (Servadio et al., 1995). Mutant ataxin-1 aggregates in nuclear inclusions in *post mortem* brains from SCA1 patients and in SCA1 transgenic mice (Skinner et al., 1997; Duyckaerts et al., 1999). Cell culture studies have revealed that mutant ataxin-1 alters the distribution of nuclear matrix–associated domains and may be involved in the ubiquitin-proteasomal pathway for clearance of abnormally folded proteins (Skinner et al., 2001). Transgenic mouse models demonstrate that mutant ataxin-1 exhibits a toxic gain of function as mice with expanded alleles develop ataxia and Purkinje cell neuronal inclusions (Burright et al., 1995). These findings support the hypothesis that polyglutamine disorders lead to protein misfolding and aggregation, with subsequent neuronal dysfunction and cell death. However, the neuronal inclusions do not necessarily cause disease.

Studies investigating the biological function of ataxin-1 in murine models suggest a role in cerebellar development and spatial learning (Banfi et al., 1996). Ataxin-1 also may regulate genetic programs involved in motor function in mice, and abnormal ataxin-1 may contribute to SCA1 pathogenesis through dysregulation of signaling pathways (Matilla-Dueñas et al., 2008).

Clinical Features

SCA1 is characterized by cerebellar ataxia, pyramidal tract signs, and neuropathy, as well as later ophthalmoplegia and bulbar dysfunction (Burk et al., 1996; Schols et al., 1997; Matilla-Dueñas et al., 2008). Age at onset varies from adolescence to late adulthood (age 4–74), with an average around the third to fourth decades. The course of SCA1 is progressive, with many patients requiring a wheelchair within 10 years of disease onset; death occurs after 10–20 years. Cerebellar features include predominantly gait ataxia with a lesser degree of limb ataxia, dysarthria, and nystagmus. Spasticity occurs in the lower extremities in about 75% of patients, often accompanied by hyperreflexia and extensor plantar responses. A sensory or sensorimotor neuropathy with axonal loss occurs in about 40%, especially with increased CAG repeats, and may be apparent on nerve conduction studies. Later clinical features include abnormal eye movements, bulbar dysfunction, and movement disorders. Abnormal saccades with decreased velocity or increased amplitude may be seen, and ophthalmoplegia occurs in about 50%. Bulbar dysfunction includes dysphagia, tongue fasciculations, vocal cord paralysis, and stridor. Cognitive impairment with executive dysfunction occurs in about 50%, but dementia is rare.

Brain MRI reveals atrophy of the cerebellum, brainstem, and cervical spinal cord. Neuropathology reveals marked cerebellar atrophy with loss of Purkinje cells in the cerebellar cortex and vermis and atrophy of the pons and inferior olives, spinal cord, spinocerebellar tracts, and posterior columns. In addition, neuronal loss of the nuclei of cranial nerves III, X, and XII is seen; and ubiquitin-positive nuclear inclusions can be found.

Chorea

Chorea has been variably reported in SCA1, usually as a feature in late stages of the disease. The chorea has been described as athetoid movements in most reported cases (Currier et al., 1972; Haines et al., 1984; Sasaki et al., 1996; Namekawa et al., 2001), as orolingual chorea in another report (Iwabuchi et al., 1999), and as arm chorea accompanied by neck dystonia in another case (Kameya et al., 1995). Although not all cases reported in the literature were genetically confirmed, the earlier cases stem from the two large families from whom linkage to HLA was established and are considered SCA1 kindreds. Little is known about the pathophysiology of chorea or choreoathetosis in SCA1, such as whether it reflects basal ganglia dysfunction or underlying neuropathic, sensory changes. Electromyography was reported in a 51-year-old, genetically confirmed SCA1 patient with a 13-year history of disease by Namekawa et al. (2001). This patient had choreiform movements in her fingers, arms, feet, and legs bilaterally, with greater severity in her lower extremities. Sensation was normal, but electromyography revealed neurogenic changes.

Treatment

Presently, there is no cure for SCA1. Research strategies may target transcriptional regulation, alter protein misfolding or aggregation of ataxin-1, silence mutant SCA1 alleles using RNA interference, or modify signaling pathways. In SCA1 transgenic mice, a creatine-supplemented diet resulted in maintenance of Purkinje cell numbers but did not improve the ataxia or delay its development (Kaemmerer et al., 2001). SCA1 knock-in mice receiving lithium demonstrated improved motor coordination, learning, and memory; and neuropathologically, lithium treatment attenuated the reduction of dendritic branching in mutant hippocampal pyramidal neurons (Watase et al., 2007). Pilot studies of lithium in SCA1 humans are currently under way.

SCA17

SCA17 is a rare autosomal dominant neurodegenerative disorder with heterogeneous clinical features including ataxia, dementia, chorea, parkinsonism, and psychiatric disturbances. The clinical phenotype of SCA17, particularly with prominent dementia and chorea, may overlap with that of HD; SCA17 also has been known as "Huntington disease-like 4" (HDL4). Also a polyglutamine disorder, SCA17 is caused by a CAG/CAA repeat expansion on chromosome 6q27 in the coding region of the TATA-binding protein (TBP) gene. In their review, Stevanin and Brice (2008) cite reports of about 55 SCA17 families or cases worldwide, representing about 130 patients. The majority of the families are German or Japanese, while others are from western Europe and Taiwan. The frequency of SCA17 ranges 0.3%–3% of ADCA families. Occasional sporadic cases have been detected.

Genetics

The expansion of the CAG repeat in the TBP gene was first described by Koide et al. (1999) in a sporadic case of a young Japanese female with gait disturbance and intellectual deterioration. Subsequently, other groups reported expansions in the TBP gene in families with an autosomal dominant ataxia (Fujigasaki et al., 2001; Nakamura et al., 2001; Zuhlke et al., 2001). Mutant alleles range about 45–63 repeats (normal 25–44 repeats). Compared to other polyglutamine disorders, SCA17 does not typically exhibit anticipation, and repeat sizes are relatively stable between generations. The stability may relate to the presence of CAA interruptions, similar to the CAT interruptions in SCA1. In addition, the correlation between repeat size and age of onset is not as strong in SCA17 compared to other ADCAs. Several sporadic cases have been detected, resulting from either *de novo* expansions or incomplete penetrance. Thus, testing for the SCA17 genetic mutation in patients with the appropriate phenotype but lacking a family history may detect additional cases.

Pathophysiology

TBP is an important general transcription initiator factor. It is ubiquitously expressed from a single gene on chromosome 6q27 and forms part of the transcription initiation complexes of the three RNA polymerases (Rigby, 1993; Imbert et al., 1994; Lescure et al., 1994). TBP is the DNA-binding subunit of RNA polymerase II transcription factor D and is involved in mRNA transcription. Proposed pathogenic mechanisms of the CAG repeat expansion include effects on transcriptional initiator factor. In addition, intranuclear inclusions in *post mortem* brains of SCA17 cases suggest a toxic gain-of-function mechanism as in other polyglutamine diseases.

Clinical Features

The clinical phenotype of SCA17 is varied but predominantly features ataxia and dementia. Presenting symptoms differ, with some pedigrees manifesting greater initial dementia. Ataxic, DRPLA-like, HD-like, or parkinsonian phenotypes of SCA17 may be evident. The age of onset ranges 19–48 years, with a mean in the third decade. Initial symptoms are primarily gait ataxia or movement disorders such as focal dystonia or chorea (Bruni et al., 2004; Hagenah et al., 2004; Stevanin et al., 2003; Bauer et al., 2004). Cognitive symptoms frequently occur early in the disease course and include slowed thinking, impaired memory, and intellectual decline. Dementia has been reported in about 77% of subjects and psychiatric disturbances with depression, behavioral changes, or psychosis in about 67%. Parkinsonism occurs in about 50%, and epilepsy with atypical absence or generalized tonic–clonic seizures occurs in about 35%. Eye-movement abnormalities have been variably reported and include nystagmus, hypometric saccades, normal saccade velocity, and impaired smooth pursuit. Brain MRI reveals marked cerebellar atrophy and mild cortical atrophy. Positron emission tomography (PET) and SPECT imaging studies performed on two unrelated SCA17 patients by Minnerop et al. (2005) demonstrated significantly reduced glucose metabolism in the putamen, with reduced dopamine transporter activity in the basal ganglia, most pronounced in the putamen. An MRI voxel-based morphometric study by Lasek et al. (2006) in 12 patients with SCA17, six of whom had dementia, revealed gray matter atrophy in the cerebellum, basal ganglia, and frontal and temporal lobes compared to normal controls. Neuropathology reveals moderate cerebellar degeneration, neuronal intranuclear inclusions, and mild to moderate changes in the basal ganglia and cortical regions. The widespread cortical and subcortical involvement depicted on imaging and pathological studies likely underscores the cognitive deterioration and other neurological manifestations.

Chorea

About 36% of SCA17 patients have been reported to exhibit chorea or choreoathetosis. In these reports, chorea has been generalized, involving the extremities as well as the face. Phenotypically, the chorea appears similar to HD. SCA17 mutations have been detected in families with an HD-like syndrome but who have been negative for the expanded CAG repeat in the *IT15* gene on chromosome 4 for HD (Toyoshima et al., 2004; Schneider et al., 2006). However, SCA17 accounts for <1% of HD-like cases with cerebellar ataxia. As mentioned, neuroimaging studies reveal abnormal dopamine transporter binding and altered glucose metabolism in the striatum and cerebellum; these changes may play a role in the manifestation of parkinsonism, dystonia, and chorea in SCA17.

Treatment

To date, there is no specific treatment for SCA17. Supportive therapies, such as physical, occupational, and speech therapies, may be helpful. Seizures should be treated with antiepileptic medications. Medications often used to treat parkinsonism, dystonia, or chorea that act on dopaminergic or cholinergic systems may be considered. However, controlled studies are lacking, and these medications may require cautious use in patients with dementia and/or psychosis.

Dentatorubral-Pallidoluysian Atrophy

DRPLA is a rare, autosomal dominant, neurodegenerative disorder with phenotypic similarities to progressive myoclonic epilepsy, SCA, or HD depending upon the age at onset. DRPLA was initially described by Smith (1958) as an unusual form of cerebellar ataxia with pathological findings of combined dentatorubral and pallidoluysian degeneration. The familial form of DRPLA was first reported by Naito et al. (1972) and further characterized by Naito and Oyanagi (1982). Also a member of the polyglutamine disorder family, DRPLA is caused by a trinucleotide CAG repeat mapped to chromosome 12p and marked by a cytoplasmic protein, atrophin-1. DRPLA is relatively common in Japan, with a prevalence rate of 0.2–0.7/100,000 and is present in the United States as a variant, Haw River syndrome, which has been reported in African American kindreds in North Carolina (Inazuki et al., 1990; Burke et al., 1994). DRPLA has been reported in four families in south Wales (Wardle et al., 2008).

Genetics

In 1990, Kondo et al. reported that despite a similar clinical phenotype, the disorder now known as DRPLA was not linked to the HD locus. The disease was mapped to chromosome 12p by Nagafuchi et al. (1994) and further defined by Kuwano et al. (1996), localizing to chromosome 12p13.1-p12.3. Using cDNA clones, Koide et al. (1994) and Nagafuchi et al. (1994) independently discovered that the CAG repeat on chromosome 12 was expanded in patients with DRPLA. Abnormal alleles in DRPLA range 49–88 repeats (normal alleles <30 repeats). There is a strong inverse correlation between age at onset and CAG repeat length. This inverse correlation also determines clinical phenotype, with younger patients manifesting myoclonic epilepsy and older patients exhibiting predominantly ataxia and chorea. Anticipation occurs, particularly with paternal transmission. Paternal transmission may increase the CAG repeat length by five or more, whereas maternal transmission may decrease the repeat length or increase it by less than five.

Pathophysiology

The DRPLA protein, or atrophin-1, is widely expressed in various tissues, such as brain, skeletal muscle, heart, lung, and kidney. However, regional or cell type–specific factors may be responsible for the predilection for neuronal degeneration. Mutant DRPLA proteins with polyglutamine expansions may act by toxin gain of function. Transgenic mice demonstrate ataxia, tremors, abnormal movements, seizures, and early death as well as intranuclear accumulation of atrophin-1 and intranuclear inclusion bodies (Sato et al., 1999; Schilling et al, 1999). The transgenic mouse models suggest that DRPLA involves abnormal protein processing and nuclear accumulation of truncated fragments. In *post mortem* human DRPLA brains, immunoreactive, intranuclear inclusions have been found in neurons and glia (Hayashi et al., 1998), thereby suggesting an association between the CAG repeat expansion and neurodegenerative pathology.

Clinical Features

The clinical features of DRPLA overlap with progressive myoclonic epilepsy, SCA, and HD depending on the onset age. Clinical features of ataxia and dementia are present regardless in all patients. Age of onset is variable, ranging from childhood to late adulthood, but on average symptoms occur at around age 30. Patients with symptom onset at age less than 20 share a phenotype with progressive myoclonic epilepsy as seizures and myoclonus are present in addition to ataxia and dementia. The frequency of seizures decreases with age after age 20, and seizures are rare in those patients with older age at onset. Seizure types may include absence or atonic seizures, generalized seizures, or myoclonic epilepsy. Those patients with symptom onset after age 20 are more likely to resemble either SCA or HD with chorea and neuropsychiatric symptoms. Cognitive features are generally similar to a subcortical dementia with psychomotor retardation, executive dysfunction, and mild memory deficits. Psychiatric symptoms include mood disorders, apathy, irritability, childish behavior, and occasionally hallucinations or psychosis. Neuropathological examination reveals degeneration in the dentate, red, and subthalamic nuclei and globus pallidus, with accumulation of atrophin-1 in neuronal nuclei. Useful laboratory studies, besides genetic testing, include brain MRI and electroencephalography.

Chorea

Chorea is a common feature in those DRPLA patients with symptom onset after age 20. The chorea may be generalized and involve the face, trunk, and extremities. In some series, choreoathetoid movements of the extremities have been described. As suggested by the south Wales study (Wardle et al., 2008), DRPLA should be considered in the differential diagnosis for chorea and ataxia, especially if genetic testing is negative for HD, regardless of ethnicity.

Treatment

There is no cure for DRPLA. Epilepsy should be appropriately treated, but other therapies are supportive. Chorea may be managed with dopamine-blocking or dopamine-depleting agents. In one case report, Watarai et al. (2003) report beneficial effects of bilateral pallidotomy in a young patient with DRPLA and severe generalized chorea. At 8-month follow-up, only trace choreiform movements persisted.

REFERENCES

Agamanolis DP, Greenstein JI (1979) Ataxia-telangiectasia. Report of a case with Lewy bodies and vascular abnormalities within cerebral tissue. J Neuropathol Exp Neurol 38(5):475–489.

Aicardi J, Barbosa C, Andermann E, et al. (1988) Ataxia-ocular motor apraxia: a syndrome mimicking ataxia-telangiectasia. Ann Neurol 24(4):497–502.

Al-Mahdawi S, Pinto RM, Varshney D, et al. (2006) GAA repeat expansion mutation mouse models of Friedreich ataxia exhibit oxidative stress leading to progressive neuronal and cardiac pathology. Genomics 88(5):580–590.

Anheim M, Fleury MC, Franques J, et al. (2008) Clinical and molecular findings of ataxia with oculomotor apraxia type 2 in 4 families. Arch Neurol 65(7):958–962.

Anheim M, Monga B, Fleury M, et al. (2009) Ataxia with oculomotor apraxia type 2: clinical, biological and genotype/phenotype correlation study of a cohort of 90 patients. Brain 132(10):2688–2698.

Babcock M, Silva D, Oaks R, et al. (1997) Regulation of mitochondrial iron accumulation by Yfh1p, a putative homolog of frataxin. Science 276:1709–1712.

Banfi S, Servadio A, Chung M, et al. (1996) Cloning and developmental expression analysis of the murine homolog of the spinocerebellar ataxia type 1 gene. Hum Mol Genet 5:33–40.

Banfi S, Servadio A, Chung M, et al. (1994) Identification and characterization of the gene causing type 1 spinocerebellar ataxia. Nat Genet 7:513–520.

Barbot C, Coutinho P, Chorão R, et al. (2001) Recessive ataxia with ocular apraxia: review of 22 Portuguese patients. Arch Neurol 58(2):201–205.

Barlow C, Hirotsune S, Paylor R, et al. (1996) Atm-deficient mice: a paradigm of ataxia telangiectasia. Cell 86(1):159–171.

Bauer P, Laccone F, Rolfs A, et al. (2004) Trinucleotide repeat expansion in SCA17/TBP in white patients with Huntington's disease-like phenotype. J Med Genet 41:230–232.

Beamish H, Williams R, Chen P, Lavin MF (1996) Defect in multiple cell cycle checkpoints in ataxia-telangiectasia postirradiation. J Biol Chem 271(34):20486–20493.

Bidichandani SI, Ashizawa T, Patel PI (1998) The GAA triplet-repeat expansion in Friedreich ataxia interferes with transcription and may be associated with an unusual DNA structure. Am J Hum Genet 62(1):111–121.

Bodensteiner JB, Goldblum RM, Goldman AS (1980) Progressive dystonia masking ataxia in ataxia-telangiectasia. Arch Neurol 37(7):464–465.

Bomont P, Watanabe M, Gershoni-Barush R, et al. (2000) Homozygosity mapping of spinocerebellar ataxia with cerebellar atrophy and peripheral neuropathy to 9q33±34, and with hearing impairment and optic atrophy to 6p21±23. Eur J Hum Genet 8:986–990.

Bruni AC, Takahashi-Fujigasaki J, Maltecca F, et al. (2004) Behavioral disorder, dementia, ataxia, and rigidity in a large family with TATA box-binding protein mutation. Arch Neurol 61:1314–1320.

Bulteau AL, O'Neill HA, Kennedy MC, Ikeda-Saito M, Isaya G, Szweda LI (2004) Frataxin acts as an iron chaperone protein to modulate mitochondrial aconitase activity. Science 305(5681):242–245.

Burk K, Abele M, Fetter M, et al. (1996) Autosomal dominant cerebellar ataxia type I: clinical features and MRI in families with SCA1, SCA2 and SCA3. Brain 119: 1497–1505.

Burke JR, Ikeuchi T, Koide R, et al. (1994) Dentatorubral-pallidoluysian atrophy and Haw River syndrome. Lancet 344:1711–1712.

Burright EN, Clark HB, Servadio A, et al. (1995) SCA1 transgenic mice: a model for neurodegeneration caused by an expanded CAG trinucleotide repeat. Cell 82:937–948.

Campuzano V, Montermini L, Lutz Y, et al. (1997) Frataxin is reduced in Friedreich ataxia patients and is associated with mitochondrial membranes. Hum Mol Genet 6(11):1771–1780.

Campuzano V, Montermini L, Moltò MD, et al. (1996) Friedreich's ataxia: autosomal recessive disease caused by an intronic GAA triplet repeat expansion. Science 271 (5254):1423–1427.

Cancel G, Abbas N, Stevanin G, et al. (1995) Marked phenotypic heterogeneity associated with expansion of a CAG repeat sequence at the spinocerebellar ataxia 3/Machado-Joseph disease locus. Am J Hum Genet 57:809–816.

Cavadini P, Gellera C, Patel PI, Isaya G (2000) Human frataxin maintains mitochondrial iron homeostasis in Saccharomyces cerevisiae. Hum Mol Genet 9(17):2523–2530.

Chen YZ, Bennett CL, Huynh HM, et al. (2004) DNA/RNA helicase gene mutations in a form of juvenile amyotrophic lateral sclerosis (ALS4). Am J Hum Genet 74(6):1128–1135.

Chung MY, Ranum LP, Duvick LA, et al. (1993) Evidence for a mechanism predisposing to intergenerational CAG repeat instability in spinocerebellar ataxia type 1. Nat Genet 5(3):254–258.

Cossée M, Puccio H, Gansmuller A, et al. (2000) Inactivation of the Friedreich ataxia mouse gene leads to early embryonic lethality without iron accumulation. Hum Mol Genet 9(8):1219–1226.

Crawford TO, Skolasky RL, Fernandez R, Rosquist KJ, Lederman HM (2006) Survival probability in ataxia telangiectasia. Arch Dis Child 91:610–611.

Criscuolo C, Chessa L, Di Giandomenico S, et al. (2006) Ataxia with oculomotor apraxia type 2: a clinical, pathologic, and genetic study. Neurology 66(8):1207–1210.

Criscuolo C, Mancini P, Menchise V, et al. (2005) Very late onset in ataxia oculomotor apraxia type I. Ann Neurol 57(5):777.

Criscuolo C, Mancini P, Saccà F, et al. (2004) Ataxia with oculomotor apraxia type 1 in southern Italy: late onset and variable phenotype. Neurology 63(11):2173–2175.

Currier RD, Glover G, Jackson JF, Tipton AC (1972) Spinocerebellar ataxia: study of a large kindred. I. General information and genetics. Neurology 22:1041–1043.

Date H, Onodera O, Tanaka H, et al. (2001) Early-onset ataxia with ocular motor apraxia and hypoalbuminemia is caused by mutations in a new HIT superfamily gene. Nat Genet 29(2):184–188.

Delatycki MB, Knight M, Koenig M, Cossée M, Williamson R, Forrest SM (1999) G130V, a common FRDA point mutation, appears to have arisen from a common founder. Hum Genet 105:343–346.

De Michele G, Mainenti PP, Soricelli A, et al. (1998) Cerebral blood flow in spinocerebellar degenerations: a single photon emission tomography study in 28 patients. J Neurol 245(9):603–608.

Di Prospero NA, Baker A, Jeffries N, Fischbeck KH (2007). Neurological effects of high-dose idebenone in patients with Friedreich's ataxia: a randomised, placebo-controlled trial. Lancet Neurol 6(10):878–886.

Duquette A, Roddier K, McNabb-Baltar J, et al. (2005) Mutations in senataxin responsible for Quebec cluster of ataxia with neuropathy. Ann Neurol 57(3):408–414.

Dürr A, Cossee M, Agid Y, et al. (1996) Clinical and genetic abnormalities in patients with Friedreich's ataxia. N Engl J Med 335(16):1169–1175.

Duyckaerts C, Durr A, Cancel G, Brice A (1999) Nuclear inclusions in spinocerebellar ataxia type 1. Acta Neuropathol 97:201–207.

Elson A, Wang Y, Daugherty CJ, et al. (1996) Pleiotropic defects in ataxia-telangiectasia protein-deficient mice. Proc Natl Acad Sci USA 93(23):13084–13089.

Filla A, De Michele G, Cavalcanti F, et al. (1996) The relationship between trinucleotide (GAA) repeat length and clinical features in Friedreich ataxia. Am J Hum Genet 59(3):554–560.

Filla A, De Michele G, Marconi R, et al. (1992) Prevalence of hereditary ataxias and spastic paraplegias in Molise, a region of Italy. J Neurol 239(6):351–353.

Fogel BL, Perlman S (2006) Novel mutations in the senataxin DNA/RNA helicase domain in ataxia with oculomotor apraxia 2. Neurology 67(11):2083–2084.

Fujigasaki H, Martin JJ, De Deyn PP, et al. (2001) CAG repeat expansion in the TATA box–binding protein gene causes autosomal dominant cerebellar ataxia. Brain 123 :1939–1947.

Geschwind DH, Perlman S, Figueroa CP, et al. (1997) The prevalence and wide clinical spectrum of the spinocerebellar ataxia type 2 trinucleotide repeat in patients with autosomal dominant cerebellar ataxia. Am J Hum Genet 60:842–850.

Gilad S, Khosravi R, Shkedy D, et al. (1996) Predominance of null mutations in ataxia-telangiectasia. Hum Mol Genet 5(4):433–439.

Gueven N, Becherel OJ, Kijas AW, et al. (2004) Aprataxin, a novel protein that protects against genotoxic stress. Hum Mol Genet 13(10):1081–1093.

Hagenah JM, Zuhlke C, Hellenbroich Y, et al. (2004) Focal dystonia as a presenting sign of spinocerebellar ataxia 17. Mov Disord 19:217–220.

Haines JL, Schut LJ, Weitkamp LR, et al. (1984) Spinocerebellar ataxia in a large kindred: age at onset, reproduction, and genetic linkage studies. Neurology 34:1542–1548.

Hanna MG, Davis MB, Sweeney MG, et al. (1998) Generalized chorea in two patients harboring the Friedreich's ataxia gene trinucleotide repeat expansion. Mov Disord 13(2):339–340.

Harding AE (1981) Friedreich's ataxia: a clinical and genetic study of 90 families with an analysis of early diagnostic criteria and intrafamilial clustering of clinical features. Brain 104(3):589–620.

Harding AE (1982) The clinical features and classification of the late onset autosomal dominant cerebellar ataxias: a study of 11 families, including descendants of: the Drew family of Walworth." Brain 105:1–28.

Hausse AO, Aggoun Y, Bonnet D, et al. (2002) Idebenone and reduced cardiac hypertrophy in Friedreich's ataxia. Heart 87:346–349.

Hayashi Y, Kakita A, Yamada M, et al. (1998) Hereditary dentatorubral-pallidoluysian atrophy: detection of widespread ubiquitinated neuronal and glial intranuclear inclusions in the brain. Acta Neuropathol 96:547–552.

Imbert G, Trottier Y, Beckmann J, Mandel JL (1994) The gene for the TATA binding protein (TBP) that contains a highly polymorphic protein coding CAG repeat maps to 6q27. Genomics 21:667–668.

Inazuki G, Kumagai K, Naito H (1990) Dentatorubral-pallidoluysian atrophy (DRPLA): its distribution in Japan and prevalence rate in Niigata. Seishin Igaku 32:1135–1138.

Iwabuchi K, Tsuchiya K, Uchihara T, Yagishita S (1999) Autosomal dominant spinocerebellar degenerations: clinical, pathological, and genetic correlations. Rev Neurol 155:255–270.

Jackson JF, Currier RD, Terasaki P, Morton N (1977) Spinocerebellar ataxia and HLA linkage: risk prediction by HLA typing. N Engl J Med 296:1138–1141.

Juvonen V, Kulmala SM, Ignatius J, Penttinen M, Savontaus ML (2002) Dissecting the epidemiology of a trinucleotide repeat disease—example of FRDA in Finland. Hum Genet 110:36–40.

Kaemmerer WF, Rodriques CM, Steer CJ, Low WC (2001) Creatine-supplemented diet extends Purkinje cell survival in spinocerebellar ataxia type 1 transgenic mice but does not prevent the ataxic phenotype. Neuroscience 103:713–724.

Kameya T, Abe K, Aoki M, et al. (1995) Analysis of spinocerebellar ataxia type 1–related CAG trinucleotide expansion in Japan. Neurology 45(8):1587–1594.

Kamsler A, Daily D, Hochman A, et al. (2001) Increased oxidative stress in ataxia telangiectasia evidenced by alterations in redox state of brains from Atm-deficient mice. Cancer Res 61(5):1849–1854.

Klein C, Stewart GS, Quinn NP, Malcolm A, Taylor R (2001) Ataxia without telangiectasia revisited: update on genetic findings in two brothers with an ataxia-telangiectasia-like disorder. Mov Disord 16(4):788–789.

Klockgether T, Petersen D, Grodd W, Dichgans J (1991) Early onset cerebellar ataxia with retained tendon reflexes. Clinical, electrophysiological and MRI observations in comparison with Friedreich's ataxia. Brain 114(4):1559–1573.

Koepp M, Schelosky L, Cordes I, Cordes M, Poewe W (1994) Dystonia in ataxia telangiectasia: report of a case with putaminal lesions and decreased striatal [123I]iodobenzamide binding. Mov Disord 9(4):455–459.

Koide R, Ikeuchi T, Onodera O, et al. (1994) Unstable expansion of CAG repeat in hereditary dentatorubral-pallidoluysian atrophy (DRPLA). Nat Genet 6:9–13.

Koide R, Kobayashi S, Shimohata T, et al. (1999) A neurological disease caused by an expanded CAG trinucleotide repeat in the TATA-binding protein gene: a new polyglutamine disease? Hum Mol Genet 8:2047–2053.

Kondo I, Ohta H, Yazaki M, et al. (1990) Exclusion mapping of the hereditary dentatorubropallidoluysian atrophy gene from the Huntington's disease locus. J Med Genet 27:105–108.

Kuwano A, Morimoto Y, Nagai T, et al. (1996) Precise chromosomal locations of the genes for dentatorubral-pallidoluysian atrophy (DRPLA), von Willebrand factor (F8vWF) and parathyroid hormone-like hormone (PTHLH) in human chromosome 12p by deletion mapping. Hum Genet 97:95–98.

Labuda M, Labuda D, Miranda C, et al. (2000) Unique origin and specific ethnic distribution of the Friedreich ataxia GAA expansion. Neurology 54(12):2322–2324.

Lamarche JB, Lemieux B, Lieu HB (1984) The neuropathology of "typical" Friedreich's ataxia in Quebec. Can J Neurol Sci 11(4 Suppl):592–600.

Lasek K, Lencer R, Gaser C, et al. (2006) Morphological basis for the spectrum of clinical deficits in spinocerebellar ataxia 17 (SCA17). Brain 129:2341–2352.

Le Ber I, Bouslam N, Rivaud-Péchoux S, et al. (2004) Frequency and phenotypic spectrum of ataxia with oculomotor apraxia 2: a clinical and genetic study in 18 patients. Brain 127(4):759–767.

Le Ber I, Moreira MC, Rivaud-Péchoux S, et al. (2003) Cerebellar ataxia with oculomotor apraxia type 1: clinical and genetic studies. Brain 126(12):2761–2772.

Lee Y, McKinnon PJ (2000) ATM dependent apoptosis in the nervous system. Apoptosis 5:523–529.

Lescure A, Lutz Y, Eberhard D, et al. (1994) The N-terminal domain of the human TATA-binding protein plays a role in transcription from TATA-containing RNA polymerase II and III promotors. EMBO J 13:1166–1175.

Mantovan MC, Martinuzzi A, Squarzanti F, et al. (2006) Exploring mental status in Friedreich's ataxia: a combined neuropsychological, behavioral and neuroimaging study. Eur J Neurol 13(8):827–835.

Matilla T, Volpini V, Genis D, et al. (1993) Presymptomatic analysis of spinocerebellar ataxia type 1 (SCA1) via the expansion of the SCA1 CAG-repeat in a large pedigree displaying anticipation and parental male bias. Hum Mol Genet 2:2123–2128.

Matilla-Dueñas A, Goold R, Guinti P (2008) Clinical, genetic, molecular, and pathophysiological insights into spinocerebellar ataxia type 1. Cerebellum 7(2):106–114.

McConville CM, Stankovic T, Byrd PJ, et al. (1996) Mutations associated with variant phenotypes in ataxia-telangiectasia. Am J Hum Genet 59(2):320–330.

Minnerop M, Joe A, Lutz M, et al. (2005) Putamen dopamine transporter and glucose metabolism are reduced in SCA17. Ann Neurol 58:490–491.

Monrós E, Moltó MD, Martínez F, et al. (1997) Phenotype correlation and intergenerational dynamics of the Friedreich ataxia GAA trinucleotide repeat. Am J Hum Genet 61(1):101–110.

Moreira MC, Barbot C, Tachi N, et al. (2001a) Homozygosity mapping of Portuguese and Japanese forms of ataxia-oculomotor apraxia to 9p13, and evidence for genetic heterogeneity. Am J Hum Genet 68(2):501–508.

Moreira MC, Barbot C, Tachi N, et al. (2001b) The gene mutated in ataxia-ocular apraxia 1 encodes the new HIT/Zn-finger protein aprataxin. Nat Genet 29(2):189–193.

Moreira MC, Klur S, Watanabe M, et al. (2004) Senataxin, the ortholog of a yeast RNA helicase, is mutant in ataxia-ocular apraxia 2. Nat Genet 36(3):225–227.

Nagafuchi S, Yanagisawa H, Sato K, et al. (1994) Dentatorubral and pallidoluysian atrophy expansion of an unstable CAG trinucleotide on chromosome 12p. Nat Genet 6:14–18.

Naito H, Izawa K, Kurosaki T, et al. (1972) Two families of progressive myoclonic epilepsy with Mendelian dominant heredity. Psychiatr Neurol Jpn 74:871–897.

Naito H, Oyanagi S (1982) Familial myoclonus epilepsy and choreoathetosis: hereditary dentatorubral-pallidoluysian atrophy. Neurology 32:798–807.

Nakamura K, Jeong SY, Uchihara T, et al. (2001) SCA17, a novel autosomal dominant cerebellar ataxia caused by an expanded polyglutamine in TATA-binding protein. Hum Mol Genet 10:1441–1448.

Namekawa M, Takiyama Y, Ando Y, et al. (2001) Choreiform movements in spinocerebellar ataxia type I. J Neurol Sci 187:103–106.

Nemeth AH, Bochukova E, Dunne E, et al. (2000) Autosomal recessive cerebellar ataxia with oculomotor apraxia (ataxia telangiectasia-like syndrome) is linked to chromosome 9q34. Am J Hum Genet 67:1320–1326.

Nowak-Wegrzyn A, Crawford TO, Winkelstein JA, Carson KA, Lederman HM (2004) Immunodeficiency and infections in ataxia-telangiectasia. J Pediatr 144(4):505–511.

Orr HT, Chung M, Banfi S, et al. (1993) Expansion of an unstable trinucleotide CAG repeat in spinocerebellar ataxia type 1. Nat Genet 4:221–226.

Pineda M, Arpa J, Montero R, et al. (2008) Idebenone treatment in paediatric and adult patients with Friedreich ataxia: long-term follow-up. Eur J Paediatr Neurol 12(6): 470–475.

Puccio H, Simon D, Cossée M, et al. (2001) Mouse models for Friedreich ataxia exhibit cardiomyopathy, sensory nerve defect and Fe-S enzyme deficiency followed by intramitochondrial iron deposits. Nat Genet 27(2):181–186.

Ranum LPW, Duvick L A, Rich SS, et al. (1991) Localization of the autosomal dominant HLA-linked spinocerebellar ataxia (SCA1) locus, in two kindreds, within an 8-cM subregion of chromosome 6p. Am J Hum Genet 49:31–41.

Rigby PW (1993) Three in one and one in three: it all depends on TBP. Cell 72:7–10.

Rottnek M, Riggio S, Byne W, et al. (2008) Schizophrenia in a patient with spinocerebellar ataxia 2: coincidence of two disorders or a neurodegenerative disease presenting with psychosis? Am J Psychiatry 165:964–967.

Rustin P, von Kleist-Retzow JC, Chantrel-Groussard K, Sidi D, Munnich A, Rötig A (1999) Effect of idebenone on cardiomyopathy in Friedreich's ataxia: a preliminary study. Lancet 354:477–479.

Salvatore E, Varrone A, Criscuolo C, et al. (2008) Nigrostriatal involvement in ataxia with oculomotor apraxia type 1. J Neurol 255(1):45–48.

Sano Y, Date H, Igarashi S, et al. (2004) Aprataxin, the causative protein for EAOH is a nuclear protein with a potential role as a DNA repair protein. Ann Neurol 55(2): 241–249.

Sasaki H, Fukazawa T, Yanagihara T, et al. (1996) Clinical features and natural history of spinocerebellar ataxia type 1. Acta Neurol Scand 93:64–71.

Sato T, Oyake M, Nakamura K, et al. (1999) Transgenic mice harboring a full-length mutant DRPLA gene exhibit age-dependent intergenerational and somatic instabilities of CAG repeats comparable with those in DRPLA patients. Hum Mol Genet 8:99–106.

Savitsky K, Bar-Shira A, Gilad S, et al. (1995) A single ataxia telangiectasia gene with a product similar to PI-3 kinase. Science 268(5218):1749–1753.

Schilling G, Wood JD, Duan K, et al. (1999) Nuclear accumulation of truncated atrophin-1 fragments in a transgenic mouse model of DRPLA. Neuron 24:275–286.

Schmitz-Hübsch T, Coudert M, Bauer P, et al. (2008) Spinocerebellar ataxia types 1, 2, 3, and 6: disease severity and nonataxia symptoms. Neurology 71:982–989.

Schneider SA, van de Warrenburg BPC, Hughes TD, et al. (2006) Phenotypic homogeneity of the Huntington disease-like presentation in a SCA17 family. Neurology 67:1701–1703.

Schols L, Amoiridis G, Buttner T, et al. (1997) Autosomal dominant cerebellar ataxia: phenotypic differences in genetically defined subtypes? Ann Neurol 42:924–932.

Sekijima Y, Ohara S, Nakagawa S, et al. (1998) Hereditary motor and sensory neuropathy associated with cerebellar atrophy (HMSNCA): clinical and neuropathological features of a Japanese family. J Neurol Sci 158(1):30–37.

Servadio A, Koshy B, Armstrong D, et al. (1995) Expression analysis of the ataxin-1 protein in tissues from normal and spinocerebellar ataxia type 1 individuals. Nat Genet 10:94–98.

Seznec H, Simon D, Monassier L, et al. (2004) Idebenone delays the onset of cardiac functional alteration without correction of Fe-S enzymes deficit in a mouse model for Friedreich ataxia. Hum Mol Genet 13(10):1017–1024.

Shimazaki H, Takiyama Y, Sakoe K, et al. (2002) Early-onset ataxia with ocular motor apraxia and hypoalbuminemia: the aprataxin gene mutations. Neurology 59(4):590–595.

Simon D, Seznec H, Gansmuller A, et al. (2004) Friedreich ataxia mouse models with progressive cerebellar and sensory ataxia reveal autophagic neurodegeneration in dorsal root ganglia. J Neurosci 24(8):1987–1995.

Skinner PJ, Koshy B, Cummings CJ, et al. (1997) Ataxin-1 with an expanded glutamine tract alters nuclear matrix-associated structures. Nature 389:971–974.

Skinner PJ, Vierra-Green CA, Clark HB, et al. (2001) Altered trafficking of membrane proteins in Purkinje cells of SCA1 transgenic mice. Am J Pathol 159:905–913.

Smith JK, Gonda VE, Malamud N. (1958). Unusual form of cerebellar ataxia; combined dentato-rubral and pallido-Luysian degeneration. Neurology 8(3):205–9.

Spacey SD, Szczygielski BI, Young SP, Hukin J, Selby K, Snutch TP (2004) Malaysian siblings with Friedreich ataxia and chorea: a novel deletion in the frataxin gene. Can J Neurol Sci 31(3):383–386.

Stevanin G, Brice A (2008) Spinocerebellar ataxia 17 (SCA17) and Huntington's disease-like 4 (HDL4). Cerebellum 7(2):170–178.

Stevanin G, Fujigasaki H, Lebre AS, et al. (2003) Huntington's disease–like phenotype due to trinucleotide repeat expansions in the TBP and JPH3 genes. Brain 126:1599–1603.

Sun X, Becker-Catania SG, Chun HH, et al. (2002) Early diagnosis of ataxia-telangiectasia using radiosensitivity testing. J Pediatr 140(6):724–731.

Suraweera A, Becherel OJ, Chen P, et al. (2007) Senataxin, defective in ataxia oculomotor apraxia type 2, is involved in the defense against oxidative DNA damage. J Cell Biol 177(6):969–979.

Swift M, Morrell D, Cromartie E, Chamberlin AR, Skolnick MH, Bishop DT (1986) The incidence and gene frequency of ataxia-telangiectasia in the United States. Am J Hum Genet 39(5):573–583.

Tang B, Liu C, Shen L, et al. (2000) Frequency of SCA1, SCA2, SCA3/MJD, SCA6, SCA7, and DRPLA CAG trinucleotide repeat expansion in patients with hereditary spinocerebellar ataxia from Chinese kindreds. Arch Neurol 57:540–544.

Taylor AM, Metcalfe JA, Thick J, Mak YF (1996) Leukemia and lymphoma in ataxia telangiectasia. Blood 87(2):423–438.

Tazir M, Ali-Pacha L, M'zahem A, et al. (2009) Ataxia with oculomotor apraxia type 2: a clinical and genetic study of 19 patients. J Neurol Sci 278(1–2):77–81.

Toyoshima Y, Yamada M, Onodera O, et al. (2004) SCA17 homozygote showing Hunting-ton's disease–like phenotype. Ann Neurol 55:281–286.

Wardle M, Majounie E, Williams NM, et al. (2008) Dentatorubral pallidoluysian atrophy in south Wales. J Neurol Neurosurg Psychiatry 79:804–807.

Watarai M, Hashimoto T, Yamamoto K, et al. (2003) Pallidotomy for severe generalized chorea of juvenile-onset dentatorubral-pallidoluysian atrophy. Neurology 61(10): 1452–1454.

Watase K, Gatchel JR, Sun Y, et al. (2007) Lithium therapy improves neurological function and hippocampal dendritic arborization in a spinocerebellar ataxia type 1 mouse model. PLoS Med 4:3182.

Watters D, Khanna KK, Beamish H, et al. (1997) Cellular localisation of the ataxia-telangiectasia (ATM) gene product and discrimination between mutated and normal forms. Oncogene 14(16):1911–1921.

Woods CG, Bundey SE, Taylor AM (1990) Unusual features in the inheritance of ataxia telangiectasia. Hum Genet 84(6):555–562.

Wüllner U, Klockgether T, Petersen D, Naegele T, Dichgans J (1993) Magnetic resonance imaging in hereditary and idiopathic ataxia. Neurology 43(2):318–325.

Xu Y, Ashley T, Brainerd EE, Bronson RT, Meyn MS, Baltimore D (1996) Targeted disrup-tion of ATM leads to growth retardation, chromosomal fragmentation during meiosis, immune defects, and thymic lymphoma. Genes Dev 10(19):2411–2422.

Yakura H, Wakisaka A, Fujimoto S, Itakura K (1974) Hereditary ataxia and HL-A geno-types. N Engl J Med 291:154–155.

Zhu D, Burke C, Leslie A, Nicholson GA (2002) Friedreich's ataxia with chorea and myo-clonus caused by a compound heterozygosity for a novel deletion and the trinucleotide GAA expansion. Mov Disord 17(3):585–589.

Zoghbi HY, Jodice C, Sandkuijl LA, et al. (1991) The gene for autosomal dominant spinoc-erebellar ataxia (SCA1) maps telomeric to the HLA complex and is closely linked to the D6S89 locus in three large kindreds. Am J Hum Genet 49:23–30.

Zuhlke C, Hellenbroich Y, Dalski A, et al. (2001) Different types of repeat expansion in the TATA-binding protein gene are associated with a new form of inherited ataxia. Eur J Hum Genet 9:160–164.

13

Inherited Metabolic Diseases Causing Chorea in Childhood

Donald L. Gilbert, MD, MS

INTRODUCTION AND OVERVIEW

The primary aim of this chapter is to discuss clinical features and diagnosis of children and, to a much lesser extent, adults with the hyperkinetic phenomenologies chorea, athetosis, choreoathetosis, and ballismus due to hereditary metabolic diseases (HMDs). In general, the term "chorea" will be emphasized rather than "choreoathetosis" (Sanger et al., 2009). However, in the literature on HMDs, the terms "choreoathetosis" and "chorea" are often used interchangeably, in part because of overlap between slower, athetoid movements and faster, choreic movements and in part because most movement disorders related to metabolic diseases are mixed. Combinations of chorea with myoclonus, ataxia, or parkinsonism lead to phenomenological confusion even among experts (Schrag et al., 2000).

For the purpose of this chapter, metabolic diseases causing chorea will encompass predominantly conditions having onset before adulthood. Most are inherited in an autosomal recessive manner (Garcia-Cazorla et al., 2009; Lyon et al., 2006). The emphasis here will be on diseases affecting enzymes for processing proteins, carbohydrates, or lipids. The term "metabolic disease" can be used broadly to refer to almost any cellular process, including disorders of purine or pyrimidine metabolism, disorders of steroid metabolism, disorders of lysosome or peroxisomal function or storage, disorders of porphyrin metabolism, neurotransmitter diseases (e.g., diseases of tetrahydrobiopterin), disorders of mineral accumulation (e.g., copper), and other degenerative disorders involving other intracellular accumulations. These other diseases will be discussed when they are in the differential diagnosis or manifest with prominent childhood chorea; however, most are covered in more detail elsewhere in this book. Other resources available on metabolic diseases affecting the nervous system include excellent textbooks on pediatric movement disorders in general (Nardocci and Fernandez-Alvarez, 2007; Singer et al., 2010) and the neurology of hereditary metabolic diseases in children (Lyon et al., 2006). In addition, vast amounts of information are available online through the U.S. National Institutes of Health and National Library of Medicine's Web sites, particularly Online Mendelian Inheritance in Man (OMIM, http://www.ncbi.nlm.nih.gov/omim/) and Genetests Gene Reviews (http://www.ncbi.nlm.nih.gov/sites/GeneTests/). For general physicians, patients, and families, excellent resources include Worldwide Education and Awareness for Movement Disorders (http://www.wemove.org/), the Genetics Home Reference pages (http://ghr.nlm.nih.gov/), as well as disease-based Web sites.

This chapter begins with two sections. The first discusses situations when a clinician should consider metabolic diseases. The second discusses an approach for narrowing the differential diagnosis using the OMIM and Genetests Web pages. Subsequently, specific diseases are discussed, organized by age at presentation.

WHEN IS CHOREA LIKELY TO BE CAUSED BY A METABOLIC DISEASE?

Chorea in childhood is usually not caused by metabolic diseases. Most acquired chorea is autoimmune, particularly poststreptococcal, Sydenham chorea (Chapter 17). However, in certain cases of delayed or progressively impaired motor and cognitive function, the presence of choreiform movements can be a clue to the presence of a metabolic disease. With regard to the common presentation of developmental delay in children under age 6 years, there is no current consensus about whether testing for metabolic diseases should be part of the diagnostic work-up (Engbers et al., 2008; McDonald et al., 2006; Shevell, 2009; Shevell et al., 2003). It is relatively easy for any clinician to obtain a broad spectrum of blood and urine tests. Expert consultation and targeted, rather than broad, work-ups may yield diagnostically and therapeutically important results (Engbers et al., 2008; Miles et al., 2006).

There are four main clinical features of metabolic diseases which, when present together, strongly suggest the presence of a hereditary metabolic etiology of a neurological disease: (1) heritability; (2) the appearance of a neurological sign which was not previously present; (3) loss of neurologically based skills or function over time; and (4) the presence, outside the nervous system, of symptoms or signs that tend to occur in metabolic diseases. These pose major challenges to clinicians and will be discussed in turn.

Heritability

Metabolic diseases are typically heritable, with the most common mode being autosomal recessive. This is unfortunate because there may not be any affected siblings at presentation, or ever, to clarify this mode of inheritance. In any case, a careful three-generation pedigree should be drawn out by the clinician in every new case. It is incumbent upon the clinician to be familiar with the basic modes of inheritance: autosomal recessive, autosomal dominant, X-linked, mitochondrial. The Genetics Home Reference page online (http://ghr.nlm.nih.gov/handbook/inheritance/inheritancepatterns) and a page available through the Wellcome Trust (http://genome.wellcome.ac.uk/doc_WTD020848.html) are recommended. Other, more advanced and recent topics such as copy number variants, variable expressivity, and reduced penetrance are also defined and discussed in the Genetics Home Reference page online handbook.

New Neurological Signs

Persons with HMDs may be affected by a new neurological symptom or sign prenatally, in the first week of life, or at any time thereafter throughout life, although adult onset is less common. Prior to the onset, the individual may appear healthy and normal. A significant stress, such as fasting, febrile illness, trauma, or a medical procedure, may unmask the genetic problem. This poses several diagnostic challenges.

First, death or disability may occur due to the triggering stressor. For example, trauma, hypotension, infection, or autoimmune disease may damage the nervous system and simultaneously trigger metabolic disease that damages the nervous system. Therefore, the presence or contribution of an HMD may be difficult or impossible to sort out. However, when a metabolic disease is suspected, a childhood death of an older sibling may be a clue.

Second, new signs often emerge during development due to the combination of a remote static process and neurological maturation. For example, a stroke present since birth may be asymptomatic until a sufficient level of myelination or neuroplasticity allows the gliotic brain region to act as a locus for a neurological sign, with spasticity and weakness becoming apparent between 2 and 8 months and chorea and ataxia becoming apparent between 9 and 14 months after birth. Similarly, cortical dysplasias present since birth may become a locus for epilepsy in childhood, adolescence, or even adulthood. Thus, there are situations during neurological maturation where an old lesion, not a metabolic decompensation, produces a new neurological sign. Complicating this interpretation further, some remote static processes (i.e., structural brain lesions) may have metabolic causes (Chow and Thorburn, 2000; Keng et al., 2003; Miller et al., 2004).

Third, the child may not have any prior carefully documented neurological examination. A primary physician may fail to note or document eye movement apraxia, gaze limitation, weakness, reflex or sensory abnormalities, tremor, or dyskinesias during routine well-care visits. With regard to cognitive function, academic performance functions to some extent as a quantitative measure in school-age children. However, neurologically meaningful declines may not be reflected in a child's grades. Development of attentional or emotional difficulties is nonspecific and as an isolated finding is only rarely due to new neuropathology.

Fourth, with regard to a new sign of chorea specifically, the most common pathophysiology of acquired chorea and recurring chorea in childhood is autoimmune, which can have fairly rapid onset (Chapter 17). Thus, while clinicians need to remain vigilant for metabolic disease in acute/subacute chorea, in many cases metabolic testing is unnecessary. In many cases careful clinical follow-up, with judicious use of neuroimaging, clarifies the need to consider metabolic diseases in the differential diagnosis.

Loss of Skills

The basal ganglia structures that underlie chorea also interface with cognitive and emotional circuits (DeLong and Wichmann, 2007). Thus, determining that a child with chorea has an HMD involves understanding and assessing neurodevelopment broadly. When an HMD is suspected, the most important question to ask a parent of a child, particularly a pre-school-age child, is, "Is there anything your child cannot do now that she or he could previously?" Even this response may be unreliable, as when a static encephalopathy affects motor skills or language in a way that parents interpret as a loss of function but which actually represents increasing divergence from normally maturing peers. Compounding this, high-level cognitive functions mature at variable rates, and the range of what is healthy for cognitive functions is quite broad in children. At the first clinic visit, the question of regression may be especially difficult. Sometimes a sequence of home videos, from prior birthday celebrations, for example, allows for more rapid clarification of progressive vs. static processes. If the child is in special education, serial cognitive, speech, physical, and occupational therapy evaluations through the schools, if competently performed, can also provide useful data. Parents usually readily consent to have these forwarded to the clinician from the school.

Nonneurological Symptoms and Signs

Unfortunately, nearly any chief complaint in any organ system could be caused by a metabolic disease. However, clues in some key areas may suggest the presence of a metabolic disease (Table 13–1).

TABLE 13–1. Prominent Nonneurological Manifestations of Metabolic Diseases in Children

SYSTEM	FEATURE
Growth	Short stature, failure to thrive, weight loss
Gastrointestinal	Recurrent vomiting, hepato- or splenomegaly
Respiratory	Hyperventilation
Endocrine	Delayed puberty, multi-endocrine organ problems
Dermatological	Abnormal pigmentation or hair growth
Hematological	Anemia, thrombocytopenia
Immunological	Deficiency
Orthopedic	Bony anomalies in face, trunk, limbs

EFFICIENT DIAGNOSIS OF METABOLIC CAUSES OF CHOREA

The focus of this section is on the diagnosis of the rare metabolic diseases that cause acute, paroxysmal, and chronic progressive chorea. Metabolic diseases do not cause chorea in isolation. Usually, there is a mixed movement disorder with some degree of encephalopathy or other nonneurological findings (as discussed earlier in "Nonneurological Symptoms and Signs"). Some children may present in emergent clinical situations, where hyperkinesia (ballismus/chorea, status dystonicus/dystonia) is new, life-threatening, and typically accompanied by encephalopathy. In these cases emergent management often involves supportive care, reversal of acidosis, and arrest of catabolism with administration of dextrose. In situations where metabolic diseases are suspected but not confirmed, an acute crisis may be a window for narrowing the differential diagnosis, for example, by identifying lactic acidosis in this setting. In other chronic settings, such as developmental delay, the emergence of a movement disorder over time may be a clue that a metabolic disease should be investigated. In such cases the clinician may have to put in a great deal of extra work to come to the correct diagnosis in the context of an ever-expanding field of metabolic disease. In this sense, having a good approach is paramount.

Neuroimaging

When, based on factors discussed earlier (under "When Is Chorea Likely to Be Caused by a Metabolic Disease?"), an HMD is suspected, brain magnetic resonance imaging (MRI) sequences may disclose focal symmetric processes in basal ganglia, gray matter disease, white matter disease, or structural malformations; and these findings may confirm a clinical diagnosis or efficiently guide further

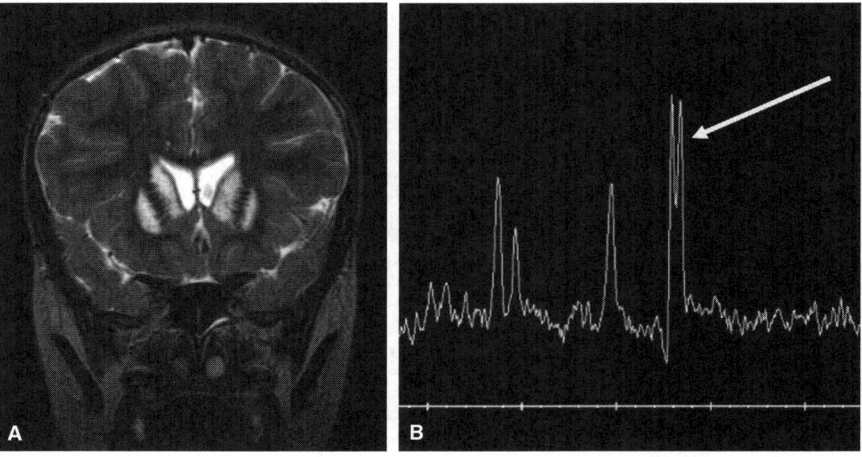

FIGURE 13–1. **A** Magnetic resonance image showing a characteristic striatal signal change in a patient with electron transport complex I deficiency. **B** Magnetic resonance spectroscopy reveals a lactate peak (*arrow*). Courtesy of A. Dinopolous.

work-up (Dinopoulos et al., 2005) (Figure 13–1). The addition of magnetic resonance spectroscopy (MRS) allows for quantitative assessment of important metabolites. For example, reduction of *N*-acetylaspartate indicates neuronal loss, and elevation of lactate can indicate the presence of a mitochondrial disorder (Haas et al., 2008; Zafeiriou et al., 2008). Abnormally elevated lactate may be identified in voxels placed in either gray or white matter (Dinopoulos et al., 2005).

Neuroimaging findings may be nonspecific however, and subtle changes in basal ganglia volumes, in the absence of changes in signal intensity, may not be apparent. While overall less useful, brain computed tomographic (CT) scanning may be more helpful for clarifying whether a signal change represents calcification.

Laboratory Testing

Blood, urine, and sometimes cerebrospinal fluid metabolic laboratory testing may be critical for confirming the diagnosis or narrowing the differential diagnosis before obtaining highly expensive genetic testing. Clinicians often cast a broad net, particularly in dire, infantile, or complex cases. Table 13–2 shows some commonly used tests, patterns of results, and underlying disease categories. Note that most of these patterns of laboratory abnormality, when present in infancy, occur in the context of hypotonia, encephalopathy, and seizures, not movement disorders. Further information is provided in the context of specific diseases.

TABLE 13–2. Patterns of Laboratory Abnormalities in Metabolic Diseases

LABORATORY ABNORMALITIES	METABOLIC DISEASE CATEGORY
Acidosis, ketosis +/– hypoglycemia, +/– hyperammonemia	Aminoacidopathies, organic acidopathies, defects of biotin metabolism, some disorders of carbohydrate metabolism
Hyperammonemia, respiratory alkalosis	Urea cycle disorders
Lactic acidosis (blood, CSF), no hypoglycemia, no organic aciduria	Mitochondrial disorders of pyruvate metabolism or respiratory chain, Leigh syndrome
Hypoglycemia, low ketone bodies	Mitochondrial fatty acid oxidation disorders, ketogenesis and ketolysis disorders
High very long chain fatty acids	Peroxisomal disease
Abnormal pattern of serum sialotransferrins by isoelectrofocusing	Disorders of glycosylation

CSF, cerebrospinal fluid; +/–, with or without.

Online Search Strategy for Genetic Movement Disorders

The expanding number of identified genetic diseases and the diverse but overlapping phenotypes means that considerable time may be spent pursuing a molecular diagnosis. The following is a search strategy that may be considered for use of the two Web sites OMIM (http://www.ncbi.nlm.nih.gov/omim/) and Genetests (http://www.ncbi.nlm.nih.gov/sites/GeneTests/).

OMIM can be searched using one or more terms, separated by a space, similar to searching for medical publications using MEDLINE PubMed (http://www.ncbi.nlm.nih.gov/PubMed). OMIM is fully integrated and linked to the PubMed and GENETESTS databases to identify availability of clinical genetic testing. OMIM searches can be limited in several important and helpful ways. For example, the search can be limited by chromosomal location, including the X chromosome, or by mitochondrial DNA. Thus, combining phenotype and information about the inheritance pattern can rapidly narrow the search. Searches can also be restricted based on other genetic information. OMIM uses a series of abbreviations for its entries as follows:

- * for genes with known sequence
- + for genes with known sequence and phenotype
- # for entries where there is phenotype description and known molecular basis
- % for Mendelian phenotype but unknown molecular basis

This genetic information classification can be selected to limit searches as well.

To understand the efficiency of using this strategy, it is helpful to look at the following example, based on OMIM entries at the time of this writing. A search for "chorea" yields 63 entries, and a search for "choreoathetosis" yields 74. Combining these, "chorea OR choreoathetosis," yields 123 entries. Limiting this to X chromosome reduces the hits to 11—a much more manageable list upon which to focus.

It is important to recognize that OMIM disease entries have some very useful subsections. At the initial stage, the most useful of these is the "Clinical Synopsis," which describes each entry with an outline by organ system so that one can easily see the typical dermatological, ophthalmological, orthopedic, etc. features as well as the neurological. By resetting the display to "Clinical Synopsis," one can scan through search "hits" in a clinically useful and efficient way. Note that if one employs the presence of chorea in the clinical synopsis as a "limit," this reduces "chorea OR choreoathetosis" entries from 123 to 60.

In summary, optimizing search strategies can save substantial clinician time and may enhance diagnostic capabilities without requiring an extremely expensive genetic testing panel.

Once the differential diagnosis is narrowed, there is additional text in OMIM that may be worth reading. In addition, the references to PubMed and to Genetests are linked for further consideration and to arrange for diagnostic testing from laboratories worldwide that test for over 1,000 diseases. Genetests also has up-to-date expert reviews on many disease topics.

The increasing availability of specific genetic tests has been critical for families but as yet has made little specific impact on treatment. For example, evidence of the utility of supplementation with mitochondrial cofactors is lacking in the majority of mitochondrial diseases. Often, as in the case of galactosemia (Ridel et al., 2005), specific lifesaving dietary interventions do not normalize cognitive or motor function.

Making a precise genetic, molecular diagnosis, even in the absence of rational and clinically useful therapy, narrows the prognostic landscape and opens up social and emotional resources for affected families. As new treatment studies come online, families using Internet resources such as disease-based Web sites, e-mail lists, or the clinical trials registry Web site (http://clinicaltrials.gov/) may become aware of options before the primary physician.

METABOLIC DISEASES CAUSING CHOREA OR CHOREOATHETOSIS, BY AGE AT PRESENTATION

Neonatal Presentations

As discussed in earlier (see "When Is Chorea Likely to Be Caused by a Metabolic Disease?"), the brain of the neonate will generally not generate hyperkinetic movement disorders, even when the substrate for subsequent disease is already present. Nevertheless, a few key entities bear mention based on their tendency to induce hyperkinetic movements.

"Post-Pump Chorea"—Chorea After Neonatal and Infant Cardiac Surgery

Clinical Features.   Although the incidence has decreased markedly, chorea has long been described as a neurological complication of cardiac surgery in neonates and infants (Brunberg et al., 1974). Dyskinetic movements, either transient or prolonged, are usually accompanied by subnormal intellectual outcomes (du Plessis et al., 2002; Medlock et al., 1993).

Pathophysiology.   There is selective striatal injury, with reactive gliosis and neuronal loss particularly in the external globus pallidus (Kupsky et al., 1995).

Treatment.   The best treatment is prevention through improved surgical and anesthetic techniques.

Dyskinetic/Choreoathetoid Cerebral Palsy

Clinical Features.   Choreoathetoid movements emerge in late infancy.

Pathophysiology.   There is injury to the basal ganglia during the third trimester of pregnancy or the perinatal period.

Treatment.   Treatment is supportive and nonspecific. Anticholinergics such as trihexyphenidyl should be tried, but they may reduce dystonia at the expense of increasing chorea. Carbidopa/levodopa, baclofen, diazepam, and, with caution, dopamine receptor–blocking agents may be considered. Use of deep brain stimulation (DBS) is increasing (Vidailhet et al., 2009).

Kernicterus/Chronic Bilirubin Encephalopathy

Clinical Features.   The three classic neurological sequelae in children with chronic encephalopathy due to damage from neonatal exposure to unconjugated bilirubin are hearing loss, hyperkinetic movement disorder, and impaired upgaze. Cognitive impairment is variable. Brain MRI may appear normal in the first year or may have subtle T1 signal hyperintensity in the globus pallidus interna (GPi) (Govaert et al., 2003). Subsequently, scarring in the GPi is more obvious, with increased T2 signal and volume loss.

Pathophysiology.   Bilirubin staining accompanies neuronal damage in the globus pallidus, subthalamic nucleus, hippocampus, substantia nigra pars reticulata, and brainstem and cerebellar nuclei (Ahdab-Barmada and Moossy, 1984; Volpe, 2001).

Treatment.   Treatment is mainly supportive. Anticholinergic agents may reduce choreoathetosis (Merhar and Gilbert, 2005). There are few published data regarding surgical intervention. Pallidotomy with current stereotactic techniques has yielded at best minimal benefit.

Metabolic Diseases Presenting in the First 2 Years of Life

There are a large number of metabolic diseases that present in the first year of life but after the neonatal period. These tend to produce a variety of neurological symptoms which are nonspecific, including hypotonia and developmental delay. Two keys to the possibility of a metabolic diagnosis are developmental regression or arrest and acute remitting episodes. Characteristic MRI, ocular/ophthalmological, or nonneurological findings may narrow the differential diagnosis. Most neurological diseases presenting in the first 9 months do not produce chorea. Alternatively, there may be a mixed movement disorder, described variously in the literature as ataxia, dystonia, choreoathetosis, or extrapyramidal symptoms. At age 9–24 months the child is mastering aspects of control of trunk, limbs, and locomotion. The more complex, highly developed cerebral cortex and cortical–striatal circuits can, when diseased, generate more complex abnormal movements.

X-Linked Pyruvate Dehydrogenase Complex Deficiency

Clinical Features.   These are highly variable. There can be hypotonia and weakness, episodic ataxia, episodic dystonia, or chorea. Adult-onset cases have been described.

Pathophysiology.   The mechanism of injury involves lactic acidosis produced because of mutations in the E1 subunit of the pyruvate dehydrogenase complex (Dahl et al., 1990).

Treatment.   Treatment options include thiamine and the ketogenic diet. These can be helpful in some patients.

Glutaric Aciduria, Type I

Clinical Features.   These can be highly variable (Gitiaux et al., 2008; Hedlund et al., 2006; Strauss et al., 2003). One presentation involves a child with early macrocephaly and rapid deterioration. These infants are prone to subdural bleeds after mild head injury. Hypotonia and irritability may occur in infancy, with progressive hyperkinetic movements. Typically, an illness between the age of

6 and 18 months leads to an acute decompensation with striatal injury, followed by dystonia and/or chorea. Some children may survive infancy without developing symptoms. Imaging shows severe striatal degeneration, atrophy of the fronto-temporal cortex, enlarged subdural fluid spaces, and dilation of sylvian fissures (Strauss et al., 2007).

Pathophysiology.   The disease is caused by mutations in the gene that codes for glutaryl-coenzyme A dehydrogenase. The mechanism of disease is unclear but may involve 3-hydroxyglutaric acid stimulated, glutamate-mediated excitotoxicity in the striatum.

Treatment.   Therapy is supportive. Restricting dietary proteins to reduce the glutarigenic amino acids lysine, tryptophan, and hydroxylysine has been used, along with riboflavin and L-carnitine. In the Amish, dietary treatment has been used with mixed success. Benefits are probably limited once striatal injury has already occurred. In this population, after newborn screening, dietary treatment and urgent intravenous fluid therapy with dextrose during febrile illnesses prior to age 2 have markedly reduced the incidence of basal ganglia injury.

Brain Creatine Deficiency Syndromes: Guanidinoacetate Methyltransferase Deficiency, Arginine:Glycine Amidinotransferase Deficiency (Autosomal Recessive), and X-Linked Creatine Transporter Deficiency

Clinical Features.   Children with these diseases have developmental delay/regression, mental retardation, severe language disturbances, autistic behavior, and dyskinetic movements (Bianchi et al., 2000; deGrauw et al., 2002; Stockler et al., 2007). In guanidinoacetate methyltransferase deficiency, seizures are prominent. Diagnoses are based on elevated guanidinoacetate in urine; absence of enzyme activity in fibroblasts. MRS (Figure 13–2) shows cerebral creatine deficiency.

Pathophysiology.   The pathophysiology relates to reduction in creatine as a substrate for creatine kinase and, therefore, reduced availability of phospho-creatine as a source for adenosine triphosphate (ATP) production.

Treatment.   Treatment with creatine supplementation is helpful for both guanidinoacetate methyltransferase and arginine:glycine amidinotransferase deficiencies (Stockler et al., 2007) but not for creatine transporter deficiency (deGrauw et al., 2003).

Leigh Syndrome

Clinical Features.   This disease is a progressive encephalopathy which presents before age 2 in approximately 80% of cases. Key features include respiratory

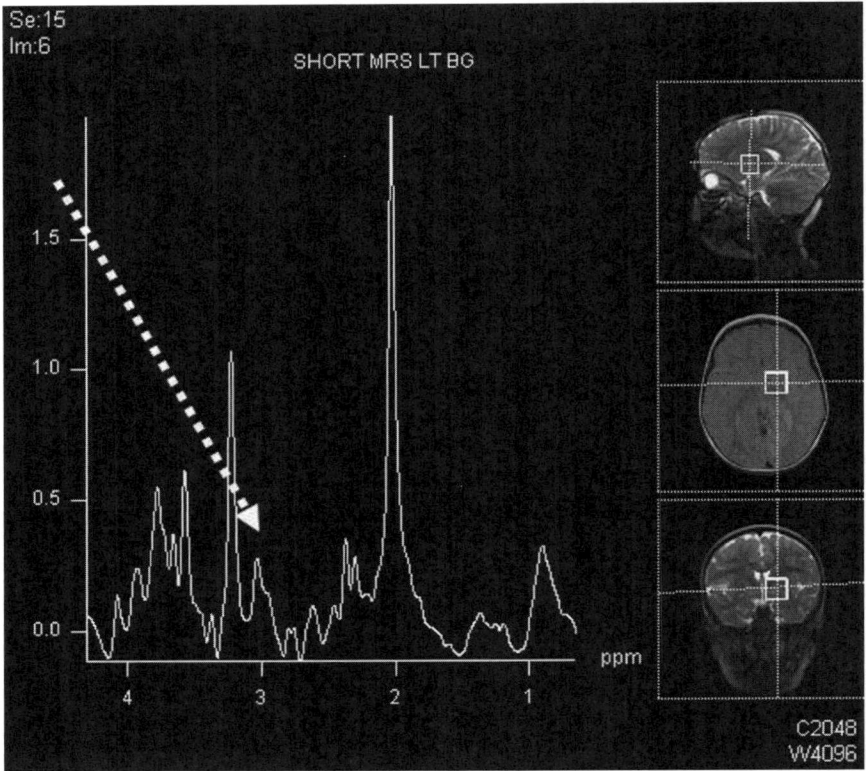

FIGURE 13–2. Magnetic resonance spectroscopy from a child with guanidinoacetate methyltransferase deficiency shows absence of creatine peak to the right of the choline peak. Courtesy of T. Degrauw.

disorders such as unexplained hyperventilation; nuclear or supranuclear oculomotor paralyses; movement disorders including chorea, optic atrophy, and pigmentary retinal degeneration; and a remitting or (rarely) a fulminant, rapidly fatal course (Lyon et al., 2006). The movement disorder may be ataxia, tremor, chorea, dystonia, or athetosis and may be chronic and progressive or may present during episodes of physiological decompensation with lactic acidosis. Mixed hyperkinesias after diffuse brain injury may also be seen. Death usually occurs in fewer than 5 years from disease onset. Diagnosis is made based on clinical findings, elevated lactate and pyruvate in cerebrospinal fluid, and typical pattern seen on MRI of symmetric foci of necrosis in basal ganglia, thalamus, cerebellum, brainstem, spinal cord, or optic nerves (Arii and Tanabe, 2000; Finsterer, 2008).

Pathophysiology. This disease is related to genes affecting mitochondrial function. These are nuclear genes causing deficiencies in respiratory chain complexes I, II, IV, or V in most cases. Inheritance is usually autosomal recessive. A smaller proportion of cases are due to mutation in mitochondrially encoded genes or mtDNA. Deletions in multiple mitochondrial genes have been associated with Leigh syndrome.

Treatment.   Treatment is primarily supportive, with sodium citrate or bicarbonate for acute acidosis, antiseizure medications, and symptomatic treatment of movement disorders.

Ataxia-Telangiectasia (see also Chapter 12)

Clinical Features.   The main diagnostic entity presenting between ages 1 and 2 with chorea is ataxia-telangiectasia (AT). Although not a metabolic disease, it is discussed here because it is in the differential diagnosis of the child with chorea. It is important to diagnose this disorder early because immune deficiencies are treatable. The diagnosis may be missed because chorea may appear before ataxia and neurological manifestations precede the telangiectasias by several years (Cabana et al., 1998). Unsteadiness of trunk control and gait are noted, usually between 12 and 14 months of age, with mixed manifestations of chorea and ataxia (Lavin et al., 2007). Slow choreic movements of the neck and trunk with involuntary dystonic posturing of the limbs may occur. In cases where chorea predominates, the gait may not be consistently broad-based, but rather, intrusive choreic movements of the trunk or limbs may cause the gait to lurch, without loss of balance. Abnormal oculomotor control, similar to oculomotor apraxia, then ensues. Immune deficiency occurs in approximately two-thirds of cases, causing sinopulmonary infections. Risk of lymphoreticular neoplasms is also increased.

Pathophysiology.   AT is autosomal recessive, caused by mutations in the *ATM* (ataxia-telangiectasia mutated) gene (Savitsky et al., 1995). This gene is phosphorylated and activated in the presence of DNA damage, signaling cell cycle checkpoints to facilitate DNA repair (Lavin et al., 2007). Absence of function leads to sensitivity to ionizing radiation and chromosomal aberrations. The primary pathology noted *post mortem* is death of Purkinje and granule cells in the cerebellum. Blood alpha-fetoprotein levels are elevated, confirming the diagnosis in most cases. Due to the length of the gene and the large number of possible mutations, genetic sequencing is expensive and not always standard practice.

Treatment.   Therapy is with intravenous immune globulins for symptomatic immune deficiency. Treatment of neurological symptoms is supportive. Clinical trials to arrest neurodegeneration have been directed toward reducing the effects of oxidative stress (Lavin et al., 2007). Median survival is approximately 25 years (Crawford et al., 2006).

A summary of the key metabolic diseases which may present with chorea or athetosis at this age is presented in Table 13–3.

TABLE 13–3. Diseases Presenting with Chorea in the First 2 Years of Life

DISEASE	INHERITANCE	GENE	ADDITIONAL FEATURES	LABORATORY FINDINGS	MRI FINDINGS
Pyruvate dehydrogenase complex deficiency	X-Linked	E1-alpha subunit of the pyruvate dehydrogenase complex (PDHA1, 300502.0001)	Variable age at onset, paroxysmal ataxia and chorea, may have facial dysmorphisms, some respond to thiamine or to ketogenic diet	Increased blood lactate, pyruvate, alanine, ammonia	Variable: absent corpus callosum, cystic basal ganglia lesions similar to Leigh syndrome
Glutaric aciduria type 1	AR	Glutaryl-CoA dehydrogenase (GCDH, 608801)	May present in crisis, dystonia predominates	Episodic ketoacidosis	Striking striatal degeneration
Methylglutaconic aciduria type 1	AR	*AUH* gene (600529), which encodes 3-methylglutaconyl-CoA hydratase	Extremely rare, spasticity, blindness, optic atrophy, asymptomatic diagnosis possible, adult cases described	3-Methylglutaconic aciduria, 3-methylglutaric aciduria	Cerebral, basal ganglia atrophy, progressive
Ethylmalonic encephalopathy	AR	*ETHE1* gene, which encodes a mitochondrial matrix protein	Extremely rare, with chronic diarrhea and early death	Ethylmalonic and methylsuccinic aciduria and lactic acidemia	Increased T2 signal in basal ganglia
Ataxia-telangiectasia	AR	Mutations in *ATM* gene	Immune deficiency, hematological malignancies	Elevated alpha-fetoprotein	None or atrophy

AR, autosomal recessive.

Metabolic Diseases Presenting in Childhood, Usually After Age 2 Years

Pantothenate Kinase–Associated Neurodegeneration (See Chapter 8)

Clinical Features. Onset is usually in childhood, with progressive problems with walking, dystonia, choreic movements, dysarthria, and leg spasticity. Progressive intellectual deterioration usually occurs. MRI shows bilateral hypointensity of the globus pallidus (iron accumulation), with central necrosis, leading to the "eye of the tiger" sign (Hayflick et al., 2006). The disease course is relentlessly progressive if onset is prior to age 10 years.

Pathophysiology. Inheritance is autosomal recessive, due to mutations in the gene encoding pantothenate kinase 2 (*PANK2*) (Zhou et al., 2001), a protein essential to mitochondrial coenzyme A synthesis. Deficiency may cause accumulation of cysteine and oxidative stress via iron in the globus pallidus (Johnson et al., 2004; Kotzbauer et al., 2005).

Treatment. Treatment is supportive. Two case series describe benefit from DBS (Castelnau et al., 2005; Timmermann et al., 2010).

Chorea-Acanthocytosis (see Chapter 6)

Clinical Features. Onset can occasionally be seen in patients as young as 8 years but is more typically in adulthood. Chorea and orofaciolingual and pharyngeal dystonia are prominent. Seizures may occur. Psychiatric and behavioral changes are common and may predate the hyperkinetic movements. MRI may show atrophy or signal change in the striatum, and *post mortem* studies show neuronal loss and scarring in the basal ganglia and substantia nigra pars reticulata. Acanthocytosis (spiculation) of red blood cells, with normal serum lipoprotein levels, supports the diagnosis, although occasionally this may be absent.

Pathophysiology. The disorder is caused by autosomal recessively inherited mutations in the *VPS13A* gene, which encodes the protein chorein (Ueno et al., 2001). The function of chorein in humans is not known.

Treatment. Treatment is supportive.

Bilateral Striatal Necrosis or Calcinoses

Clinical Features. Most cases are poorly understood and probably heterogenous syndromes (Basel-Vanagaite et al., 2006; Medina et al., 1990; Murakami et al., 2005) with dystonia or slow choreic movements (Straussberg et al., 2002).

In cases with striatal necrosis, there may be infancy- or early childhood–onset chorea or dystonia, with cognitive impairment variably present.

Pathophysiology. The cause in autosomal recessive cases appears to be mutations in the *nup62* gene, which encodes a nuclear pore complex protein (Basel-Vanagaite et al., 2006).

Treatment. Therapy is supportive.

Niemann-Pick Disease, Type C

Clinical Features. Usual onset of Niemann Pick type C is between ages 2 and 10. The infantile form results in encephalopathy and early death. Childhood/adolescent-onset cases develop supranuclear vertical gaze paralysis (particularly downward) (Breen et al., 1981), dysarthria, ataxia, tremor, dystonia and/or chorea, and often cataplexy and seizures. MRI findings are nonspecific. Fibroblasts show accumulation of cholesterol in lysosomes. Bone marrow testing shows characteristic "sea-blue histocytes."

Pathophysiology. The cause is autosomal recessive mutations in the *NPC1* (Carstea et al., 1997) or *NPC2* (Naureckiene et al., 2000) gene. Abnormal intracellular processing of dietary cholesterol, affecting glycolipids, leads to lysosomal accumulations (Vanier, 1999).

Treatment. Treatment is supportive.

Hyperglycemia/Diabetes-Associated Subacute Hemichorea or Hemiballism (See Chapter 15)

Clinical Features. Hemiballismus or hemichorea can be seen in adults with chorea during an episode of nonketotic hyperglycemia. MRI shows increased signal in the putamen on T1 imaging (Ahlskog et al., 2001; Lai et al., 1996; Oh et al., 2002). Chorea has been described in a diabetic adolescent with similar neuroimaging findings, with a polymerase gamma I (*POLG1*) mutation (Hopkins et al., 2009).

Pathophysiology. A spectrum of focal striatal pathology may be responsible as there are reports of focal microhemorrhage and of striatal gliosis (Mestre et al., 2007; Ohara et al., 2001). Acute/subacute disruption of function of frontostriatal pallidothalamic circuits, particularly due to putaminal pathology, appears likely.

Treatment. Acute treatment of hyperglycemia may improve the chorea. In some cases, symptomatic treatment with dopamine receptor–blocking agents is needed.

TABLE 13–4. Differential Diagnosis of Heritable Neurologic Diseases in which Chorea is a Feature.*

DISEASE	INHERITANCE	NEUROLOGIC FEATURES	OTHER MEDICAL FEATURES	GENETICS
17-beta-hydroxysteroid dehydrogenase X deficiency	X-linked Dominant	Onset infancy, hearing loss, retinal degeneration, nystagmus, neurodegeneration, hypotonia, chorea, seizures, mental retardation; frontotemporal atrophy	Lactic acidosis, metabolic acidosis; favorable response to isoleucine restriction	Mutation in the 17-beta-hydroxysteroid dehydrogenase gene
Aceruloplasminemia (Chapter 10)	AR	Onset 30–50 years: Ataxia, chorea, dystonia, rigidity, dementia, retinal degeneration; iron deposition in basal ganglia	Diabetes, anemia; iron deposition liver, pancreas; decreased or absent serum ceruloplasmin, decreased serum iron, increased ferritin	Mutations in the ceruloplasmin gene (CP)
Alternating Hemiplegia of Childhood	AD	Onset before 18 months, Episodes of hemidystonia, hemiplegia, chorea, upward eye deviation, nystagmus with progressive cognitive decline; mental retardation		Mutation in the ATPase Na$^+$K$^+$ transporting, alpha-2 polypeptide gene; allelic to familial hemiplegic migraine 2
Aromatic L-amino acid decarboxylase deficiency	AR	Ptosis, oculogyric crises, miosis, myoclonus, hypotonia, dystonia, choreoathetosis, sleep disturbances, behavioral irritability	Hypotension, poor feeding, bowel dysmotility, paroxysmal sweating	Mutation in the dopa decarboxylase gene DDC

(continued)

TABLE 13–4. (continued)

DISEASE	INHERITANCE	NEUROLOGIC FEATURES	OTHER MEDICAL FEATURES	GENETICS
Ataxia, early-onset, with oculomotor apraxia and hypoalbuminemia (EAOH) (Chapter 12)	AR	Oculomotor apraxia, hypometric saccades, nystagmus, distal weakness and atrophy, muscle CoQ deficiency, severe ataxia, chorea, tremor, dystonia; cerebellar atrophy, nerve axon degeneration	Scoliosis, low albumin, high cholesterol	Mutation in the aprataxin gene (APTX)
Ataxia-Telangiectasia: AT (Chapter 12)	AR	Chorea, ataxia, dysarthria, oculomotor abnormalities, seizures	Sinopulmonary infections, telangiectasias, hypogonadism, progeric skin changes; immune deficiency, hematologic malignancies, diabetes	Mutations in the ataxia-telangiectasia mutated gene (ATM)
Basal Ganglia Calcification, Idiopathic 1 (IBGC1) (Chapter 16)	AD	Onset 30–50 years, parkinsonism, dysarthria, chorea, memory impairment/deterioration, depression, psychosis; dense calcium in basal ganglia, dentate nucleus	Urinary incontinence	
Basal Ganglia Disease, Adult onset (Chapter 9)	AD	Onset 19–55; Parkinsonism, chorea, dystonia, spasticity, ataxia, cognitive deficits; cavitation and iron aggregates in the basal ganglia, forebrain, cerebellum; decreased serum ferritin		Mutation in the ferritin light-chain gene (FTL)

Disease	Inheritance	Clinical features	Gene/Mutation
Benign Hereditary Chorea (Chapter 4)	AD	Chorea onset before age 5, delayed motor development, no dementia; peak 2nd decade	Mutation in the thyroid transcription gene TITF1
Choreoacanthocytosis (ChAc) (Chapter 6)	AR	Progressive chorea, orofacial dyskinesia, dysphagia, seizures, tics, dystonia, parkinsonism, neuropathy, mood changes, psychosis, aggression; striatal atrophy	Acanthocytes	Mutation in the chorein gene (VPS13A)
Choreoathetosis, hypothyroidism, and neonatal respiratory distress (Chapter 4)	AD	Global developmental delay, chorea, ataxia, hypotonia, dysarthria;	Neonatal respiratory distress and recurrent infections; hypothyroidism	Mutation in the thyroid transcription gene TITF1; allelic to Benign Hereditary Chorea
Chromosome 18q Deletion Sydrome	AD	Mental retardation, chorea, tremor, seizures; Dysmyelination, cerebellar hypoplasia	Short stature, flat small midface, short dysmorphic ears, cardiac malformations, asthma; micropenis/hypospadias; joint laxity, limb dysmorphisms, eczema, immunoglobulin deficiency	Interstitial or terminal deletion of chromosome 18q
Congenital cataracts, facial dysmorphism, and neuropathy	AR	Mental retardation, chorea, ataxia, neuropathy; rhabdomyolysis; cerebral and spinal cord atrophy	Short stature, prominent midface, mandibular retrognathism, cataracts, microcorneas, abnormal teeth protrusion; hypogonadism, scoliosis	Mutation in the subunit1 phosphatase of the C-terminal domain of RNA polymerase II subunit A gene (CTD P1)

(continued)

TABLE 13–4. (continued)

DISEASE	INHERITANCE	NEUROLOGIC FEATURES	OTHER MEDICAL FEATURES	GENETICS
Convulsions, infantile, with paroxysmal choreoathetosis; ICCA (Chapter 19)	AD	Seizures infancy, chorea age 6–23 years;		May be allelic to benign infantile convulsions and paroxysmal kinesigenic dyskinesia
De Sanctis-Cacchione Syndrome	AR	Neurodegeneration, microcephaly, deafness, hyporeflexia, spasticity, ataxia, chorea; cerebral and olivopontocerebellar atrophy	Skin photosensitivity, early skin cancers, skin atrophy/ pigmentary changes, telangiectasias, conjunctivitis; dwarfism, gonadal hypoplasia	Complementation Group in DNA radiation damage repair
Dentatorubral-pallidoluysian Atrophy (DRPLA) (Chapter 12)	AD	Ataxia, myoclonus, seizures, chorea, dementia		Trinucleotide repeat expansion (CAG)n in the DRPLA gene (DRPLA)
Epileptic Encephalopathy, Early Infantile, 1	X-linked recessive	Intractable seizures/infantile spasms, developmental arrest, mental retardation, dystonia, chorea, spasticity; cerebral atrophy; T2 signal change in basal ganglia	Dyspnea, dysphagia	Mutation in the X-linked aristaless-related homeobox gene (ARX)

Disease	Inheritance	Clinical features	Laboratory features	Gene/Mutation
Glucose Transport Defect, Blood brain barrier (Chapter 19)	AD	Infantile seizures, acquired microcephaly, developmental delay, ataxia, spasticity, myoclonus, paroxysmal eye movements, some chorea; response to ketogenic diet; hypoglychorrhachia		Mutations in the solute carrier family 2 (facilitated glucose transporter) member 1 gene (SLC2 A1)
Glutaric Acidemia I (this chapter)	AR	Dystonia, hypotonia, chorea, opisthotonus, encephalopathy, diplegia; dilation of ventricals and widening of cortical sulci; hypodensity of striatum;	Macrocrania, failure to thrive, hepatomegaly; acidosis, ketonemia, ketonuria, hypoglycemia	Mutation in the glutaryl-CoA dehydrogenase gene (GA1)
Huntington Disease (Chapter 3)	AD	Personality/behavioral changes, chorea, parkinsonism, dementia,		Trinucleotide repeat expansion (CAG)n in the huntingtin gene (HTT)
Huntington Disease-like 1; HDL1 (Chapter 11)	AD	Mean onset 28, dementia, parkinsonism, ataxia, chorea; anxiety, aggression, depression, delusions; diffuse basal ganglia and brain atrophy and gliosis		Insertion of 8 extra octapeptide repeats in the prion protein gene (PRNP)
Huntington Disease-like 2;HDL2 (Chapter 5)	AD	Mean onset 30's; Dystonia, chorea, rigidity, hyperreflexia, parkinsonism; depression, hallucinations; striatal atrophy	Weight loss	Trinucleotide repeat expansion (CAG)n in the junctophilin-3 gene (JPH3)

(continued)

TABLE 13–4. (continued)

DISEASE	INHERITANCE	NEUROLOGIC FEATURES	OTHER MEDICAL FEATURES	GENETICS
Huntington Disease-Like 3; HDL3	AR	Onset 3-5 years; Chorea, dystonia, ataxia, spasticity, seizures, dementia; frontal cortical and caudate atrophy	GI and bladder incontinence, limb contractures	
Hypogonadism, alopecia, diabetes, mental retardation, and extrapyramidal syndrome	AR	Deafness, mental retardation, dystonia, dysarthria, chorea; MRI white matter lesions and signal change basal ganglia	Hypogonadism, alopecia/fine hair, loss of eyebrows, diabetes; decreased testosterone and estradiol	
Karak Syndrome (Chapter 8)	AR	Childhood onset ataxia, chorea, tremor, dystonia, spasticity, impaired eye movement, cognitive decline; cerebellar atrophy and basal ganglia iron deposition	Dysphagia	Mutation in the phospholipase A2, group V1 gene (PLA2G6); allelic to infantile neuroaxonal dystrophy
Leigh Syndrome, X-Linked	X-linked recessive	Hypotonia, neurodegeneration, spasticity, chorea, nystagmus; lesions in basal ganglia, brainstem, thalamus, spinal cord	Respiratory difficulties; lactic acidosis	Mutation in the E1-alpha complex gene (PDHA1)

Lesch-Nyhan Syndrome; LNS	X-linked recessive	Mental retardation, self injurious behavior, dystonia, chorea, spasticity, opisthotonus, dysphagia	Short stature, growth retardation, vomiting, testicular atrophy, nephrolithiasis, gout, anemia, hyperuricemia	Mutation in the hypoxanthine phosphoribox-syltransferase gene (HPRT1)
Leukodystrophy, hypomyelinating, 2	AR	Global developmental delay, chorea, ataxia, hypotonia, progressive spasticity, tremor, nystagmus, seizures, mild to moderate mental impairment, neuropathy; T2 hyperintense white matter		Mutation in the gap junction alpha-12 gene (GJA12)
Leukodystrophy, hypomyelinating, 4	AR	Hypotonia, profound mental retardation, seizures, progressive spasticity, choreoathetosis, nystagmus, microcephaly acquired	Apnea, shallow breathing, feeding difficulty; joint contractures; symptoms exacerbation during fevers; fatal first 2 decades usual	Mutation in the heat-shock 60-kd protein 1 gene (HSPD1); allelic to AD SPG13
Mental retardation, X-Linked Syndromic 10; MRXS10	X-linked recessive	Mental retardation, chorea, hypotonia, spasticity, dysarthria, aggression, psychosis, self injurious behavior	Lumbar lordosis, arachnodactyly	Mutation in the 17-beta-hydroxysteroid dehydrogenase X gene (HSD17B10)
Mental retardation, X-Linked Syndromic 13; MRXS13	X-linked recessive	Mental retardation, spasticity, tremor, ataxia, parkinsonism, chorea, seizures, psychosis	Micrognathia, microcephaly, large ears, high palate, short neck	Mutation in the methyl-CpG-binding protein 2 gene (MECP2), allelic to Rett Syndrome

(continued)

TABLE 13–4. (continued)

DISEASE	INHERITANCE	NEUROLOGIC FEATURES	OTHER MEDICAL FEATURES	GENETICS
Metachromatic Leukodystrophy	AR	Optic atrophy, neurodegeneration, dystonia, chorea, ataxia, seizures, spasticity, polyneuropathy; adult onset form psychiatric	Biliary tract dysfunction, incontinence; decreased arylsulfatase A activity in urine, leukocytes, fibroblasts	Mutation in the arylsulfatase A gene (ARSA)
Neurodegeneration with Brain Iron Accumulation, NBIA1 (Chapter 8)	AR	Retinal degeneration, optic atrophy, facial grimacing, blepharospasm, apraxia of eyelid opening, dystonia, chorea, ataxia, spasticity, parkinsonism, cognitive decline; iron deposition in globus pallidus (eye of tiger), caudate, substantia nigra	Feeding difficulty, dysphagia, incontinence,	Mutation in the pantothenate kinase-2 gene (PANK2); allelic to HARP syndrome
Oculorenocerebellar Syndrome	AR	Retinal degeneration, mental retardation, chorea, spastic diplegia; absent cerebellar granular cell layer	Glomerulosclerosis	
Paroxysmal Nonkinesigenic Dyskinesia 1 (PNKD1) (Chapter 19)	AD	Infancy/childhood onset episodes facial grimacing, dystonia neck/trunk/face, chorea; last minutes to hours several times per week; precipitated by stress, caffeine, fatigue, exertion, alcohol		Mutation in the myofibrillogenesis regulator 1 gene (MR1)

Pelizaeus-Merzbacher Disease, PMD	X-linked recessive	Hypotonia, rotary head/eye movements, ataxia, spasticity, dystonia, chorea, mental retardation, seizures; dysmyelination; severe form death in childhood; classic form survives to adulthood	Stridor	Mutation in the proteolipid protein 1 gene (PLP1); allelic with Spastic paraplegia SPG2
Pyruvate Decarboxylase Deficiency	X-linked Dominant	Mental retardation (some), hyptonia, lethargy, seizures, episodic ataxia after stress; cerebral atrophy, basal ganglia cystic lesions, increased lactate on MRS	Low birth weight, 35% dysmorphic face/head	Mutation in the E1-alpha subunit of the pyruvate dehydrogenase complex
Spinocerebellar Ataxia 1 (SCA1) (Chapter 12)	AD	Onset 30s, optic atrophy, slow saccades, opthalmoplegia – supranuclear, amyotrophy, ataxia, hyperreflexia early, hyporeflexia and neuropathy late, chorea	Sphincter problems	Expanded CAG trinucleotide repeats in the ataxin-1 gene

(continued)

TABLE 13–4. (continued)

DISEASE	INHERITANCE	NEUROLOGIC FEATURES	OTHER MEDICAL FEATURES	GENETICS
Spinocerebellar Ataxia 17; SCA17 (Chapter 12)	AD	Progressive ataxia, dystonia, tremor, chorea, myoclonus, nystagmus and abnormal eye movement, frontal lobe dementia, seizures; diffuse cerebral and cerebellar atrophy; basal ganglia inclusions; median onset 23 years	Bladder incontinence	Trinucleotide repeat expansion (CAG)n in the TATA box-binding protein gene TBP
Spinocerebellar Ataxia 7 (SCA7)	AD	Onset 32 years, pigmentary retinal degeneration, slow saccades, progressive ataxia, dysarthria, spasticity, orofacial dyskinesia, chorea		Mutations in the ataxin 7 gene
Striatonigral Degeneration, Infantile, Mitochondrial	Mitochondrial	Developmental delay, intermittent chorea; Caudate/ putamen lesions, ragged red fibers in muscle		Mutation in the mitochondrial-encoded ATP synthase 6 gene (MTATP6)

Striatonigral degeneration, infantile, SNDI	AR	Onset 7-15 months; Nystagmus, optic atrophy, regression, chorea, spasticity, dystonia, mental retardation; progressive symmetric degeneratino of the caudate, putamen, sometimes globus pallidus	Failure to thrive, dysphagia	Mutation in the 62-kd nucleoporin gene (NUP62)
Sulfocysteinuria	AR	Infantile hemiplegia, hypotonia, dystonia, chorea, seizures, ataxia; death in infancy	Ectopia lentis, delayed teething, mild eczema, fine hair; increased urinary sulfite, decreased urinary sulfate	Mutation in sulfite oxidase gene (SUOX)
Xeroderma Pigmentosum, Complementation Group A, XPA	AR	See De Sanctis-Cacchione Syndrome	See De Sanctis-Cacchione Syndrome	Complementation Group in DNA radiation damage repair
Xeroderma Pigmentosum, Complementation Group D, XPD	AR	See De Sanctis-Cacchione Syndrome	See De Sanctis-Cacchione Syndrome	Complementation Group in DNA radiation damage repair

* This table was generated through extracting information from a CLINICAL SYNOPSIS search of "Chorea or Choreoathetosis" from the National Library of Medicine's Online Mendelian Inheritance in Man.

SUMMARY: HERITABLE METABOLIC DISEASES PRESENTING WITH CHOREA

Children presenting with acute chorea which is not immune-mediated may have a metabolic disease. When chorea is present in a child with developmental delay or regression, metabolic diseases are an important part of the differential diagnosis. Inheritance pattern is important but not always informative, for example, in isolated cases which may be autosomal recessive.

Table 13–4 was generated through extracting information from a clinical synopsis search of "chorea OR choreoathetosis" from the National Library of Medicine's OMIM, an extremely useful tool for the complex task of diagnosing heritable diseases. This database is of particular utility for disorders in which chorea is a minor or rare feature, which are not addressed in this volume. For others (e.g., Karak syndrome), classification and definition are in evolution as causative genes are identified. Nevertheless, this is a valuable resource for the diagnosis of these disorders.

REFERENCES

Ahdab-Barmada M, Moossy J (1984) The neuropathology of kernicterus in the premature neonate: diagnostic problems. J Neuropathol Exp Neurol 43(1):45–56.

Ahlskog JE, Nishino H, Evidente VG, Tulloch JW, Forbes GS, Caviness JN, et al. (2001) Persistent chorea triggered by hyperglycemic crisis in diabetics. Mov Disord 16(5): 890–898.

Arii J, Tanabe Y (2000) Leigh syndrome: serial MR imaging and clinical follow-up. AJNR Am J Neuroradiol 21(8):1502–1509.

Basel-Vanagaite L, Muncher L, Straussberg R, Pasmanik-Chor M, Yahav M, Rainshtein L, et al. (2006) Mutated nup62 causes autosomal recessive infantile bilateral striatal necrosis. Ann Neurol 60(2):214–222.

Bianchi MC, Tosetti M, Fornai F, Alessandri MG, Cipriani P, De Vito G, et al. (2000) Reversible brain creatine deficiency in two sisters with normal blood creatine level. Ann Neurol 47(4):511–513.

Breen L, Morris HH, Alperin JB, Schochet SS Jr (1981) Juvenile Niemann-Pick disease with vertical supranuclear ophthalmoplegia. Two cases reports and review of the literature. Arch Neurol 38(6):388–390.

Brunberg JA, Doty DB, Reilly EL (1974) Choreoathetosis in infants following cardiac surgery with deep hypothermia and circulatory arrest. J Pediatr 84(2):232–235.

Cabana MD, Crawford TO, Winkelstein JA, Christensen JR, Lederman HM (1998) Consequences of the delayed diagnosis of ataxia-telangiectasia. Pediatrics 102(1 Pt 1):98–100.

Carstea ED, Morris JA, Coleman KG, Loftus SK, Zhang D, Cummings C, et al. (1997) Niemann-Pick C1 disease gene: homology to mediators of cholesterol homeostasis. Science 277(5323):228–231.

Castelnau P, Cif L, Valente EM, Vayssiere N, Hemm S, Gannau A, et al. (2005) Pallidal stimulation improves pantothenate kinase–associated neurodegeneration [see comment]. Ann Neurol 57(5):738–741.

Chow CW, Thorburn DR (2000) Morphological correlates of mitochondrial dysfunction in children. Hum Reprod 15(Suppl 2):68–78.

Crawford TO, Skolasky RL, Fernandez R, Rosquist KJ, Lederman HM (2006) Survival probability in ataxia telangiectasia. Arch Dis Child 91(7):610–611.

Dahl HH, Maragos C, Brown RM, Hansen LL, Brown GK (1990) Pyruvate dehydrogenase deficiency caused by deletion of a 7-bp repeat sequence in the E1 alpha gene. Am J Hum Genet 47(2):286–293.

deGrauw TJ, Cecil KM, Byars AW, Salomons GS, Ball WS, Jakobs C (2003) The clinical syndrome of creatine transporter deficiency. Mol Cell Biochem 244(1–2):45–48.

deGrauw TJ, Salomons GS, Cecil KM, Chuck G, Newmeyer A, Schapiro MB, et al. (2002) Congenital creatine transporter deficiency. Neuropediatrics 33(5):232–238.

DeLong MR, Wichmann T (2007) Circuits and circuit disorders of the basal ganglia. Arch Neurol 64(1):20–24.

Dinopoulos A, Cecil KM, Schapiro MB, Papadimitriou A, Hadjigeorgiou GM, Wong B, et al. (2005) Brain MRI and proton MRS findings in infants and children with respiratory chain defects. Neuropediatrics 36(5):290–301.

du Plessis AJ, Bellinger DC, Gauvreau K, Plumb C, Newburger JW, Jonas RA, et al. (2002) Neurologic outcome of choreoathetoid encephalopathy after cardiac surgery. Pediatr Neurol 27(1):9–17.

Engbers HM, Berger R, van Hasselt P, de Koning T, de Sain-van der Velden MG, Kroes HY, et al. (2008) Yield of additional metabolic studies in neurodevelopmental disorders. Ann Neurol 64(2):212–217.

Finsterer J (2008) Leigh and Leigh-like syndrome in children and adults. Pediatr Neurol 39(4):223–235.

Garcia-Cazorla A, Wolf NI, Serrano M, Perez-Duenas B, Pineda M, Campistol J, et al. (2009) Inborn errors of metabolism and motor disturbances in children. J Inherit Metab Dis 32(5):618–629.

Gitiaux C, Roze E, Kinugawa K, Flamand-Rouviere C, Boddaert N, Apartis E, et al. (2008) Spectrum of movement disorders associated with glutaric aciduria type 1: a study of 16 patients. Mov Disord 23(16):2392–2397.

Govaert P, Lequin M, Swarte R, Robben S, De Coo R, Weisglas-Kuperus N, et al. (2003) Changes in globus pallidus with (pre)term kernicterus. Pediatrics 112(6 Pt 1): 1256–1163.

Haas RH, Parikh S, Falk MJ, Saneto RP, Wolf NI, Darin N, et al. (2008) The in-depth evaluation of suspected mitochondrial disease. Mol Genet Metab 94(1):16–37.

Hayflick SJ, Hartman M, Coryell J, Gitschier J, Rowley H (2006) Brain MRI in neurodegeneration with brain iron accumulation with and without PANK2 mutations. AJNR Am J Neuroradiol 27(6):1230–1233.

Hedlund GL, Longo N, Pasquali M (2006) Glutaric acidemia type 1. Am J Med Genet C Semin Med Genet 142C(2):86–94.

Hopkins SE, Somoza A, Gilbert DL (2009) Rare autosomal dominant *POLG1* mutation in a family with metabolic strokes, posterior column spinal degeneration, and multi-endocrine disease. J Child Neurol. doi:10.1177/0883073809343313.

Johnson MA, Kuo YM, Westaway SK, Parker SM, Ching KH, Gitschier J, et al. (2004) Mitochondrial localization of human PANK2 and hypotheses of secondary iron accumulation in pantothenate kinase–associated neurodegeneration. Ann N Y Acad Sci 1012:282–298.

Keng WT, Pilz DT, Minns B, FitzPatrick DR (2003) A3243G mitochondrial mutation associated with polymicrogyria. Dev Med Child Neurol 45(10):704–708.

Kotzbauer PT, Truax AC, Trojanowski JQ, Lee VM (2005) Altered neuronal mitochondrial coenzyme A synthesis in neurodegeneration with brain iron accumulation caused by abnormal processing, stability, and catalytic activity of mutant pantothenate kinase 2. J Neurosci 25(3):689–698.

Kupsky WJ, Drozd MA, Barlow CF (1995) Selective injury of the globus pallidus in children with post-cardiac surgery choreic syndrome. Dev Med Child Neurol 37(2): 135–144.

Lai PH, Tien RD, Chang MH, Teng MM, Yang CF, Pan HB, et al. (1996) Chorea-ballismus with nonketotic hyperglycemia in primary diabetes mellitus. AJNR Am J Neuroradiol 17(6):1057–1064.

Lavin MF, Gueven N, Bottle S, Gatti RA (2007) Current and potential therapeutic strategies for the treatment of ataxia-telangiectasia. Br Med Bull 81–82:129–147.

Lyon G, Kolodny EH, Pastores GM (2006) Neurology of Hereditary Metabolic Diseases of Children, 3rd ed. McGraw-Hill, New York.

McDonald L, Rennie A, Tolmie J, Galloway P, McWilliam R (2006) Investigation of global developmental delay. Arch Dis Child 91(8):701–705.

Medina L, Chi TL, DeVivo DC, Hilal SK (1990) MR findings in patients with subacute necrotizing encephalomyelopathy (Leigh syndrome): correlation with biochemical defect. AJNR Am J Neuroradiol 11(2):379–384.

Medlock MD, Cruse RS, Winek SJ, Geiss DM, Horndasch RL, Schultz DL, et al. (1993) A 10-year experience with postpump chorea. Ann Neurol 34(6):820–826.

Merhar SL, Gilbert DL (2005) Clinical (video) findings and cerebrospinal fluid neurotransmitters in 2 children with severe chronic bilirubin encephalopathy, including a former preterm infant without marked hyperbilirubinemia. Pediatrics 116(5):1226–1130.

Mestre TA, Ferreira JJ, Pimentel J (2007) Putaminal petechial haemorrhage as the cause of non-ketotic hyperglycaemic chorea: a neuropathological case correlated with MRI findings. J Neurol Neurosurg Psychiatry 78(5):549–550.

Miles L, Wong BL, Dinopoulos A, Morehart PJ, Hofmann IA, Bove KE (2006) Investigation of children for mitochondriopathy confirms need for strict patient selection, improved morphological criteria, and better laboratory methods. Hum Pathol 37(2): 173–184.

Miller C, Saada A, Shaul N, Shabtai N, Ben-Shalom E, Shaag A, et al. (2004) Defective mitochondrial translation caused by a ribosomal protein (MRPS16) mutation. Ann Neurol 56(5):734–738.

Murakami A, Morimoto M, Adachi S, Ishimaru Y, Sugimoto T (2005) Infantile bilateral striatal necrosis associated with human herpes virus-6 (HHV-6) infection. Brain Dev 27(7):527–530.

Nardocci N, Fernandez-Alvarez E (2007) Movement Disorders in Children: A Clinical Update with Video Recordings. John Libbey Eurotext, Montrouge, France.

Naureckiene S, Sleat DE, Lackland H, Fensom A, Vanier MT, Wattiaux R, et al. (2000) Identification of *HE1* as the second gene of Niemann-Pick C disease. Science 290 (5500):2298–2301.

Oh SH, Lee KY, Im JH, Lee MS (2002) Chorea associated with non-ketotic hyperglycemia and hyperintensity basal ganglia lesion on T1-weighted brain MRI study: a meta-analysis of 53 cases including four present cases. J Neurol Sci 200(1–2):57–62.

Ohara S, Nakagawa S, Tabata K, Hashimoto T (2001) Hemiballism with hyperglycemia and striatal T1-MRI hyperintensity: an autopsy report. Mov Disord 16(3):521–525.

Fidel KR, Leslie ND, Gilbert DL (2005) An updated review of the long-term neurological effects of galactosemia. Pediatr Neurol 33(3):153–161.

Sanger TD, Chen D, Fehling DL, Hallett M, Lang AE, Mink JW, et al. (2010) Definition and classification of hyperkinetic movements in childhood. Mov Disord (in press).

Savitsky K, Bar-Shira A, Gilad S, Rotman G, Ziv Y, Vanagaite L, et al. (1995) A single ataxia telangiectasia gene with a product similar to PI-3 kinase. Science 268(5218): 1749–1753.

Schrag A, Quinn NP, Bhatia KP, Marsden CD (2000) Benign hereditary chorea—entity or syndrome? Mov Disord 15(2):280–288.

Shevell M (2009) Metabolic evaluation in neurodevelopmental disabilities [author reply]. Ann Neurol 65(4):483–484.

Shevell M, Ashwal S, Donley D, Flint J, Gingold M, Hirtz D, et al. (2003) Practice parameter: evaluation of the child with global developmental delay: report of the Quality Standards Subcommittee of the American Academy of Neurology and the Practice Committee of the Child Neurology Society [see comment]. Neurology 60(3):367–380.

Singer HS, Mink JW, Gilbert DL, Jankovic J (2010) Movement Disorders in Childhood. Elsevier, Philadelphia, 2010.

Stockler S, Schutz PW, Salomons GS (2007) Cerebral creatine deficiency syndromes: clinical aspects, treatment and pathophysiology. Subcell Biochem 46:149–166.

Strauss KA, Lazovic J, Wintermark M, Morton DH (2007) Multimodal imaging of striatal degeneration in Amish patients with glutaryl-CoA dehydrogenase deficiency. Brain 130(Pt 7):1905–1920.

Strauss KA, Puffenberger EG, Robinson DL, Morton DH (2003) Type I glutaric aciduria, part 1: natural history of 77 patients. Am J Med Genet C Semin Med Genet 121(1): 38–52.

Straussberg R, Shorer Z, Weitz R, Basel L, Kornreich L, Corie CI, et al. (2002) Familial infantile bilateral striatal necrosis: clinical features and response to biotin treatment. Neurology 59(7):983–989.

Timmermann L, Pauls KA, Wieland K, Jech R, Kurlemann G, Sharma N, et al. (2010) Dystonia in neurodegeneration with brain iron accumulation: outcome of bilateral pallidal stimulation. Brain 133(Pt 3):701–712.

Ueno S, Maruki Y, Nakamura M, Tomemori Y, Kamae K, Tanabe H, et al. (2001) The gene encoding a newly discovered protein, chorein, is mutated in chorea-acanthocytosis. Nat Genet 28(2):121–122.

Vanier MT (1999) Lipid changes in Niemann-Pick disease type C brain: personal experience and review of the literature. Neurochem Res 24(4):481–489.

Vidailhet M, Yelnik J, Lagrange C, Fraix V, Grabli D, Thobois S, et al. (2009) Bilateral pallidal deep brain stimulation for the treatment of patients with dystonia-choreoathetosis cerebral palsy: a prospective pilot study. Lancet Neurol 8(8):709–717.

Volpe JJ (2001) Bilirubin and brain injury. In: Neurology of the Newborn, 4th ed. Saunders, Philadelphia, 2001, pp 521–546.

Zafeiriou DI, Rodenburg RJ, Scheffer H, van den Heuvel LP, Pouwels PJ, Ververi A, et al. (2008) MR spectroscopy and serial magnetic resonance imaging in a patient with mitochondrial cystic leukoencephalopathy due to complex I deficiency and NDUFV1 mutations and mild clinical course. Neuropediatrics 39(3):172–175.

Zhou B, Westaway SK, Levinson B, Johnson MA, Gitschier J, Hayflick SJ (2001) A novel pantothenate kinase gene (PANK2) is defective in Hallervorden-Spatz syndrome [see comment]. Nat Genet 28(4):345–349.

14

Medication-Induced Chorea

Marta San Luciano, MD and
Rachel Saunders-Pullman, MD, MPH

INTRODUCTION

Chorea, a hyperkinetic movement disorder characterized by involuntary, spontaneous, irregular flowing movements, may be caused by medications and drugs.
Medication-induced chorea is most often observed as a side effect of dopaminergic medications (primarily levodopa [L-dopa]) used to treat Parkinson's disease
(PD) or as a sequela of treatment with antidopaminergic medications. It is seen
much less frequently as an adverse effect from other medications, although a wide
variety of medications may induce chorea (see Table 14–1).

In this chapter we will focus primarily on the phenomenology, pathophysiology, and management of L-dopa-induced chorea (dyskinesias) and neuroleptic-
induced tardive chorea. We will then review other medications most commonly
associated with chorea as a side effect occurring at the time of administration,
including dopaminomimetic stimulant agents such as cocaine, amphetamines, and
methylphenidate.

L-DOPA-INDUCED CHOREA

Development of Dyskinesias in PD

In 1960 Hornykiewicz demonstrated a marked depletion of dopamine in the caudate nucleus and putamen of patients with postencephalitic parkinsonism and PD

TABLE 14-1. Medications and Drugs of Abuse Which Cause Chorea

Most frequently cause chorea

- *Dopaminergic drugs*: L-Dopa and dopamine agonists, as well as other antiparkinsonian drugs
- *Antidopaminergic agents:*
  - Neuroleptics (typical and atypical antipsychotics, some are now also used as adjunct therapy for depression)
  - Gastrointestinal medications; metoclopramide, prochloperazine

Also may cause chorea

- *Steroids*: Estrogen-containing oral contraceptives
- *Antiepileptic medications:*
  - Phenytoin
  - Valproate
  - Carbamazepine
  - Gabapentin
- Lithium
- *Dopaminomimetic stimulant agents:*
  - Cocaine
  - Amphetamines
  - Methylphenidate and pemoline

Additional

Antihistamines, cimetidine, cyclizine, diazoxide, digoxin, isoniazide, methadone, tricyclic antidepressants

(Ehringer and Hornykiewicz, 1960; Hornykiewicz, 1966). Together with Birkmayer, he subsequently reported a dramatic, although transient, improvement in parkinsonian symptoms after intravenous injection of L-dihydroxyphenylalanine (L-dopa) (Birkmayer and Hornykiewicz, 1961). In 1967, Cotzias et al. administered oral D,L-dihydroxyphenylalanine (dopa) to several patients and showed marked amelioration of the motor features of PD. Already in this report, there is mention of "exaggerated facial expression and gesticulation on talking" and "athetoid movements" but only in those patients receiving D,L-dopa after a few weeks of treatment and at doses high enough to improve symptoms, thus first describing dopa-induced dyskinesias. Such movements would disappear when lowering the L-dopa dose and were absent in the nonparkinsonian control patients receiving the drug. Despite the tremendous gains with dopaminergic therapy, clinicians continue to be challenged by the emergence of dopa-induced dyskinesia in many patients with PD.

In an early series, 37 out of 60 patients treated with L-dopa developed dyskinesias (Yahr et al., 1969). One case was described as follows: "Choreiform involuntary movements gradually became more prominent involving the head and trunk as well as the extremities, but remained at the same level of intensity after the third month of treatment (Page 348)." The authors also noted a frequent clinical feature, that the patient might be oblivious to the adventitious movements unless brought to his or her attention or when the chorea was severe. By the early 1970s it was evident that while L-dopa was the most effective agent to treat the parkinsonian syndrome, such choreic movements were as common as the gastrointestinal side effects, appeared later with chronic use, and were the most common dose-limiting adverse effect (McDowell et al., 1970; Schwarz and Fahn, 1970; Calne et al., 1971; Mones et al., 1971). Dyskinesias may cause significant morbidity and decrease quality of life for PD patients (Pechevis et al., 2005).

Relationship of Dyskinesias to L-Dopa Dosing

Dyskinesias are a common occurrence, estimated to affect ~40% of PD patients treated chronically with L-dopa after 5 years of therapy and about 90% of patients with treatment duration longer than 9 years (Nutt, 1990, 2008; Ahlskog and Muenter, 2001). Initial reports from the time of introduction of L-dopa showed a much higher incidence of dyskinesia within the first year of therapy than is currently observed. It has been postulated that these differences may have been due to a longer disease duration prior to L-dopa treatment, more aggressive dosing in the early stages, and the later introduction of dopa-decarboxylase inhibitor/L-dopa combinations (Mones et al., 1971; Ahlskog and Muenter, 2001). Younger age at PD diagnosis also appears to be an important risk factor (Rascol et al., 2006).

Dyskinesias usually appear at the peak concentration of L-dopa dose (peak-dose dyskinesia), but they may occur throughout the duration of the "on" period (square-wave dyskinesia, considered part of the spectrum of peak-dose dyskinesias) or at the beginning and end of the clinical benefit, with minimal presence during the period of best motor function (diphasic dyskinesia, also called "dyskinesia or dystonia-improvement-dyskinesia or dystonia," D-I-D) (Nutt, 1990; Marconi et al., 1994; Fox and Lang, 2008).

Phenomenology

L-Dopa-induced abnormal movements are usually referred to as "dyskinesias" as they encompass a mixture of abnormal movements that include chorea, ballism, dystonia, and myoclonus. However, chorea affecting facial, neck, trunk, and limb muscles is the most common presentation. Involvement of the respiratory and/or abdominal muscles has also been described (Calne et al., 1971). Dyskinesias tend to start on the most affected parkinsonian side (Marconi et al., 1994). Peak-dose dyskinesias are generally choreic in nature and commonly affect the face, neck, and less often the limbs but may affect any muscle group. They are commonly action- or movement-induced and are not always apparent at rest. Diphasic dyskinesias, or dyskinesias during "off" periods or "on–off" transitions, are predominantly dystonic, are less likely choreic, and affect predominantly the legs. This biphasic pattern is considerably less common than peak-dose dyskinesias and is also observed in the 1-methyl-4-phenyl-1,2,3,6-tetrahydropyridine (MPTP)-treated monkey on chronic apomorphine (Clarke et al., 1989). However, there is no absolute dichotomy between diphasic dyskinesias and peak-dose dyskinesias but rather a continuum between dystonic movements on the background of the parkinsonian "off" state and choreic movements during the period of maximal improvement (Marconi et al., 1994).

These adventitious movements do not appear after the first administration, and chronic administration is necessary. The latency may be related to disease duration, with movements appearing sooner with more advanced disease and with higher L-dopa doses.

Pathophysiology

The pathophysiology of L-dopa-induced dyskinesias is not well understood. Most of the current knowledge derives from studies on animal models, predominantly 6-hydroxydopamine (6-OHDA)–lesioned rats (Dekundy et al., 2007) and MPTP-treated primates (Clarke et al., 1989). For the abnormal movements to appear, a dopamine-denervated striatum is generally required, although dyskinesias have been described in nonparkinsonian individuals and nonhuman primates at very high L-dopa doses (Goodwin et al., 1970; Calne et al., 1971; Sassin et al., 1972). In addition, dyskinesia appears in those parkinsonian patients who show a good response to L-dopa, and it is usually absent in patients with atypical parkinsonisms who respond poorly to dopaminergic therapies (Cotzias et al., 1967; Mones et al., 1971; Nutt, 1990). An intact striatal outflow appears also to be necessary for dyskinesia to develop. Dyskinesias are uncommon in dopa-responsive dystonia, a condition due to metabolic dopamine deficiency.

The method of drug delivery plays a pivotal role in the development of the abnormal movements. Repeated "pulsatile" subcutaneous administration of the short-acting D_1/D_2 dopamine receptor agonist apomorphine induces dramatic dyskinesias in MPTP-parkinsonian primates but only very mild movements when administered by subcutaneous continuous infusion (Bibbiani et al., 2005). Nonphysiological intermittent stimulation of dopamine receptors is thought to underlie the pathophysiology of such movements (Calabresi et al., 2008). Intermittent oral administration produces pathological maladaptive changes pre- and postsynaptically in the already molecularly altered denervated striatum (Klawans et al., 1977; Zigmond et al., 1990). Continuous administration (so-called continuous dopaminergic stimulation) appears to raise the threshold for clinical response and dyskinesias, possibly through dopamine receptor subsensitivity or downregulation. However, this theory of continuous dopaminergic stimulation as a therapeutic approach has been challenged. It has not emerged that early treatment with catechol-O-methyltransferase inhibitors, which lead to a more prolonged dopaminergic response, decrease dyskinesias, as might be expected from this hypothesis (Nutt, 2007). The exact mechanism through which different dopaminergic and nondopaminergic pathways change as a consequence of chronic and pulsatile administration of L-dopa, in potentially genetically predisposed parkinsonian individuals, resulting in the development of dyskinesias, remains to be elucidated.

Long-term potentiation, a long-lasting form of synaptic plasticity at corticostriatal synapses, is thought to underlie both motor learning and striatum-dependent cognitive tasks. This is muted in the 6-OHDA-lesioned rat model but can be restored by chronic L-dopa treatment. However, only neurons from lesioned animals that developed abnormal movements on chronic L-dopa lose the ability to "forget" irrelevant synaptic signals ("depotentiation") (Picconi et al., 2003). The effect on synaptic depotentiation appears to be in part mediated by D_1 dopamine receptors and leads to the development of nonphysiological basal ganglia motor circuits (Picconi et al., 2003). D_1 receptor blockade has been shown to improve dyskinesias in MPTP-treated monkeys (Grondin et al., 1999) and in patients (Durif et al., 2004).

Other receptor systems have been implicated in the pathophysiology of dyskinesias, such as the glutamatergic system, adenosine A2A receptors, and others. In particular, D_1 dopamine receptors and N-methyl-D-aspartate (NMDA) glutamate receptors are known to interact with each other in many brain regions. The corticostriatal glutamatergic excitatory pathway in the nigrostriatal dopaminergic-depleted state undergoes molecular changes that result in glutamatergic overactivity (Picconi et al., 2004), and chronic L-dopa treatment also causes further adaptive changes in the corticostriatal glutamatergic pathways. NMDA receptor blockade diminishes L-dopa-induced dyskinesias in animal models (Papa and Chase, 1996), and it is thought to underlie the antidyskinetic effect of amantadine in PD patients without reemergence of parkinsonian symptoms (Del Dotto et al., 2001).

Whether the molecular changes in the glutamate receptors represent compensatory mechanisms or the primary molecular trigger of the movements remains to be elucidated.

More recently, adenosine A2A receptor antagonists have been proposed as potential antidyskinetic agents in PD. Drugs acting at adenosine A2A receptors oppose the action of dopamine at D_2 dopamine receptors on GABAergic striatopallidal neurons; thus, adenosine A2A receptor antagonists might have an antiparkinsonian effect (Schwarzschild et al., 2006). Although A2A antagonists do not suppress preexisting dyskinesia, preclinical findings raise the possibility that A2A blockade may prevent their development in drug-naive patients (Xu et al., 2005; Schwarzschild et al., 2006).

Cannabinoid receptors are widespread in the basal ganglia. Motor effects following the activation or inhibition of cannabinoid receptors in laboratory animals and the capacity of cannabinoids to modulate key neurotransmitter systems within the basal ganglia support a potential role for this system in modulating dyskinesias (Fox et al., 2002a; Fernandez-Ruiz, 2009; Morgese et al., 2009; Perez-Rial et al., 2009).

Dopamine D_2 agonists (ropinirole, pramipexole, cabergoline, pergolide) as monotherapy are also capable of producing dyskinesias, although less frequently than L-dopa (Pearce et al., 1998; Rinne et al., 1998; Oertel et al., 2006). A 5-year prospective, randomized, controlled study compared the incidence of dyskinesias in two groups of PD patients, receiving initial ropinirole or L-dopa monotherapy, in which patients could subsequently receive open-label L-dopa supplementation: 20% of patients in the ropinirole group vs. 45% of the L-dopa group developed dyskinesias (Rascol et al., 2000). However, the ropinirole group was more likely to receive open L-dopa supplementation (Rascol et al., 2006). A similar study comparing pramipexole to L-dopa as monotherapy resulted in a lower incidence of dyskinesia in the pramipexole group, but initial treatment with L-dopa resulted in better symptomatic control and tolerability (Holloway et al., 2004).

Longer half-lives and an L-dopa-sparing effect of dopamine agonists, as well as differences in D_1 vs. D_2 receptor activation, may underlie this discrepancy. Pure D_1 agonists, on the other hand, appear to produce dyskinesias with chronic administration similar to L-dopa (Rascol et al., 2001), further supporting the role of D_1 receptors in the pathophysiology of dyskinesias.

Treatment

The treatment of L-dopa-induced dyskinesias in PD patients is challenging. Strategies to prevent the development of dyskinesia are hence important and include the early use of long-acting dopamine agonists (Rascol et al., 2000). However, delaying treatment with L-dopa to prevent dyskinesia can be justified only if the underlying symptoms of PD are sufficiently controlled. Treatment of dyskinesias includes reduction of dopaminergic medication with potential reemergence of parkinsonian symptoms, introduction of amantadine (Del Dotto et al., 2001) with significant risk of poor tolerability and lack of efficacy, and surgical approaches (pallidotomy [Laitinen et al., 1992; Dogali et al., 1995; Lozano et al., 1995] and deep brain stimulation [Krack et al., 2003; Schupbach et al., 2005; Simonin et al., 2009]) in selected patients, with the subsequent inherent surgical risk.

While there is significant evidence to support the use of amantadine, including double-blind, placebo-controlled studies with long follow-up periods (Metman et al., 1999; Luginger et al., 2000; Snow et al., 2000; Del Dotto et al., 2001; Paci et al., 2001), the evidence for the efficacy of other agents in the treatment of dyskinesias is limited to very few studies and case reports, for example, of buspirone (Kleedorfer et al., 1991; Bonifati et al., 1994), clonidine (Nishikawa et al., 1984), fluoxetine (Durif et al., 1995), propranolol (Carpentier et al., 1996), and riluzole (Merims et al., 1999).

Dopamine Antagonists

Clozapine, an atypical antipsychotic agent with a relatively weak potency at brain dopaminergic receptors and equal or greater potency at blocking brain D_1 receptors compared to D_2 receptors, is known to cause little or no parkinsonism in psychotic patients and is used for the treatment of psychosis in PD (Factor and Brown, 1992). Anecdotal data exist for its dyskinesia-ameliorating and long-lasting effects from single patient reports (Factor and Brown, 1992) and small open-label studies (Bennett et al., 1993, 1994; Durif et al., 1997). A 10-week, double-blind, parallel-group, placebo-controlled study showed reductions in the "on" time with dyskinesias in the clozapine group (Durif et al., 2004). However, the occurrence of sedation, orthostatic hypotension, sialorrhea, and the need for close monitoring for agranulocytosis limit its clinical applicability.

Cannabinoid Agonists

Based on the basic data and case reports, cannabinoid receptor agonists have been advocated for the treatment of hyperkinetic movement disorders (Fernandez-Ruiz, 2009). A small pilot study significantly reduced total L-dopa-induced dyskinesias compared to placebo without affecting the "on" period, although side effects of vertigo and orthostatic hypotension were common (Sieradzan et al., 2001). A randomized, double-blind, placebo-controlled trial, however, failed to demonstrate benefit in patients with dystonia (Fox et al., 2002b) despite anecdotal evidence of benefit (Farooq et al., 2009).

Glutamate Receptor Antagonists

More recent therapeutic strategies targeting glutamatergic pathways include a selective NMDA glutamate receptor antagonist (CP-101,606), which in a randomized, double-blind, placebo-controlled trial improved L-dopa-induced dyskinesias but caused dose-related dissociation and amnesia (Nutt et al., 2008). The anticonvulsant topiramate, as an attenuator of α-amino-3-hydroxy-5-methyl-4-isoxazole propionic acid (AMPA) receptor–mediated transmission, has been shown to be effective in an animal model (Silverdale et al., 2005) but is poorly tolerated in older adults. Metabotropic mGluR5 receptor antagonists to date have been extensively tested only in animal models (Levandis et al., 2008; Ouattara et al., 2009; Marin et al., 2009).

Serotonin Agonists

Serotonin receptors as pharmacological targets for potential therapies have also been considered. With progressive degeneration of dopaminergic neurons in PD, dopamine formation from exogenous L-dopa increasingly takes place in striatal serotonergic nerve terminals (Bibbiani et al., 2001; Gregoire et al., 2009). Sarizotan is a 5-hydroxytryptamine 1A (5-HT1A) receptor agonist that showed effectiveness in reducing dyskinesias in parkinsonian monkeys (Gregoire et al., 2009). In a 3-week, double-blind, placebo-controlled trial, the higher-dose group had a 40% reduction in L-dopa-induced dyskinesias (Bara-Jimenez et al., 2005); however, a more recent study did not demonstrate improvement in the primary outcome of "on" time without dyskinesias (Goetz et al., 2007).

Continuous Dopamine Stimulation

Continuous infusion of L-dopa or apomorphine is a therapeutic option for the treatment of dyskinesias in advanced PD as this approach provides constant dopaminergic stimulation with potential lowering of the L-dopa dose (Antonini and Tolosa, 2009). While subcutaneous apomorphine provides a similar level of motor benefit to L-dopa, its long-term use is limited by compliance and injection-site skin reactions. The administration of L-dopa/carbidopa by continuous duodenal infusion allows for replacement of all oral medications and permits achievement of a satisfactory therapeutic response paralleled by a reduction in motor complication severity. However, compared with apomorphine, it is more invasive as it requires a percutaneous endoscopic gastrostomy.

Other Mechanisms

Several studies have suggested that repetitive transcranial magnetic stimulation may improve L-dopa-induced dyskinesias; however, in others, the benefit was short-lived and the outcomes were variable (Koch et al., 2005; Brusa et al., 2006; Wagle-Shukla et al., 2007).

Conclusion

In summary, L-dopa-induced dyskinesia in PD is the most common cause of drug-induced chorea. Despite advances in the understanding of its pathophysiology, mechanisms and pathways are still poorly understood, and treatment of these dyskinesias remains a significant clinical problem. Improved therapeutic strategies for prevention and suppression of L-dopa-induced dyskinesias are needed and, if successful, would significantly decrease the need for dopamine-sparing strategies.

ANTIDOPAMINERGIC-INDUCED TARDIVE CHOREA

Chorea may arise as a complication of chronic use of dopamine-blocking medications. Long-term use of these medications may lead to stereotypic movements involving oral, buccal, and lingual areas; however, other movements, such as distal limb chorea, dystonia, and myoclonus, may appear. The syndrome is collectively known as "tardive dyskinesia" (TD).

Development of TD

In the 1950s dopamine-blocking agents were introduced for the treatment of psychosis and other psychiatric diagnoses (Delay and Deniker, 1955). While this was a major breakthrough in medicine and a tremendous advance in the field of psychiatry, the emergence of abnormal movements, including chorea, after sustained treatment led to a more cautious use of such medications.

Several years after the first reports on the use of chlorpromazine for psychiatric conditions, TD was described in the U.S. literature (Kruse, 1960). Three schizophrenic women in their 50s were treated with different neuroleptics (chlorpromazine, trifluoperazine, fluphenazine, and thioridazine) and developed bothersome muscular restlessness (akathisia) predominantly in the legs, associated with occasional involuntary jerky movements of both arms and involuntary lip and tongue movements. In this report, persistence of the abnormal movements as well as an increase in severity after discontinuation of the offending drug are described (Kruse, 1960), features now considered classic in TD. In 1964, after surveying their chronic mental hospital population, Hunter et al. reported 13 female patients with persistent choreiform movements in the limbs and prominent involvement of the face, jaw, and tongue. Their results were compared to similar reports in the European literature, in which the syndrome developed after at least a few months of therapy with neuroleptics, was irreversible or persisted for many months after discontinuation of the medication, and involved female gender and preexisting brain damage as risk factors (Hunter et al., 1964). By the late 1960s and early 1970s, TD was well recognized as a complication of phenothiazines, thioxanthenes, and butyrophenones (Tarsy and Baldessarini, 1976), and the first therapeutic trials took place (Kazamatsuri et al., 1972a–c; Kazamatsuri and Cole, 1972). Reports in young adults (Tarsy et al., 1977) as well as severe and disabling forms (Tarsy and Baldessarini, 1976; Casey and Rabins, 1978) were also described.

Since its first descriptions, TD has also been noted in patients without psychiatric diagnoses who had other indications for use of dopamine receptor–blocking agents, such as those with gastrointestinal complaints (Casey, 1983) or Gilles de la Tourette syndrome (Riddle et al., 1987).

Estimates of the prevalence of TD range 0.5%–65% in the literature (Kane and Smith, 1982; Yassa and Jeste, 1992). These estimates are complicated by differences in diagnostic criteria, assessment methods, gender, psychiatric diagnosis, comorbid medical and neurological illnesses, and duration and type of neuroleptic use as well as the difficulty in differentiating between the spontaneous dyskinesias described in schizophrenia and TD in individual patients. The prevalence of TD was noticed to increase from 5% before 1965 to 25% in the late 1970s (Kane and Smith, 1982), although mean prevalence rates agreed on ~20% (Kane and

Smith, 1982; Yassa and Jeste, 1992). More recent studies estimate the average prevalence to be about 30% with typical neuroleptics (Kane et al., 1985; Chouinard et al., 1988). Data from large-scale prospective studies have yielded an incidence rate of 0.053 per year of developing TD and a cumulative 5-year incidence of 20% (Morgenstern and Glazer, 1993). The demographic risk factors identified with the development of TD are increased age, mood disorders (as a psychiatric diagnosis), female gender in the older age groups, presence of diabetes, schizophrenic negative symptoms, and preexisting brain damage; the treatment variables associated with increased risk include higher neuroleptic doses, number of medication-free periods, and history of drug-induced parkinsonism (Tarsy and Baldessarini, 1976; Kane and Smith, 1982; Kane et al., 1985; Chouinard et al., 1988; Yassa and Jeste, 1992; Morgenstern and Glazer, 1993).

TD with Atypical Neuroleptics

The newer antipsychotics (known as "atypical" neuroleptics or antipsychotics), which include risperidone, olanzapine, quetiapine, sertindole, ziprasidone, and aripiprazole, appear to cause less drug-induced parkinsonism and acute dystonia as well as to have a lower incidence of TD with long-term use (Glazer, 2000; Jeste, 2004). A double-blind randomized trial of olanzapine vs. haloperidol over a 2-year period revealed a markedly lower incidence of TD in the olanzapine-treated subjects (0.52% vs. 7.45%) (Beasley et al., 1999). While several reports of TD arising from risperidone use have been published (Campbell, 1999; Hong et al., 1999), systematic studies found lower rates when compared to haloperidol (Chouinard, 1995; Lemmens et al., 1999; Jeste, 2000, 2004). However, there is still a risk of TD with these medications.

Clozapine, a highly effective newer atypical antipsychotic agent, and quetiapine appear to carry the lowest risk of development of TD or drug-induced parkinsonism (Kane et al., 1993; Glazer, 2000). Unfortunately, clozapine use is limited by its potentially serious side effects of agranulocytosis and seizures. There are two reports of quetiapine-induced TD (Ghelber and Belmaker, 1999; Rizos et al., 2009); however, in both cases the patients had been previously exposed to high-potency typical antipsychotic agents.

Phenomenology

The phenomenology of TD is quite distinct from that of other movement disorders. In its classic presentation, continuous lower facial grimacing with mouth, jaw, and tongue movements, ranging from writhing movements of the tongue with mouth opening and closing or lateral chewing movements, sucking movements of the lips, and bulging of the cheeks, to continuous rapid protrusion and withdrawal of the tongue ("fly-catcher tongue"), are observed. Tongue involvement may interfere significantly with feeding and speech and frequently results in muscular hypertrophy (Fahn, 1984). Similar to other choreas, respiratory muscles (Hunter et al., 1964; Yassa and Jeste, 1992) as well as esophageal musculature (Horiguchi et al., 1999) may also be involved. Dystonic involvement of neck and trunk muscles in the form of retrocollis, backward arching of the torso, and forward thrusting movements of the abdomen and pelvis are classical manifestations of TD, although they may be observed in other dystonic syndromes as well (Fahn, 1984). Distal limbs tend to be affected by more classic choreiform movements in TD (Tarsy et al., 1977).

Several important distinctions should be made between the choreiform movements seen in TD and the classic chorea resulting from Huntington disease, for example. This distinction is important as movement disorders arising in patients with psychiatric symptoms from basal ganglia disease (Chapter 20) may erroneously be attributed to TD. First, the involuntary movements of the mouth in TD are more readily volitionally suppressed, as well as when an object is placed in the mouth or lips. Second, involvement of the lower face with relative sparing of the upper face is more common in TD. Third, the phenomenon of motor impersistence, or the inability to maintain a protruded tongue, seen in Huntington disease patients, is less likely to be observed in TD (Fahn, 1984). However, discrimination of Huntington disease from TD may not be possible on clinical grounds alone.

Pathophysiology

Although TD is an iatrogenic condition with established etiological links to dopamine receptor antagonism, its pathophysiology is not well understood. Several theories have been hypothesized, including dopamine supersensitivity, based upon the similarities between L-dopa-induced dyskinesias and TD and the fact that subjects with drug-induced parkinsonism seem to be at higher risk for TD (Klawans, 1973). Involvement of dopaminergic systems in animal models appears to support this hypothesis (Nielsen and Lyon, 1978; Benes et al., 1985; Turrone et al., 2003). Dysfunction or depletion of the GABAergic system as the main inhibitory neurotransmitter in the basal ganglia has also been implicated in the development of TD (Fibiger and Lloyd, 1984; Gunne et al., 1984; Andersson et al., 1989; Thaker et al., 1987). Studies have also sought evidence of neuronal damage resulting from neurotoxicity of long-term neuroleptic treatment, although results have been inconsistent and many had methodological drawbacks (Christensen et al., 1970; Pakkenberg et al., 1973; Nielsen, 1977; Nielsen and Lyon, 1978).

Treatment

The many theories regarding TD have led to a wide variety of medication trials, many of which had serious deficiencies and none of which was clearly successful in the majority of patients. As a result, the current practice calls for a slow taper and discontinuation of the offending drug and empiric medication trials. The selection is guided by the underlying psychiatric diagnosis, comorbidities, potential side effects, and interactions with other medications.

Typical Neuroleptics

Typical neuroleptics are effective in suppressing the abnormal movements, although the improvement may be most pronounced in the short term (Roxburgh, 1970; Kazamatsuri et al., 1972c; Jeste and Wyatt, 1979, 1982; Doongaji et al., 1982). One concern is the potential of typical neuroleptics to worsen TD, but in severe cases with life-threatening situations, increasing the dose or switching to a high-potency typical neuroleptic may be the only option to provide fast relief. While potentially helpful, the safety and efficacy of increased neuroleptic dose for long-term suppression have been questioned.

Atypical Neuroleptics

Atypical antipsychotics have been tried as potential suppressive agents for TD. Case reports, open-label trials, and two out of four double-blind controlled trials have shown beneficial effects of clozapine use (Simpson et al., 1978; Meltzer and Luchins, 1984; Small et al., 1987; Lamberti and Bellnier, 1993; Friedman, 1994; Trugman et al., 1994; Tamminga et al., 1994). Risperidone has also been shown to suppress TD, although there are some conflicting reports (Kopala and Honer, 1994; Chouinard, 1995; Kooptiwoot and Settachan, 2000; Bai et al., 2005). Other atypical neuroleptics may be used as alternatives. Olanzapine, sertindole, quetiapine, and ziprasidone have been shown to be effective and are postulated to carry less risk of side effects compared to the typical neuroleptics (Seeger et al., 1995; Beasley et al., 1996; Schulz et al., 1996; Borison et al., 1996; Tollefson et al., 1997).

Dopamine-Depleting Agents

Dopamine-depleting agents including reserpine, tetrabenazine (now commercially available in the United States), alpha-methyl-dopa, and alpha-methyl-p-tyrosine (AMPT) are effective agents for the treatment of TD. Unfortunately, major side effects including hypotension, impotence, severe depression, parkinsonism, and akathisia considerably limit their use (Jeste and Wyatt, 1979; Huang et al., 1981; Nasrallah et al., 1986; Lang and Marsden, 1982; Fahn, 1985; Jeste et al., 1988).

Dopaminergic Agents

Dopamine agonists downregulate dopamine receptors and theoretically can help ameliorate TD. However, fear exists of potentially exacerbating both the movements and the underlying psychosis with use of these agents. Anecdotal data exist of their benefit in TD (Smith et al., 1977; Fuller et al., 1982; Jeste et al., 1988; Lieberman et al., 1989); among them, L-dopa appears to be the most effective (Ludatscher, 1989).

Other Agents

Other nondopaminergic medications with evidence of therapeutic benefit in TD include noradrenergic blocking agents such as propranolol (Schrodt et al., 1982) and clonidine (Freedman et al., 1982; Browne et al., 1986), GABA agonists (the most studied and effective include diazepam, clonazepam, and baclofen) (Sedman, 1976; Jeste and Wyatt, 1979, 1982; Stewart et al., 1982; Singh et al., 1983b; Jeste et al., 1988; Thaker et al., 1990; Soares et al., 2004), antioxidants such as vitamin E (Egan et al., 1992; Shriqui et al., 1992; Adler et al., 1993a, b; Lam et al., 1994; Lohr and Caligiuri, 1996), and calcium channel blockers (Barrow and Childs, 1986; Ross et al., 1987; Adler et al., 1988; Buck and Havey, 1988; Falk et al., 1988; Leys et al., 1988; Reiter et al., 1989; Kushnir and Ratner, 1989; Duncan et al., 1990; Stedman et al., 1991; Loonen et al., 1992), among others. Most data indicate that long-term treatment with anticholinergic agents does not ameliorate TD; therefore, with the exception of tardive dystonia, which may improve with anticholinergics, they are not generally recommended (Jeste and Wyatt, 1982; Fahn, 1983; Friis et al., 1983; Jeste et al., 1988; Yassa, 1988). Botulinum toxin injections into selected muscle groups can be helpful in treating focal spasms, although they are usually reserved for the treatment of tardive dystonia (especially cervical dystonia) and are less commonly used for facial movements associated with TD (van Harten and Hovestadt, 2006; Slotema et al., 2008; Hennings et al., 2008; Tschopp et al., 2009). Lastly, neurosurgical interventions, previously pallidotomy or thalamotomy (Wang et al., 1997; Weetman et al., 1997; Hillier et al., 1999; Lenders et al., 2005) and more recently deep brain stimulation, remain an option for severe intractable cases (Franzini et al., 2005; Trottenberg et al., 2005; Cohen et al., 2007; Damier et al., 2007; Sun et al., 2007; Sako et al., 2008; Gruber et al., 2009; Kefalopoulou et al., 2009).

Conclusion

Despite the introduction of the atypical antipsychotics and the lower incidence rates, TD remains an important therapeutic dilemma. Prevention is an important issue that clinicians should take into consideration when choosing dopaminergic blocking agents for different conditions, especially in the treatment of depression without psychotic features where other medications may be available.

CENTRAL NERVOUS SYSTEM STIMULANTS ASSOCIATED WITH CHOREA

Chorea is one of the many different movement disorders that may result from the direct effect of central nervous system stimulants, both nonprescription and prescription. This discussion will focus on the drugs of abuse cocaine, amphetamine and amphetamine-related compounds, the medications for attention-deficit/hyperactivity disorder (ADHD) methylphenidate and pemoline, as well as related dopaminomimetic stimulant agents.

Cocaine

Cocaine use has been a recognized social and medical problem in our society since the early 1970s (Boghdadi and Henning, 1997; Williams et al., 2006), affecting millions of people worldwide. Cocaine blocks the dopamine transporter, preventing the reuptake of dopamine at the presynaptic nerve terminal and increasing the extracellular levels of this neurotransmitter. The increase in extracellular levels of dopamine in the circuits controlling reward, movement, and cognition are thought to underlie the euphoric effects of cocaine as well as to explain its motoric effects (Geracitano et al., 2006; Nakagawa and Kaneko, 2008).

Apart from the known medical and neurological complications of cocaine, a variety of movement disorders may be associated with its use, many of which are transient in nature. It is known to cause motor and vocal tics, tremors, and acute dystonia (Pascual-Leone and Dhuna, 1990; Hegarty et al., 1991; Fines et al., 1997); but possibly one of the most bizarre movement disorders caused by this drug is the transient chorea and buccolingual dykinesia known in the streets as "crack dancing" or "boca torcida." This consists of self-limiting choreoathetoid movements involving orofacial and limb musculature that can be associated with akathisia and may last for one or several days (Daras et al., 1994; Bartzokis et al., 1999). Prior neuroleptic use or preexisting organic brain disease appear to be risk factors for the choreoathetoid movements (Daras et al., 1994; Kamath and Bajaj, 2007); however, in a study with imaging, no structural lesions were observed and genetic screening for inherited causes of chorea was negative (Kamath and Bajaj, 2007). The epidemiology of this condition is not well known and is likely to be underreported due to the self-limiting and benign nature of the movements and because family members are usually more disturbed than the patient.

Amphetamine

Amphetamine was first synthesized in the nineteenth century and introduced into clinical practice in the 1930s as a nasal decongestant and appetite suppressant. At therapeutic doses, amphetamine produces elevated mood, increased alertness, and decreased fatigue. At high doses, it can produce agitation, dysphoria, psychosis, and seizures (Gray et al., 2007). Its stimulant effects are mediated through the release of biogenic amines stored in nerve terminals, by blocking dopamine reuptake and by inhibiting monoamine oxidase enzymes (Nakagawa and Kaneko, 2008). The related compound 3,4-methylenedioxymethamphetamine (MDMA, "Ecstasy"), with increased street use, has similar stimulant effects (Hall and Henry, 2006).

Apart from the known stereotypic behaviors and "punding" (complex, prolonged, purposeless and stereotyped behaviors) commonly recognized as motor effects of these drugs (Rylander, 1972; Schiorring, 1981), chorea is also reported.

Individuals with preexisting basal ganglia damage, even if subtle, may be at higher risk and develop such movements after single doses. Amphetamine and related compounds have indeed been shown to enhance chorea from other etiologies such as Sydenham chorea, Huntington disease, and systemic lupus erythematosus (Klawans and Weiner, 1974; Waugh et al., 2008). Although chronic high-dose use of amphetamines alone may cause dyskinesias in subjects previously presumed "normal," given the widespread use of these medications and the limited reports of amphetamine-induced chorea, it is probably an infrequent side effect in subjects without preexisting basal ganglia damage (Morgan et al., 2004).

Stimulants Used for ADHD

Methylphenidate is a piperidine derivate structurally related to amphetamine with mild central nervous system stimulant effects with more prominent mental rather than motor activities. Pemoline is another medication used for the treatment of ADHD. Similarly to amphetamine, both methylphenidate and pemoline produce their effect through the release of stored dopamine at nerve terminal vesicles. There have been several case reports of methylphenidate-induced chorea, some of them in the setting of neuroleptic use and most with preexisting brain disease (Palatucci, 1974; Weiner et al., 1978; Boogerd and Beijnen, 2000).

Pemoline-induced chorea has rarely been reported. In two case reports, patients were treated with neuroleptics prior to its administration (Bonthala and West, 1983; Singh et al., 1983a). In patients without prior neuroleptic exposure or other predisposing condition, the ability of pemoline to induce chorea is unclear. A 3-year-old twin pair with ADHD previously treated with methylphenidate developed choreoathetosis after a pemoline overdose (Stork and Cantor, 1997). A 2-year-old who also overdosed on pemoline developed encephalopathy and chorea (Nausieda et al., 1981), indicating little evidence of pemoline-induced chorea in patients without a history of a movement disorder except in cases of significant overdose.

OTHER MEDICATION-INDUCED CHOREA

In addition to the already discussed L-dopa and the tardive syndromes caused by dopamine-blocking agents, many prescription medications have been associated with the development of chorea; the commonest are shown in Table 14–1. Such reactions are infrequent, and most remit on stopping the offending medication with the exception of the tardive syndromes. The exact mechanism through which the different medications cause chorea in many instances is not well understood, although previous basal ganglia damage may be a predisposing factor.

Oral Contraceptives

The use of oral contraceptives is a well-known, although uncommon, cause of chorea. In this particular case, it has been hypothesized that the condition is due to reactivation of childhood Sydenham chorea (Lewis and Harrison, 1969; Green, 1980) (see Chapter 17), to the presence of other autoimmune disorders such as systemic lupus erythematosus (Mathur and Gatter, 1988), or to the development of anti-basal ganglia antibodies (Miranda et al., 2004) (see Chapter 18). In 1966 the first report of chorea associated with oral contraceptive use was published (Fernando, 1966), followed over the years by other case reports and small case series (Lewis and Harrison, 1969; Gamboa et al., 1971; Nausieda et al., 1979; Dove, 1980; Green, 1980; Mathur and Gatter, 1988). While in some cases the link to childhood Sydenham chorea was clear, in many others no clear relationship was established to a prior history of Sydenham chorea, streptococcal infection, or autoimmune disorders (Dove, 1980). The occurrence of chorea during pregnancy (*chorea gravidarum*) in rare cases suggests a role for estrogen (Cardoso, 2002). Immunologically mediated disorders such as systemic lupus erythematosus and antiphospholipid antibody syndrome must be ruled out in any patient presenting with chorea induced by oral contraceptives.

Anticonvulsants

With some exceptions (ataxia related to phenytoin and tremor with valproate), chorea and other movement disorders are relatively rare in patients taking antiepileptic drugs. In fact, some antiepileptics are used to ameliorate some movement disorders (primidone and gabapentin in essential tremor). It is important, however, to recognize that movement disorders may occur during treatment with these agents, particularly in the setting of polypharmacy.

Among the antiepileptic medications, phenytoin is the most commonly associated with the development of chorea or choreoathetosis (Harrison et al., 1993). From the case reports and series published, structural brain disease appears to be a recognized risk factor (Harrison et al., 1993; Koukkari et al., 1996; Shulman et al., 1996; Saito et al., 2001). Choreoathetosis can occur in patients treated with nontoxic levels of phenytoin, although most patients who develop choreoathetosis are often on multiple antiepileptic agents (Harrison et al., 1993). Phenytoin may aggravate preexisting TD (DeVeaugh-Geiss, 1978).

There are a few reports of chorea caused by valproate (Lancman et al., 1994; Gunal et al., 2002). In contrast, valproate has been used to treat chorea from different etiologies, such as Sydenham chorea (Daoud et al., 1990), postanoxic choreoathetosis (Chandra et al., 1982, 1983; Giroud and Dumas, 1986), chorea from lupus (Song et al., 1997), and kernicterus-associated choreiform movements (Kulkarni, 1992).

Carbamazepine (Bimpong-Buta and Froescher, 1982; Weaver et al., 1988), phenobarbital (Lightman, 1978; Wiznitzer and Younkin, 1984; Sechi et al., 1988), ethosuximide (Kirschberg, 1975), and methsuximide (Dooley et al., 1991) have also been reported to very infrequently cause chorea; carbamazepine and phenobarbital, similarly to valproate, have also proven useful for the treatment of some forms of chorea (Garello et al., 1983; Roig et al., 1988; Roulet and Deonna, 1989; Harel et al., 2000). Among the new antiepileptics, gabapentin (Buetefisch et al., 1996; Chudnow et al., 1997), zonisamide (Shimizu et al., 1997), lamotrigine (Miller and Levsky, 2008), and felbamate (Kerrick et al., 1995) have been associated with the development of choreiform movements in case reports. To our knowledge, there are no reports of levetiracetam-induced choreoathetosis.

Benzodiazepines

Orofacial dyskinesias have occasionally been reported in individuals treated with a variety of benzodiazepines (Kaplan and Murkofsky, 1978; Rosenbaum and de la Fluente, 1979; van der Kroef, 1979; Sandyk, 1986). In most cases, however, patients were treated with antipsychotic drugs or antidepressants, and the benzodiazepine was presumed to have either exacerbated a preexisting tardive syndrome or contributed to unmasking a subclinical dyskinesia. Benzodiazepines much more commonly ameliorate acute or chronic hyperkinetic movement disorders than precipitate or aggravate them (Shoulson and Chase, 1975; Bressman, 2006).

Lithium

Lithium carbonate is a standard therapy for the treatment of acute mania and bipolar disorders. Its narrow therapeutic window predisposes this drug to common potential side effects. At high concentrations ataxia, hypertonia, and confusion may arise; seizures, coma, and irreversible brain damage may occur. It is a drug well known to cause tremor, thought to represent an enhanced physiological tremor, although parkinsonism may also be seen. Chorea has also been associated with lithium use, possibly as a result of anticholinergic effects, although far less frequently than tremor (Peters, 1949; Coats et al., 1957; Sachdeva and Paruthi, 1980; Zorumski and Bakris, 1983; Walevski and Radwan, 1986; Reed et al., 1989; Helmuth et al., 1989; Matsis et al., 1989; Podskalny and Factor, 1996; Jimenez-Jimenez et al., 1997; Higes-Pascual et al., 1998; Stemper et al., 2003). Some cases were confused by the concomitant or prior use of dopamine receptor–blocking agents (Zorumski and Bakris, 1983); in most, chorea appeared in the context of drug intoxication (Peters, 1949; Coats et al., 1957; Sachdeva and Paruthi, 1980; Zorumski and Bakris, 1983; Walevski and Radwan, 1986; Reed et al., 1989; Helmuth et al., 1989; Matsis et al., 1989; Podskalny and Factor, 1996; Stemper et al., 2003).

Antidepressants

Antidepressants have only very rarely been associated with the development of choreiform movements, while other movement disorders are more commonly described.

Two cases of tricyclic antidepressant–induced chorea are well described (Burks et al., 1974). In both cases, physostigmine improved the symptomatology, suggesting that the abnormal movements were mediated by an anticholinergic effect.

The newer selective serotonin reuptake inhibitors (SSRIs) have been reported to cause TD (Botsaris and Sypek, 1996; Gill et al., 1997) among other movement disorders, most frequently tremor. Buspirone, which has been used to treat TD and L-dopa-induced dyskinesias with mixed results, has been reported to paradoxically induce akathisia, dystonia, and oral dyskinesias (Patterson, 1988; Strauss, 1988; Boylan, 1990; LeWitt et al., 1993; Detweiler and Harpold, 2002).

Trazodone has been linked to a reaction consisting of oromandibular and lingual dyskinesias associated with dystonic posturing of the limbs, which resolved upon drug discontinuation (Kramer et al., 1986), and bupropion caused attacks of ballism in a 42-year-old woman (de Graaf et al., 2003).

Anticholinergic drugs (benztropine, trihexyphenidyl) are an uncommon but well-established cause of reversible chorea and can exacerbate L-dopa-induced dyskinesias in PD patients (Mano, 1973; Birket-Smith, 1974; Warne and Gubbay, 1979) and tardive dyskinesias and dystonia from other causes (Nomoto et al., 1987). Rarely, anticholinergic medications may trigger chorea in neurologically normal older individuals (Birket-Smith, 1974).

SUMMARY

Medication-induced chorea is most frequently due to dopaminergic and antidopaminergic medications; however, other medication types may also induce chorea. While dysfunction of the dopamine system is clearly implicated, the precise mechanism is far from apparent. The mechanism of action by which nondopaminergic agents cause chorea is likewise unclear. Insights into the pathophysiology of medication-induced chorea may shed light upon treatments both for these disorders and for chorea of other etiologies.

REFERENCES

Adler L, Duncan E, Reiter S, Angrist B, Peselow E, Rotrosen J (1988) Effects of calcium-channel antagonists on tardive dyskinesia and psychosis. Psychopharmacol Bull 24: 421–425.

Adler LA, Peselow E, Duncan E, Rosenthal M, Angrist B (1993a) Vitamin E in tardive dyskinesia: time course of effect after placebo substitution. Psychopharmacol Bull 29: 371–374.

Adler LA, Peselow E, Rotrosen J, Duncan E, Lee M, Rosenthal M, et al. (1993b) Vitamin E treatment of tardive dyskinesia. Am J Psychiatry 150:1405–1407.

Ahlskog JE, Muenter MD (2001) Frequency of levodopa-related dyskinesias and motor fluctuations as estimated from the cumulative literature. Mov Disord 16:448–458.

Andersson U, Haggstrom JE, Levin ED, Bondesson U, Valverius M, Gunne LM (1989) Reduced glutamate decarboxylase activity in the subthalamic nucleus in patients with tardive dyskinesia. Mov Disord 4:37–46.

Antonini A, Tolosa E (2009) Apomorphine and levodopa infusion therapies for advanced Parkinson's disease: selection criteria and patient management. Expert Rev Neurother 9:859–867.

Bai YM, Yu SC, Chen JY, Lin CY, Chou P, Lin CC (2005) Risperidone for pre-existing severe tardive dyskinesia: a 48-week prospective follow-up study. Int Clin Psychopharmacol 20:79–85.

Bara-Jimenez W, Bibbiani F, Morris MJ, Dimitrova T, Sherzai A, Mouradian MM, et al. (2005) Effects of serotonin 5-HT1A agonist in advanced Parkinson's disease. Mov Disord 20:932–936.

Barrow N, Childs A (1986) An anti-tardive-dyskinesia effect of verapamil. Am J Psychiatry 143:1485.

Bartzokis G, Beckson M, Wirshing DA, Lu PH, Foster JA, Mintz J (1999) Choreoathetoid movements in cocaine dependence. Biol Psychiatry 45:1630–1635.

Beasley CM Jr, Tollefson G, Tran P, Satterlee W, Sanger T, Hamilton S (1996) Olanzapine versus placebo and haloperidol: acute phase results of the North American double-blind olanzapine trial. Neuropsychopharmacology 14:111–123.

Beasley CM, Dellva MA, Tamura RN, Morgenstern H, Glazer WM, Ferguson K, et al. (1999) Randomised double-blind comparison of the incidence of tardive dyskinesia in patients with schizophrenia during long-term treatment with olanzapine or haloperidol. Br J Psychiatry 174:23–30.

Benes FM, Paskevich PA, Davidson J, Domesick VB (1985) The effects of haloperidol on synaptic patterns in the rat striatum. Brain Res 329:265–273.

Bennett JP Jr, Landow ER, Dietrich S, Schuh LA (1994) Suppression of dyskinesias in advanced Parkinson's disease: moderate daily clozapine doses provide long-term dyskinesia reduction. Mov Disord 9:409–414.

Bennett JP Jr, Landow ER, Schuh LA (1993) Suppression of dyskinesias in advanced Parkinson's disease. II. Increasing daily clozapine doses suppress dyskinesias and improve parkinsonism symptoms. Neurology 43:1551–1555.

Bibbiani F, Costantini LC, Patel R, Chase TN (2005) Continuous dopaminergic stimulation reduces risk of motor complications in parkinsonian primates. Exp Neurol 192:73–78.

Bibbiani F, Oh JD, Chase TN (2001) Serotonin 5-HT1A agonist improves motor complications in rodent and primate parkinsonian models. Neurology 57:1829–1834.

Bimpong-Buta K, Froescher W (1982) Carbamazepine-induced choreoathetoid dyskinesias. J Neurol Neurosurg Psychiatry 45:560.

Birket-Smith E (1974) Abnormal involuntary movements induced by anticholinergic therapy. Acta Neurol Scand 50:801–811.

Birkmayer W, Hornykiewicz, O (1961) The L-3,4-dioxyphenylalanine (DOPA)-effect in Parkinson-akinesia. Wien Klin Wochenschr 73:787–788.

Boghdadi MS, Henning RJ (1997) Cocaine: pathophysiology and clinical toxicology. Heart Lung 26:466–483, quiz 484–485.

Bonifati V, Fabrizio E, Cipriani R, Vanacore N, Meco G (1994) Buspirone in levodopa-induced dyskinesias. Clin Neuropharmacol 17:73–82.

Bonthala CM, West A (1983) Pemoline induced chorea and Gilles de la Tourette's syndrome. Br J Psychiatry 143:300–302.

Boogerd W, Beijnen JH (2000) Methylphenidate for cerebral palsy with choreoathetosis. Ann Intern Med 132:510.

Borison RL, Arvanitis LA, Miller BG (1996) A comparison of five fixed doses of "seroquel" (ICI 204,636) with haloperidol and placebo in patients with schizophrenia. Schizophr Res 18:132–132.

Botsaris SD, Sypek JM (1996) Paroxetine and tardive dyskinesia. J Clin Psychopharmacol 16:258–259.

Boylan K (1990) Persistent dystonia associated with buspirone. Neurology 40:1904.

Bressman S (2006) Genetics of dystonia. J Neural Transm Suppl 70:489–495.

Browne J, Silver H, Martin R, Hart R, Mergener M, Williams P (1986) The use of clonidine in the treatment of neuroleptic-induced tardive dyskinesia. J Clin Psychopharmacol 6:88–92.

Brusa L, Versace V, Koch G, Iani C, Stanzione P, Bernardi G, et al. (2006) Low frequency rTMS of the SMA transiently ameliorates peak-dose LID in Parkinson's disease. Clin Neurophysiol 117:1917–1921.

Buck OD, Havey P (1988) Treatment of tardive dyskinesia with verapamil. J Clin Psychopharmacol 8:303–304.

Buetefisch CM, Gutierrez A, Gutmann L (1996) Choreoathetotic movements: a possible side effect of gabapentin. Neurology 46:851–852.

Burks JS, Walker JE, Rumack BH, Ott JE (1974) Tricyclic antidepressant poisoning. Reversal of coma, choreoathetosis, and myoclonus by physostigmine. JAMA 230:1405–1407.

Calabresi P, Di Filippo M, Ghiglieri V, Picconi B (2008) Molecular mechanisms underlying levodopa-induced dyskinesia. Mov Disord 23(Suppl 3):S570–S579.

Calne DB, Reid JL, Vakil SD, Pallis C (1971) Problems with levodopa therapy. Clin Med 78:21–23.

Campbell M (1999) Risperidone-induced tardive dyskinesia in first-episode psychotic patients. J Clin Psychopharmacol 19:276–277.

Cardoso F (2002) *Chorea gravidarum*. Arch Neurol 59:868–870.

Carpentier AF, Bonnet AM, Vidailhet M, Agid Y (1996) Improvement of levodopa-induced dyskinesia by propranolol in Parkinson's disease. Neurology 46:1548–1551.

Casey DE (1983) Metoclopramide side effects. Ann Intern Med 98:673–674.

Casey DE, Rabins P (1978) Tardive dyskinesia as a life-threatening illness. Am J Psychiatry 135:486–488.

Chandra V, Spunt AL, Rusinowitz MS (1983) Treatment of post-traumatic choreo-athetosis with sodium valproate. J Neurol Neurosurg Psychiatry 46:963.

Chandra V, Wharton S, Spunt AL (1982) Amelioration of hemiballismus with sodium valproate. Ann Neurol 12:407.

Chouinard G (1995) Effects of risperidone in tardive dyskinesia: an analysis of the Canadian multicenter risperidone study. J Clin Psychopharmacol 15:36S–44S.

Chouinard G, Annable L, Ross-Chouinard A, Mercier P (1988) A 5-year prospective longitudinal study of tardive dyskinesia: factors predicting appearance of new cases. J Clin Psychopharmacol 8:21S–26S.

Christensen E, Moller JE, Faurbye A (1970) Neuropathological investigation of 28 brains from patients with dyskinesia. Acta Psychiatr Scand 46:14–23.

Chudnow RS, Dewey RB Jr, Lawson CR (1997) Choreoathetosis as a side effect of gabapentin therapy in severely neurologically impaired patients. Arch Neurol 54: 910–912.

Clarke CE, Boyce S, Robertson RG, Sambrook MA, Crossman AR (1989) Drug-induced dyskinesia in primates rendered hemiparkinsonian by intracarotid administration of 1-methyl-4-phenyl-1,2,3,6-tetrahydropyridine (MPTP). J Neurol Sci 90:307–314.

Coats DA, Trautner EM, Gershon S (1957) The treatment of lithium poisoning. Australas Ann Med 6:11–15.

Cohen OS, Hassin-Baer S, Spiegelmann R (2007) Deep brain stimulation of the internal globus pallidus for refractory tardive dystonia. Parkinsonism Relat Disord 13:541–544.

Cotzias GC, Van Woert MH, Schiffer LM (1967) Aromatic amino acids and modification of parkinsonism. N Engl J Med 276:374–379.

Damier P, Thobois S, Witjas T, Cuny E, Derost P, Raoul S, et al. (2007) Bilateral deep brain stimulation of the globus pallidus to treat tardive dyskinesia. Arch Gen Psychiatry 64:170–176.

Daoud AS, Zaki M, Shakir R, al-Saleh Q (1990) Effectiveness of sodium valproate in the treatment of Sydenham chorea. Neurology 40:1140–1141.

Daras M, Koppel BS, Atos-Radzion E (1994) Cocaine-induced choreoathetoid movements ("crack dancing"). Neurology 44:751–752.

de Graaf L, Admiraal P, van Puijenbroek EP (2003) Ballism associated with bupropion use. Ann Pharmacother 37:302–303.

Dekundy A, Lundblad M, Danysz W, Cenci MA (2007) Modulation of L-DOPA-induced abnormal involuntary movements by clinically tested compounds: further validation of the rat dyskinesia model. Behav Brain Res 179:76–89.

Del Dotto P, Pavese N, Gambaccini G, Bernardini S, Metman LV, Chase TN, et al. (2001) Intravenous amantadine improves levadopa-induced dyskinesias: an acute double-blind placebo-controlled study. Mov Disord 16:515–520.

Delay J, Deniker P (1955) Neuroleptic effects of chlorpromazine in therapeutics of neuro-psychiatry. Int Rec Med Gen Pract Clin 168:318–326.

Detweiler MB, Harpold GJ (2002) Bupropion-induced acute dystonia. Ann Pharmacother 36:251–254.

DeVeaugh-Geiss J (1978) Aggravation of tardive dyskinesia by phenytoin. N Engl J Med 298:457–458.

Dogali M, Fazzini E, Kolodny E, Eidelberg D, Sterio D, Devinsky O, et al. (1995) Stereotactic ventral pallidotomy for Parkinson's disease. Neurology 45:753–761.

Dooley J, Camfield P, Buckley D, Gordon K, Wirrell E, Camfield C (1991) Methsuximide-induced movement disorder. Pediatrics 88:1291–1292.

Doongaji DR, Jeste DV, Jape NM, Sheth AS, Apte JS, Vahia VN, et al. (1982) Effects of intravenous metoclopramide in 81 patients with tardive dyskinesia. J Clin Psychopharmacol 2:376–379.

Dove DJ (1980) Chorea associated with oral contraceptive therapy. Am J Obstet Gynecol 137:740–742.

Duncan E, Adler L, Angrist B, Rotrosen J (1990) Nifedipine in the treatment of tardive dyskinesia. J Clin Psychopharmacol 10:414–416.

Durif F, Debilly B, Galitzky M, Morand D, Viallet F, Borg M, et al. (2004) Clozapine improves dyskinesias in Parkinson disease: a double-blind, placebo-controlled study. Neurology 62:381–388.

Durif F, Vidailhet M, Assal F, Roche C, Bonnet AM, Agid Y (1997) Low-dose clozapine improves dyskinesias in Parkinson's disease. Neurology 48:658–662.

Durif F, Vidailhet M, Bonnet AM, Blin J, Agid Y (1995) Levodopa-induced dyskinesias are improved by fluoxetine. Neurology 45:1855–1858.

Egan MF, Hyde TM, Albers GW, Elkashef A, Alexander RC, Reeve A, et al. (1992) Treatment of tardive dyskinesia with vitamin E. Am J Psychiatry 149:773–777.

Ehringer H, Hornykiewicz O (1960) Distribution of noradrenaline and dopamine (3-hydroxytyramine) in the human brain and their behavior in diseases of the extrapyramidal system. Klin Wochenschr 38:1236–1239.

Factor SA, Brown D (1992) Clozapine prevents recurrence of psychosis in Parkinson's disease. Mov Disord 7:125–131.

Fahn S (1985) A therapeutic approach to tardive dyskinesia. J Clin Psychiatry 46:19–24.

Fahn S (1983) High dosage anticholinergic therapy in dystonia. Neurology 33:1255–1261.

Fahn S (1984) The tardive dyskinesias. In: Mathews WB, Glaser GH (eds.) Recent Advances in Clinical Neurology. Churchill Livingstone, Edinburgh, pp 229–260.

Falk WE, Wojick JD, Gelenberg AJ (1988) Diltiazem for tardive dyskinesia and tardive dystonia. Lancet 1:824–825.

Farooq MU, Ducommun E, Goudreau J (2009) Treatment of a hyperkinetic movement disorder during pregnancy with dronabinol. Parkinsonism Relat Disord 15:249–251.

Fernandez-Ruiz J (2009) The endocannabinoid system as a target for the treatment of motor dysfunction. Br J Pharmacol 156:1029–1040.

Fernando SJ (1966) An attack of chorea complicating oral contraceptive therapy. Practitioner 197:210–211.

Fibiger HC, Lloyd KG (1984) Neurobiological substrates of tardive dyskinesia: the GABA hypothesis. Trends Neurosci 7:462–464.

Fines RE, Brady WJ, DeBehnke DJ (1997) Cocaine-associated dystonic reaction. Am J Emerg Med 15:513–515.

Fox SH, Henry B, Hill M, Crossman A, Brotchie J (2002a) Stimulation of cannabinoid receptors reduces levodopa-induced dyskinesia in the MPTP-lesioned nonhuman primate model of Parkinson's disease. Mov Disord 17:1180–1187.

Fox SH, Kellett M, Moore AP, Crossman AR, Brotchie JM (2002b) Randomised, double-blind, placebo-controlled trial to assess the potential of cannabinoid receptor stimulation in the treatment of dystonia. Mov Disord 17:145–149.

Fox SH, Lang AE (2008) Levodopa-related motor complications—phenomenology. Mov Disord 23(Suppl 3):S509–S514.

Franzini A, Marras C, Ferroli P, Zorzi G, Bugiani O, Romito L, et al. (2005) Long-term high-frequency bilateral pallidal stimulation for neuroleptic-induced tardive dystonia. Report of two cases. J Neurosurg 102:721–725.

Freedman R, Kirch D, Bell J, Adler LE, Pecevich M, Pachtman E, et al. (1982) Clonidine treatment of schizophrenia. Double-blind comparison to placebo and neuroleptic drugs. Acta Psychiatr Scand 65:35–45.

Friedman JH (1994) Clozapine treatment of psychosis in patients with tardive dystonia: report of three cases. Mov Disord 9:321–324.

Friis T, Christensen TR, Gerlach J (1983) Sodium valproate and biperiden in neuroleptic-induced akathisia, parkinsonism and hyperkinesia. A double-blind cross-over study with placebo. Acta Psychiatr Scand 67:178–187.

Fuller RW, Clemens JA, Hynes MD 3rd (1982) Degree of selectivity of pergolide as an agonist at presynaptic versus postsynaptic dopamine receptors: implications for prevention or treatment of tardive dyskinesia. J Clin Psychopharmacol 2:371–375.

Gamboa ET, Isaacs G, Harter DH (1971) Chorea associated with oral contraceptive therapy. Arch Neurol 25:112–114.

Garello L, Ottonello GA, Regesta G, Tanganelli P (1983) Familial paroxysmal kinesigenic choreoathetosis. Report of a pharmacological trial in 2 cases. Eur Neurol 22:217–221.

Geracitano R, Federici M, Bernardi G, Mercuri NB (2006) On the effects of psychostimulants, antidepressants, and the antiparkinsonian drug levodopa on dopamine neurons. Ann N Y Acad Sci 1074:320–329.

Ghelber D, Belmaker RH (1999) Tardive dyskinesia with quetiapine. Am J Psychiatry 156:796–797.

Gill HS, DeVane CL, Risch SC (1997) Extrapyramidal symptoms associated with cyclic antidepressant treatment: a review of the literature and consolidating hypotheses. J Clin Psychopharmacol 17:377–389.

Giroud M, Dumas R (1986) Valproate sodium in postanoxic choreoathetosis. J Child Neurol 1:80.

Glazer WM (2000) Expected incidence of tardive dyskinesia associated with atypical antipsychotics. J Clin Psychiatry 61(Suppl 4):21–26.

Goetz CG, Damier P, Hicking C, Laska E, Muller T, Olanow CW, et al. (2007) Sarizotan as a treatment for dyskinesias in Parkinson's disease: a double-blind placebo-controlled trial. Mov Disord 22:179–186.

Goodwin FK, Murphy DL, Brodie HK, Bunney WE, Jr (1970) L-DOPA, catecholamines, and behavior: a clinical and biochemical study in depressed patients. Biol Psychiatry 2:341–366.

Gray SD, Fatovich DM, McCoubrie DL, Daly FF (2007) Amphetamine-related presentations to an inner-city tertiary emergency department: a prospective evaluation. Med J Aust 186:336–339.

Green PM (1980) Chorea induced by oral contraceptives. Neurology 30:1131.

Gregoire L, Samadi P, Graham J, Bedard PJ, Bartoszyk GD, Di Paolo T (2009) Low doses of sarizotan reduce dyskinesias and maintain antiparkinsonian efficacy of L-dopa in parkinsonian monkeys. Parkinsonism Relat Disord 15:445–452.

Grondin R, Doan VD, Gregoire L, Bedard PJ (1999) D_1 receptor blockade improves L-dopa-induced dyskinesia but worsens parkinsonism in MPTP monkeys. Neurology 52:771–776.

Gruber D, Trottenberg T, Kivi A, Schoenecker T, Kopp UA, Hoffmann KT, et al. (2009) Long-term effects of pallidal deep brain stimulation in tardive dystonia. Neurology 73:53–58.

Gunal DI, Guleryuz M, Bingol CA (2002) Reversible valproate-induced choreiform movements. Seizure 11:205–206.

Gunne LM, Haggstrom JE, Sjoquist B (1984) Association with persistent neuroleptic-induced dyskinesia of regional changes in brain GABA synthesis. Nature 309:347–349.

Hall AP, Henry JA (2006) Acute toxic effects of "Ecstasy" (MDMA) and related compounds: overview of pathophysiology and clinical management. Br J Anaesth 96:678–685.

Harel L, Zecharia A, Straussberg R, Volovitz B, Amir J (2000) Successful treatment of rheumatic chorea with carbamazepine. Pediatr Neurol 23:147–151.

Harrison MB, Lyons GR, Landow ER (1993) Phenytoin and dyskinesias: a report of two cases and review of the literature. Mov Disord 8:19–27.

Hegarty AM, Lipton RB, Merriam AE, Freeman K (1991) Cocaine as a risk factor for acute dystonic reactions. Neurology 41:1670–1672.

Helmuth D, Ljaljevic Z, Ramirez L, Meltzer HY (1989) Choreoathetosis induced by verapamil and lithium treatment. J Clin Psychopharmacol 9:454–455.

Hennings JM, Krause E, Botzel K, Wetter TC (2008) Successful treatment of tardive lingual dystonia with botulinum toxin: case report and review of the literature. Prog Neuropsychopharmacol Biol Psychiatry 32:1167–1171.

Higes-Pascual F, de Arriba de la Fuente G, de Pedro-Esteban F (1998) Choreoathetosis: an uncommon sign of lithium poisoning. Rev Neurol 26:841.

Hillier CE, Wiles CM, Simpson BA (1999) Thalamotomy for severe antipsychotic induced tardive dyskinesia and dystonia. J Neurol Neurosurg Psychiatry 66:250–251.

Holloway RG, Shoulson I, Fahn S, Kieburtz K, Lang A, Marek K, et al. (2004) Pramipexole vs levodopa as initial treatment for Parkinson disease: a 4-year randomized controlled trial. Arch Neurol 61:1044–1053.

Hong KS, Cheong SS, Woo JM, Kim E (1999) Risperidone-induced tardive dyskinesia. Am J Psychiatry 156:1290.

Horiguchi J, Shingu T, Hayashi T, Kagaya A, Yamawaki S, Horikawa Y, et al. (1999) Antipsychotic-induced life-threatening "esophageal dyskinesia." Int Clin Psychopharmacol 14:123–127.

Hornykiewicz O (1966) Dopamine (3-hydroxytyramine) and brain function. Pharmacol Rev 18:925–964.

Huang CC, Wang RI, Hasegawa A, Alverno L (1981) Reserpine and alpha-methyldopa in the treatment of tardive dyskinesia. Psychopharmacology (Berl) 73:359–362.

Hunter R, Earl CJ, Thronicroft S (1964) An apparently irreversible syndrome of abnormal movements following phenothiazine medication. Proc R Soc Med 57:758–762.

Jeste DV (2000) Tardive dyskinesia in older patients. J Clin Psychiatry 61(Suppl 4):27–32.

Jeste DV (2004) Tardive dyskinesia rates with atypical antipsychotics in older adults. J Clin Psychiatry 65(Suppl 9):21–24.

Jeste DV, Lohr JB, Clark K, Wyatt RJ (1988) Pharmacological treatments of tardive dyskinesia in the 1980s. J Clin Psychopharmacol 8:38S–48S.

Jeste DV, Wyatt RJ (1982) Therapeutic strategies against tardive dyskinesia. Two decades of experience. Arch Gen Psychiatry 39:803–816.

Jeste DV, Wyatt RJ (1979) In search of treatment for tardive dyskinesia: review of the literature. Schizophr Bull 5:251–293.

Jimenez-Jimenez FJ, Garcia-Ruiz PJ, Molina JA (1997) Drug-induced movement disorders. Drug Saf 16:180–204.

Kamath S, Bajaj N (2007) Crack dancing in the United Kingdom: apropos a video case presentation. Mov Disord 22:1190–1191.

Kane JM, Smith JM (1982) Tardive dyskinesia: prevalence and risk factors, 1959 to 1979. Arch Gen Psychiatry 39:473–481.

Kane JM, Woerner M, Lieberman J (1985) Tardive dyskinesia: prevalence, incidence, and risk factors. In: Casey DE, Chase TN, Christensen AV, Gerlach J (eds.) Dyskinesia Research and Treatment (Psychopharmacology Suppl 2). Springer, Berlin, pp 72–78.

Kane JM, Woerner MG, Pollack S, Safferman AZ, Lieberman JA (1993) Does clozapine cause tardive dyskinesia? J Clin Psychiatry 54:327–330.

Kaplan SR, Murkofsky C (1978) Oral-buccal dyskinesia symptoms associated with low-dose benzodiazepine treatment. Am J Psychiatry 135:1558–1559.

Kazamatsuri H, Cole (1972) Treatment of tardive dyskinesia. 3. Clinical efficacy of a dopamine competing agent, methyldopa. Arch Gen Psychiatry 27:824–827.

Kazamatsuri H, Chien C, Cole JO (1972a) Therapeutic approaches to tardive dyskinesia. A review of the literature. Arch Gen Psychiatry 27:491–499.

Kazamatsuri H, Chien C, Cole JO (1972b) Treatment of tardive dyskinesia. I. Clinical efficacy of a dopamine-depleting agent, tetrabenazine. Arch Gen Psychiatry 27:95–99.

Kazamatsuri H, Chien C, Cole JO (1972c) Treatment of tardive dyskinesia. II. Short-term efficacy of dopamine-blocking agents haloperidol and thiopropazate. Arch Gen Psychiatry 27:100–103.

Kefalopoulou Z, Paschali A, Markaki E, Vassilakos P, Ellul J, Constantoyannis C (2009) A double-blind study on a patient with tardive dyskinesia treated with pallidal deep brain stimulation. Acta Neurol Scand 119:269–273.

Kerrick JM, Kelley BJ, Maister BH, Graves NM, Leppik IE (1995) Involuntary movement disorders associated with felbamate. Neurology 45:185–187.

Kirschberg GJ (1975) Dyskinesia—an unusual reaction to ethosuximide. Arch Neurol 32:137–138.

Klawans HL Jr (1973) The pharmacology of tardive dyskinesias. Am J Psychiatry 130: 82–86.

Klawans HL, Goetz C, Nausieda PA, Weiner WJ (1977) Levodopa-induced dopamine receptor hypersensitivity. Trans Am Neurol Assoc 102:80–83.

Klawans HL, Weiner WJ (1974) The effect of d-amphetamine on choreiform movement disorders. Neurology 24:312–318.

Kleedorfer B, Lees AJ, Stern GM (1991) Buspirone in the treatment of levodopa induced dyskinesias. J Neurol Neurosurg Psychiatry 54:376–377.

Koch G, Brusa L, Caltagirone C, Peppe A, Oliveri M, Stanzione P, et al. (2005) rTMS of supplementary motor area modulates therapy-induced dyskinesias in Parkinson disease. Neurology 65:623–625.

Kooptiwoot S, Settachan T (2000) Improvement of tardive dyskinesia with risperidone: a case report. J Med Assoc Thai 83:1430–1432.

Kopala LC, Honer WG (1994) Schizophrenia and severe tardive dyskinesia responsive to risperidone. J Clin Psychopharmacol 14:430–431.

Koukkari MW, Vanefsky MA, Steinberg GK, Hahn JS (1996) Phenytoin-related chorea in children with deep hemispheric vascular malformations. J Child Neurol 11: 490–491.

Krack P, Batir A, Van Blercom N, Chabardes S, Fraix V, Ardouin C, et al. (2003) Five-year follow-up of bilateral stimulation of the subthalamic nucleus in advanced Parkinson's disease. N Engl J Med 349:1925–1934.

Kramer MS, Marcus DJ, DiFerdinando J, Dewey D (1986) Atypical acute dystonia associated with trazodone treatment. J Clin Psychopharmacol 6:117–118.

Kruse W (1960) Persistent muscular restlessness after phenothiazine treatment: report of 3 cases. Am J Psychiatry 117:152–153.

Kulkarni ML (1992) Sodium valproate controls choreoathetoid movements of kernicterus. Indian Pediatr 29:1029–1030.

Kushnir SL, Ratner JT (1989) Calcium channel blockers for tardive dyskinesia in geriatric psychiatric patients. Am J Psychiatry 146:1218–1219.

Laitinen LV, Bergenheim AT, Hariz MI (1992) Leksell's posteroventral pallidotomy in the treatment of Parkinson's disease. J Neurosurg 76:53–61.

Lam LC, Chiu HF, Hung SF (1994) Vitamin E in the treatment of tardive dyskinesia: a replication study. J Nerv Ment Dis 182:113–114.

Lamberti JS, Bellnier T (1993) Clozapine and tardive dystonia. J Nerv Ment Dis 181: 137–138.

Lancman ME, Asconape JJ, Penry JK (1994) Choreiform movements associated with the use of valproate. Arch Neurol 51:702–704.

Lang AE, Marsden CD (1982) Alpha methylparatyrosine and tetrabenazine in movement disorders. Clin Neuropharmacol 5:375–387.

Lemmens P, Brecher M, Van Baelen B (1999) A combined analysis of double-blind studies with risperidone vs. placebo and other antipsychotic agents: factors associated with extrapyramidal symptoms. Acta Psychiatr Scand 99:160–170.

Lenders MW, Buschman HP, Vergouwen MD, Steur EN, Kolling P, Hariz M (2005) Long term results of unilateral posteroventral pallidotomy for antipsychotic drug induced tardive dyskinesia. J Neurol Neurosurg Psychiatry 76:1039.

Levandis G, Bazzini E, Armentero MT, Nappi G, Blandini F (2008) Systemic administration of an mGluR5 antagonist, but not unilateral subthalamic lesion, counteracts l-DOPA-induced dyskinesias in a rodent model of Parkinson's disease. Neurobiol Dis 29:161–168.

Lewis PD, Harrison MJ (1969) Involuntary movements in patients taking oral contraceptives. Br Med J 4:404–405.

LeWitt PA, Walters A, Hening W, McHale D (1993) Persistent movement disorders induced by buspirone. Mov Disord 8:331–334.

Leys D, Vermersch P, Danel T, Comayras S, Goudemand M, Caron J, et al. (1988) Diltiazem for tardive dyskinesia. Lancet 1:250–251.

Lieberman JA, Alvir J, Mukherjee S, Kane JM (1989) Treatment of tardive dyskinesia with bromocriptine. A test of the receptor modification strategy. Arch Gen Psychiatry 46:908–913.

Lightman SL (1978) Phenobarbital dyskinesia. Postgrad Med J 54:114–115.

Lohr JB, Caligiuri MP (1996) A double-blind placebo-controlled study of vitamin E treatment of tardive dyskinesia. J Clin Psychiatry 57:167–173.

Loonen AJ, Verwey HA, Roels PR, van Bavel LP, Doorschot CH (1992) Is diltiazem effective in treating the symptoms of (tardive) dyskinesia in chronic psychiatric inpatients? A negative, double-blind, placebo-controlled trial. J Clin Psychopharmacol 12:39–42.

Lozano AM, Lang AE, Galvez-Jimenez N, Miyasaki J, Duff J, Hutchinson WD, et al. (1995) Effect of GPi pallidotomy on motor function in Parkinson's disease. Lancet 346:1383–1387.

Ludatscher JI (1989) Stable remission of tardive dyskinesia by l-dopa. J Clin Psychopharmacol 9:39–41.

Luginger E, Wenning GK, Bosch S, Poewe W (2000) Beneficial effects of amantadine on l-dopa-induced dyskinesias in Parkinson's disease. Mov Disord 15:873–878.

Mano T (1973) Drug-induced dyskinesia—an electrophysiological analysis of dyskinesia induced by l-DOPA and anticholinergic drugs. Nagoya J Med Sci 36:29–48.

Marconi R, Lefebvre-Caparros D, Bonnet AM, Vidailhet M, Dubois B, Agid Y (1994) Levodopa-induced dyskinesias in Parkinson's disease phenomenology and pathophysiology. Mov Disord 9:2–12.

Marin C, Bonastre M, Aguilar E, Jimenez A (2009) Effect of metabotropic glutamate antagonist MPEP on levodopa-induced dyskinesias and the striatal regulation of vesicular glutamate transporters. Mov Disord 24:S356–S357.

Mathur AK, Gatter RA (1988) Chorea as the initial presentation of oral contraceptive induced systemic lupus erythematosus. J Rheumatol 15:1042–1043.

Matsis PP, Fisher RA, Tasman-Jones C (1989) Acute lithium toxicity—chorea, hypercalcemia and hyperamylasemia. Aust N Z J Med 19:718–720.

McDowell F, Lee JE, Swift T, Sweet RD, Ogsbury JS, Kessler JT (1970) Treatment of Parkinson's syndrome with L-dihydroxyphenylalanine (levodopa). Ann Intern Med 72:29–35.

Meltzer HY, Luchins DJ (1984) Effect of clozapine in severe tardive dyskinesia: a case report. J Clin Psychopharmacol 4:286–287.

Merims D, Ziv I, Djaldetti R, Melamed E (1999) Riluzole for levodopa-induced dyskinesias in advanced Parkinson's disease. Lancet 353:1764–1765.

Metman LV, Del Dotto P, LePoole K, Konitsiotis S, Fang J, Chase TN (1999) Amantadine for levodopa-induced dyskinesias: a 1-year follow-up study. Arch Neurol 56:1383–1386.

Miller MA, Levsky ME (2008) Choreiform dyskinesia following isolated lamotrigine overdose. J Child Neurol 23:243.

Miranda M, Cardoso F, Giovannoni G, Church A (2004) Oral contraceptive induced chorea: another condition associated with anti-basal ganglia antibodies. J Neurol Neurosurg Psychiatry 75:327–328.

Mones RJ, Elizan TS, Siegel GJ (1971) Analysis of L-dopa induced dyskinesias in 51 patients with Parkinsonism. J Neurol Neurosurg Psychiatry 34:668–673.

Morgan JC, Winter WC, Wooten GF (2004) Amphetamine-induced chorea in attention deficit-hyperactivity disorder. Mov Disord 19:840–842.

Morgenstern H, Glazer WM (1993) Identifying risk factors for tardive dyskinesia among long-term outpatients maintained with neuroleptic medications. Results of the Yale Tardive Dyskinesia Study. Arch Gen Psychiatry 50:723–733.

Morgese MG, Cassano T, Gaetani S, Macheda T, Laconca L, Dipasquale P, et al. (2009) Neurochemical changes in the striatum of dyskinetic rats after administration of the cannabinoid agonist WIN55,212-2. Neurochem Int 54:56–64.

Nakagawa, Kaneko S (2008) Neuropsychotoxicity of abused drugs: molecular and neural mechanisms of neuropsychotoxicity induced by methamphetamine, 3,4-methylenedioxymethamphetamine (ecstasy), and 5-methoxy-N,N-diisopropyltryptamine (foxy). J Pharmacol Sci 106:2–8.

Nasrallah HA, Dunner FJ, McCalley-Whitters M, Smith RE (1986) Pharmacologic probes of neurotransmitter systems in tardive dyskinesia: implications for clinical management. J Clin Psychiatry 47:56–59.

Nausieda PA, Koller WC, Weiner WJ, Klawans HL (1981) Pemoline-induced chorea. Neurology 31:356–360.

Nausieda PA, Koller WC, Weiner WJ, Klawans HL (1979) Chorea induced by oral contraceptives. Neurology 29:1605–1609.

Nielsen EB (1977) Long-term behavioural and biochemical effects following prolonged treatment with a neuroleptic drug (flupenthixol) in rats. Psychopharmacology (Berl) 54:203–208.

Nielsen EB, Lyon M (1978) Evidence for cell loss in corpus striatum after long-term treatment with a neuroleptic drug (flupenithixol) in rats. Psychopharmacology (Berl) 59:85–89.

Nishikawa T, Tanaka M, Tsuda A, Koga I, Uchida Y (1984) Clonidine therapy for tardive dyskinesia and related syndromes. Clin Neuropharmacol 7:239–245.

Nomoto M, Thompson PD, Sheehy MP, Quinn NP, Marsden CD (1987) Anticholinergic-induced chorea in the treatment of focal dystonia. Mov Disord 2:53–56.

Nutt JG (2007) Continuous dopaminergic stimulation: is it the answer to the motor complications of levodopa? Mov Disord 22:1–9.

Nutt JG (1990) Levodopa-induced dyskinesia: review, observations, and speculations. Neurology 40:340–345.

Nutt JG (2008) Pharmacokinetics and pharmacodynamics of levodopa. Mov Disord 23(Suppl 3):S580–S584.

Nutt JG, Gunzler SA, Kirchhoff T, Hogarth P, Weaver JL, Krams M, et al. (2008) Effects of a NR2B selective NMDA glutamate antagonist, CP-101,606, on dyskinesia and Parkinsonism. Mov Disord 23:1860–1866.

Oertel WH, Wolters E, Sampaio C, Gimenez-Roldan S, Bergamasco B, Dujardin M, et al. (2006) Pergolide versus levodopa monotherapy in early Parkinson's disease patients: the PELMOPET study. Mov Disord 21:343–353.

Ouattara B, Gregoire L, Morisette M, Gasparini F, Rajput A, Hornykiewicz O, et al. (2009) Brain metabotropic glutamate receptor 5 in Parkinson's disease with motor complications. Mov Disord 24:S349–S350.

Paci C, Thomas A, Onofrj M (2001) Amantadine for dyskinesia in patients affected by severe Parkinson's disease. Neurol Sci 22:75–76.

Pakkenberg H, Fog R, Nilakantan B (1973) The long-term effect of perphenazine enanthate on the rat brain. Some metabolic and anatomical observations. Psychopharmacologia 29:329–336.

Palatucci DM (1974) Iatrogenic dyskinesia. A unique reaction to parenteral methylphenidate. J Nerv Ment Dis 159:73–76.

Papa SM, Chase TN (1996) Levodopa-induced dyskinesias improved by a glutamate antagonist in Parkinsonian monkeys. Ann Neurol 39:574–578.

Pascual-Leone A, Dhuna A (1990) Cocaine-associated multifocal tics. Neurology 40: 999–1000.

Patterson JF (1988) Akathisia associated with buspirone. J Clin Psychopharmacol 8:296–297.

Pearce RK, Banerji T, Jenner P, Marsden CD (1998) De novo administration of ropinirole and bromocriptine induces less dyskinesia than L-dopa in the MPTP-treated marmoset. Mov Disord 13:234–241.

Pechevis M, Clarke CE, Vieregge P, Khoshnood B, Deschaseaux-Voinet C, Berdeaux G, et al. (2005) Effects of dyskinesias in Parkinson's disease on quality of life and health-related costs: a prospective European study. Eur J Neurol 12:956–963.

Perez-Rial S, Garcia-Gutierrez MS, Molina JA, Perez-Nievas BG, Ledent C, Leiva C, et al. (2009) Increased vulnerability to 6-hydroxydopamine lesion and reduced development of dyskinesias in mice lacking CB1 cannabinoid receptors. Neurobiol Aging (in press). d.o.i:10.1016/j.neurobiolaging.2009.03.017

Peters HA (1949) Lithium intoxication producing chorea athetosis with recovery. Wis Med J 48:1075.

Picconi B, Centonze D, Hakansson K, Bernardi G, Greengard P, Fisone G, et al. (2003) Loss of bidirectional striatal synaptic plasticity in L-DOPA-induced dyskinesia. Nat Neurosci 6:501–506.

Picconi B, Centonze D, Rossi S, Bernardi G, Calabresi P (2004) Therapeutic doses of L-dopa reverse hypersensitivity of corticostriatal D_2-dopamine receptors and glutamatergic overactivity in experimental parkinsonism. Brain 127:1661–1669.

Podskalny GD, Factor SA (1996) Chorea caused by lithium intoxication: a case report and literature review. Mov Disord 11:733–737.

Rascol O, Brooks DJ, Korczyn AD, De Deyn PP, Clarke CE, Lang AE (2000) A five-year study of the incidence of dyskinesia in patients with early Parkinson's disease who were treated with ropinirole or levodopa. 056 Study Group. N Engl J Med 342:1484–1491.

Rascol O, Brooks DJ, Korczyn AD, De Deyn PP, Clarke CE, Lang AE, et al. (2006) Development of dyskinesias in a 5-year trial of ropinirole and L-dopa. Mov Disord 21: 1844–1850.

Rascol O, Nutt JG, Blin O, Goetz CG, Trugman JM, Soubrouillard C, et al. (2001) Induction by dopamine D$_1$ receptor agonist ABT-431 of dyskinesia similar to levodopa in patients with Parkinson disease. Arch Neurol 58:249–254.

Reed SM, Wise MG, Timmerman I (1989) Choreoathetosis: a sign of lithium toxicity. J Neuropsychiatry Clin Neurosci 1:57–60.

Reiter S, Adler L, Angrist B, Peselow E, Rotrosen J (1989) Effects of verapamil on tardive dyskinesia and psychosis in schizophrenic patients. J Clin Psychiatry 50:26–27.

Riddle MA, Hardin MT, Towbin KE, Leckman JF, Cohen DJ (1987) Tardive dyskinesia following haloperidol treatment in Tourette's syndrome. Arch Gen Psychiatry 44: 98–99.

Rinne UK, Bracco F, Chouza C, Dupont E, Gershanik O, Marti Masso JF, et al. (1998) Early treatment of Parkinson's disease with cabergoline delays the onset of motor complications. Results of a double-blind levodopa controlled trial. The PKDS009 Study Group. Drugs 55(Suppl 1):23–30.

Rizos E, Douzenis A, Gournellis R, Christodoulou C, Lykouras LP (2009) Tardive dyskinesia in a patient treated with quetiapine. World J Biol Psychiatry 10:54–57.

Roig M, Montserrat L, Gallart A (1988) Carbamazepine: an alternative drug for the treatment of nonhereditary chorea. Pediatrics 82:492–495.

Rosenbaum AH, de la Fluente JR (1979) Benzodiazepines and tardive dyskinesia. Lancet 2:900.

Ross JL, Mackenzie TB, Hanson DR, Charles CR (1987) Diltiazem for tardive dyskinesia. Lancet 1:268.

Roulet E, Deonna T (1989) Successful treatment of hereditary dominant chorea with carbamazepine. Pediatrics 83:1077.

Roxburgh PA (1970) Treatment of persistent phenothiazine-induced oral dyskinesia. Br J Psychiatry 116:277–280.

Rylander G (1972) Psychoses and the punding and choreiform syndromes in addiction to central stimulant drugs. Psychiatr Neurol Neurochir 75:203–212.

Sachdeva JR, Paruthi SC (1980) Chorea—a complication of lithium. J Indian Med Assoc 75:37–38.

Saito Y, Oguni H, Awaya Y, Hayashi K, Osawa M (2001) Phenytoin-induced choreoathetosis in patients with severe myoclonic epilepsy in infancy. Neuropediatrics 32: 231–235.

Sako W, Goto S, Shimazu H, Murase N, Matsuzaki K, Tamura T, et al. (2008) Bilateral deep brain stimulation of the globus pallidus internus in tardive dystonia. Mov Disord 23:1929–1931.

Sandyk R (1986) Orofacial dyskinesias associated with lorazepam therapy. Clin Pharm 5:419–421.

Sassin JF, Taub S, Weitzman ED (1972) Hyperkinesia and changes in behavior produced in normal monkeys by L-dopa. Neurology 22:1122–1125.

Schiorring E (1981) Psychopathology induced by "speed drugs." Pharmacol Biochem Behav 14(Suppl 1):109–122.

Schrodt GR Jr, Wright JH, Simpson R, Moore DP, Chase S (1982) Treatment of tardive dyskinesia with propranolol. J Clin Psychiatry 43:328–331.

Schulz SC, Mack R, Zborowski J, Morris D, Sebree T, Wallin B (1996) Efficacy, safety, and dose response of three doses of sertindole and three doses of haldol in schizophrenic patients. Schizophr Res 18:133–134.

Schupbach WM, Chastan N, Welter ML, Houeto JL, Mesnage V, Bonnet AM, et al. (2005) Stimulation of the subthalamic nucleus in Parkinson's disease: a 5 year follow-up. J Neurol Neurosurg Psychiatry 76:1640–1644.

Schwarz GA, Fahn S (1970) Newer medical treatment in parkinsonism. Med Clin North Am 54:773–785.

Schwarzschild MA, Agnati L, Fuxe K, Chen JF, Morelli M (2006) Targeting adenosine A2A receptors in Parkinson's disease. Trends Neurosci 29:647–654.

Sechi GP, Piras MR, Rosati G, Zuddas M, Ortu R, Tanca S, et al. (1988) Phenobarbital-induced buccolingual dyskinesia in oral apraxia. Eur Neurol 28:139–141.

Sedman G (1976) Clonazepam in treatment of tardive oral dyskinesia [letter]. Br Med J 2:583.

Seeger TF, Seymour PA, Schmidt AW, Zorn SH, Schulz DW, Lebel LA, et al. (1995) Ziprasidone (CP-88,059): a new antipsychotic with combined dopamine and serotonin receptor antagonist activity. J Pharmacol Exp Ther 275:101–113.

Shimizu T, Yamashita Y, Satoi M, Togo A, Wada N, Matsuishi T, et al. (1997) Heat stroke-like episode in a child caused by zonisamide. Brain Dev 19:366–368.

Shoulson I, Chase TN (1975) Huntington disease. Annu Rev Med 26:419–436.

Shriqui CL, Bradwejn J, Annable L, Jones BD (1992) Vitamin E in the treatment of tardive dyskinesia: a double-blind placebo-controlled study. Am J Psychiatry 149:391–393.

Shulman LM, Singer C, Weiner WJ (1996) Phenytoin-induced focal chorea. Mov Disord 11:111–114.

Sieradzan KA, Fox SH, Hill M, Dick JP, Crossman AR, Brotchie JM (2001) Cannabinoids reduce levodopa-induced dyskinesia in Parkinson's disease: a pilot study. Neurology 57:2108–2111.

Silverdale MA, Nicholson SL, Crossman AR, Brotchie JM (2005) Topiramate reduces levodopa-induced dyskinesia in the MPTP-lesioned marmoset model of Parkinson's disease. Mov Disord 20:403–409.

Simonin C, Tir M, Devos D, Kreisler A, Dujardin K, Salleron J, et al. (2009) Reduced levodopa-induced complications after 5 years of subthalamic stimulation in Parkinson's disease: a second honeymoon. J Neurol 256(10):1736–1741.

Simpson GM, Lee JH, Shrivastava RK (1978) Clozapine in tardive dyskinesia. Psychopharmacology (Berl) 56:75–80.

Singh BK, Singh A, Chusid E (1983a) Chorea in long-term use of pemoline. Ann Neurol 13:218.

Singh MM, Becker RE, Pitman RK, Nasrallah HA, Lal H (1983b) Sustained improvement in tardive dyskinesia with diazepam: indirect evidence for corticolimbic involvement. Brain Res Bull 11:179–185.

Slotema CW, van Harten PN, Bruggeman R, Hoek HW (2008) Botulinum toxin in the treatment of orofacial tardive dyskinesia: a single blind study. Prog Neuropsychopharmacol Biol Psychiatry 32:507–509.

Small JG, Milstein V, Marhenke JD, Hall DD, Kellams JJ (1987) Treatment outcome with clozapine in tardive dyskinesia, neuroleptic sensitivity, and treatment-resistant psychosis. J Clin Psychiatry 48:263–267.

Smith RC, Tamminga CA, Haraszti J, Pandey GN, Davis JM (1977) Effects of dopamine agonists in tardive dyskinesia. Am J Psychiatry 134:763–768.

Snow BJ, Macdonald L, Mcauley D, Wallis (2000) The effect of amantadine on levodopa-induced dyskinesias in Parkinson's disease: a double-blind, placebo-controlled study. Clin Neuropharmacol 23:82–85.

Soares K, Rathbone J, Deeks J (2004) Gamma-aminobutyric acid agonists for neuroleptic-induced tardive dyskinesia. Cochrane Database Syst Rev 4:CD000203.

Song CH, Oftadeh LC, Oh C, Louie J, Yu KT (1997) Successful treatment of steroid-resistant chorea associated with lupus by use of valproic acid and clonidine-HCL patch. Clin Pediatr (Phila) 36:659-662.

Stedman TJ, Whiteford HA, Eyles D, Welham JL, Pond SM (1991) Effects of nifedipine on psychosis and tardive dyskinesia in schizophrenic patients. J Clin Psychopharmacol 11:43–47.

Stemper B, Thurauf N, Neundorfer B, Heckmann JG (2003) Choreoathetosis related to lithium intoxication. Eur J Neurol 10:743–744.

Stewart RM, Rollins J, Beckham B, Roffman M (1982) Baclofen in tardive dyskinesia patients maintained on neuroleptics. Clin Neuropharmacol 5:365–373.

Stork CM, Cantor R (1997) Pemoline induced acute choreoathetosis: case report and review of the literature. J Toxicol Clin Toxicol 35:105–108.

Strauss A (1988) Oral dyskinesia associated with buspirone use in an elderly woman. J Clin Psychiatry 49:322–323.

Sun B, Chen S, Zhan S, Le W, Krahl SE (2007) Subthalamic nucleus stimulation for primary dystonia and tardive dystonia. Acta Neurochir Suppl 97:207–214.

Tamminga CA, Thaker GK, Moran M, Kakigi T, Gao XM (1994) Clozapine in tardive dyskinesia: observations from human and animal model studies. J Clin Psychiatry 55(Suppl B):102–106.

Tarsy D, Baldessarini RJ (1976) The tardive dyskinesia syndrome. In: Klawans HL (ed.) Clinical Neuropharmacology. Raven Press, New York, pp 29–61.

Tarsy D, Granacher R, Bralower M (1977) Tardive dyskinesia in young adults. Am J Psychiatry 134:1032–1034.

Thaker GK, Nguyen JA, Strauss ME, Jacobson R, Kaup BA, Tamminga CA (1990) Clonazepam treatment of tardive dyskinesia: a practical GABAmimetic strategy. Am J Psychiatry 147:445–451.

Thaker GK, Tamminga CA, Alphs LD, Lafferman J, Ferraro TN, Hare TA (1987) Brain gamma-aminobutyric acid abnormality in tardive dyskinesia. Reduction in cerebrospinal fluid GABA levels and therapeutic response to GABA agonist treatment. Arch Gen Psychiatry 44:522–529.

Tollefson GD, Beasley CM Jr, Tran PV, Street JS, Krueger JA, Tamura RN, et al. (1997) Olanzapine versus haloperidol in the treatment of schizophrenia and schizoaffective and schizophreniform disorders: results of an international collaborative trial. Am J Psychiatry 154:457–465.

Trottenberg T, Volkmann J, Deuschl G, Kuhn AA, Schneider GH, Muller J, et al. (2005) Treatment of severe tardive dystonia with pallidal deep brain stimulation. Neurology 64:344–346.

Trugman JM, Leadbetter R, Zalis ME, Burgdorf RO, Wooten GF (1994) Treatment of severe axial tardive dystonia with clozapine: case report and hypothesis. Mov Disord 9:441–446.

Tschopp L, Salazar Z, Micheli F (2009) Botulinum toxin in painful tardive dyskinesia. Clin Neuropharmacol 32:165–166.

Turrone P, Remington G, Kapur S, Nobrega JN (2003) The relationship between dopamine D_2 receptor occupancy and the vacuous chewing movement syndrome in rats. Psychopharmacology (Berl) 165:166–171.

van der Kroef C (1979) Reactions to triazolam. Lancet 2:526.

van Harten PN, Hovestadt A (2006) Botulinum toxin as a treatment for tardive dyskinesia. Mov Disord 21:1276–1277.

Wagle-Shukla A, Angel MJ, Zadikoff C, Enjati M, Gunraj C, Lang AE, et al. (2007) Low-frequency repetitive transcranial magnetic stimulation for treatment of levodopa-induced dyskinesias. Neurology 68:704–705.

Walevski A, Radwan M (1986) Choreoathetosis as toxic effect of lithium treatment. Eur Neurol 25:412–415.

Wang Y, Turnbull I, Calne S, Stoessl AJ, Calne DB (1997) Pallidotomy for tardive dyskinesia. Lancet 349:777–778.

Warne RW, Gubbay SS (1979) Choreiform movements induced by anticholinergic therapy. Med J Aust 1:465.

Waugh JL, Miller VS, Chudnow RS, Dowling MM (2008) Juvenile Huntington disease exacerbated by methylphenidate: case report. J Child Neurol 23:807–809.

Weaver DF, Camfield P, Fraser A (1988) Massive carbamazepine overdose: clinical and pharmacologic observations in five episodes. Neurology 38:755–759.

Weetman J, Anderson IM, Gregory RP, Gill SS (1997) Bilateral posteroventral pallidotomy for severe antipsychotic induced tardive dyskinesia and dystonia. J Neurol Neurosurg Psychiatry 63:554–556.

Weiner WJ, Nausieda PA, Klawans HL (1978) Methylphenidate-induced chorea: case report and pharmacologic implications. Neurology 28:1041–1044.

Williams J, Pacula RL, Chaloupka FJ, Wechsler H (2006) College students' use of cocaine. Subst Use Misuse 41:489–509.

Wiznitzer M, Younkin D (1984) Phenobarbital-induced dyskinesia in a neurologically-impaired child. Neurology 34:1600–1601.

Xu K, Bastia E, Schwarzschild M (2005) Therapeutic potential of adenosine A_{2A} receptor antagonists in Parkinson's disease. Pharmacol Ther 105:267–310.

Yahr MD, Duvoisin RC, Schear MJ, Barrett RE, Hoehn MM (1969) Treatment of parkinsonism with levodopa. Arch Neurol 21:343–354.

Yassa R (1988) Tardive dyskinesia and anticholinergic drugs. A critical review of the literature. Encephale 14(Spec No):233–239.

Yassa R, Jeste DV (1992) Gender differences in tardive dyskinesia: a critical review of the literature. Schizophr Bull 18:701–715.

Zigmond MJ, Abercrombie ED, Berger TW, Grace AA, Stricker EM (1990) Compensations after lesions of central dopaminergic neurons: some clinical and basic implications. Trends Neurosci 13:290–296.

Zorumski CF, Bakris GL (1983) Choreoathetosis associated with lithium: case report and literature review. Am J Psychiatry 140:1621–1622.

15

Metabolic Causes of Chorea

S. Elizabeth Zauber, MD and Katie Kompoliti, MD

INTRODUCTION

Chorea can result from several metabolic causes, most commonly disruptions in glucose, thyroid, and renal function. Although metabolic etiologies are relatively rare causes of chorea, they should be considered in the differential diagnosis of chorea because they are usually reversible.

ELECTROLYTES

Glucose Metabolism

Hyperglycemia

Clinical. Chorea associated with hyperglycemia has several distinctive clinical features, as well as interesting imaging findings (Tables 15–1, 15–2). All patients have marked hyperglycemia, although many lack a known history of diabetes. One reported nondiabetic patient developed chorea after excessive sucrose ingestion (Jung et al., 2009). Elderly women appear to be affected most commonly. In one meta-analysis, the average age was 71, average glucose was 481 mg/dl, and average hemoglobin A_{1c} was 14% (Oh et al., 2002). Hyperglycemia-induced chorea

294

TABLE 15–1. Imaging Characteristics of Metabolic Choreas

	HYPERGLYCEMIA	HYPOGLYCEMIA	UREMIA
T1	Increased	Decreased	Decreased
T2	Decreased	Increased	Increased
SPECT	Increased	Increased	Increased
PET	Decreased	N/A	N/A
Chorea	Unilateral	Unilateral or bilateral	Generalized

N/A, not available; PET, positron emission tomography; SPECT, single-photon emission computed tomography; T1, T1-weighted magnetic resonance image (MRI); T2, T2-weighted MRI.

accounted for 4% of sporadic choreas in one hospital-based series (Piccolo et al., 2003).

Chorea is usually of acute onset but can be delayed by weeks after blood sugar elevation (Nguyen, 2007). The majority of patients (88%) have hemichorea and asymmetric imaging findings. This asymmetry is unexpected for a metabolic problem (Chang et al., 2007) and suggests that other etiological factors may contribute to the pathophysiology (see later, "Pathophysiology").

Treatment consists of blood sugar control, and in some patients this alone leads to resolution of chorea. Occasionally, patients require temporary treatment with dopamine receptor–blocking drugs. In a meta-analysis of 53 cases, 73% of patients had full resolution by 6-month follow-up, while the remainder had

TABLE 15–2. Clinical Characteristics of Metabolic Choreas

	PRESENTATION	COURSE	IMAGING
Hyperglycemia	Usually hemichorea	Most resolve or improve in weeks	Increased signal on T1
Hyperthyroidism	Generalized > focal	Reversible	Normal
Hypocalcemia	Often paroxysmal	All resolve with treatment of hypocalcemia	Often have basal ganglia calcifications
Uremia	Patients on hemodialysis who have diabetes	Resolve, although many patients critically ill	Increased T2 signal, can occur with mass effect and contrast enhancement

T1, T1-weighted magnetic resonance image (MRI); T2, T2-weighted MRI.

some improvement. Rarely, cases of persistent chorea are reported; however, these cases differ in their clinical features. Patients with persistent chorea have more extensive neuroimaging changes and the onset of chorea is delayed, occurring 1–4 weeks after glucose is normalized (Ahlskog et al., 2001).

Imaging.   The distinctive magnetic resonance imaging (MRI) findings in hyperglycemia-induced chorea have been the subject of significant discussion in the literature. Brain computed tomography (CT) shows increased signal in the contralateral basal ganglia (Nguyen, 2007). MRI shows increased signal on T1-weighted images and decreased signal on T2-weighted images (Figure 15–1, Table 15–1). Diffusion-weighted imaging findings vary. Some cases have restricted diffusion, usually without a corresponding apparent diffusion coefficient change to suggest acute infarct (Hsu et al., 2004; Wintermark et al., 2004; Nath et al., 2006). The putamen is always involved (Oh et al., 2002; Kandiah et al., 2009), although other basal ganglia regions may also be affected. The changes in imaging are usually reversible, but clinical symptoms resolve before imaging (Lai et al., 1996).

Pathophysiology.   Despite extensive literature on the topic, the exact nature of the imaging findings has not been elucidated. The finding of increased signal

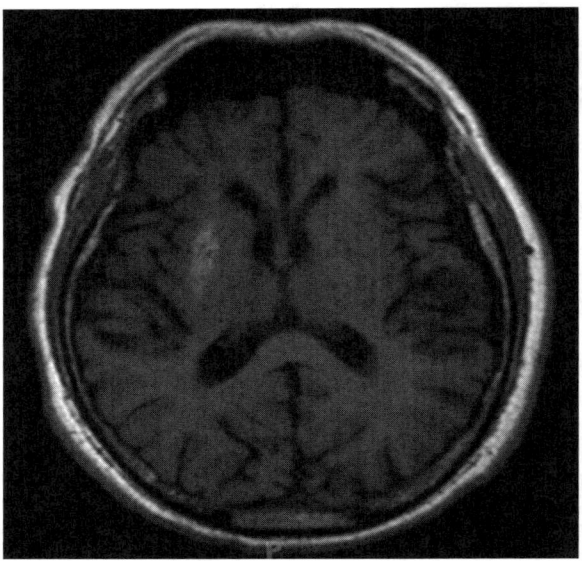

FIGURE 15–1. T1-weighted magnetic resonance image of the brain in a patient with left-sided hemichorea and nonketotic hyperglycemia demonstrates right putaminal hyperintensity.

on T1-weighted images and on CT led some to hypothesize that petechial hemorrhage is responsible for the findings. However, gradient echo, an MRI sequence sensitive to iron and, thus, hemorrhage, is normal (Chu et al., 2002; Kandiah et al., 2009). Further, most pathological studies do not show evidence of hemorrhage (Shan et al., 1998).

A combination of functional neuroimaging and pathological data has been used to investigate the etiology of this disorder. Single-photon emission computed tomographic (SPECT) scans typically show increased perfusion of the basal ganglia contralateral to the chorea (Hsu et al., 2004). Despite increased perfusion, positron emission tomography (PET) studies of glucose metabolism reveal decreased glucose metabolism in the same areas (Nguyen, 2007). The combination of decreased glucose metabolism with increased blood flow argues against a simple metabolic or vascular explanation. Some have suggested that a combination of metabolic and vascular derangements contributes to metabolic failure (Hsu et al., 2004).

Autopsy and biopsy results are limited but show a combination of infarcts and reactive astrocytes (Ohara et al., 2001; Nath et al., 2006). Despite these pathological data, infarct is thought to be an unlikely cause in most patients. Instead, transient, reversible ischemia without infarct is more consistent with the neuroimaging and clinical findings. Animal models of transient ischemia produce similar imaging changes. In addition, transient ischemia in animal models results in gliosis and reactive astrocytes, both of which are seen in pathological samples of patients with hyperglycemia-induced chorea. The high protein content in these reactive astrocytes is thought to be responsible for the increased T1 signal seen on MRI.

Furthermore, dysfunction of gamma-aminobutyric acid (GABA)-ergic neurons in the basal ganglia may have an etiological role in producing chorea. Reduced regional blood flow caused by hyperglycemia (and/or hyperviscosity) leads to anaerobic metabolism, which damages GABA neurons in the striatum. Magnetic resonance spectroscopy provides further evidence for both gliosis and neuronal dysfunction (Lai et al., 2001).

Hypoglycemia

Clinical/Imaging.   Less commonly, hypoglycemia can cause both chorea and paroxysmal kinesigenic dyskinesia (PKD). Several cases of patients with diabetes and chronic renal failure on hemodialysis are reported. In these patients chorea was either focal or generalized. The abnormal movements usually began 1–2 days after hypoglycemia and were reversible in 1–2 weeks, although most patients required transient treatment with neuroleptics. MRI showed increased basal ganglia signal on T2 and fluid-attenuated inversion recovery (FLAIR) and decreased signal on T1, with hyperperfusion on SPECT (Lai et al., 2004) (Table 15–1).

Hypoglycemia-induced chorea can also occur in patients without a history of diabetes. One patient developed episodes of abnormal movements consisting of choreic and dystonic posturing of her limbs and trunk. The attacks occurred after exertion and improved after eating. She was found to have hypoglycemia, and further evaluation revealed an insulinoma. Following surgical resection of the tumor, she had no recurrent attacks of abnormal movements (Shaw et al., 1996).

Paroxysmal exercise–induced chorea can occur in patients with normal serum glucose but low cerebral spinal fluid glucose, due to a mutation in the glucose transporter 1 gene (Weber et al., 2008) (Chapter 19).

Pathophysiology. The pathophysiology of hypoglycemia-induced chorea has not been fully elucidated. Some hypothesize that hypoglycemia causes temporary striatal dysfunction, which may lead to reduced pallidal and subthalamic nucleus inhibitory outflow to the thalamus. This loss of thalamocortical inhibition then results in hyperkinetic movements (Shaw et al., 1996).

Calcium Metabolism

Hypocalcemia

Clinical. Hypocalcemia affects both the central and peripheral nervous systems. Common symptoms include tetany, confusion, paresthesias, and seizures. Chorea is a less common manifestation of hypocalcemia. Interestingly, sustained chorea is less often reported than paroxysmal chorea mimicking PKD or paroxysmal nonkinesigenic dyskinesia (PNKD) (Table 15–2) (Chapter 19). Correction of calcium leads to resolution of the movement disorder in all reported cases.

A variety of causes of hypocalcemia are described. Generalized chorea as well as tetany, confusion, and seizures were observed in a 54-year-old woman with basal ganglia calcifications from idiopathic hypoparathyroidism (Hossain, 1970). Hypocalcemia can also result from elevated parathyroid hormone (PTH) in pseudohypoparathyroidism. In this condition patients have end-organ resistance to PTH (Mahmud et al., 2005), low calcium, high phosphorus, and high PTH. One patient had abnormal movements consisting of both PKD and PNKD. The same patient also had extensive calcifications (Figure 15–2) of the basal ganglia and thalamus (Dure and Mussell, 1998).

Other causes of hypocalcemia have resulted in chorea. An 85-year-old patient with prostate cancer and extensive bone metastases received intravenous bisphosphonate, resulting in paroxysmal choreic movements of both arms, triggered by movement. He had associated tetany and paresthesias. Calcium was markedly low at 0.7 (normal 2.15–2.6) (Topakian et al., 2006). Hemichorea has been reported to result from hypocalcemia due to vitamin D deficiency in a child with protein-losing enteropathy (Fernandez et al., 2007).

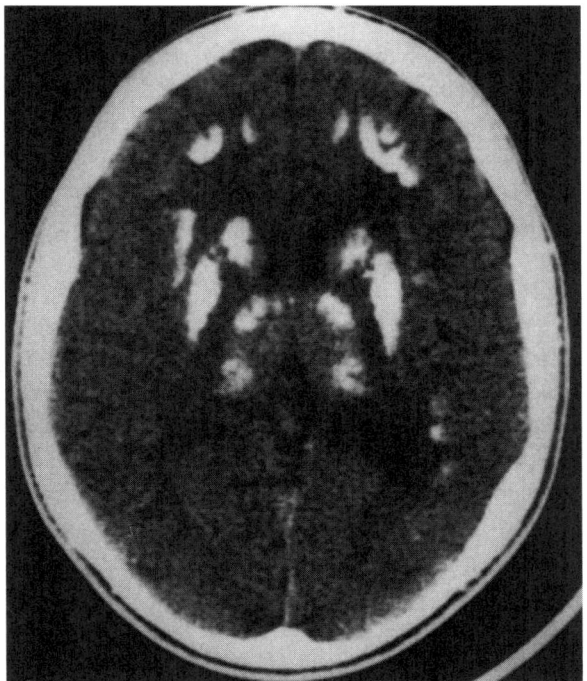

FIGURE 15–2. Axial computed tomogram of the head shows calcium in the basal ganglia, thalamus, and cortex in a patient with pseudohypoparathyroidism. From Dure and Mussell (1998). Reprinted with permission of John Wiley & Sons, Inc.

Imaging/Pathophysiology.   Two cases of idiopathic hypoparathyroidism were investigated with PET imaging. Both patients had low calcium, low PTH, and marked intracerebral calcifications. One patient had attacks of PKD and PNKD and the other just PKD (Kato et al., 1987; Volonté et al., 2001). PET showed bilateral hypometabolism in the ventral striatum. Repeat PET imaging after the movements resolved and calcium normalized showed normal basal ganglia metabolism (Volonté et al., 2001). The basal ganglia calcifications were unchanged, suggesting that hypocalcemia, not basal ganglia calcifications, was responsible for the abnormal PET findings and abnormal movements. It is hypothesized that, as in other forms of chorea, reduced function of the indirect pathway leads to disinhibition of the thalamus and allows for involuntary movements.

Sodium Metabolism

Compared to the electrolyte disturbances already described, sodium alterations are rarely reported to cause chorea.

Hypernatremia

Rare reports describe hypernatremia-induced chorea occurring in the setting of dehydration. However, other electrolyte disturbances associated with dehydration, which are known to cause chorea, were also present in those reports, such as hypocalcemia, metabolic acidosis, and elevated blood urea nitrogen. Similarly, other neurological signs of dehydration such as myoclonus and somnolence were observed. Chorea in these patients was generalized and resolved several days after correction of serum sodium (Sparacio et al., 1976).

Hyponatremia

Chorea has also been reported in patients who presented with hyponatremia. However, the onset of chorea occurred months to years after correction of serum sodium. These patients had prominent dystonia as well as chorea and clinical and imaging evidence of central pontine myelinolysis. Chorea and dystonia are thought to result from extrapontine myelinolysis affecting the basal ganglia (Tison et al., 1991).

SYSTEMIC METABOLIC DISORDERS

Renal Failure

Clinical

The majority of patients with uremia who develop movement disorders and basal ganglia lesions have parkinsonism. Only a minority of patients present with chorea. Affected patients have end-stage renal disease on regular hemodialysis. Chorea is usually of acute onset and generalized, and may be accompanied by other neurological signs of uremia, such as impaired level of consciousness and dysarthria (Wang and Cheng, 2003). Asians appear to be affected more commonly. Laboratory findings include elevated blood urea nitrogen, creatinine, and acidosis. While nearly all affected patients have diabetes, glucose is usually normal at the time of onset. Chorea often improves with more frequent dialysis; however, many patients in these series died of sepsis or other complications of their medical illnesses (Wang and Cheng, 2003).

Imaging

Imaging findings consist of bilateral symmetric basal ganglia lesions which are hypointense on CT and have low signal on T1-weighted and high signal on T2-weighted MRIs (Table 15–1). Some patients also have mass effect and contrast enhancement, which is thought to be due to vasogenic edema (Lee et al., 2007). Imaging changes usually resolve as the chorea does, but permanent cystic changes in basal ganglia may occur, perhaps corresponding to small areas of cytotoxic edema (Kim et al., 2006; Lee et al., 2007; Park et al., 2007). The globus pallidus is the most common site for these cystic changes (Park et al., 2007).

Pathophysiology

The mechanism is hypothesized to be a combination of microvascular dysfunction from long-standing diabetes and uremic toxins. Increased levels of PTH and aluminum have been hypothesized to be pathophysiological toxins but are not consistently elevated in affected patients (Wang and Cheng, 2003; Park et al., 2007).

Hepatic Failure

Aquired hepatocerebral degeneration (AHCD) is a mixed movement disorder that occurs in some patients with end-stage liver disease. It has been named to distinguish it from the *inherited* hepatocerebral degeneration, Wilson's disease (WD). Like WD, AHCD causes a variety of abnormal movements including parkinsonism, tremor, and chorea. Unlike Wilson's disease which affects young people, AHCD usually presents in the 5th or 6th decade, and can result from any type of liver failure, as long as porto-systemic shunting is present.

AHCD should be clinically distinguished from hepatic encephalopathy. Patients with AHCD do not have significant cognitive dysfunction; and treatments aimed at lowering serum ammonia, are not effective for treating the abnormal movements. Parkinsonism and action tremor occur more commonly than chorea. When hyperkinetic movements are present, they often take the form of oral-bucal-lingual movements resembling tardive dyskinesia. Patients may have tongue protrusion and facial grimacing leading to dysphagia (Ferrara and Jankovic, 2009).

Distinct imaging findings consist of increased T1 signal in the pallidum (Jog and Lang, 1995). This T1 signal is hypothesized to represent manganese, since severity of imaging findings parallel serum manganese (Ferrara and Jankovic, 2009). However, manganese is likely not the pathological agent since the imaging findings and serum manganese levels do not correlate with disease severity. AHCD is thought to be irreversible, however, some patients may improve following liver transplantation (Stracciari et al., 2001).

Vitamin B$_{12}$

A 71-year-old man with a history of resected gastric cancer developed subacute onset of right hemichorea. Symptoms worsened despite treatment with a dopamine antagonist. He developed generalized chorea with blepharospasm and dysarthria. After vitamin B$_{12}$ replacement, the movements resolved, the dopamine antagonist was withdrawn, and he had a normal neurological exam at 6-month follow-up (Pacchetti et al., 2002). The authors hypothesize that low vitamin B_{12} levels lead to increased homocystine, which excites N-methyl-D-aspartic acid (NMDA) receptors and produces excitatory activity in the basal ganglia (Pacchetti et al., 2002; Shyambabu et al., 2008).

Acidosis

There are a few reports linking acidosis and chorea. In one case report, a 5-year-old girl with refractory epilepsy developed focal dystonia, then generalized chorea, 3 weeks after starting the ketogenic diet. Brain MRI showed hyperintense T2/FLAIR signal in bilateral putamina; MR spectroscopy showed a lactate peak in the putamen (Erickson et al., 2003). After stopping the diet, the MRI findings resolved and she improved clinically.

ENDOCRINE

Thyroid Disease

Hyperthyroidism is a rare metabolic cause of chorea. The movements are usually generalized but can be focal or intermittent (Drake, 1987) (Table 15–2). Chorea can result from hyperthyroidism due to an endogenous source, such as a goiter, or an exogenous source, as in thyroid-replacement therapy (Drake, 1987; Isaacs et al., 2005). When chorea occurs with Hashimoto's thyroiditis, it is often in the setting of Hashimoto's encephalopathy (Taurin et al., 2002). Imaging studies are normal (Baba et al., 1992).

Treatment of hyperthyroidism leads to improvement in chorea (Marks et al., 1979). The abnormal movements usually resolve within 2 weeks of normalization of thyroid levels, although they may occasionally persist for weeks (Isaacs et al., 2005). Rarely, chorea can be persistent (Javaid et al., 1988). Just as tremor from hyperthyroidism improves with beta-blockers, propranolol has been reported to be effective symptomatic treatment for hyperthyroid-induced chorea (Hayashi et al., 2003).

Chorea in hyperthyroidism is thought to result from enhanced catecholamine activity in the striatum (Hayashi et al., 2003) as hyperthyroidism can increase dopamine receptor sensitivity (Klawans and Shenker, 1972; Ristić et al., 2004).

Chorea Gravidarum and Reproductive Hormone–Related Chorea

Both estrogen and progesterone can influence the development of a variety of movement disorders. Chorea has been associated with the use of oral contraceptives as well as pregnancy.

Clinical

Oral contraceptive–induced chorea is rare, with reports of fewer than 100 cases in the literature. Chorea develops subacutely, several months after initiation of estrogen-containing oral contraceptives, and is often unilateral. The movements resolve after stopping estrogen (Kompoliti, 1999). Many patients have a prior history of Sydenham's chorea or other autoimmune disease, such as systemic lupus erythematosus or antiphospholipid antibody syndrome; but some patients have no such history. There is one report of exacerbation of chorea by a progesterone-containing contraceptive pill in a patient with chorea-acanthocytosis, but this has not been reported in other neurodegenerative choreas (Munhoz et al., 2009).

"*Chorea gravidarum*" refers to chorea which begins during pregnancy. The abnormal movements usually begin in the first or second trimester, improve during pregnancy, and remit after delivery. Most affected patients have a history of Sydenham's chorea (Cardoso, 2002).

Imaging/Pathophysiology

The exact mechanism of estrogen-induced chorea is not fully elucidated but likely involves a combination of a focal lesion from autoimmune disease and enhanced striatal dopaminergic tone by the estrogen and/or progesterone.

Vela et al. (2004) used PET to study the pathophysiology of oral contraceptive–induced chorea in a 27-year-old woman with hemichorea who had no history of autoimmune disease or prior chorea. Huntington's disease and other neurodegenerative causes of chorea show decreased metabolism, while autoimmune causes show increased metabolism. This patient had hypermetabolism of the contralateral caudate nucleus (Vela et al., 2004), which provides indirect evidence of an autoimmune-mediated etiology. Further evidence for autoimmunity comes from the report of anti-basal ganglia antibodies in a patient with oral contraceptive–induced chorea and no prior history of rheumatic fever or other autoimmune disease (Miranda et al., 2004).

Estrogen and/or progesterone exert a complex modulatory effect on the dopaminergic system, and both pro- and antidopaminergic effects have been proposed, with a plethora of different mechanisms of action (Van Hartesveldt and Joyce, 1986). Prodopaminergic effects of estrogen are mediated through an increase in tyrosine hydroxylase activity as well as by increased dopamine release in the striatum (Kompoliti, 1999) and likely contribute to the pathophysiology of oral contraceptive–induced chorea and *chorea gravidarum* (Caviness and Muenter, 1991).

CONCLUSION

Chorea may occur in the setting of several metabolic disturbances including electrolyte abnormalities (sodium, glucose, calcium), systemic disorders (renal failure), and hormonal changes (hyperthyroidism, pregnancy). These metabolic changes can cause focal, generalized, or paroxysmal chorea and are often associated with typical neuroimaging characteristics. Since chorea usually improves with treatment of the underlying metabolic disturbance, metabolic etiologies should be considered in the differential diagnosis of sporadic chorea.

REFERENCES

Ahlskog JE, Nishino H, Evidente VG, Tulloch JW, Forbes GS, Caviness JN, Gwinn-Hardy KA (2001) Persistent chorea triggered by hyperglycemic crisis in diabetics. Mov Disord 16:890–898.

Baba M, Terada A, Hishida R, Matsunaga M, Kawabe Y, Takebe K (1992) Persistent hemichorea associated with thyrotoxicosis. Intern Med 31:1144–1146.

Cardoso F (2002) *Chorea gravidarum*. Arch Neurol 59:868–870.

Caviness JN, Muenter MD (1991) An unusual cause of recurrent chorea. Mov Disord 6(4):355–357.

Chang CV, Felicio AC, Godeiro Cde O Jr, Matsubara LS, Duarte DR, Ferraz HB, Okoshi MP (2007) Chorea-ballism as a manifestation of decompensated type 2 diabetes mellitus. Am J Med Sci 333:175–177.

Chu K, Kang DW, Kim DE, Park SH, Roh JK (2002) Diffusion-weighted and gradient echo magnetic resonance findings of hemichorea-hemiballismus associated with diabetic hyperglycemia: a hyperviscosity syndrome? Arch Neurol 59(3):448–452.

Drake ME Jr (1987) Paroxysmal kinesigenic choreoathetosis in hyperthyroidism. Postgrad Med J 63:1089–1090.

Dure LS 4th, Mussell HG (1998) Paroxysmal dyskinesia in a patient with pseudohypoparathyroidism. Mov Disord 13:746–748.

Erer S, Yilmazlar S, Zarifoglu M, Guclu M (2008) A case report on pituitary macroadenoma presented as hemichorea hemiballism syndrome. Neurol Sci 29:289–290.

Erickson JC, Jabbari B, Difazio MP (2003) Basal ganglia injury as a complication of the ketogenic diet. Mov Disord 18:448–451.

Fernandez R, Ashraf A, Dure LS (2007) Nutritional vitamin D deficiency presenting as hemichorea. J Child Neurol 22:74–76.

Ferrara J, Jankovic J (2009) Acquired hepatocerebral degeneration. J Neurol. 256:320–332.

Hayashi R, Hashimoto T, Tako K (2003) Efficacy of propranolol in hyperthyroid-induced chorea: a case report. Mov Disord 18(9):1073–1076.

Hossain M (1970) Neurological and psychiatric manifestations in idiopathic hypoparathyroidism: response to treatment. J Neurol Neurosurg Psychiatry 33:153–156.

Hsu JL, Wang HC, Hsu WC (2004) Hyperglycemia-induced unilateral basal ganglion lesions with and without hemichorea. A PET study. J Neurol 251:1486–1490.

Isaacs JD, Rakshi J, Baker R, Brooks DJ, Warrens AN (2005) Chorea associated with thyroxine replacement therapy. Mov Disord 20:1656–1657.

Javaid A, Hilton DD (1988) Persistent chorea as a manifestation of thyrotoxicosis. Postgrad Med J. 64: 789–790.

Jog MS, Lang AE. (1995) Chronic acquired hepatocerebral degeneration: case reports and new insights. Mov Disord. 10: 714–722.

Jung S, Hwang S, Kang S, Kwon S (2009) Bilateral choreiform movements induced by excessive sucrose ingestion. Mov Disord 24:1247–1249.

Kandiah N, Tan K, Lim CC, Venketasubramanian N (2009) Hyperglycemic choreoathetosis: role of the putamen in pathogenesis. Mov Disord 24:915–919.

Kato H, Kobayashi K, Kohari S, Okita N, Iijima K (1987) Paroxysmal kinesigenic choreoathetosis and paroxysmal dystonic choreoathetosis in a patient with familial idiopathic hypoparathyroidism. Tohoku J Exp Med 151:233–239.

Kim TK, Seo SI, Kim JH, Lee NJ, Seol HY (2006) Diffusion-weighted magnetic resonance imaging in the syndrome of acute bilateral basal ganglia lesions in diabetic uremia. Mov Disord 21:1267–1270.

Klawans HL, Shenker DM (1972) Observations on the dopaminergic nature of hyperthyroid chorea. J Neural Transm 33:73–81.

Kompoliti K (1999) Estrogen and movement disorders. Clin Neuropharmacol 22:318–326.

Lai PH, Chen PC, Chang MH, Pan HB, Yang CF, Wu MT, Li JY, Chen C, Liang HL, Chen WL (2001) *In vivo* proton MR spectroscopy of chorea-ballismus in diabetes mellitus. Neuroradiology 43:525–531.

Lai PH, Tien RD, Chang MH, Teng MM, Yang CF, Pan HB, Chen C, Lirng JF, Kong KW (1996) Chorea-ballismus with nonketotic hyperglycemia in primary diabetes mellitus. AJNR Am J Neuroradiol 17:1057–1064.

Lai SL, Tseng YL, Hsu MC, Chen SS (2004) Magnetic resonance imaging and single-photon emission computed tomography changes in hypoglycemia-induced chorea. Mov Disord 19:475–478.

Lee EJ, Park JH, Ihn Y, Kim YJ, Lee SK, Park CS (2007) Acute bilateral basal ganglia lesions in diabetic uraemia: diffusion-weighted MRI. Neuroradiology 49:1009–1013.

Mahmud FH, Linglart A, Bastepe M, Jüppner H, Lteif AN (2005) Molecular diagnosis of pseudohypoparathyroidism type Ib in a family with presumed paroxysmal dyskinesia. Pediatrics 115:e242–e244.

Marks P, Anderson J, Vincent R (1979) Choreo-athetosis with severe thyrotoxicosis. Postgrad Med J 55:830–831.

Miranda M, Cardoso F, Giovannoni G, Church A (2004) Oral contraceptive induced chorea: another condition associated with anti-basal ganglia antibodies. J Neurol Neurosurg Psychiatry 75:327–328.

Munhoz RP, Kowacs PA, Soria MG, Raskin S, Teive HA, Ducci RD (2009) Catamenial and oral contraceptive–induced exacerbation of chorea in chorea-acanthocytosis: case report. Mov Disord 24:S69.

Nath J, Jambhekar K, Rao C, Armitano E (2006) Radiological and pathological changes in hemiballism-hemichorea with striatal hyperintensity. J Magn Reson Imaging 23:564–568.

Nguyen BD (2007) Brain and upper extremity PET/CT findings of hyperglycemia-induced hemiballism-hemichorea. Clin Nucl Med 32:643–645.

Oh SH, Lee KY, Im JH, Lee MS (2002) Chorea associated with non-ketotic hyperglycemia and hyperintensity basal ganglia lesion on T1-weighted brain MRI study: a meta-analysis of 53 cases including four present cases. J Neurol Sci 200:57–62.

Ohara S, Nakagawa S, Tabata K, Hashimoto T (2001) Hemiballism with hyperglycemia and striatal T1-MRI hyperintensity: an autopsy report. Mov Disord 16:521–525.

Pacchetti C, Cristina S, Nappi G (2002) Reversible chorea and focal dystonia in vitamin B_{12} deficiency. N Engl J Med 347:295.

Park JH, Kim HJ, Kim SM (2007) Acute chorea with bilateral basal ganglia lesions in diabetic uremia. Can J Neurol Sci 34:248–250.

Piccolo I, Defanti CA, Soliveri P, Volontè MA, Cislaghi G, Girotti F (2003) Cause and course in a series of patients with sporadic chorea. J Neurol 250:429–435.

Ristić AJ, Svetel M, Dragasević N, Zarković M, Koprivsek K, Kostić VS (2004) Bilateral chorea-ballism associated with hyperthyroidism. Mov Disord 19:982–983.

Shan DE, Ho DM, Chang C, Pan HC, Teng MM (1998) Hemichorea-hemiballism: an explanation for MR signal changes. AJNR Am J Neuroradiol 19:863–870.

Shaw C, Haas L, Miller D, Delahunt J (1996) A case report of paroxysmal dystonic choreoathetosis due to hypoglycaemia induced by an insulinoma. J Neurol Neurosurg Psychiatry 61:194–195.

Shyambabu C, Sinha S, Taly AB, Vijayan J, Kovoor JM (2008) Serum vitamin B$_{12}$ deficiency and hyperhomocystinemia: a reversible cause of acute chorea, cerebellar ataxia in an adult with cerebral ischemia. J Neurol Sci 273:152–154.

Sparacio RR, Anziska B, Schutta HS (1976) Hypernatremia and chorea. A report of two cases. Neurology 26:46–50.

Stracciari A, Guarino M, Pazzaglia P, Marchesini G, Pisi P (2001) Acquired hepatocerebral degeneration: full recovery after liver transplantation. J Neurol Neurosurg Psychiatry. 70:136–137.

Taurin G, Golfier V, Pinel JF, et al. (2002) Choreic syndrome due to Hashimoto's encephalopathy. Mov Disord 17(5):1091–1092.

Tison FX, Ferrer X, Julien J (1991) Delayed onset movement disorders as a complication of central pontine myelinolysis. Mov Disord 6:171–173.

Topakian R, Stieglbauer K, Rotaru J, Haring HP, Aichner FT, Pichler R (2006) Hypocalcemic choreoathetosis and tetany after bisphosphonate treatment. Mov Disord 21:2026–2027.

Van Hartesveldt C, Joyce JN (1986) Effects of estrogen on the basal ganglia. Neurosci Biobehav Rev 10:1–14.

Vela L, Sfakianakis GN, Heros D, Koller W, Singer C (2004) Chorea and contraceptives: case report with pet study and review of the literature. Mov Disord 19:349–352.

Volonté MA, Perani D, Lanzi R, Poggi A, Anchisi D, Balini A, Comi G, Fazio F (2001) Regression of ventral striatum hypometabolism after calcium/calcitriol therapy in paroxysmal kinesigenic choreoathetosis due to idiopathic primary hypoparathyroidism. J Neurol Neurosurg Psychiatry 71:691–695.

Wang HC, Cheng SJ (2003) The syndrome of acute bilateral basal ganglia lesions in diabetic uremic patients. J Neurol 250:948–955.

Weber YG, Storch A, Wuttke TV, et al. (2008) GLUT1 mutations are a cause of paroxysmal exertion-induced dyskinesias and induce hemolytic anemia by a cation leak. J Clin Invest 118:2157–2168.

Wintermark M, Fischbein NJ, Mukherjee P, Yuh EL, Dillon WP (2004) Unilateral putaminal CT, MR, and diffusion abnormalities secondary to nonketotic hyperglycemia in the setting of acute neurologic symptoms mimicking stroke. AJNR Am J Neuroradiol 2004;25:975–976.

16

Structural Causes of Chorea

Nora L. Chan, MD and Winona Tse, MD

INTRODUCTION

Chorea consists of involuntary, brief, continuous, irregular movements that flow randomly from one body part to another. The spectrum ranges from small twitches to large-amplitude jerks and may affect the entire body, half of the body, or only a specific part of the body. The mechanisms causing chorea are still unknown but involve disruption of the basal ganglia and its connections. Classically, it is postulated that disruption of the indirect pathway of the basal ganglia, which normally inhibits cortical activity, results in disinhibition of the thalamocortical outflow and resultant hyperkinetic movement disorders (Chapter 2). In theory, virtually any structural lesion situated in the right location has the potential to cause chorea directly or indirectly through ischemia, alterations in blood flow, compression, and destruction of neurons. Accordingly, a wide variety of structural lesions have been associated with chorea, including ischemic and hemorrhagic strokes, vascular malformations, traumatic intracranial hemorrhages, infections, demyelinating plaques, neoplasms, and basal ganglia calcifications (Table 16–1).

VASCULAR ETIOLOGIES

Ischemic and Hemorrhagic Stroke

The most common cause of sporadic chorea is cerebrovascular disease, with an estimated incidence ranging 26%–41% of neurology department admissions for

TABLE 16–1. Structural Causes of Chorea

Cerebrovascular
  Hemorrhagic stroke
  Ischemic stroke
  Ischemia secondary to hypotension
  Moyamoya disease
  Carotid stenosis
  Subdural hematoma
  Epidural hematoma
  Vascular malformations: AVM, venous angioma, cavernous angioma

Infectious Disease
  Neurocysticercosis
  Tuberculosis
  Bacterial endocarditis
  Neurosyphilis, meningovascular syphilis

HIV-Related
  HIV-1
  Toxoplasmosis
  Cryptococcocal granuloma
  Primary CNS lymphoma
  Progressive multifocal leukoencephalopathy

Neoplastic
  Primary brain tumor
  Metastatic brain tumor
  Primary CNS lymphoma

Other Neurological and Miscellaneous Disorders
  Basal ganglia calcification
  Tuberous sclerosis
  Demyelinating disease: multiple sclerosis, central pontine and extrapontine myelinolysis
  Sarcoidosis
  Congenital brain disease: semilobar holoprosencephaly

AVM, arteriovenous malformation; CNS, central nervous system; HIV, human immunodeficiency virus.

nongenetic etiologies of chorea (Piccolo et al., 1994, 2003). However, although chorea is the most common movement disorder following stroke, it is a rare complication of acute vascular lesions and accounts for only 1% of acute stroke symptoms (Ghika-Schmid et al., 1997).

The usual presentation is an abrupt onset of hemichorea/ballismus (HCHB) which typically spares the face (Video 16–1 Poststroke Hemichorea). Most patients recover spontaneously within 2–4 weeks, but some patients may experience intermittent or continuous movements for longer periods. In the acute phase, if the movements interfere significantly with normal functioning, they respond well to a trial of neuroleptics and dopamine depletors. However, persistent, medically refractory cases may require surgical intervention, including thalamotomy or posteroventral pallidotomy (Choi et al., 2003; Jankovic and Tolosa, 2007).

Historically, lesions affecting the subthalamic nucleus (STN) have been implicated in HCHB. However, most cases of hemichorea from stroke originate from outside the STN. In fact, ischemia of various nuclei of the basal ganglia, thalamus, midbrain, and adjacent white matter involved in the afferent and efferent subthalamopallidal pathways may result in chorea; and it is often difficult to determine the corresponding anatomical lesion (Figure 16–1). Up to 76% of acute stroke patients presenting with chorea have neuroimaging that reveals numerous lacunae in the basal ganglia, thalamus, and cerebral white matter (Chung et al., 2004; Piccolo et al., 2003).

In addition to focal ischemic or hemorrhagic lesions, chorea may be associated with diffuse cerebral hypoxia and accounts for 3.9% of patients with sporadic chorea. Chorea from hypoxia may be due to selective hypoperfusion of the vascular territories of the basal ganglia and their intrinsic susceptibility from increased oxidative metabolism. Chorea may also be delayed after hypoxic injury, probably reflecting the time required for reactive events such as remyelination, inflammatory changes, aberrant synaptic reorganization, trans-synaptic neuronal degeneration, or the development of denervation by hypersensitivity to occur (Scott and Jankovic, 1996).

Moyamoya Disease and Carotid Stenosis

Moyamoya disease is an idiopathic cerebral vasculopathy characterized by steno-occlusive changes in the terminal portions of the bilateral internal carotid arteries and the formation of abnormal collateral vascular networks (Figure 16–2A). Moyamoya disease has a bimodal distribution of age of onset, with peaks in the first and fourth decades of life. Neurological manifestations usually occur as headaches, seizures, transient ischemic attacks, and ischemic or hemorrhagic strokes. However, patients may also present with chorea. An analysis of 1,500 moyamoya cases in Japan revealed that 2.6% of the initial symptoms and 3.3% of the neurological symptoms on hospital admission were due to involuntary movements (Li et al., 2007; Watanabe et al., 1990). When present, chorea is more often seen in children than adults. The etiology of chorea in moyamoya disease includes ischemic or hemorrhagic strokes involving the basal ganglia and possibly reversible ischemia or compression of the striatum and pallidum and their connections by abnormal vasculature. Support for this theory comes from case reports in which

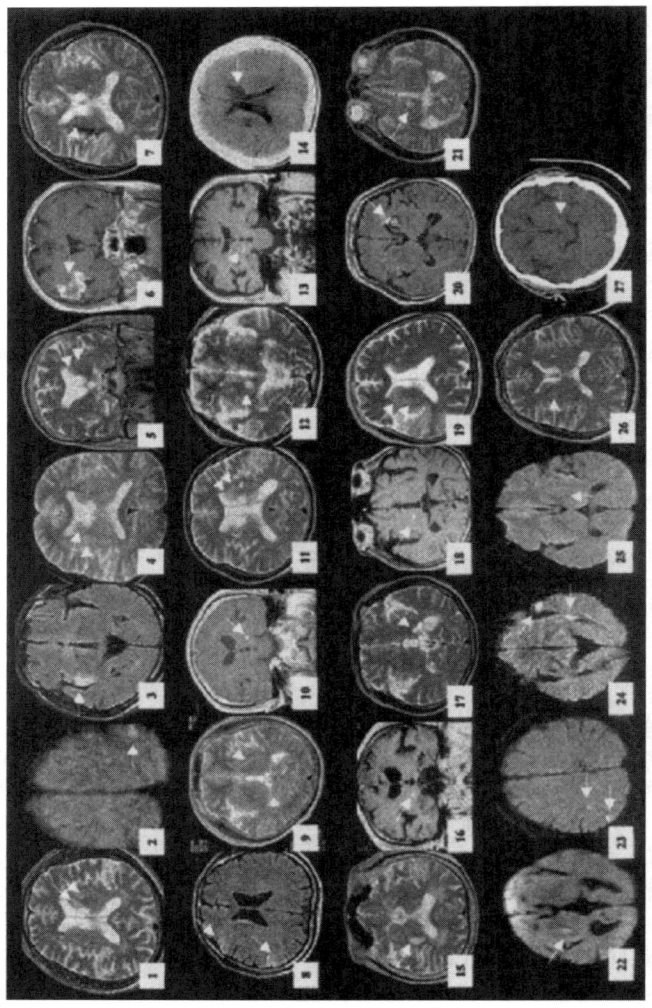

FIGURE 16–1. Ischemic stroke. T2-weighted magnetic resonance image (MRI; patients 1, 4, 5, 7, 9, 11, 12, 15, 17, 19, 21, and 26), gadolinium-enhanced T1-weighted MRI (patients 6 and 10), T1-weighted MRI without enhancement (patients 13, 16, and 18), fluid-attenuated inversion recovery MRI (patients 3, 8, and 20), diffusion MRI (patients 2, 22, 23, 24, and 25), and computed tomographic scan (patients 14 and 27) show the lesions responsible for hemichorea. Lesions are indicated by *arrows. Numbers* are patient identification numbers. From Chung et al. (2004) © Springer, 2004, with permission of Springer Science and Business Media.

patients with chorea show hypoperfusion to their basal ganglia structures. After successful cerebral bypass surgery, these patients had both improved blood flow to these regions and clinical improvement (Hong et al., 2002; Kim et al., 2006) (Figure 16–2B).

Hypoperfusion due to severe internal carotid artery stenosis independent of moyamoya disease has also been associated with chorea (Morigaki et al., 2006; Shimizu et al., 2006). A few case reports have been identified in which patients presented with transient ischemic attacks of hemiparesis and shaking limbs that gradually progressed to hemichorea. In one study, hemichorea appeared to be directly related to decreased contralateral hemispheric cerebral blood flow; single-photon emission computed tomographic (SPECT) scanning pre- and post–carotid endarterectomy demonstrated hypoperfusion of the anterior border zone affecting the frontal lobe and its associated motor and premotor cortices. After revascularization, these patients demonstrated both radiographic and clinical improvement (Kowacs et al., 2004).

Subdural and Epidural Hematoma

Subdural hematomas as a cause of chorea have been described only in case reports (Vincent, 1980; Young et al., 2008). Unilateral hematomas usually result in contralateral chorea, and bilateral hematomas may manifest in generalized movements. However, there are also reports of unilateral hematomas resulting in bilateral and ipsilateral symptoms. In most cases, evacuation of the hematoma resulted in improvement or complete resolution of symptoms. Presumably, mechanisms of pathology include ischemia to basal ganglia structures from herniation, edema, and/or alteration of neurotransmitter pathways. Interestingly, chorea may also present as a delayed complication of chronic subdural hematomas. The exact mechanism is unclear, but it has been proposed that chronic subdural hematomas, over time, may exert a cumulative pressure on the surrounding brain parenchyma, which affects initially cortical function and subsequently the function of deeper subcortical structures including the basal ganglia. Eventually, the pressure induces ischemic change in the basal ganglia and results in chorea (Sung et al., 2004). Even more rarely, chorea can be seen as an acute manifestation and late sequela of epidural hematomas (Adler and Winston, 1984).

Vascular Malformations

Cerebrovascular malformations are categorized as arteriovenous malformation (AVM), cavernous angioma, venous angioma, and capillary telangiectasia. They may cause headaches, seizures, intracranial hemorrhages, and focal neurological deficits, depending on location and size. With the exception of capillary telangiectasia, vascular malformations have also been rarely associated with a variety of

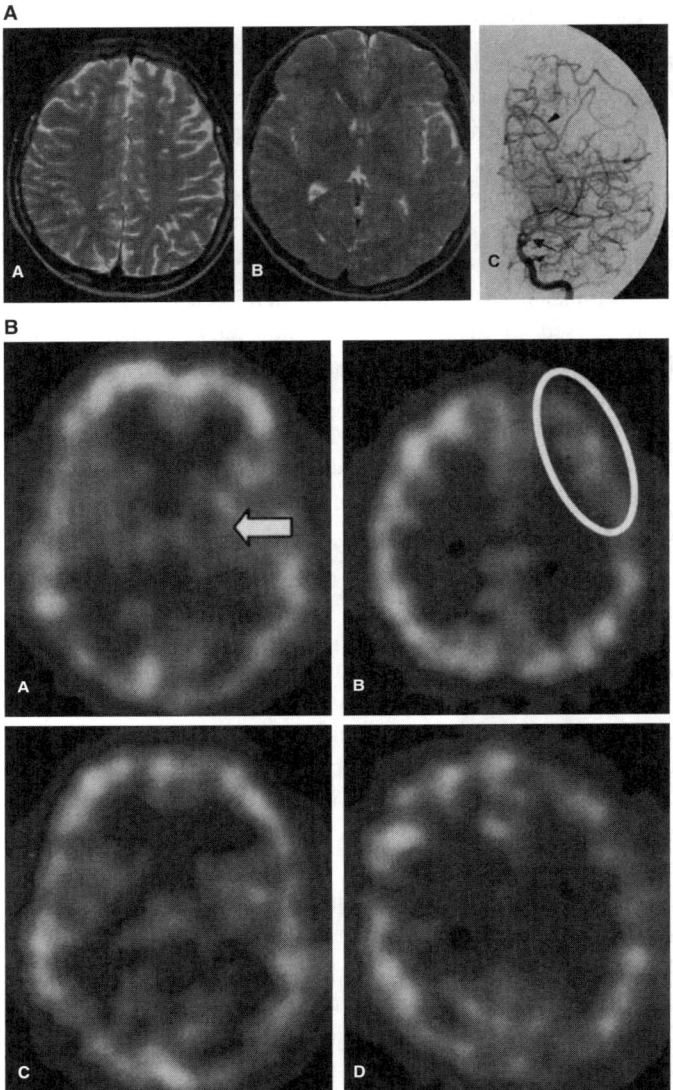

FIGURE 16–2. Moyamoya disease. **A** T2-weighted magnetic resonance image showing multiple, small, high signal–intensity lesions in the centrum semiovale in the left frontal lobe (*a*). There was no basal ganglia lesion (*b*). Left internal carotid angiogram (*c*), antero-posterior projection, demonstrating near complete occlusion of the internal carotid artery at the supraclinoid portion (*arrow*). Note the fine scanty basal collaterals suggestive of moyamoya vessels and the leptomeningeal collateral flow from the PCA (*arrowhead*). **B** [99mTc]-Hexamethylpropyleneamine oxime (HMPAO) brain basal (*a*) and post-acetazolamide (*b*) single-photon emission computed tomogram (SPECT) showing a perfusion defect in the left basal ganglia (*arrow*) and decreased vascular reserve in the left frontal lobe (*oval*) in moyamoya. Postoperative follow-up basal (*c*) and post-acetazolamide (*d*) SPECT demonstrated no significant perfusion defect in the left basal ganglia and little change of vascular reserve in the left frontal lobe. From Hong et al. (2002) © John Wiley & Sons, 2002, reprinted with permission of John Wiley & Sons, Inc.

movement disorders, including HCHB. They may exert their effect by direct compression of basal ganglia structures and their connections, alteration in the vasculature resulting in hypoperfusion, ischemia, and spontaneous hemorrhage.

The estimated incidence of AVMs is 0.14%, and they represent approximately 14%–20% of all cerebral vascular malformations. Cerebral AVMs most frequently present with spontaneous hemorrhage or seizure. The annual bleeding risk has been estimated to be 2%–3%, and hemorrhage into the basal ganglia and their connections is most often associated with the development of movement disorders. AVM-related movement disorders are rare, but there have been several reports of AVM-related chorea (Krauss et al., 1999; Tamaoka et al., 1987) due to direct hemorrhage or mass effect within the basal ganglia and connections.

The estimated incidence of cavernous angiomas ranges 0.5%–1% and accounts for 5%–13% of cerebrovascular malformations. Many cavernous angiomas are incidental findings, with approximately 10%–25% of lesions being asymptomatic. However, they may also present with hemorrhage, mass effect, and seizures. They have also been reported to cause hemichorea when located within the caudate nucleus and putamen (Donmez et al., 2004) (Figure 16–3).

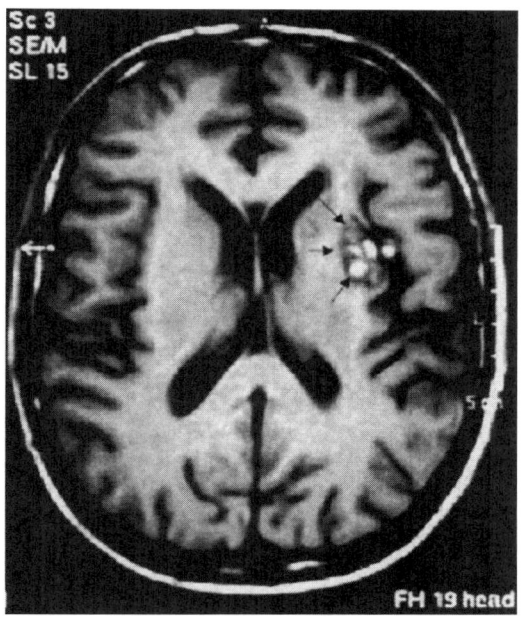

FIGURE 16–3. Cavernous angioma. Transverse T1-weighted magnetic resonance image demonstrating a cavernous angioma located within the putamen (*arrows*). From Donmez et al. (2004) © John Wiley & Sons, 2004, reprinted with permission of John Wiley & Sons, Inc.

Rarely, venous angiomas in the caudate nucleus and putamen have been reported as causing hemichorea (Burke et al., 1984).

INFECTION-RELATED CAUSES

Human Immunodeficiency Virus

Although movement disorders originally accounted for only a small proportion of the neurological problems associated with human immunodeficiency virus (HIV), progression of HIV appears to increase the frequency of movement disorders. The exact frequency of HCHB is not well established, but some studies suggest it is the most commonly seen hyperkinetic movement disorder in HIV-positive patients (Cardoso, 2002; Navia et al., 1986). However, other studies have found that tremor may be more common, seen in 5% of HIV patients and up to 44% of patients with progressive HIV encephalopathy. Other clinically relevant movement disorders including parkinsonism, dystonia, tremor, myoclonus, tics, and paroxysmal dyskinesias are also identified in up to 3% of patients (Piccolo et al., 1999).

The majority of hyperkinetic movement disorders in HIV patients are due to opportunistic infections that cause destructive lesions affecting the basal ganglia and connections. Management of chorea therefore involves treatment of the underlying infections and the use of highly active antiretroviral therapy (HAART).

Toxoplasma gondii is a parasitic protozoan that commonly affects immunocompromised individuals. In HIV-positive patients, cerebral toxoplasmosis is a common etiology of chorea. In fact, it has been suggested that the presence of HCHB in an acquired immunodeficiency syndrome (AIDS) patient is pathognomonic of cerebral toxoplasmosis. The majority of patients have multiple lesions throughout the brain. However, *T. gondii* has a propensity to localize to the basal ganglia, and the most common site involved is the STN. Interestingly, pathological studies have demonstrated that although 50% of HIV patients have toxoplasmic abscesses within their basal ganglia, only 7.4% of patients with cerebral toxoplasmosis develop chorea. The reasons for this discrepancy remain unclear (Tse et al., 2004) (Figures 16–4, 16–5, and 16–6).

Chorea in HIV patients is usually focal or limited to one-half of the body. Generalized chorea is rare, as is chorea involving the face. Generalized movements may be associated with bilateral toxoplasmic lesions but may also be associated with HIV-associated dementia. Chorea usually presents acutely or subacutely. In most cases, patients already carry a diagnosis of HIV, but chorea may occasionally be the presenting symptom. Therefore, all patients with new-onset hyperkinetic movement disorders should undergo testing for HIV infection.

Less common causes of chorea in the HIV patient include lesions associated with *Treponema pallidum*, *Cryptococcus neoformans*, progressive multifocal

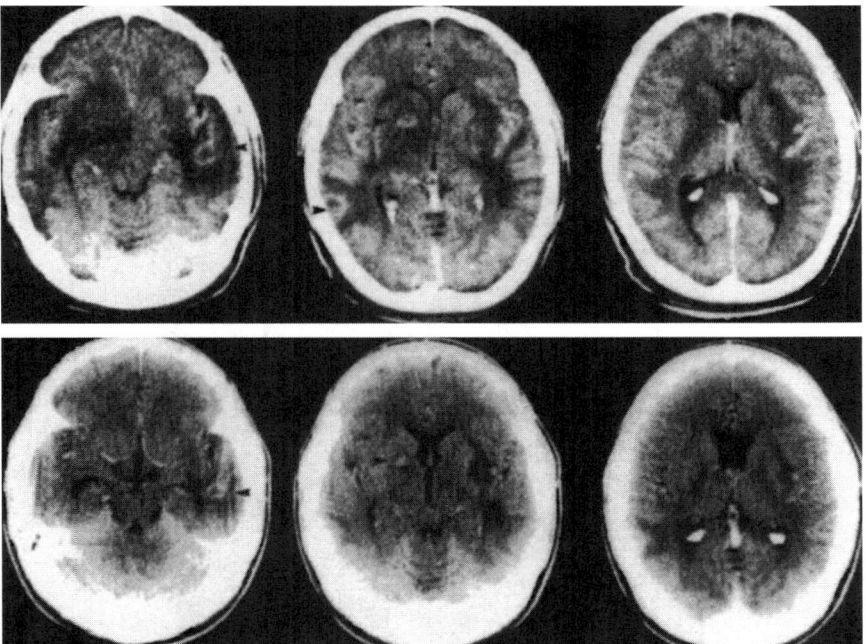

FIGURE 16–4. Toxoplasmosis. **A** Single-dose, contrast-enhanced scan at initial presentation showing ring-enhancing lesions in the right globus pallidus, right parietal, and left temporal regions with surrounding edema. **B** Double-dose, contrast-enhanced scan 10 days after antitoxoplasmosis therapy shows marked reduction in surrounding edema and partial resolution of the lesions. From Nath et al. (1993) © John Wiley and Sons, 1993, reprinted with permission of John Wiley and Sons, Inc.

encephalopathy, primary lymphoma of the central nervous system, vacuolar myelopathy, and HIV encephalopathy.

Most cases of chorea improve after treatment of the underlying infection. HAART in general may also reduce the rate of neurological complications. However, some patients may continue to have disabling movements and require additional symptomatic treatment. In these cases, dopamine receptor–blocking drugs may be helpful; but they have a tendency to produce other movement disorders, such as parkinsonism and dystonia on the contralateral side (Cardoso, 2002). This may be due to a concurrent alteration in dopamine systems by HIV infection itself and, therefore, increased susceptibility to extrapyramidal medication side effects.

Other Infectious Masses

Neurocysticercosis is one of the most common neurological parasitic infections worldwide. It is caused by infestation of the larval stage of the tapeworm

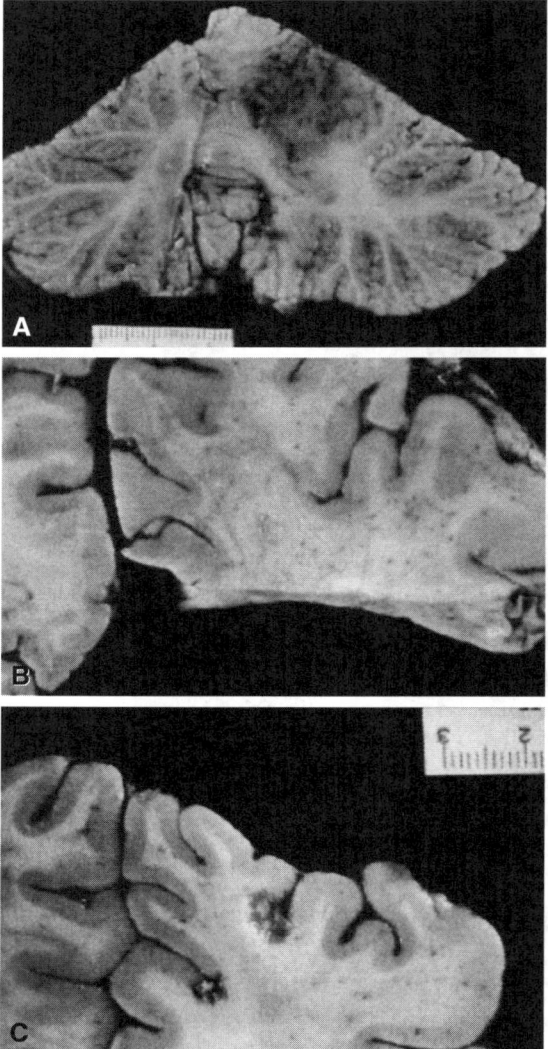

FIGURE 16–5. Toxoplasma gondii abscess. **A** Untreated, right cerebellum. **B** Organizing, left thalamus. **C** Cystic lesions in cerebral cortex, communicating with overlying subarachnoid space. From Petito (2003) © Oxford University Press, 2003, with permission of Oxford University Press, Inc.

Taenia solium, which infects the brain and meninges. The neurological manifestations vary from none to sudden death, but neurocysticercosis is a leading cause of acquired epilepsy in endemic areas. Rarely, neurocysticercosis may present with movement disorders such as parkinsonism and hemichorea, and there are only a few case reports of neurocysticercosis causing HCHB (Cosentino et al.,

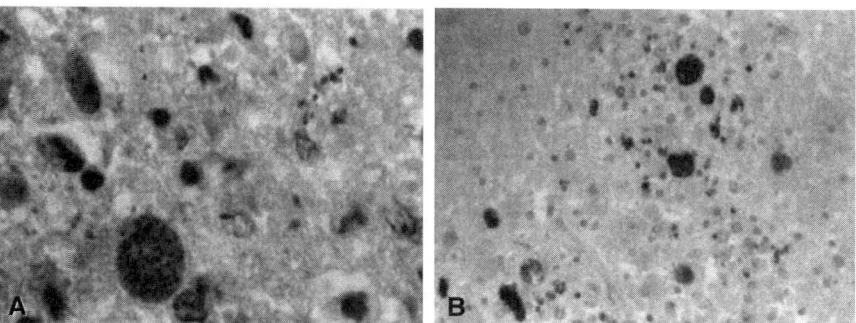

FIGURE 16–6. Toxoplasmosis. **A** Encysted bradyzoites and extracellular tachyzoites. **B** Positive immunoreactivity of cysts and tachyzoite. From Petito (2003) © Oxford University Press, 2003, with permission of Oxford University Press, Inc.

2002, 2006). The cysts localize to the basal ganglia in 25% of cases, more frequently affecting the caudate nucleus and putamen. The proposed mechanisms of pathology include direct neuronal destruction of basal ganglia structures, increased intracranial pressure and hydrocephalus, inflammation, ischemia, and vasculitis.

Central nervous system manifestations of tuberculosis occur diffusely as leptomeningeal disease and as localized tuberculoma, abscess, or cerebritis. Focal walled-off tuberculomas can occur anywhere within the brain but have a predilection for the corticomedullary junction and periventricular white matter. These may be single or multiple and present with symptoms referrable to their mass effect. Tubercular abscesses may also occur in the subarachnoid, subdural, and epidural spaces. Very rarely, tuberculomas located within the basal ganglia may present with contralateral HCHB. Treatment with antituberculosis medications results in radiographic, serological, and clinical improvement over weeks to months (Kalita et al., 2003; Ozer et al., 2006). Chorea may occur with tubercular meningitis. A case series examining 30 cases of movement disorders following tubercular meningitis revealed seven with choreiform movements. These patients tended to be younger, developed abnormal movements more rapidly in their disease course, and improved more rapidly after initiating antitubercular treatment. The etiology of chorea in these patients included contralateral basal ganglia hemorrhage or infarction, basal exudates, cortical and subcortical atrophy, and hydrocephalus (Alarcón et al., 2000).

NEOPLASTIC CAUSES

Neoplasms may cause movement disorders by a variety of mechanisms. They may act directly through tumor infiltration and alterations in the regional cerebral blood supply, resulting in ischemia or hemorrhage. In addition, they may act indirectly through paraneoplastic mechanisms (Chapter 18), metabolic derangements, and changes in coagulability, which increase the risk of acute stroke and spontaneous hemorrhage.

Tumors of the basal ganglia and thalamus are relatively rare and account for only 1%–2.5% of intracranial tumors. Most of these are benign or malignant astrocytomas. In a review of 225 patients with histologically verified astrocytomas involving the basal ganglia and thalamus, 9% of patients displayed movement disorders. Most patients present with tremor or parkinsonism, but chorea has also been documented. In these cases, chorea was a transient phenomenon which disappeared during long-term follow-up (Krauss et al., 1992).

Primary central nervous system lymphoma is a rare condition, accounting for 0.8%–1.5% of intracranial tumors. Involvement of the basal ganglia is a common radiographic and pathological finding and may be seen in up to 15.7% of cases. However, signs of extrapyramidal dysfunction are rarely reported. There are only case reports of hemichorea resulting from contralateral basal ganglia infiltration (Karempelas et al., 2008; Poewe et al., 1988; Tan et al., 2003) (Figure 16–7).

Extracranial neoplasms may also present with movement disorders. These can directly metastasize to the brain via hematogenous and nodal spread. There are rare case reports of brain metastasis from breast, lung, and hematological cancer (Hengstman et al., 2005) to basal ganglia structures presenting as HCHB.

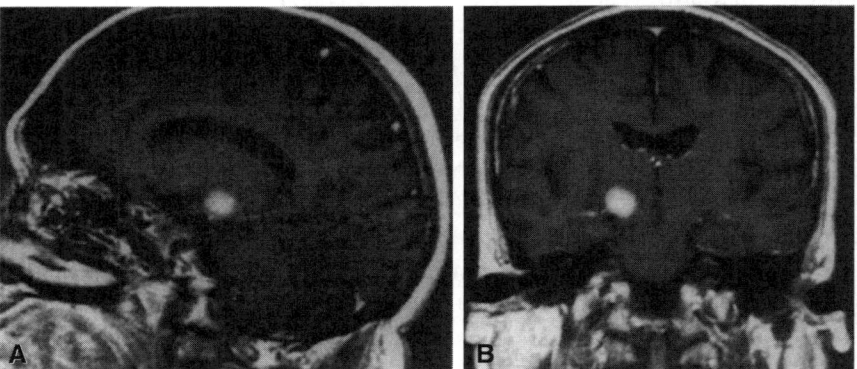

FIGURE 16–7. Central nervous system (CNS) lymphoma. Primary CNS lymphoma involving the region of the subthalamic nucleus in a patient with contralateral hemichorea/ballismus. **A** Midsagittal view on T1-weighted magnetic resoance image (MRI). **B** Coronal view on T1-weighted MRI. From Tolosa et al. (1998) © Butterworth-Heinemann, 1998, with permission of Butterworth-Heinemann.

OTHER MISCELLANEOUS

Basal Ganglia Mineralization

Basal ganglia calcifications are found in 0.6%–1.2% of normal brains and are common in patients older than 50 years. More extensive calcifications throughout the brain may rarely be seen, with a predilection for the dentate nuclei and basal ganglia structures. Although often referred to as "Fahr disease," "bilateral striato-pallidodentate calcinosis" may be a more appropriate descriptive name. In a combined data set of reported cases and those recruited through a registry, the most common clinical presentation was a movement disorder, seen in 55% of patients. Fifty-seven percent of patients displayed parkinsonian features, but 19% also had chorea. A smaller number of patients have tremor, athetosis, dystonia, and orofacial dyskinesia (Manyam et al., 2004) (Figure 16–8).

Demyelination

Movement disorders other than tremor are rare in multiple sclerosis (MS). However, HCHB can occasionally be caused by demyelinating lesions. It usually develops during the course of established MS and improves or resolves with an acute exacerbation. From a case series of six patients with MS and chorea with available neuroimaging, four were found to have demyelinating plaques in the STN; the other cases revealed no basal ganglia lesions (Tranchant et al., 1995). There are also rare case reports of movement disorders following rapid correction

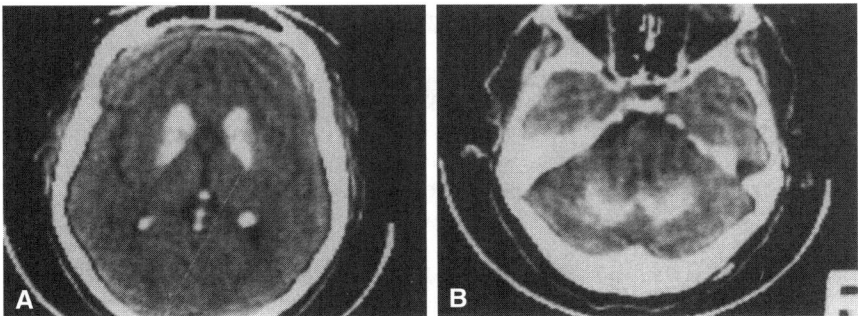

FIGURE 16–8. Bilateral striatopallidodentate calcinosis. **A, B** Noncontrast computed tomographic (CT) images of the brain. The axial CT images show extensive calcifications of the bilateral basal ganglia, bilateral thalami, and extensive calcification of the dentate nuclei and white matter of the cerebellum. From Hathout (2009) © Cambridge University Press, 2009, with permission of Cambridge University Press.

of hyponatremia resulting in central pontine and extrapontine myelinolysis. Patients have been described with parkinsonian features and choreoathetosis.

CONCLUSION

As evidenced by the present discussion, the structural etiologies of chorea are diverse and include vascular, neoplastic, inflammatory, and infectious processes. In fact, any structural lesion, if situated in an opportune location, may potentially derange basal ganglion outflow connections and lead to chorea.

REFERENCES

Adler JR, Winston KR (1984) Chorea as a manifestation of epidural hematoma. Case report. J Neurosurg 60(4):856–857.

Alarcón F, Dueñas G, Cevallos N, Lees AJ (2000) Movement disorders in 30 patients with tuberculous meningitis. Mov Disord 15(3):561–569.

Burke L, Berenberg RA, Kim KS (1984) Choreoballismus: a nonhemorrhagic complication of venous angiomas. Surg Neurol 21(3):245–248.

Cardoso F (2002) HIV-related movement disorders: epidemiology, pathogenesis and management. CNS Drugs 16(10):663–668.

Choi SJ, Lee SW, Kim MC, Kwon JY, Park CK, Sung JH, Hong JT, Woo HK (2003) Posteroventral pallidotomy in medically intracatble postapoplectic monochorea: case report. Surg Neurol 59(6):486–490.

Chung SJ, Im JH, Lee MC, Kim JS (2004) Hemichorea after stroke: clinical–radiological correlation. J Neurol 251(6):725–729.

Cosentino C, Vélez M, Torres L, Garcia HH (2006) Neurocysticercosis-induced hemichorea. Mov Disord 21(2):286–287.

Cosentino C, Velez M, Torres L, Garcia HH; Cysticercosis Working Group in Perú (2002) Cysticercosis lesions in basal ganglia are common but clinically silent. Clin Neurol Neurosurg 104(1):57–60.

Donmez B, Cakmur R, Uysal U, Men S (2004) Putaminal cavernous angioma presenting with hemichorea. Mov Disord 19(11):1379–1380.

Ghika-Schmid F, Ghika J, Regli F, Bogousslavsky J (1997) Hyperkinetic movement disorders during and after acute stroke: the Lausanne Stroke Registry. J Neurol Sci 146(2):109–116. Erratum in: J Neurol Sci 1997;152(2):234–235.

Hathout GM (2009) Clinical Neuroradiology: A Case-Based Approach. Cambridge University Press, Cambridge.

Hengstman GJ, van Rossum MM, van der Kerkhof PC, Bloem BR (2005) Chorea due to mycosis fungoides metastasis. J Neurooncol 73(1):87–88.

Hong YH, Ahn TB, Oh CW, Jeon BS (2002) Hemichorea as an initial manifestation of moyamoya disease: reversible striatal hypoperfusion demonstrated on single photon emission computed tomography. Mov Disord 17(6):1380–1383.

Jankovic J, Tolosa E (eds.) (2007) Parkinson's Disease and Movement Disorders, 5th ed. Lippincott Williams & Wilkins, Philadelphia.

Kalita J, Ranjan P, Misra UK, Das BK (2003) Hemichorea: a rare presentation of tuberculoma. J Neurol Sci 208(1–2):109–111.

Karampelas I, Podgorsak MB, Plunkett RJ, Fenstermaker RA (2008) Subthalamic nucleus metastasis causing hemichorea-hemiballism treated by gamma knife stereotactic radiosurgery. Acta Neurochir (Wien) 150(4):395–396, discussion 397.

Kim YO, Kim TS, Woo YJ, Kim CJ, Oh CK (2006) Moyamoya disease–induced hemichorea corrected by indirect bypass surgery. Pediatr Int 48(5):504–506.

Kowacs PA, Troiano AR, Mendon YF, Ma HI, Hsu YD (2004) Carotid transient ischemic attacks presenting as limb-shaking syndrome: report of two cases. Eur Neurol 51(4): 227–230.

Krauss JK, Kiriyanthan GD, Borremans JJ (1999) Cerebral arteriovenous malformations and movement disorders. Clin Neurol Neurosurg 101(2):92–99.

Krauss JK, Nobbe F, Wakhloo AK, Mohadjer M, Vach W, Mundinger F (1992) Movement disorders in astrocytomas of the basal ganglia and the thalamus. J Neurol Neurosurg Psychiatry 55(12):1162–1167.

Li JY, Lai PH, Peng NJ (2007) Moyamoya disease presenting with hemichoreoathetosis and hemidystonia. Mov Disord 22(13):1983–1984.

Manyam BV, Walters AS, Narla KR (2001) Bilateral striopallidodentate calcinosis: clinical characteristics of patients seen in a registry. Mov Disord 16(2):258–264.

Morigaki R, Uno M, Suzue A, Nagahiro S (2006) Hemichorea due to hemodynamic ischemia associated with extracranial carotid artery stenosis. Report of two cases. J Neurosurg 105(1):142–147.

Nath A, Hobson DE, Russell A (1993) Movement disorders with cerebral toxoplasmosis and AIDS. Mov Disord 8(1):107–112.

Navia BA, Petito CK, Gold JW, Cho ES, Jordan BD, Price RW (1986) Cerebral toxoplasmosis complicating the acquired immune deficiency syndrome: clinical and neuropathological findings in 27 patients. Ann Neurol 19(3):224–238.

Ozer F, Meral H, Aydemir T, Ozturk O (2006) Hemiballism-hemichorea in presentation of cranial tuberculoma. Mov Disord 21(8):1293–1294.

Petito C (2003) Neuropathology of acquired immunodeficiency syndrome. In: Nelson J, Mena H, Parisi JE, Schochet SS (eds.) Principles and Practice of Neuropathology, 2nd ed. Oxford University Press, Oxford.

Piccolo I, Causarano R, Sterzi R, Sberna M, Oreste PL, Moioli C, Caggese L, Girotti F (1999) Chorea in patients with AIDS. Acta Neurol Scand 100(5):332–336.

Piccolo I, Defanti CA, Soliveri P, Volontè MA, Cislaghi G, Girotti F (2003) Cause and course in a series of patients with sporadic chorea. J Neurol 250(4):429–435.

Piccolo I, Sterzi R, Thiella G, Minazzi MS, Caraceni T (1994) Sporadic choreas: analysis of a general hospital series. Eur Neurol 41(3):142–149.

Poewe WH, Kleedorfer B, Willeit J, Gerstenbrand F (1988) Primary CNS lymphoma presenting as a choreic movement disorder followed by segmental dystonia. Mov Disord 3(4):320–325.

Scott BL, Jankovic J (1996) Delayed-onset progressive movement disorders after static brain lesions. Neurology 46(1):68–74.

Shimizu T, Hiroki M, Yamaoka Y, Kato S, Suda M, Ide K, Yagishita A, Hirai S (2001) Alternating paroxysmal hemiballism-hemichorea in bilateral internal carotid artery stenosis. Intern Med 40(8):808–812.

Sung YF, Ma HI, Hsu YD (2004) Generalized chorea associated with bilateral chronic subdural hematoma. Eur Neurol 51(4):227–230.

Tamaoka A, Sakuta M, Yamada H (1987) Hemichorea-hemiballism caused by arteriovenous malformations in the putamen. J Neurol 234(2):124–125.

Tan EK, Chan LL, AuchusAP, Wong MC (2003) Reversible choreoathetosis in primary cerebral lymphoma: clinicoradiologic correlation. Eur Neurol 50(1):53–54.

Tolosa E, Koller WC, Gershanik OS (eds.) (1998) Differential Diagnosis and Treatment of Movement Disorders. Butterworth-Heinemann, Boston.

Tranchant C, Bhatia KP, Marsden CD (1995) Movement disorders in multiple sclerosis. Mov Disord 10(4):418–423.

Tse W, Cersosimo MG, Gracies JM, Morgello S, Olanow CW, Koller W (2004) Movement disorders and AIDS: a review. Parkinsonism Relat Disord 10(6):323–334.

Vincent FM (1980) Chorea: a late complication of a subdural hematoma. Neurology 30(3):335–336.

Watanabe K, Negoro T, Maehara M, Takahashi I, Nomura K, Miura K (1990) Moyamoya disease presenting with chorea. Pediatr Neurol 6(1):40–42.

Young VE, Pickett G, Richardson PL, Leach P (2008) Choreathetoid movement as an unusual presentation of subdural haematoma. Acta Neurochir (Wien) 50(7):733–735.

17

Sydenham Chorea

Esther Cubo, MD, PhD

INTRODUCTION

Sydenham chorea, still referred to as "St. Vitus chorea" or "St. Vitus dance" (Krack, 1999), "rheumatic chorea," or "chorea minor," is the most frequent childhood chorea and is considered a consequence of infection with group A β hemolytic streptococcal pharyngitis (Swedo, 1994; Cardoso et al., 1997; Cardoso, 2004; Zomorrodi and Wald, 2006). Sydenham chorea was first described as postinfectious choreic movements of children in 1686, but the causal relationship of this form of chorea with streptococcal infection was firmly established only in 1956 (Taranta and Stollerman, 1956). Sydenham chorea is considered an important health problem in developing countries because of its resurgence in the United States and Australia in the 1990s, and the recent hypothesis that streptococcus-induced antibodies targeted at basal ganglia neurons might account for tics and behavioral abnormalities among children (Ryan et al., 2000; Cardoso, 2002a; Cardoso et al., 2002, 2006).

EPIDEMIOLOGY

Sydenham chorea occurs in about 26% of patients with rheumatic fever (Cardoso et al., 1997) and has remained a significant public health problem in developing areas, particularly within the low-income population. However, despite the lack of community-based studies, a gradual decline in the incidence of Sydenham chorea has been observed. In this regard, the incidence of rheumatic fever and Sydenham chorea in the United States and western Europe has declined since World War II as the result of improved health care, increased antibiotic usage, and lower virulence of streptococcal strains (Quinn, 1989). This fall is demonstrated by the finding that the annual age-adjusted incidence rate of initial attacks of rheumatic fever per 100,000 children declined from 3.0 in 1970 to 0.5 in 1980 in Fairfax County, Virginia, United States (Schwartz et al., 1983). Despite this fall in incidence, Sydenham chorea remains the most common cause of acute chorea in children. Outbreaks of rheumatic fever with occurrence of chorea have been identified in the United States and Australia (Ayoub, 1992; Ryan et al., 2000). The importance of Sydenham chorea even in developed areas is shown by a recent study performed in the pediatrics unit of a university hospital in Pennsylvania, in which it accounted for 96% of all patients with chorea seen from 1980 to 2004 (Zomorrodi and Wald, 2006).

CLINICAL FEATURES

Sydenham chorea is the most common movement disorder associated with bacterial infection. The usual age at onset of chorea is 8–9 years; but there are reports on patients who developed chorea during the third decade of life, and variable manifestations may occur among people of differing ethnic backgrounds (Carapetis and Currie, 1999). In most series there is a female preponderance (Cardoso et al., 1997). Typically, patients develop chorea 4–8 weeks after an episode of group A β hemolytic streptococcal pharyngitis. In some patients, unlike arthritis and carditis, which occur soon after streptococcal infection, chorea and various neurobehavioral symptoms may be delayed for 6 months or longer and may be the sole manifestation of rheumatic fever (Stollerman, 1997). Sydenham chorea is characterized by a random and continuous flow of contractions, spreads rapidly, and becomes generalized with bilateral involvement (Video 17–1 Sydenham Chorea), but 20% of patients manifest only hemichorea (Nausieda et al., 1980; Cardoso et al., 1997). The contractions seen in this particular form of chorea are slightly longer compared to those seen in patients with Huntington disease (Hallett and Kaufman, 1981). Patients display motor impersistence, particularly noticeable during tongue protrusion and ocular fixation. The muscle tone is usually decreased, and in severe, rare cases this is so pronounced that the patient may become bedridden (*chorea paralytica*).

Patients often display other neurological and nonneurological symptoms and signs. There are reports of the common occurrence of tics, especially vocal, in Sydenham chorea (Mercadante et al., 1997), along with dystonia of the pharynx and larynx. However, in contrast to true tics, patients with Sydenham chorea lack the subjective feeling (premonitory urge or sensory tic) so characteristic of idiopathic tic disorders such as Tourette syndrome. These findings suggest that involuntary sounds present in a few patients with Sydenham chorea result from choreic contractions of the upper respiratory tract muscles rather than true tics (Teixeira et al., 2009). Dysarthria is also common. There is evidence that many patients with active chorea have hypometric saccades, and a few patients show oculogyric crises. Other reported features include decreased verbal output, papilledema, central retinal occlusion, migraine, and seizures.

Sydenham chorea is usually a monophasic, self-limited illness, which tends to resolve spontaneously in 3–4 months, although persistence and recurrence (in 20%) have been reported during a 3-year follow-up (Cardoso et al., 1999). In approximately 20% of patients, chorea is the sole finding (Cardoso et al., 1997). Female gender and carditis may be risk factors for persistent disease. It is important to note that survivors of Sydenham chorea may be at increased risk of developing chorea associated with pregnancy, oral contraceptives, or other drugs (Miranda et al., 2004; Cardoso, 2002a). However, recurrences of chorea are not associated with anti-basal ganglia antibodies (Harrison et al., 2004).

The most worrisome problem in patients with Sydenham chorea is the occurrence of valvulopathy and other cardiac problems. In approximately 80% of cases, Sydenham chorea is associated with carditis, particularly mitral valve dysfunction. A prospective follow-up of patients with Sydenham chorea with and without cardiac involvement during the first episode of chorea suggests that the heart remains spared in those without a lesion at the onset of the rheumatic fever (Panamonta et al., 2007). Arthritis seems to be less common, occurring in approximately 30% of patients.

Behavioral problems associated with Sydenham chorea include irritability, emotional lability, obsessive–compulsive disorder, hyperactivity, learning disorders, and others, similar to those seen in patients with Tourette syndrome (Swedo et al., 1988; Mercadante et al., 2000; Maia et al., 2005). The neurobehavioral manifestations typically occur within 2–4 weeks after the onset of the choreic movements. These behavioral problems are consistent with dysfunction of the dorsolateral prefrontal–basal ganglia circuit, causing a dysexecutive syndrome (Cardoso, 2005). Obsessive–compulsive disorder seems to be most frequent in the group of patients with chorea related to Sydenham chorea compared to the group of patients with rheumatic fever (Swedo et al., 1988; Asbahr et al., 1998; Mercadante et al., 2000). However, the obsessive–compulsive behavior seems to display little interference in the performance of activities of daily living. In another study of 30 patients with Sydenham chorea, Asbahr and colleagues (1998) demonstrated that 70% of the subjects presented with obsessions and compulsions, whereas 16.7% of them met the criteria for obsessive–compulsive disorder. Mercadante and colleagues (2000) also tackled the issue of attention-deficit hyperactivity disorder in Sydenham chorea and found that 45% of their 22 patients met the criteria for this condition. Maia and colleagues (2005) investigated behavioral abnormalities in 50 healthy subjects, 50 patients with rheumatic fever without chorea, and 56 patients with Sydenham chorea. They found that obsessive–compulsive behavior, obsessive–compulsive disorder, and attention–deficit/hyperactivity disorder were more frequent in the Sydenham chorea group (19%, 23.2%, 30.4%) than in the healthy controls (11%, 4%, 8%) or the patients with rheumatic fever without chorea (14%, 6%, 8%) and that attention-deficit/hyperactivity disorder was significantly more common in persistent cases than in acute cases of Sydenham chorea (50% vs. 16%). There was also a trend toward more obsessive–compulsive behavior and obsessive–compulsive disorder among patients with more prolonged forms of Sydenham chorea, but the difference failed to reach statistical significance. As there is no biological marker used in the current diagnostic criteria (*Diagnostic and Statistical Manual of Mental Disorders*, fourth edition [DSM-IV]), it is not always easy to differentiate restlessness associated with chorea from the true hyperactivity of attention-deficit/hyperactivity disorder. A recent investigation comparing healthy controls to patients with rheumatic fever showed that obsessive–compulsive behavior is more commonly seen in patients with Sydenham chorea with relatives who also have obsessions and compulsions (Hounie et al., 2007). This study makes clear that there is an interplay between genetic factors and environment in the development of behavioral problems in Sydenham chorea. Also, it has been reported that, although rare, Sydenham chorea may induce psychosis during the acute phase of the illness (Teixeira et al., 2007b).

The current diagnostic criteria for the chorea seen in Sydenham chorea are a modification of the Jones criteria, where chorea with acute or subacute onset and lack of clinical and laboratory evidence of an alternative cause are mandatory findings. The diagnosis is further supported by the presence of additional major or minor manifestations of rheumatic fever (Special Writing Group, 1992; Cardoso et al., 1997, 1999). Recently, the first validated scale to rate Sydenham chorea was published. The Universidade Federal de Minas Gerais Sydenham Chorea Rating Scale was designed to provide a detailed quantitative description of the performance of activities of daily living, behavioral abnormalities, and motor function of patients with Sydenham chorea. It comprises 27 items, and each is scored from 0 (no symptoms or signs) to 4 (severe disability or findings) (Teixeira et al., 2005a).

The observation that behavioral problems are common in patients with rheumatic fever and chorea has contributed to the notion that Sydenham chorea is a model for childhood autoimmune neuropsychiatric disorders (Swedo, 1994). The existence of pediatric autoimmune neuropsychiatric disorders associated with streptococcus (PANDAS) is a controversial hypothesis. This proposes that infection with group A β hemolytic streptococci may induce tics, obsessive–compulsive behavior, and other neuropsychiatric disturbances. The following working diagnostic criteria for

PANDAS have been proposed: (1) presence of obsessive–compulsive disorder or a tic disorder, (2) prepubertal symptom onset, (3) episodic course of symptom severity, (4) association with group A β hemolytic streptococcal infections, and (5) association with neurological abnormalities.

There is also a growing list of neurological symptoms and signs related to streptococcal infection; dementia, dystonia, encephalitis lethargica-like syndrome, motor stereotypies, myoclonus, opsoclonus, parkinsonism, paroxysmal dyskinesia, restless leg syndrome, and tremor (Cardoso, 2005; Walker et al., 2005). At the present time, however, there is no conclusive evidence that anti-basal ganglia antibodies induced by streptococcus play a significant role in the pathogenesis of tic disorders (Kurlan et al., 2008; Singer et al., 2008).

DIFFERENTIAL DIAGNOSIS

Several conditions may present with clinical manifestations similar to Sydenham chorea (Cardoso, 2004) (Table 17–1). The most important differential diagnosis is of systemic lupus erythematosus (SLE), where 2% of patients develop chorea and in 22% of patients choreic movements precede the diagnosis of SLE (Chapter 18). Chorea in SLE has been associated with the presence of antiphospholipid antibodies, a heterogeneous group of antibodies that produce platelet endothelial dysfunction and promote thrombogenesis. From a clinical point of view, the majority of subjects with SLE will have other nonneurological manifestations, such as arthritis, pericarditis, and other serositis, as well as skin abnormalities. Moreover, the neurological picture of SLE tends to be more complex and may include psychosis, seizures, other movement disorders, and even mental status and consciousness level changes. Only in rare instances will chorea, with a tendency for spontaneous remissions and recurrences, be an isolated manifestation of SLE. The difficulty in distinguishing these two conditions is increased by the finding that up to 20% of patients with Sydenham chorea display recurrence of the movement disorder. Eventually, most patients with SLE will develop other features, meeting the diagnostic criteria for this condition (Bakdash et al., 1999). Anticardiolipin antibodies, frequently found in SLE, are absent in patients with Sydenham chorea. Primary antiphospholipid antibody syndrome is also differentiated from Sydenham chorea by the absence of other clinical and laboratory features of rheumatic fever as well as the usual association with repeated abortions, venous thrombosis, other vascular events, and the presence of typical laboratory abnormalities.

A variety of infections that affect the central nervous system have been associated with chorea. Acute manifestations of bacterial meningitis, encephalitis, tuberculous meningitis, and aseptic meningitis include movement disorders, such as chorea, athetosis, dystonia, and hemiballismus (Alarcon et al., 2000). Encephalitis, as a result of either direct viral invasion or an immune-mediated postinfectious

TABLE 17–1. Differential Diagnosis for Infectious and Immune-Mediated Chorea

Immune-mediated chorea:

- Systemic lupus erythematosus
- Antiphospholipid antibody syndrome
- *Chorea gravidarum*
- Henoch-Schönlein purpura
- Behçet disease
- Polyarteritis nodosa
- Paraneoplastic chorea
- Multiple sclerosis
- Sarcoidosis
- Postvaccinial meningoencephalitis
- Acquired immune deficiency syndrome (AIDS)

Infections

Bacterial

- Subacute bacterial endocarditis
- Neurosyphilis
- Tuberculosis
- Scarlet fever (streptococcal erythrogenic toxin)
- Diphtheria
- Pertussis
- Typhoid fever
- Mononucleosis
- Legionnaire disease
- Lyme disease

Viral

- Measles
- Influenza
- Varicella
- Cytomegalovirus
- Human immunodeficiency virus
- Epstein-Barr virus (mononucleosis)
- Mumps
- Echovirus
- Herpes zoster

Prion

- Creutzfeldt-Jakob disease
- New variant Creutzfeldt-Jakob disease

Postinfectious

- Chickenpox
- Measles
- Mumps
- Rubella

process, can cause chorea. This usually happens in younger children, and the clinical picture is more diversified to include seizures, pyramidal signs, and impairment of psychomotor development, with laboratory abnormalities suggestive of the underlying condition.

Drug-induced choreas (dopaminergic or antidopaminergic drugs, anticonvulsants, and other drugs) are readily distinguished by a careful history demonstrating the temporal relationship between onset of the movement disorder and exposure to the agent (Chapter 14). In children, chorea may be the chief manifestation with withdrawal emergent syndrome (Jankovic, 1995). Chorea in children has also been reported as a sequela to cardiac surgery (Robinson et al., 1988), as a consequence of prolonged time on pump, deep hypothermia, and circulatory arrest (Medlock et al., 1993; Du Plessis et al., 2002) (Chapter 13). However, the incidence of this complication has declined after the modification of treatment strategies during the perioperative period.

Choreic movements associated with pregnancy (*chorea gravidarum*) (Chapter 15) and with birth control pills (Chapter 14) probably result from a common pathogenesis. *Chorea gravidarum* may be the first manifestation of SLE or may represent a variant of Sydenham chorea.

DIAGNOSTIC TESTS

Children and young adults with chorea should undergo complete neurological examination and diagnostic testing to assess the various causes of chorea because there is no specific biological marker of Sydenham chorea. The diagnostic work-up of patients suspected of having rheumatic chorea should include (1) identification of recent streptococcal infection or acute-phase reactant, (2) a search for cardiac injury associated with rheumatic fever, and (3) the ruling out of alternative causes. Due to the usual long latency between the infection and onset of chorea, diagnostic tests are much less helpful in patients with Sydenham chorea than in other forms of rheumatic fever. If positive, the following tests support the diagnosis: acute-phase reactants (erythrocyte sedimentation rate and C-reactive protein), leukocytosis, rheumatoid factor, mucoproteins, protein electrophoresis, and evidence of preceding streptococcal infection (increased antistreptolysin-O, anti-DNase-B, or other antistreptococcal antibodies; positive throat culture for group A *Streptococcus*; or recent scarlet fever). An elevated antistreptolysin O titer may be found in populations with a high prevalence of streptococcal infection. Furthermore, the antistreptolysin O titer declines if the interval between infection and rheumatic fever is greater than 2 months. Anti-DNase-B titers, however, may remain elevated up to 1 year after streptococcal pharyngitis. Cardiac evaluation (i.e., Doppler echocardiography) is mandatory because of the association of Sydenham chorea with carditis in up to 80% of patients, which is the main source of serious morbidity in Sydenham chorea. Serological studies for SLE and primary antiphospholipid antibody syndrome must be ordered to rule out these conditions. Electroencephalography may show generalized slowing acutely or after clinical recovery. Spinal fluid analysis is usually normal, but it may show a slightly increased lymphocyte count.

In general, neuroimaging will help rule out structural causes. Computed tomography (CT) of the brain invariably fails to display abnormalities. Similarly, magnetic resonance imaging (MRI) is often normal, although there are case reports of enlargement of the basal ganglia and reversible signal changes in the basal ganglia, suggestive of vasculitis. Positron emission tomography (PET) and single-photon emission CT (SPECT) may prove to be useful tools in the evaluation, revealing transient increases in striatal metabolism (Goldman et al., 1993; Weindl et al., 1993; Lee et al., 1999). Barsottini and colleagues (2002) showed that six of 10 patients with Sydenham chorea have hyperperfusion of the basal ganglia. This contrasts with other choreic disorders (such as Huntington disease) that are associated with hypometabolism. Increasing interest is now directed to autoimmune markers that may be useful for diagnosis. The test for antineuronal antibodies is not commercially available and, at present, is performed only for research purposes. Moreover, preliminary evidence suggests that these antibodies are not specific for Sydenham chorea. Similarly, the low sensitivity and specificity of the alloantigen D8/17 render it unsuitable for the diagnosis of this condition (Feldman et al., 1993).

PATHOGENESIS AND PATHOPHYSIOLOGY

Taranta and Stollerman (1956) established the causal relationship between infection with group A β hemolytic streptococci and the occurrence of Sydenham chorea. However, high antistreptolysin titers are not specific for group A streptococcal infections and can also reflect group G. In addition to elevated titers of antistreptolysin, the majority of patients have immunoglobulin G (IgG) antibodies, which react with neurons in the caudate and subthalamic nuclei (Kiessling et al., 1993; Swedo et al., 1993). Currently, the weight of evidence suggests that the pathogenesis of Sydenham chorea is related to circulating cross-reactive antibodies. It has been demonstrated that streptococcus-induced antibodies can be associated with a form of acute disseminated encephalomyelitis characterized by a high frequency of dystonia and other movement disorders as well as basal ganglia lesions on neuroimaging (Dale et al., 2001).

Based on the assumption of molecular mimicry between streptococcal and central nervous system antigens, it has been proposed that the bacterial infection in genetically predisposed subjects leads to formation of cross-reactive antibodies that disrupt basal ganglia function. Several studies have demonstrated the presence of such circulating antibodies in 50%–90% of patients with Sydenham chorea (Husby et al., 1976; Cardoso, 2002b). Antineural and antinuclear antibodies have also been found in patients with Tourette syndrome, but their relationship to prior streptococcal infection remains equivocal (Morshed et al., 2001). In this regard, a specific epitope of streptococcal M proteins that cross-reacts with basal ganglia has been identified (Bronze and Dale, 1993). In subjects with persistent Sydenham chorea (duration of disease >2 years despite best medical treatment) the positivity was about 60% (Church et al., 2002). A linear correlation has also been reported between the increase of intracellular calcium levels in PC12 cells and anti-basal ganglia antibody titers in the serum from Sydenham chorea patients, suggesting a possible pathogenic role of these antibodies (Teixeira et al., 2005b). However, it must be emphasized that the biological significance of anti-basal ganglia antibodies and their interference with normal neuronal function remain to be determined.

Although some investigations suggest that susceptibility to rheumatic chorea is linked to human leukocyte antigen (HLA) expression (Ayoub et al., 1986), other studies failed to identify any relationship between Sydenham chorea and HLA class I and II alleles (Donadi et al., 2000). One recent investigation reported an association between HLA-DRB1*07 and recurrent streptococcal pharyngitis and rheumatic heart disease (Haydardedeoglu et al., 2006).

Because of the difficulties with the molecular mimicry hypothesis in accounting for the pathogenesis of Sydenham chorea, there have been studies that address the role of immune cellular mechanisms in this condition. Some evidence suggests that Th1 (cell-mediated) mechanisms may also be involved. Investigating sera and cerebrospinal fluid (CSF) samples of patients of the Movement Disorders of the Federal University of Minas Gerais, Church and colleagues (2003) found elevations of cytokines that take part in the Th2 (antibody-mediated) response, interleukins 4 (IL-4) and 10 (IL-10), in the serum of acute Sydenham chorea in comparison to persistent Sydenham chorea. They described elevation of CSF IL-4 in 31% of acute Sydenham chorea and 50% of persistent Sydenham chorea cases. CSF IL-10 was also elevated in 31% of acute but 0% of persistent cases. Serum IL-4, IL-10, and IL-12 were elevated in acute compared to persistent Sydenham chorea. Oligoclonal bands were found in 46% of acute Sydenham chorea cases. Anti-basal ganglia antibodies of IgG1 and IgG3 subclasses were found in 93% of acute and in 50% of persistent Sydenham chorea cases. The authors concluded that Sydenham chorea is characterized by a Th2 response. In addition, elevation of IL-12 and increased concentrations of the chemokines CXCL9 and CXCL10 have been found in acute Sydenham chorea (Teixeira et al., 2004). The rheumatic B-cell alloantigen D8/17 is frequently found in patients with acute and persistent Sydenham chorea, providing further evidence that the disease is antibody-mediated (Church et al., 2002).

Some authors have suggested that streptococcal infection induces vasculitis of medium-sized vessels, leading to neuronal dysfunction. Such vascular lesions could be produced by antiphospholipid antibodies. Interestingly, although essentially all patients with Sydenham chorea are negative for antiphospholipid antibodies, one study demonstrated many immunological similarities between primary antiphospholipid antibody syndrome and Sydenham chorea (Blank et al., 2006). There is also a suggestion that cellular immune mechanisms participate in the pathogenesis of streptococcus-related movement disorders. However, most of these findings have not been replicated to date.

TREATMENT

Prompt treatment of streptococcal pharyngitis with appropriate antibiotics has lowered the incidence of Sydenham chorea. Penicillin prophylaxis is advisable in all patients for at least 10 years after rheumatic fever (Fahn and Jankovic, 2007). Although cephalosporins are equally effective, 500–1,000 mg of penicillin G four times per day or one intramuscular injection of 600,000–1.2 million U of benzathine penicillin is considered the drug of choice for pharyngitis caused by A β hemolytic streptococcal infection (Garvey and Swedo, 1997). Despite an adequate (10-day) course, the bacteriological failure rate is as high as 15%; and some patients develop rheumatic fever. Therefore, oral rifampin 20 mg/kg every 24 hours for four doses is recommended during the last 4 days of the 10-day course of penicillin therapy. Another choice is oral rifampin 20 mg/kg every 12 hours for eight doses, with one dose of intramuscular benzathine penicillin B. Another alternative is oral clindamycin 10 mg/kg daily in three doses for 10 days. Once the diagnosis of rheumatic chorea is established, the patient must receive secondary prophylaxis with penicillin or, for patients with an allergy to penicillin, sulfa drugs. This has been shown to effectively decrease the risk of neurological or cardiac problems with additional streptococcal infections (Mason et al., 1991).

With regard to prevention, the recommendation of the World Health Organization is to maintain secondary antibiotic prophylaxis up to age 21 years. In instances where the diagnosis of Sydenham chorea is made after this age, the policy is less clear; but because of the potential seriousness of cardiac lesion, it is recommended to maintain prophylaxis indefinitely (Cardoso et al., 2002). Patients with a history of Sydenham chorea should be informed of the possible reemergence of chorea during pregnancy or with use of oral contraceptives.

There are few controlled studies of symptomatic treatment of the chorea associated with Sydenham chorea (Cardoso, 2008). The first choice is usually valproic acid, with an initial dosage of 250 mg/day that is increased during a 2-week period to 250 mg three times a day. If the response is not satisfactory, dosage can be increased gradually to 1,500 mg/day. As this drug has a rather slow onset of action, it is prudent to wait 2 weeks before concluding that a regimen is ineffective. If the patient fails to respond to this medication, the next option is to prescribe neuroleptics. Neuroleptics can also be prescribed as a first-line treatment in patients who present with *chorea paralytica*. Risperidone, a relatively potent dopamine D_2 receptor blocker, is usually effective at controlling the chorea. The usual initial regimen is 1 mg twice a day. If, 2 weeks later, the chorea is still troublesome, the dosage can be increased to 2 mg twice a day. Haloperidol and pimozide are also occasionally used in the management of chorea. However, they are not as well tolerated as risperidone, and in general dopamine D_2 receptor blockers must be used with great caution in patients with Sydenham chorea. A case–control study compared the response to these drugs in patients with Sydenham chorea and Tourette syndrome. It was demonstrated that 5% of 100 patients with chorea developed parkinsonism, dystonia, or both, whereas these findings were not observed among patients with tics matched for age and neuroleptic dosage (Teixeira et al., 2003).

Carbamazepine (15 mg/kg daily) seems to be as effective as valproic acid (20–25 mg/kg daily) to induce remission of chorea (Genel et al., 2002). There are no published guidelines concerning the discontinuation of antichoreic agents. According to Cardoso (2002b), his general policy is to attempt a gradual decrease of the dosage (25% reduction every 2 weeks) after the patient remains free of chorea for at least 1 month.

Some controversy exists as to the role of immunosuppression in the management of Sydenham chorea. The use of immunosuppressive therapies for Sydenham chorea is usually reserved for patients with persistent, disabling chorea refractory or intolerant to other first-line therapies such as anticonvulsants and dopamine D_2 receptor blockers (Cardoso et al., 2003; Barash et al., 2005; Teixeira et al., 2005c). A proposed treatment protocol suggests methylprednisolone 1 g/kg daily in adults and 25 mg/kg daily in children for 5 days and subsequent treatment with 1 mg/kg of prednisone, which was shown to be well-tolerated and effective in open-label trials using validated Sydenham chorea scales (Cardoso et al., 2003; Teixeira et al., 2005c; Barash et al., 2005). Only one double-blind trial for steroids in Sydenham chorea exists, which demonstrated the safety and superiority of oral prednisone (2 mg/kg daily for 4 weeks, followed by a taper) compared to placebo for increasing the speed of remission of chorea in 39 patients; significant improvement was seen as soon as 1 week. However, the rate of recurrence and the severity of chorea at long-term follow-up were no different between the two groups (Paz et al., 2006). Evidence for the effectiveness of intravenous immunoglobulin or plasma exchange is limited, with few published reports demonstrating effectiveness and no clear advantage over corticosteroids (Garvey et al., 2005); for this reason, these treatments are not typically recommended, given the higher cost and possible complications (Jordan and Singer, 2003). Despite mentions of the effectiveness of prednisone at suppressing chorea, this drug is used only when there is associated severe carditis.

REFERENCES

Alarcon F, Duenas G, Ceballos N, et al. (2000) Movement disorders in 30 patients with tuberculous meningitis. Mov Disord 15:561–569.

Asbahr FR, Negrao AB, Gentil V, et al. (1998) Obsessive–compulsive and related symptoms in children and adolescents with rheumatic fever with and without chorea: a prospective 6-month study. Am J Psychiatry 155:1122–1124.

Ayoub EM (1992) Resurgence of rheumatic fever in the United States. The changing picture of a preventable illness. Postgrad Med 92:133–142.

Ayoub EM, Barrett DJ, Maclaren NK, Krischer JP (1986) Association of class II human histocompatibility leukocyte antigens with rheumatic fever. J Clin Invest 77:2019–2026.

Bakdash T, Goetz CG, Singer HS, Cardoso F (1999) A child with recurrent episodes of involuntary movements. Mov Disord 14:146–154.

Barash J, Margalith D, Matitiau A (2005) Corticosteroid treatment in patients with Sydenham's chorea. Pediatr Neurol 32:205–207.

Barsottini OG, Ferraz HB, Seviliano MM, Barbieri A (2002) Brain SPECT imaging in Sydenham's chorea. Braz J Med Biol Res 35:431–436.

Blank M, Krause I, Magrini L, et al. (2006) Overlapping humoral autoimmunity links rheumatic fever and the antiphospholipid syndrome. Rheumatology (Oxford) 45:833–841.

Bronze MS, Dale JB (1993) Epitopes of streptococcal M proteins that evoke antibodies that cross-react with human brain. J Immunol 151:2820–2828.

Carapetis JR, Currie BJ (1999) Rheumatic chorea in northern Australia: a clinical and epidemiological study. Arch Dis Child 80:353–358.

Cardoso F (2002a) *Chorea gravidarum*. Arch Neurol 59:868–870.

Cardoso F (2002b) Infectious and transmissible movement disorders. In: Jankovic J, Tolosa E (eds.) Parkinson's Disease and Movement Disorders, 4th ed. Williams and Wilkins, Baltimore, pp 930–940.

Cardoso F (2004) Chorea: non-genetic causes. Curr Opin Neurol 17:433–436.

Cardoso F (2005) Tourette syndrome: autoimmune mechanism. In: Fernández-Alvarez E, Arzimanoglou A, Tolosa E (eds.) Pediatric Movement Disorders. Progress in Understanding. John Libbey Eurotext, Montrouge, France, pp 23–46.

Cardoso F (2008) Sydenham's chorea. Curr Treat Options Neurol 10:230–235.

Cardoso F, Maia DP, Cunningham MC, Valenca G (2002) Corticosteroids in the treatment of Sydenham chorea. Mov Disord 17(Suppl):S113.

Cardoso F, Maia D, Cunningham MC, Valenca G (2003) Treatment of Sydenham chorea with corticosteroids. Mov Disord 18:1374–1377.

Cardoso F, Seppi K, Mair KJ, Wenning GK, Poewe W (2006) Seminar on choreas. Lancet Neurol 5:589–602.

Cardoso F, Silva CE, Mota CC (1997) Sydenham's chorea in 50 consecutive patients with rheumatic fever. Mov Disord 12:701–703.

Cardoso F, Vargas AP, Oliveira LD, Guerra AA, Amaral SV (1999) Persistent Sydenham's chorea. Mov Disord 14:805–807.

Church AJ, Cardoso F, Dale RC, et al. (2002) Anti-basal ganglia antibodies in acute and persistent Sydenham's chorea. Neurology 59:227–231.

Church AJ, Dale RC, Cardoso F, et al. (2003) CSF and serum immune parameters in Sydenham's chorea: evidence of an autoimmune syndrome? J Neuroimmunol 136:149–153.

Dale RC, Church AJ, Cardoso F, et al. (2001) Poststreptococcal acute disseminated encephalomyelitis with basal ganglia involvement and auto-reactive antibasal ganglia antibodies. Ann Neurol 50:588–595.

Donadi EA, Smith AG, Louzada-Junior P, Voltarelli JC, Nepom GT (2000) HLA class I and class II profiles of patients presenting with Sydenham's chorea. J Neurol 247: 122–128.

Du Plessis AJ, Belinger DC, Gauvreau K, et al. (2002) Neurologic outcome of choreoathetoid encephalopathy after cardiac surgery. Pediatr Neurol 27:9–17.

Fahn S, Jankovic J (2007) Chorea, ballism, athetosis: phenomenology and etiology. In: Principles and Practice of Movement Disorders, 1st ed. Churchill Livingstone, Philadelphia, pp 393–407.

Feldman BM, Zabriskie JB, Silverman ED, Laxer RM (1993) Diagnostic use of B-cell alloantigen D8/17 in rheumatic chorea. J Pediatr 123:84–86.

Garvey MA, Swedo SE (1997) Sydenham's chorea. Clinical and therapeutic update. Adv Exp Med Biol 418:115–120.

Garvey MA, Snider LA, Leitman SF, Werden R, Swedo SE (2005) Treatment of Sydenham's chorea with intravenous immunoglobulin, plasma exchange, or prednisone. J Child Neurol 20:424–429.

Genel F, Arslanoglu S, Uran N, Saylan B (2002) Sydenham's chorea: clinical findings and comparison of the efficacies of sodium valproate and carbamazepine regimens. Brain Dev 24:73–76.

Goldman S, Amrom D, Szliwowski HB, et al. (1993) Reversible striatal hypermetabolism in a case of Sydenham's chorea. Mov Disord 8:355–358.

Hallett M, Kaufman C (1981) Physiological observations in Sydenham's chorea. J Neurol Neurosurg Psychiatry 44:829–832.

Harrison NA, Church A, Nisbet A, Rudge P, Giovannoni G (2004) Late recurrences of Sydenham's chorea are not associated with anti-basal ganglia antibodies. J Neurol Neurosurg Psychiatry 75:1478–1479.

Haydardedeoglu FE, Tutkak H, Kose K, Duzgun N (2006) Genetic susceptibility to rheumatic heart disease and streptococcal pharyngitis: association with HLA-DR alleles. Tissue Antigens 68:293–296.

Hounie AG, Pauls DL, do Rosario-Campos MC, et al. (2007) Obsessive–compulsive spectrum disorders and rheumatic fever: a family study. Biol Psychiatry 61:266–272.

Husby G, Van De Rijn U, Zabriskie JB, Abdin ZH, Williams RC Jr (1976) Antibodies reacting with cytoplasm of subthalamic and caudate nuclei neurons in chorea and acute rheumatic fever. J Exp Med 144:1094–1110.

Jankovic J (1995) Tardive syndromes and other drug-induced movement disorders. Clin Neuropharmacol 18:197–214.

Kiessling LS, Marcotte AC, Culpepper L (1993) Antineuronal antibodies in movement disorders. Pediatrics 92:39–43.

Krack P. Relics of dancing mania: the dancing procession of Echternach. Neurology 1999;53:2169–2172.

Kurlan R, Johnson D, Kaplan EL; Tourette Syndrome Study Group (2008) Streptococcal infection and exacerbations of childhood tics and obsessive–compulsive symptoms: a prospective blinded cohort study. Pediatrics 121:1188–1197.

Lee PH, Nam HS, Lee KY, Lee BI, Lee JD (1999) Serial brain SPECT images in a case of Sydenham chorea. Arch Neurol 56:237–240.

Maia DP, Teixeira AL Jr, Quintao Cunningham MC, Cardoso F (2005) Obsessive compulsive behavior, hyperactivity, and attention deficit disorder in Sydenham chorea. Neurology 64:1799–1801.

Mason T, Fisher M, Kujala G (1991) Acute rheumatic fever in West Virginia: not just a disease of children. Arch Intern Med 151:133–136.

Medlock MD, Cruse RS, Winek SJ, et al. (1993) A 10-year experience with postpump chorea. Ann Neurol 34:820–826.

Mercadante MT, Busatto GF, Lombroso PJ, et al. (2000) The psychiatric symptoms of rheumatic fever. Am J Psychiatry 157:2036–2038.

Mercadante MT, Campos MC, Marques-Dias MJ, et al. (1997) Vocal tics in Sydenham's chorea. J Am Acad Child Adolesc Psychiatry 36:305–306.

Miranda M, Cardoso F, Giovannoni G, Church A (2004) Oral contraceptive induced chorea: another condition associated with anti-basal ganglia antibodies. J Neurol Neurosurg Psychiatry 75:327–328.

Morshed SA, Parveen S, Leckman JF, et al. (2001) Antibodies against neural, nuclear, cytoskeletal, and streptococcal epitopes in children and adults with Tourette's syndrome, Sydenham's chorea, and autoimmune disorders. Biol Psychiatry 50:566–577.

Nausieda PA, Grossman BJ, Koller WC, Weiner WJ, Klawans HL (1980) Sydenham's chorea: an update. Neurology 30:331–334.

Panamonta M, Chaikitpinyo A, Auvichayapat N, et al. (2007) Evolution of valve damage in Sydenham's chorea during recurrence of rheumatic fever. Int J Cardiol 119:73–79.

Paz JA, Silva CA, Marques-Dias MJ (2006) Randomized double-blind study with prednisone in Sydenham's chorea. Pediatr Neurol 34:264–269.

Quinn RW (1989) Comprehensive review of morbidity and mortality trends for rheumatic fever, streptococcal disease, and scarlet fever: the decline of rheumatic fever. Rev Infect Dis 11:928–953.

Robinson RO, Samuels M, Pohls KRE (1988) Choreic syndrome after cardiac surgery. Arch Dis Child 63:1466–1469.

Ryan M, Antony JH, Grattan-Smith PJ (2000) Sydenham chorea: a resurgence of the 1990s? J Pediatr Child Health 36:95–96.

Schwartz RH, Hepner SI, Ziai M (1983) Incidence of acute rheumatic fever. A suburban community hospital experience during the 1970s. Clin Pediatr 22:798–801.

Singer HS, Gause C, Morris C, Lopez P; Tourette Syndrome Study Group (2008) Serial immune markers do not correlate with clinical exacerbations in pediatric autoimmune neuropsychiatric disorders associated with streptococcal infections. Pediatrics 121:1198–1205.

Special Writing Group of the Committee of Rheumatic Fever, Endocarditis, and Kawasaki Disease of the Council on Cardio-Vascular Disease of the Young of the American Heart Association (1992) Guidelines for the diagnosis of rheumatic fever, Jones criteria, 1992 update. JAMA 268:2069–2073.

Stollerman GH (1997) Rheumatic fever. Lancet 349:935–942.

Swedo SE (1994) Sydenham's chorea. A model for childhood autoimmune neuropsychiatric disorders. JAMA 272:1788–1791.

Swedo SE, Leonard HL, Garvey M, et al. (1988) Pediatric autoimmune neuropsychiatric disorders associated with streptococcal infections: clinical description of the first 50 cases. Am J Psychiatry 155:264–271.

Swedo SE, Leonard HL, Shapiro MB, et al. (1993) Sydenham's chorea: physical and psychological symptoms of St. Vitus dance. Pediatrics 91:706–713.

Taranta A, Stollerman GH (1956) The relationship of Sydenham's chorea to infection with group A streptococci. Am J Med 20:1970.

Teixeira AL, Cardoso F, Maia DP, Cunningham MC (2003) Sydenham's chorea may be a risk factor for drug induced parkinsonism. J Neurol Neurosurg Psychiatry 74:1350–1351.

Teixeira AL Jr, Cardoso F, Souza AL, Teixeira MM (2004) Increased serum concentrations of monokine induced by interferon-gamma/CXCL9 and interferon-gamma-inducible protein 10/CXCL-10 in Sydenham's chorea patients. J Neuroimmunol 150:157–162.

Teixeira AL Jr, Maia DP, Cardoso F (2005a) UFMG Sydenham's Chorea Rating Scale (USCRS): reliability and consistency. Mov Disord 20(5):585–591.

Teixeira AL Jr, Guimaraes MM, Romano-Silva MA, Cardoso F (2005b) Serum from Sydenham's chorea patients modifies intracellular calcium levels in PC12 cells by a complement-independent mechanism. Mov Disord 20:843–845.

Teixeira AL Jr, Maia DP, Cardoso F (2005c) Treatment of acute Sydenham's chorea with methyl-prednisolone pulse-therapy. Parkinsonism Relat Disord 11(5):327–330.

Teixeira AL Jr, Maia DP, Cardoso F (2007b) Psychosis following acute Sydenham's chorea. Eur Child Adolesc Psychiatry 16:67–69.

Teixeira AL, Cardoso F, Maia DP, et al. (2009) Frequency and significance of vocalizations in Sydenham's chorea. Parkinsonism Relat Disord 15:62–63.

Walker KG, Lawrenson J, Wilmshurst JM (2005) Neuropsychiatric movement disorders following streptococcal infection. Dev Med Child Neurol 47:771–775.

Weindl A, Kuwert T, Leenders KL, et al. (1993) Increased striatal glucose consumption in Sydenham's chorea. Mov Disord 8:437–444.

Zomorrodi A, Wald ER (2006) Sydenham's chorea in western Pennsylvania. Pediatrics 117:675–679.

18

Paraneoplastic and Other Autoimmune Choreas

Michael H. Pourfar, MD

INTRODUCTION

Autoimmune disorders merit important consideration in the evaluation of cryptogenic chorea, particularly in the absence of a family history of chorea. A vast array of autoimmune disorders can be associated with chorea. Some entities, such as Sydenham chorea and pediatric autoimmune neuropsychiatric disorders associated with streptococcus (PANDAS), are addressed in other chapters (Chapter 17). This chapter focuses on chorea secondary to paraneoplastic and other systemic rheumatological disorders, such as systemic lupus erythematosus. Much remains to be learned about the underlying mechanisms of the autoimmune chorea. The heterogeneity and relative rarity of many of the syndromes, along with the lack of animal models for the chorea, all conspire to limit a full understanding. Why, for example, is chorea uncommon even within the context of autoantibodies associated with chorea? Why do imaging abnormalities (or lack of them) so rarely correlate with the presence or absence of chorea? Despite the many unanswered questions, the presence of chorea in the context of these seemingly disparate syndromes suggests a unifying mechanistic element. Indeed, though paraneoplastic and nonparaneoplastic autoimmune choreas are divided in the chapter, they share many commonalities. For the clinician, however, they represent two distinct parts of the differential diagnosis of chorea as they often follow very different treatment algorithms and prognoses depending on the underlying cause.

PARANEOPLASTIC CHOREA

Clinical features

Chorea is a relatively rare paraneoplastic phenomenon. When it does occur, it tends not to occur in isolation but rather as part of a constellation of neurological findings. With the exception of Lambert-Eaton myasthenic syndrome (LEMS), paraneoplastic syndromes (PNSs) are rare, affecting perhaps 0.01% of cancer patients (Darnell and Posner, 2003), and the incidence of paraneoplastic chorea (PNC) is smaller still. Nevertheless, PNC is an important differential to consider as its identification can have important prognostic and therapeutic implications. PNC can occur in the context of several PNSs. This section will review PNC in addition to giving more detailed consideration to specific antibody-associated etiologies. Clinical criteria for the diagnosis of a PNS can be found in Box 18–1.

Generalizations on PNC are somewhat limited, given both the rarity and heterogeneity of associated syndromes. Like most PNSs, PNC frequently predates the diagnosis of cancer and can be very disabling. The intensity of the chorea can range from mild and focal to florid and generalized. The chorea typically evolves over days to weeks but sometimes over months. It is seldom the first neurological symptom, and the debility from it, while sometimes profound, is often overshadowed by the overall neurological picture, which can include ataxia, psychosis, and dementia. The PNSs that have been most frequently associated with chorea include those with antibodies directed against CRMP-5/CV-2, NMDA receptor, and Hu (Table 18–1).

TABLE 18–1. Paraneoplastic Syndromes Associated with Chorea

AUTOANTIBODY	ASSOCIATED CANCER TYPES	ASSOCIATED CLINICAL FEATURES
CRMP-5/CV2	SCLC > thymoma	Ataxia, MG, LEMS, limbic encephalitis, uveoretinal symptoms
NMDA receptor	Teratoma (ovarian)	Neuropsychiatric prodrome followed by hyper- rather than hypokinetic movements
Hu	SCLC > prostate, gynecological	Limbic or brainstem encephalitis, peripheral neuropathy, dysautonomia

LEMS, Lambert-Eaton myasthenic syndrome; MG, myasthenia gravis;
NMDA, N-methyl-D-aspartate; SCLC, small cell lung cancer.

Box 18–1. Criteria for Probable Paraneoplastic Syndrome (Adapted from Honnorat and Antoine, 2007)

1. Classical neurological syndrome and a diagnosis of cancer within 5 years

OR

2. Nonclassical neurological syndrome that improves after cancer treatment without concomitant immunotherapy or likely spontaneous remission

OR

3. Nonclassical neurological syndrome observed with onconeural antibodies and development of cancer within 5 years of symptom onset

OR

4. A neurological syndrome with well-characterized onconeural antibodies even in the absence of an identified primary cancer.

Anti-NMDA Receptor Antibody Syndrome

Chorea is a prominent but often transient feature of the PNSs associated with antibodies against the glutamate *N*-methyl-D-aspartate (NMDA) receptor. Importantly, chorea may provide the diagnostic clue to what can be an otherwise nonspecific and disturbing clinical deterioration in a previously healthy young woman. The syndrome is most commonly—though not exclusively—associated with ovarian teratomas and often affects women in their 20s but can affect both genders and a wide spectrum of ages. It has been clinically divided into five phases; (1) a prodromal, viral-type illness accompanied or followed by (2) neuropsychiatric changes, then (3) a period of decreased responsiveness and hypoventilation that yields to (4) a hyperkinetic phase and usually concludes with (5) a period of recovery. The nature of the hyperkinetic movements is variable but often involves prominent orofacial chorea, athetoid posturing of the fingers along with jaw-opening dystonia, and choreic movements of the arms. Myoclonus, tremors, hemiballism, and seizures have also been reported (Video 18–1 Anti-NMDA Receptor Antibody Syndrome). The choreiform movements typically last between 2 and 12 months and tend not to respond well to immunotherapy or dopamine receptor blockers, often requiring sedation with benzodiazepines and/or propofol (Iizuka et al., 2008).

The clinical work-up typically reveals an initial mild pleocytosis in the cerebrospinal fluid (CSF) and often magnetic resonance imaging (MRI) hyperintensities on fluid attenuation inversion recovery (FLAIR) sequences. The largest clinical series, involving 100 cases, was reported by Dalmau et al. (2008). They reported an age range of 5–76 (mean 23), with women comprising 91 cases. Only 59% had an identifiable underlying tumor, with all being ovarian teratomas apart from one testicular cancer and one small cell lung cancer (SCLC). Most of the cases demonstrated a lymphocytic pleocytosis in the CSF. In addition, they typically had higher CSF concentrations of anti-NMDA receptor antibodies compared with levels in the sera, and titers tended to correlate with disease severity. Slightly over half had abnormal findings on their MRI, although these signal changes did not always correlate with exam findings. A limited number of brain biopsies revealed perivascular lymphocytic cuffing and microglial activation. Fourteen cases had no reported hyperkinetic movements on exam; thus, chorea, while very common, is not an absolute finding. Seventy-five patients recovered, although only 47 recovered fully, and there were seven related deaths. Most cases responded to removal of the tumor, though recalcitrant cases received added benefit from cyclophosphamide and/or rituximab.

Anti-CRMP-5/CV-2 Receptor Antibody Syndrome

The collapsin response mediator protein (CRMP) family consists of phosphoproteins important in brain development (Goshima et al., 1995), particularly relating to axon guidance, and may have a role in synaptic events (Yu et al., 2001). An antibody against CRMP-5 was first documented in 1996 (Honnorat et al., 1996), although an earlier case report (Albin et al., 1988) along with subsequent reports (Croteau et al., 2001) associated with crossveinless-2 (CV2) autoantibodies are likely related (CRMP-5 is the main antigen recognized by anti-CV2 antibodies and, given the overlap in the literature, will hereafter be referred to as "CRMP-5/CV-2" antibodies).

Chorea associated with the antibodies has been documented in at least 40 patients. The chorea can be a prominent component but often appears following personality changes and sometimes even as late as 1 year into the syndrome, which can include other neurological findings like ataxia, hyporeflexia, and uveoretinal, myasthenic, and limbic-related symptoms (Albin et al., 1988; Croteau et al., 2001; Kinirons et al., 2003; Muehlschlegel et al., 2005). Yu et al. (2001) reported a correlation between loss of smell and taste and onset of chorea. The antibodies have been most commonly associated with SCLC but have been reported also in the setting of malignant thymoma, prostate small cell sarcoma, and uterine sarcoma, with the cancer diagnosis often lagging a year behind the neurological presentation.

Presence of the antibody can be confirmed by checking sera with Western blotting. Some anti-CV2 antibody–related cases are also positive for other onconeural antibodies such as anti-Hu. In a case series by Honnorat et al. (2009), eight of 27 CV2 cases had chorea. Another report found chorea present in 11% of anti-CRMP-5 antibody cases (Vernino et al., 2002). The CSF may show a nonspecific pleocytosis in addition to antibodies against the immunoreactive protein. MRI findings vary and do not uniformly parallel clinical findings, but they can occasionally show caudate nucleus and globus pallidus involvement in the setting of chorea (Croteau et al., 2001; Muehlschlegel et al., 2005; Tani et al., 2000; Vernino et al., 2002). Brain biopsies have demonstrated cerebral amyloid angiopathy and scanty perivascular infiltrates of mature T lymphocytes.

Involvement of the basal ganglia—even in the presence of chorea—has been variable; some reports have described marked neuronal loss and/or perivascular infiltrates of mature CD8-reactive T lymphocytes limited to the striatum, whereas others have demonstrated little or patchy basal ganglia involvement (Albin et al., 1988; Muehlschlegel et al., 2005; Vernino et al., 2002).

In a review of 16 SCLC patients with anti-CRMP-5/CV2 antibodies and chorea (Vernino et al., 2002), 14 patients had additional neurological findings and most had mild CSF pleocytosis. A smaller subset had MRI scans demonstrating signal hyperintensities in the caudate nucleus and putamen, two of which resolved on follow-up. Serum titers did not correlate with severity, and CSF titers generally exceeded those seen in serum. Two autopsies showed basal ganglia neuronal loss, gliosis, microglial activation, perivascular lymphocytic infiltrate, and scant microglial nodules. Coexisting antineuronal antibodies, such as ANNA-1, were found in 50%. In nine of 15 patients, the chorea improved following either chemotherapy or steroids.

Other

Paraneoplastic chorea associated with other cancers and autoantibodies has been described, often as case reports. Chorea has occasionally been reported in anti-Hu syndromes, usually in the setting of ataxia and other neurological findings (Heckmann et al., 1997; Tremont-Lukats et al., 2002). In comparing the frequency of chorea between anti-CRMP5/CV-2 and anti-Hu-related PNSs, fewer cases with anti-Hu antibodies had chorea than cases with anti-CRMP5/CV-2 antibodies (Honnorat et al., 2009). Chorea has been present or prominent in rare cases associated with primary central nervous system (CNS) lymphoma (Poewe et al., 1988), (Tan et al., 2003), Hodgkin and non-Hodgkin lymphoma (Batchelor et al., 1998; Nuti et al., 2000), acute lymphocytic leukemia (ALL) (Schiff and Ortega, 1992), and renal cancer (Kujawa et al., 2001).

Some cryptogenic cases may be related to anti-CRMP-5/CV2 or anti-NMDA receptor antibodies that were not identified (Tani et al., 2000) or to a heretofore unidentified autoantibody. As indicated, the presence of one autoantibody does not exclude the presence of a second; and some rare cases of chorea attributed to an identified antibody may have truly been the result of a concomitant, unidentified anti-CRMP-5/CV-2 antibody or—in lymphomas, for example—an antiphospholipid antibody (Tincani et al., 2010). Nevertheless, given the heterogeneity of PNSs, it is equally plausible that chorea can be a rare manifestation of a PNS not normally associated with hyperkinetic movements. Such may be the case for an anti-Hu-associated chorea accompanied by ataxia and sensory neuropathy in which the MRI showed caudate nucleus atrophy (Heckmann et al., 1997) and one anti-Yo case with chorea and ataxia related to likely lung adenocarcinoma (Krolak-Salmon et al., 2006). There does not appear to be anything particularly unique in the constellation of clinical, imaging, and biopsy findings that distinguishes these cases with chorea from those with anti-CRMP-5/CV2 antibodies. One final consideration in PNC is the potential for metastatic disease to directly involve the basal ganglia or thalamus, as was described in a case of a woman presenting with bilateral hemichorea-hemiballism secondary to brain metastases from a primary lung tumor (Moore, 2009). Although antibodies could conceivably be present in such cases, imaging may obviate the need for an extensive paraneoplastic evaluation.

Treatment

The primary treatment for PNC is identification and removal of the underlying antibody-generating tumor. The presence of a PNS—although often devastating in and of itself—may indicate a better prognosis for the cancer as the antibody may function in some cases to suppress the tumor (Graus et al., 1997). Tumor removal often leads to significant clinical improvement but does not universally improve the chorea or other neurological features. In cases where tumor cannot be identified or where symptoms do not fully improve following resection, a number of treatment modalities have been tried, with mixed results. For most PNSs, immunotherapy is not typically effective. Plasma exchange, for example, does not significantly affect the CSF and, therefore, is generally not helpful. Use of intravenous immunoglobulin has proven similarly ineffective in most reported cases. Outcomes with other immunosuppressant therapies are generally anecdotal and have included variable responses to steroids, mycophenylate, cyclophosphamide, and other immunosuppressant agents. When these have proven ineffective, anesthetic agents like diazepam and propofol have been used as a temporizing treatment in refractory or disabling cases. There is, however, no set algorithm or preferred modality in treating the chorea associated with paraneoplastic disease compared to other forms of chorea, with the exception of the adjuvant use of chemotherapy in targeting the underlying cancer.

Specific Characteristics of Chorea

There are no specific characteristics of PNC that differentiate it from other causes of chorea. Indeed, PNC is characterized by variability of phenomenology and associated neurological findings. Focal, generalized, and hemichorea have all been described. The chorea is often mixed with dystonia or other neuropsychiatric findings and is often aggressive, although a benign course does not rule out a paraneoplastic etiology. Most cases emerge over days to weeks or months and are associated with significant disability. The chorea often follows an inexorable course, although in other cases—as described with anti-NMDA receptor antibody involvement—chorea is a transient phenomenon.

Diagnostic Tests: Laboratory and Neuroimaging Findings

A paraneoplastic etiology should be considered for any patient presenting with cryptogenic chorea. Since the cancer diagnosis frequently lags behind the neurological findings by several months, early suspicion and detection can have important prognostic implications. If chorea has been present for more than 2 years with no underlying tumor identified, the likelihood of the chorea being paraneoplastic is relatively small.

Imaging

The first priority is to identify the underlying neoplasm, most often with imaging such as computer tomography (CT) or MRI of the chest, abdomen, and pelvis or whole-body fluorodeoxyglucose-positron emission tomography (FDG-PET), as deemed appropriate. If these are unrevealing and a clinical suspicion remains, more directed testing may be performed, such as a transvaginal ultrasound for suspicion of an ovarian teratoma. Brain imaging results are highly variable and often normal or nonspecific. Findings can include atrophy, signal changes in the basal ganglia or diffusely, and edema. A normal brain MRI does not rule out PNS, but an abnormal MRI does not necessarily implicate a PNS or correlate with the clinical features. The presence of signal changes in the basal ganglia in the context of chorea suggests causality but is not specific to a paraneoplastic etiology. Imaging results can also vary over time, being abnormal for a period then returning to normal after several months, irrespective of the patient's chorea status. There are, however, cases where signal changes appear to improve following treatment intervention and corresponding resolution of chorea (Figure 18–1).

Laboratory Findings

Sera. Titers for specific antibodies can help establish the diagnosis. When the relevant antibodies are not identified, additional testing can assess for presence of antiphospholipid antibodies (present in some cancers and discussed further later, see "Systemic Lupus Erythematosus and Antiphospholipid Antibodies"). Eosinophilia has been noted in some PNC cases associated with ALL.

CSF. Specific antibody testing can be assessed in the CSF (specifically anti-Yo, anti-Hu, anti-CRMP-5/CV-2, anti-NMDA receptor). The absence of an identified antibody does not exclude the possibility of a PNS. Elevated white cells and immunoglobulins (Igs) are occasionally identified, sometimes with oligoclonal bands. Pleocytosis is usually apparent only early and often disappears within months, though IgG levels may stay elevated. The predominant CSF cell type is T (>75%), with small components of B cells and natural killer cells. Many patients have antibodies in serum and CSF that react with both the cancer and the CNS.

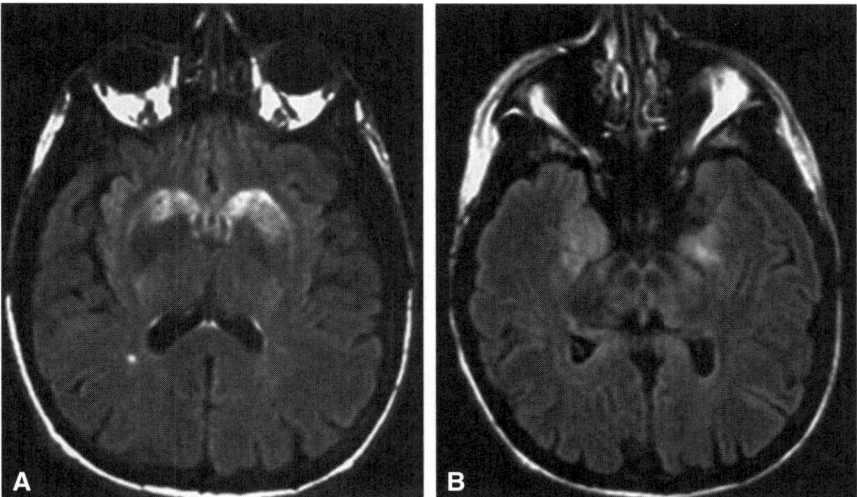

FIGURE 18–1. Magnetic resonance image (MRI) of a subject with paraneoplastic chorea associated with CRMP-5/CV-2 antibodies. Bilateral fluid attenuation inversion recovery (FLAIR) hyperintensities in the caudate and putamen (**A**) and mesial temporal lobes (**B**) 1 month after chorea onset. Chorea resolved following chemotherapy for small cell lung cancer. From Vernino et al. (2002). Reprinted with permission, © John Wiley & Sons, Inc.

Pathology

Biopsy and autopsy results have generally shown lymphocytic reactivity composed of CD-8 immunoreactive T lymphocytes compatible with T-cytotoxic/suppressor cells, while perivascular infiltrates have comprised both B and T lymphocytes (Muehlschlegel et al., 2005) (Figure 18–2). Diffuse microglial nodules, perivascular lymphocytes, neuronophagia, and atrophy have all been reported selectively or in combination. In one case of anti-CRMP-5/CV2 antibody syndrome associated with chorea, the globus pallidus showed the most severe active inflammation (Kinirons et al., 2003). Atrophy of bilateral caudate nuclei has been reported, as has severe neuronal loss and perivascular lymphocytic cuffing with proliferation of astrocytes. Involvement of the cerebellum has also been reported, with mild loss of granule cells but preserved Purkinje cells (Tani et al., 2000).

Pathophysiology (Cellular Level)

The mechanisms behind the neurological manifestations of PNSs remain speculative. Most PNSs are immune-mediated, with evidence supporting a prominent role of antibodies and cytotoxic T cells. The autoimmune hypothesis is that certain

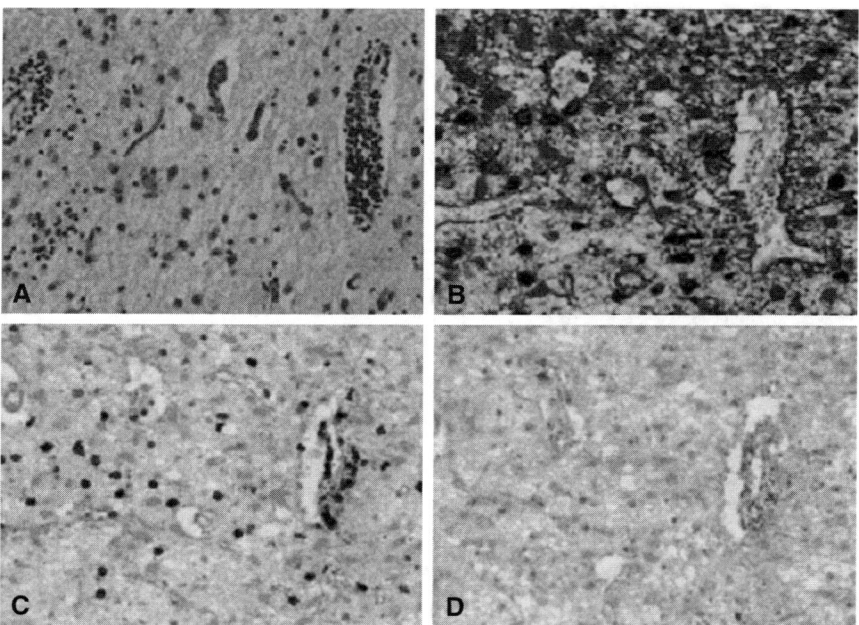

FIGURE 18–2. **A** Hematoxylin and eosin staining in a CRMP-5/CV-2 subject from the caudate nucleus showing perivascular and parenchymal infiltrates of mature lymphocytes, diffuse neuronal loss, and reactive gliosis. **B** Glial fibrillary acid protein–immunostained section showing reactive gliosis. **C** CD4 (T-helper)–immunostained section showing reactivity consistent with cytotoxic/suppressor T lymphocytes. **D** CD4-immunostained section showing rare positivity. Magnification 500×. From Muehlschlegel et al. (2005). Reprinted with permission, © John Wiley & Sons, Inc.

protein antigens are normally expressed fairly specifically in the CNS but can also be expressed in some cancers. These cancers can thus generate an immune response in which the immune system identifies the onconeural antibody as foreign, leading antibodies and cytotoxic T cells to cross the blood–brain barrier (BBB) to react with the neurons expressing these same antibodies (Darnell and Posner, 2003; Posner, 2003). Once damaged, the affected neurons reveal major histocompatibility complex (MHC) molecules, which are normally hidden, further stimulating T cells. As corroborating evidence, high titers of antibodies that react with tumor and with the CNS are found in sera, with still higher antibody titers in CSF. This provides evidence for intrathecal synthesis of antibody, presumably by specific B lymphocytes that have crossed the BBB. It is unclear, however, if these intrathecal antibodies are themselves pathogenic or whether the pathogenicity derives from the antibody reaction to the intracellular antigen (Dalmau et al., 1999). The exact role of the onconeural antibody in causing neurological symptoms remains unclear. The antibodies are likely to have some role since it has been demonstrated that autoantibodies like anti-Hu, anti-CRMP-5/CV2, and anti-Yo can be internalized into cell lines and can interact with their antigens *in vitro*. However, CRMP-5/CV-2 protein, although visualized in the cytoplasm of some tumor cells, does not itself appear sufficient to stimulate production of autoantibodies. It has been argued that these antibodies serve more as useful diagnostic markers than as the primary cause of autoimmunity and that it is the T cells that initiate the direct damage (Honnorat and Antoine, 2007). The T cell–mediated hypothesis is supported by the presence of an intense CNS monocytic infiltrate comprised of T cells specifically targeting the neuronal and tumor antigen. Another manner in which anti-CRMP-5/CV-2 antibodies could cause neurological symptoms may be through coimmunogenic tumor proteins (such as an ion channel) giving rise to plasma membrane–directed autoantibodies that could activate a complement cascade and lead to an inflammatory response (Yu et al., 2001).

Figure 18–3 outlines some of the possible mechanisms by which autoantibodies and T cells may lead to neurological findings.

Pathophysiology (Structural/Basal Ganglia Level)

Why some PNSs manifest with chorea while others do not and why imaging findings so frequently fail to correlate with the clinical picture is not known. Underscoring the mysterious variability of PNSs is the fact that some cancer patients with identified onconeural antibodies have no evident neurological syndrome at all and some patients with a PNS have no identifiable autoantibody (Graus et al., 2004; Honnorat and Antoine, 2007). No animal models have yet been developed that shed further light on the mechanisms of PNC, as immunization of animals with tumor antigens has induced serum antibodies but has not replicated neurological symptoms.

In cases of PNC, a selective attack on basal ganglia neurons by cytotoxic T cells could occur if MHC-I molecules on specific neurons preferentially displayed peptides recognized by the cytoplasmic antibody. Such appears to be the case with the anti-CRMP-5/CV-2 antibody and may explain the higher propensity for chorea with the anti-CRMP-5/CV2-related syndrome (Vernino et al., 2002). Indeed, many, if not most, paraneoplastic antibodies react preferentially with specific components of the CNS (i.e., those associated with the presenting antigen) and are thus most associated with a particular clinical syndrome (e.g., anti-Purkinje antibodies result in a predominantly cerebellar syndrome).

Nevertheless, the degree of CNS involvement is typically more widespread than the clinical syndrome, and the presence of chorea does not imply that the antigen is specific for the basal ganglia. Anti-CRMP-5/CV-2 antibodies, for example, are not associated with one specific clinical syndrome and cannot be labeled as basal ganglia–specific. In the case of the anti-NMDA receptor antibody, the clinical results are not limited to chorea and include psychosis, seizures, and

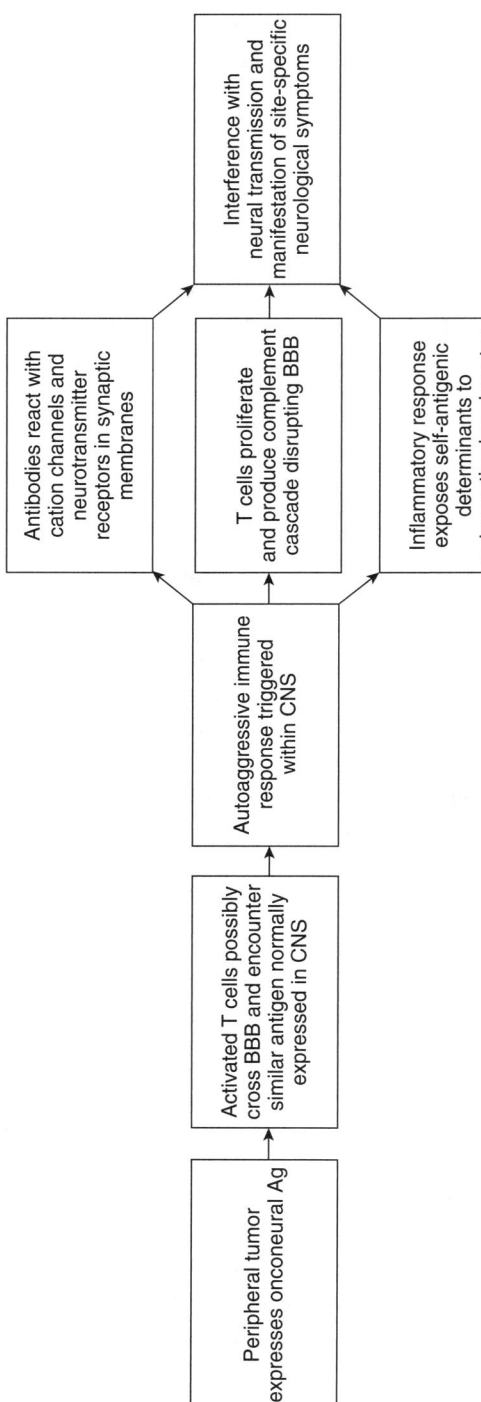

FIGURE 18–3. Possible mechanisms by which autoantibodies and T cells may lead to clinical manifestations of paraneoplastic syndrome. Ag, antigen; BBB, blood–brain barrier; CNS, central nervous system.

manifold other findings. The mechanism underlying the varied clinical findings in this syndrome may relate to the effects of a functional blockade of the NMDA receptor (Iizuka et al., 2008). Such a blockade could reduce the activation by glutamate of gamma-aminobutyric acid (GABA)-ergic interneurons in the thalamus and cortex with disinhibition of their targets, the glutamatergic projection neurons to the caudate nucleus and putamen, resulting in excessive striatal release of glutamate and possibly excitotoxicity, and could indirectly lead to dopamine dysfunction (Stone et al., 2007). The main epitope targeted by the antibodies is in the extracellular N-terminal domain of the NR1 subunit. The neuropsychiatric syndrome may be triggered by a prodromal malaise and viral-like illness, but what leads it from one stage to the next is unclear. The viral-like prodrome of the syndrome, along with the transience of the chorea, differentiates it from the other PNSs and suggests a potentially different mechanism. The paucity of inflammatory infiltrates in some cases may help to explain the reversibility of this particular autoimmune chorea.

NONPARANEOPLASTIC AUTOIMMUNE-RELATED CHOREAS

Chorea, though uncommon, can occur in a variety of autoimmune diseases. The underlying mechanisms of the chorea in these autoimmune diseases are unknown but are likely similar to those described for paraneoplastic autoimmune chorea. Chorea is most common in the setting of systemic lupus erythematosus and the often-related antiphospholipid antibody syndrome. These two entities, though not synonymous, will be covered together, followed by a brief review of some less common causes of autoimmune chorea.

Systemic Lupus Erythematosus and Antiphospholipid Antibodies

Chorea is present in <4% of patients with systemic lupus erythematosus (SLE) (Cervera et al., 1997). It can antedate other symptoms by nearly a decade or appear later in the course, sometimes precipitated by pregnancy or the use of oral contraceptives (Chapter 15). Over 20 antibodies have been described in association with SLE, at least 11 of which are reportedly specific to brain and nine of which are systemic in nature (Zandman-Goddard et al., 2007). Chorea in the context of SLE has been most strongly associated with two antiphospholipid antibodies; anticardiolipin (ACL) and lupus anticoagulant (LAC). As many as half of SLE patients with neuropsychiatric symptoms are found to be ACL[+] and one-third are LAC[+]. Other antibodies occasionally identified in SLE, such as anti-Ro and anti-NMDA receptor antibodies, may also be causative; but these appear to be rare.

Antiphospholipid syndrome (APS) can occur in the context of SLE as well as other autoimmune diseases (secondary APS) or as an independent syndrome (primary APS). In one review of 50 APS-related cases of chorea, approximately half had SLE and one-third had primary APS (Zandman-Goddard et al., 2007). The vast majority (96%) were female, with age at onset ranging 6–77 years. Chorea was more commonly a presenting sign for pediatric cases and recurred in one-third of patients. Chorea in APS can by unilateral or bilateral and alternating over the course of weeks to months. Whether with or without SLE, APL antibodies are often associated with other neuropsychiatric and autoimmune phenomena; among the most common comorbid features include thromboembolic events, polyarthritis, and cognitive dysfunction.

Brain CT imaging of APS/SLE cases with chorea is often unrevealing. Brain MRI scans, though frequently normal, may show small infarcts, occasionally involving the striatum. In one PET study of a case of alternating hemichorea due to primary APS, increased metabolism in the striatum was noted contralateral to the affected side (Furie et al., 1994) independent of any abnormalities noted on MRI (Figure 18–4). Thus, while imaging is important in excluding other possible

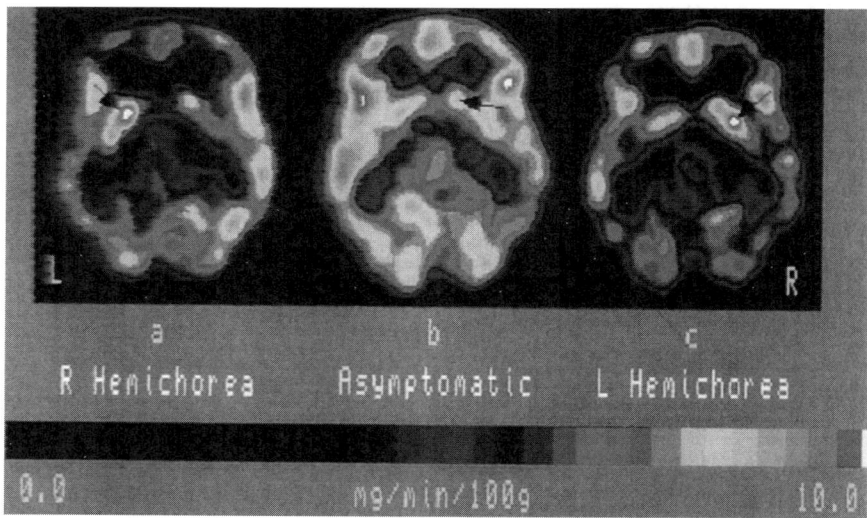

FIGURE 18–4. Fluorodeoxyglucose positron emission tomographic (FDG-PET) imaging in alternating hemichorea. Color bar (color in the original) quantifies regional cerebral metabolic rate for glucose in milligrams per milliliter per 100 g. *Left panel* Study 1: During right hemichorea, left lentiform metabolism was abnormally increased (*arrow*). *Middle panel* Study 2: During the asymptomatic period, left lentiform metabolism returned to normal but right caudate metabolism was abnormally elevated (*arrow*). *Right panel* Study 3: During left hemichorea, right caudate and lentiform metabolism (*arrow*) were abnormally elevated. Left caudate metabolism was also elevated. From Furie et al. (1994). Reprinted with permission, © Wolters Kluwer Health.

sources of neurological impairment, it is not a reliable diagnostic marker of chorea.

Laboratory testing for suspected cases of APS or SLE-related chorea should include testing for ACL (detected by enzyme-linked immunosorbent assay) and LAC (detected by clotting assays). Titers of both of these antibodies can fluctuate over time and have been reported to decrease during active prothrombotic events (Antunes et al., 2004). CSF IgG-ACL can be identified in some patients even in the absence of neurological findings (Cervera et al., 1997). In cases where SLE is suspected but has not yet been diagnosed, testing for antinuclear antibodies (ANAs) and anti-DNA antibodies may also be appropriate. When these are unremarkable, additional markers such as anti-Sm, anti-RNP, anti-Ro, anti-NMDA antibodies, and others can be considered.

Although the presence of APS tends to worsen the prognosis of SLE, chorea in SLE/APS generally has a good prognosis. Most patients recover despite the lack of any standardized treatment. Steroids and intravenous Ig have been reported to be effective, with adjuvant dopamine receptor blockers such as haloperidol for more refractory cases. Treatment with autoimmune agents such as azathioprine and cyclophosphamide has similarly been reported to improve chorea, although no controlled trials support their use in this capacity. In cases of APS, anticoagulation is generally advised and has occasionally been reported to lead to a resolution of chorea.

The etiology of chorea in the context of SLE or APS is unknown. It has been postulated to result from thrombosis of small vessels supplying the basal ganglia due to alterations in the coagulation cascade. However, the frequent presence of normal neuroimaging studies along with the response to immunosuppressant therapy (and withdrawal of oral contraceptives in some cases) supports an autoimmune mechanism. It has been postulated that the antiphospholipid component of LAC binds to phospholipid proteins within the basal ganglia (Asherson et al., 1987). The immune response, as described, may facilitate disruption of the BBB, allowing the SLE/APS antibodies to bind to targets within the basal ganglia more readily.

Other Autoimmune Syndromes

There are sufficient anecdotal reports of chorea occurring in the context of various autoimmune disorders to surmise that chorea should be considered a potential but rare manifestation of autoimmunity in general. In many instances, the underlying "culprit" may be an antiphospholipid antibody as these can occur in a host of autoimmune disorders (Gidwani et al., 2007).

Thyroid antibodies are another potential cause of chorea (Taurin et al., 2002) and should be considered even in the context of a normal thyroid-stimulating hormone level as chorea can occur in the context of hyper-, hypo-, and euthyroid states (Video 18–2 Hyperthyroidism). Presence of a goiter is a strong clinical indicator, although its absence does not rule out thyroid dysfunction. Treatment with thyroid replacement can similarly elicit chorea, suggesting that chorea may be the direct effect of thyroxine on the basal ganglia, secondary to thyroxine-induced dopamine receptor sensitivity or altered catecholamine turnover (Ristic et al., 2004) (Chapter 15).

Primary Sjögren syndrome has been reported to occasionally present with chorea, in one case with a normal brain MRI (Venegas Fanchke et al., 2005) and in another with bilateral basal ganglia lesions that resolved following treatment with steroids and haloperidol (Min and Youn, 2009). The pathophysiology of the chorea in these cases is, like those described before, unclear and likely involves cross-reactive antibodies such as anti-Ro, anti-La, anti-SSA, and anti-SSB. Neuro-Behçet syndrome is a rare cause of chorea, with chorea reported in one of 154 cases in one review (Benamour et al., 2006). The chorea can occur at disease onset or many decades later. In one case, ring-like lesions in the basal ganglia were observed and attributed to vasculitis; they improved following treatment with steroids (Kuriwaka et al., 2004).

Celiac disease can have many neurological manifestations but is only rarely associated with chorea (Hadjivassiliou et al., 2002; Pereira et al., 2004). Presence of an antigliadin antibody (as has been identified in the CSF of celiac patients with ataxia) may play an immune-mediated role in the chorea. In some cases the chorea improved following adherence to a gluten-free diet (Video 18–3 Celiac Disease).

Vasculitis has similarly been invoked as an etiology for chorea in a variety of autoimmune disorders, including giant cell arteritis (Haq and Shah, 1996) and Churg-Strauss syndrome (Kok et al., 1993). As discussed, however, it remains conjectural as to whether the chorea is the direct result of the autoimmune vasculitis affecting the basal ganglia or an epiphenomenon, such as an autoantibody-directed response.

CONCLUSION

Chorea needs to be considered in the context of a wide array of autoimmune disorders, whether paraneoplastic or rheumatological in nature. The relative rarity, myriad causes, diverse clinical presentations, and variable imaging and laboratory findings make autoimmune chorea a significant diagnostic challenge. Much remains to be learned about autoimmune chorea; the causes remain an area of conjecture, and the treatment is often by trial and error. An awareness of the differential, however, can lead to earlier diagnosis of the underlying entity; in the case of paraneoplastic chorea, in particular, this identification can occasionally be life-saving.

REFERENCES

Albin RL, Bromberg MB, Penney JB, Knapp R (1988) Chorea and dystonia: a remote effect of carcinoma. Mov Disord 3:162–169.

Antunes MC, D'Cruz D, Hughes GR (2004) Neurological manifestations of anti-phospholipid (Hughes) syndrome. Clin Exp Rheumatol 22:771–775.

Asherson RA, Derksen RH, Harris EN, Bouma BN, Gharavi AE, Kater L, et al. (1987) Chorea in systemic lupus erythematosus and "lupus-like" disease: association with antiphospholipid antibodies. Semin Arthritis Rheum 16:253–259.

Batchelor TT, Platten M, Palmer-Toy DE, Hunter GJ, Lev MH, Dalmau J, et al. (1998) Chorea as a paraneoplastic complication of Hodgkin's disease. J Neurooncol 36:185–190.

Benamour S, Naji T, Alaoui FZ, El-Kabli H, El-Aidouni S (2006) Neurological involvement in Behcet's disease. 154 cases from a cohort of 925 patients and review of the literature [in French]. Rev Neurol (Paris) 162:1084–1090.

Cervera R, Asherson RA, Font J, Tikly M, Pallares L, Chamorro A, et al. (1997) Chorea in the antiphospholipid syndrome. Clinical, radiologic, and immunologic characteristics of 50 patients from our clinics and the recent literature. Medicine (Baltimore) 76: 203–212.

Croteau D, Owainati A, Dalmau J, Rogers LR (2001) Response to cancer therapy in a patient with a paraneoplastic choreiform disorder. Neurology 57:719–722.

Dalmau J, Gleichman AJ, Hughes EG, Rossi JE, Peng X, Lai M, et al. (2008) Anti-NMDA-receptor encephalitis: case series and analysis of the effects of antibodies. Lancet Neurol 7:1091–1098.

Dalmau J, Gultekin HS, Posner JB (1999) Paraneoplastic neurologic syndromes: pathogenesis and physiopathology. Brain Pathol 9:275–284.

Darnell RB, Posner JB (2003) Paraneoplastic syndromes involving the nervous system. N Engl J Med 349:1543–1554.

Furie R, Ishikawa T, Dhawan V, Eidelberg D (1994) Alternating hemichorea in primary antiphospholipid syndrome: evidence for contralateral striatal hypermetabolism. Neurology 44:2197–2199.

Gidwani P, Segal E, Shanske A, Driscoll C (2007) Chorea associated with antiphospholipid antibodies in a patient with Kabuki syndrome. Am J Med Genet A 143A:1338–1341.

Goshima Y, Nakamura F, Strittmatter P, Strittmatter SM (1995) Collapsin-induced growth cone collapse mediated by an intracellular protein related to UNC-33. Nature 376: 509–514.

Graus F, Dalmou J, Rene R, Tora M, Malats N, Verschuuren JJ, et al. (1997) Anti-Hu antibodies in patients with small-cell lung cancer: association with complete response to therapy and improved survival. J Clin Oncol 15:2866–2872.

Graus F, Delattre JY, Antoine JC, Dalmau J, Giometto B, Grisold W, et al. (2004) Recommended diagnostic criteria for paraneoplastic neurological syndromes. J Neurol Neurosurg Psychiatry 75:1135–1140.

Hadjivassiliou M, Grunewald RA, Davies-Jones GA (2002) Gluten sensitivity as a neurological illness. J Neurol Neurosurg Psychiatry 72:560–563.

Haq N, Shah IA (1996) Chorea—a presenting feature of giant cell arteritis. J Pak Med Assoc 46:263–264.

Heckmann JG, Lang CJ, Druschky A, Claus D, Bartels O, Neundorfer B (1997) Chorea resulting from paraneoplastic encephalitis. Mov Disord 12:464–466.

Honnorat J, Antoine JC (2007) Paraneoplastic neurological syndromes. Orphanet J Rare Dis 2:22.

Honnorat J, Antoine JC, Derrington E, Aguera M, Belin MF (1996) Antibodies to a sub-population of glial cells and a 66 kDa developmental protein in patients with paraneoplastic neurological syndromes. J Neurol Neurosurg Psychiatry 61:270–278.

Honnorat J, Cartalat-Carel S, Ricard D, Camdessanche JP, Carpentier AF, Rogemond V, et al. (2009) Onco-neural antibodies and tumour type determine survival and neurological symptoms in paraneoplastic neurological syndromes with Hu or CV2/CRMP5 antibodies. J Neurol Neurosurg Psychiatry 80:412–416.

Iizuka T, Sakai F, Ide T, Monzen T, Yoshii S, Iigaya M, et al. (2008) Anti-NMDA receptor encephalitis in Japan: long-term outcome without tumor removal. Neurology 70: 504–511.

Kinirons P, Fulton A, Keoghan M, Brennan P, Farrell MA, Moroney JT (2003) Paraneoplastic limbic encephalitis (PLE) and chorea associated with CRMP-5 neuronal antibody. Neurology 61:1623–1624.

Kok J, Bosseray A, Brion JP, Micoud M, Besson G (1993) Chorea in a child with Churg-Strauss syndrome. Stroke 24:1263–1264.

Krolak-Salmon P, Androdias G, Meyronet D, Aguera M, Honnorat J, Vighetto A (2006) Slow evolution of cerebellar degeneration and chorea in a man with anti-Yo antibodies. Eur J Neurol 13:307–308.

Kujawa KA, Niemi VR, Tomasi MA, Mayer NW, Cochran E, Goetz CG (2001) Ballistic-choreic movements as the presenting feature of renal cancer. Arch Neurol 58: 1133–1135.

Kuriwaka R, Kunishige M, Nakahira H, Inoue H, Higashi T, Tokumoto Y, et al. (2004) Neuro-Behcet's disease with chorea after remission of intestinal Behcet's disease. Clin Rheumatol 23:364–367.

Min JH, Youn YC (2009) Bilateral basal ganglia lesions of primary Sjogren syndrome presenting with generalized chorea. Parkinsonism Relat Disord 15:398–399.

Moore FG (2009) Bilateral hemichorea-hemiballism caused by metastatic lung cancer. Mov Disord 24:1405–1406.

Muehlschlegel S, Okun MS, Foote KD, Coco D, Yachnis AT, Fernandez HH (2005) Paraneoplastic chorea with leukoencephalopathy presenting with obsessive–compulsive and behavioral disorder. Mov Disord 20:1523–1527.

Nuti A, Ceravolo R, Salvetti S, Gambaccini G, Bonuccelli U, Capochiani E (2000) Paraneoplastic choreic syndrome during non-Hodgkin's lymphoma. Mov Disord 15:350–352.

Pereira AC, Edwards MJ, Buttery PC, Hawkes CH, Quinn NP, Giovannoni G, et al. (2004) Choreic syndrome and coeliac disease: a hitherto unrecognised association. Mov Disord 19:478–482.

Poewe WH, Kleedorfer B, Willeit J, Gerstenbrand F (1988) Primary CNS lymphoma presenting as a choreic movement disorder followed by segmental dystonia. Mov Disord 3:320–325.

Posner JB (2003) Immunology of paraneoplastic syndromes: overview. Ann N Y Acad Sci 998:178–186.

Ristic AJ, Svetel M, Dragasevic N, Zarkovic M, Koprivsek K, Kostic VS (2004) Bilateral chorea-ballism associated with hyperthyroidism. Mov Disord 19:982–983.

Schiff DE, Ortega JA (1992) Chorea, eosinophilia, and lupus anticoagulant associated with acute lymphoblastic leukemia. Pediatr Neurol 8:466–468.

Stone JM, Morrison PD, Pilowsky LS (2007) Glutamate and dopamine dysregulation in schizophrenia—a synthesis and selective review. J Psychopharmacol 21:440–452.

Tan EK, Chan LL, Auchus AP, Wong MC (2003) Reversible choreoathetosis in primary cerebral lymphoma: clinicoradiologic correlation. Eur Neurol 50:53–54.

Tani T, Piao Y, Mori S, Ishihara N, Tanaka K, Wakabayashi K, et al. (2000) Chorea resulting from paraneoplastic striatal encephalitis. J Neurol Neurosurg Psychiatry 69:512–515.

Taurin G, Golfier V, Pinel JF, Deburghgraeve V, Poirier JY, Edan G, et al. (2002) Choreic syndrome due to Hashimoto's encephalopathy. Mov Disord 17:1091–1092.

Tincani A, Taraborelli M, Cattaneo R (2010) Antiphospholipid antibodies and malignancies. Autoimmun Rev 9:200–202.

Tremont-Lukats IW, Fuller GN, Ribalta T, Giglio P, Groves MD (2002) Paraneoplastic chorea: case study with autopsy confirmation. Neuro-oncol 4:192–195.

Venegas Fanchke P, Sinning M, Miranda M (2005) Primary Sjogren's syndrome presenting as a generalized chorea. Parkinsonism Relat Disord 11:193–194.

Vernino S, Tuite P, Adler CH, Meschia JF, Boeve BF, Boasberg P, et al. (2002) Paraneoplastic chorea associated with CRMP-5 neuronal antibody and lung carcinoma. Ann Neurol 51:625–30.

Yu Z, Kryzer TJ, Griesmann GE, Kim K, Benarroch EE, Lennon VA (2001) CRMP-5 neuronal autoantibody: marker of lung cancer and thymoma-related autoimmunity. Ann Neurol 49:146–154.

Zandman-Goddard G, Chapman J, Shoenfeld Y (2007) Autoantibodies involved in neuropsychiatric SLE and antiphospholipid syndrome. Semin Arthritis Rheum 36:297–315.

19

Paroxysmal Chorea

Camilla Kilbane, MD

INTRODUCTION

The paroxysmal dykinesias are a rare and challenging group of movement disorders. They are characterized by painless dyskinetic involuntary movements, of sudden onset and without change in consciousness. As the movements experienced can be choreiform, dystonic, ballistic, or combined in nature, these disorders are collectively called the "paroxysmal dyskinesias" (Demirkiran and Jankovic, 1995; Lance, 1977; van Rootselaar et al., 2009).

A lack of familiarity with these disorders, as well as the normal neurological exam between events, can lead to a delayed or misdiagnosis (van Rootselaar et al., 2009). Given the normal neurological exam, the diagnosis is often based on history alone. A personal history of symptoms combined with a family history of movement disorder is often the only diagnostic clue.

A review of patients at a movement disorder clinic highlights the rarity of these disorders (Blakeley and Jankovic, 2002). Over 19 years, the center examined over 12,000 patients and diagnosed only 93 cases. Not only are the paroxysmal dyskinesias a clinical challenge for physicians and general neurologists, they often are also difficult to diagnose by movement disorder specialists.

Recent research has shed light on these disorders. Genetic studies seek to find a common basis for these disorders, which when familial have autosomal dominant inheritance. However, at present there are no specific laboratory tests or radiological findings consistent with diagnosis.

Multiple classifications have been proposed since the initial description. These disorders are currently classified by precipitating factors as well as duration and frequency of attack. Response to antiepileptic drugs (AEDs) is also an important factor in classification.

HISTORICAL OVERVIEW

In 1940, Mount and Reback described a 23-year-old man with an autosomal dominant movement disorder, which clinically manifested as attacks of choreoathetoid movements involving both arms and legs. These would occur two or three times daily and were precipitated by caffeine, alcohol, tea, fatigue, or smoking. They proposed the term "familial paroxysmal choreoathetosis" (Mount and Reback, 1940). Since then, multiple attempts have been made at classifying these disorders.

Lance (1977) reviewed 100 patients reported in the literature and added 12 patients, all diagnosed with "familial paroxysmal dystonic choreoathetosis." He classified the disorders, primarily by duration, into three subtypes:

Paroxysmal dystonic choreoathetosis (PDC): characterized by long attacks, lasting 2 minutes to 4 hours

Paroxysmal kinesigenic choreoathetosis (PKC): brief events lasting seconds to 5 minutes and induced by sudden voluntary movement

Intermediate form: attacks lasting 5–30 minutes and induced by continued exercise

This classification was later disputed by Goodenough and coworkers (1978), who classified the disorders into familial and acquired. The familial included:

Kinesigenic: choreoathetotic, dystonic—lasting less than 5 minutes

Nonkinesigenic: choreoathetotic and mixed—lasting more than 5 minutes

The acquired were classified with regard to underlying etiology, whether they were related to underlying neurological diseases such as multiple sclerosis or cerebral palsy, or secondary to epileptic disorders or other metabolic abnormalities.

In 1994 Fahn proposed a new classification of paroxysmal dystonia/choreoathetosis:

1. Paroxysmal kinesigenic dystonic choreoathetosis (PKC)
2. Paroxysmal nonkinesigenic dystonic choreoathetosis (PDC)
3. Intermittent PDC

4. Paroxysmal hypnogenic dyskinesias
5. Benign paroxysmal dystonia/torticollis in infancy
6. Miscellaneous

In 1995 Demirkiran and Jankovic suggested classifying the disorders into four main categories, with short-idiopathic indicating an attack lasting less than 5 minutes in duration and long-idiopathic indicating an attack lasting greater than 5 minutes in duration:

1. Paroxysmal kinesigenic dyskinesia (PKD)
   a. short-idiopathic: familial or sporadic vs. secondary
   b. long-idiopathic: familial or sporadic vs. secondary
2. Paroxysmal nonkinesigenic dyskinesia (PNKD)
   a. short-idiopathic: familial vs. sporadic vs. secondary
   b. long-idiopathic: familial vs. sporadic vs. secondary
3. Paroxysmal exertion-induced dyskinesia (PED)
   a. short-idiopathic: familial vs. sporadic vs. secondary
   b. long-idiopathic: familial vs. sporadic vs. secondary
4. Paroxysmal hypnogenic dyskinesia (PHD)
   a. short-idiopathic: familial vs. sporadic vs. secondary
   b. long-idiopathic: familial vs. sporadic vs. secondary

PAROXYSMAL DISORDERS

Paroxysmal Kinesigenic Dyskinesia

Although rare, PKD is the most common type of paroxysmal dyskinesia. It was first described in 1941 by Smith and Heersema in three cases of brief dyskinetic episodes induced by sudden voluntary movements. Further descriptions followed, and Kertesz (1967) named the entity "paroxysmal kinesigenic choreoathetosis." As a subtype of primary dystonia, it is also called "DYT10."

PKD is characterized by brief, sudden onset of involuntary movements (duration less than 5 minutes), which are triggered by voluntary movements. Consciousness is preserved throughout, and the attacks may occur multiple times per day, up to 100 times. Remission is usually seen around age 20. Men are affected more than women, and women have a better prognosis and a higher chance of complete remission (Bruno et al., 2004; Houser et al., 1999; Tomita et al., 1999). In 27% of cases there is a positive family history with autosomal dominant inheritance. About 42% of patients reported afebrile seizures in childhood (Tomita et al., 1999).

Bruno and coworkers (2004) reviewed the symptoms of 123 patients with PKD. They found that the trigger was usually a "whole-body activity" such as standing up, walking, or running. They also found that anxiety lowers the threshold for events in 62% of patients, increasing the number of attacks. Most patients (82%) reported an aura prior to the event, such as "upset stomach," "a butterfly in my stomach," or "electricity in my head." Sixty-two percent answered a questionnaire by stating that they could potentially minimize the attack if they stopped the movement at the onset of the aura. The attacks were generally of a short duration—less than 1 minute—and 93% of subjects reported the attacks as lasting less than 30 seconds. The movements experienced during an attack included dystonia, chorea, ballismus, and combinations of these. PKD was noted to have a favorable outcome, with 27% obtaining complete remission and another 25% having marked improvement (>50% reduction in attack frequency by self-report). Most PKD patients responded to AEDs, most commonly carbamazepine and phenytoin.

PKD has been linked to infantile spasms, leading to the first linkage of PKD to chromosome 16. In 1997, the ICCA syndrome (infantile convulsions and choreoathetosis) was linked to the pericentromeric region of chromosome 16 (Szepetowski et al., 1997). Families affected by this mutation (16p12-q12) had infantile convulsions, which fully resolved; however, they later developed attacks of hyperkinetic movements. PKD and ICCA are now believed to be the same disorder. A second locus (EKD2), also on chromosome 16, was reported in 2000 in India (Valente et al., 2000).

Due to the paroxysmal nature of the disease, it has been postulated that this disorder is a channelopathy. Ion channels are a common cause of Mendelian episodic disorders, but no causative gene has been identified as of yet. The disorder has similarities to episodic ataxia-1, a potassium channel disorder, which also starts in early childhood and is triggered by voluntary muscle movements (Bhatia et al., 2000).

Based on their recent review, Bruno and colleagues (2004) suggest new diagnostic criteria for PKD:

1. identified kinesigenic trigger
2. short duration of attacks—less than 1 minute
3. no pain or loss of consciousness during attack
4. control of attacks with phenytoin or carbamazepine
5. age at onset 1–20 years, if no family history of PKD
6. exclusion of other organic diseases and a normal neurological exam

Paroxysmal Nonkinesigenic Dyskinesia

PNKD was first classified by Mount and Reback in 1940, who characterized a large family with five generations affected and labeled the disorder "familial paroxysmal choreoathetosis." It is also known as "DYT8." Males are affected twice as often as females (Lance,1977). Most patients have an autosomal dominant family history.

The dyskinesias seen in this disorder are characterized by dystonia, chorea, or combinations of the two, lasting 10 minutes to 1 hour. Typically, an attack begins with a sensation of tightness and tugging in one limb or involuntary movements of the mouth. The movements tend to start unilaterally and may generalize. In severe cases Mount and Reback reported dysarthria and even anarthria without loss of consciousness.

Attacks are usually precipitated by caffeine and alcohol consumption and less often by nicotine, hunger, fatigue, or emotional stress; but they can also occur spontaneously. They are usually increased during menses and ovulation. The onset is usually early childhood or infancy, but it has been reported up to the age of 33 (Demirkiran and Jankovic, 1995; Lance, 1977; van Rootselaar et al., 2009).

Bruno and coworkers (2007) described the genotype–phenotype correlation for PNKD. The natural history of disease is unreliable but shows a tendency toward decreasing attacks with age. In this study there was no gender difference. Alcohol and caffeine were reported as precipitants in almost 100% of subjects. Sleep benefit was also common, noted in 70%. Both prophylactic and abortive responses to benzodiazepines were experienced by 34 of 35 patients. For nonbenzodiazepine AEDs, the response was at best temporary with valproic acid and absent with carbamazepine and phenytoin. In this study, headache (including migraine) was a common associated symptom, and 47% met criteria for migraine using the International Headache Society criteria.

PNKD is usually transmitted in an autosomal dominant manner. Penetrance has been found to be approximately 80%. Linkage was found to the distal chromosome 2q33-35, to a locus named "familial paroxysmal dyskinesia type 1" (FDP1) (Hofele et al., 1997). Subsequent studies led to the discovery of the mutation of the myofibrillogenesis regulator, *MR-1*, after two separate groups found linkage to chromosome 2q31-36 (Lee et al., 2004; Rainier et al., 2004). The function of MR-1 is not known; however, it is thought to have similar activity to hydroxyacyl-glutathione hydrolase (HAGH), which is produced as a by-product of oxidative stress. HAGH functions in a pathway to detoxify methylglycoxal, a compound present in coffee and alcoholic beverages (Lee et al., 2004; Rainier et al., 2004). A further study showed that the *MR-1* mutation causes an abnormality in the mitochondrial targeting sequence, rather than an actual alteration in the mature protein (Ghezzi et al., 2009).

Bruno and colleagues (2007) contrasted the differences in symptoms in individuals with and without the *MR-1* mutation. The patient group without the *MR-1* phenotype had a later age at onset, an average of 12 years vs. infancy in the *MR-1* group. In contrast to the *MR-1* group, no patient without the mutation reported alcohol as a precipitant, whereas 40% of this group noted caffeine to be a trigger. The strong association in the *MR-1* group with alcohol is probably due to the function of the *MR-1* gene, which participates in glycolysis but degrades a product also heavily found in alcohol. This study also highlighted the fact that most of the *MR-1* group had stereotypical attacks between family members, whereas the non-*MR-1* group had more intra- and interfamily heterogeneity. PNKD has previously been shown to be poorly responsive to AEDs and is difficult to treat; however, the *MR-1* group showed almost a 100% response rate to benzodiazepines.

Electroencephalographic (EEG) recordings during an attack are usually normal; however, an invasive video-EEG study showed electrical discharges from the caudate nucleus (Lombroso and Fischman, 1999). Subsequent single-photon emission computed tomography (SPECT) images during an attack showed hyperperfusion in the caudate nucleus and thalamus (del Carmen et al., 2000). ^{18}F-Dopa positron emission tomography (PET) and ^{11}C-raclopride PET have revealed a marked reduction in the density of postsynaptic dopamine D_2 receptors, but it is still unclear whether this is a primary or compensatory mechanism (Lombroso and Fischman,1999).

Bruno et al.'s (2007) proposed diagnostic criteria for *MR-1* PNKD include the following:

1. Hyperkinetic involuntary movement attacks with dystonia, chorea, and hemiballismus, or combination of same, normally lasting 10 minutes to 1 hour but up to 4 hours
2. Normal neurological exam between attacks and exclusion of secondary causes
3. Onset of attacks in infancy or early childhood
4. Precipitation of attacks by caffeine or alcohol consumption
5. Family history of movement disorder meeting criteria 1–4

The treatment of PNKD should include the avoidance of identifiable triggers. As noted, PNKD does not tend to respond as well as the paroxysmal kinesigenic dyskinesias to AEDs, but recent evidence (Bruno et al., 2007) suggests that *MR-1*-positive individuals show a good response to benzodiazepines.

Paroxysmal Exercise-Induced Dyskinesia

PED is a rare form of paroxysmal dyskinesia, first described in 1977. Only a few cases have been described since then, mostly with autosomal dominant inheritance. Also called "DYT18," PED is precipitated by continuous exertion. Most commonly, the movements are dystonic in nature, with hemidystonia or foot involvement being most common. Generalization rarely occurs. The dyskinesia develops only in the exercised limbs (Demirkiran and Jankovic, 1995; Lance, 1977; van Rootselaar et al., 2009).

Attacks usually last from 5 minutes to 2 hours, with cessation of the abnormal movement approximately 10 minutes after cessation of exercise. Although classically associated with sustained physical activity, attacks have been associated with electric nerve stimulation as well as passive movements and muscle vibration. PED is associated with rolandic epilepsy and writer's cramp (RE-PED-WC) (Guerrini et al., 1999), which also localizes to the pericentromeric region of chromosome 16. PKD shares the same locus (Guerrini et al., 1999; Guerrini, 2001), and linkage analysis has shown a common homozygous heliotype in the same region as PKD (Weber et al., 2008). Suls and colleagues (2008) evaluated the coexistence of PED and epilepsy and found decreased transport of glucose across the blood–brain barrier. This was due to mutations in the facilitative glucose transporter type 1 (GLUT-1), which is coded by *SLC2A1*. GLUT-1 is expressed in red blood cells and at the blood–brain barrier and, hence, is associated with hemolytic anemia. It is possible that the dyskinesias seen in this disorder are caused by an energy deficiency in the basal ganglia, which occurs on exertion. This theory is supported by the response of the dyskinetic attacks to an infusion of glucose as well as the response to a ketogenic diet, which alters the main nutrient of the brain (Weber and Lerche, 2009).

EEGs are typically normal; however, hyperexcitability has been demonstrated on neurophysiological studies, including electromyography (EMG) and somatosensory-evoked potentials. Mild hypointensities have been reported in the dorsolateral putamen on magnetic resonance imaging and metabolic alteration in the same area on PET. Ictal SPECT showed hyperperfusion of the basal ganglia (Kluge et al., 1998; Margari et al., 2000).

PED does not respond well to AEDs or benzodiazepines; however, gabapentin reduced the frequency and severity of attacks (Demirkiran and Jankovic,1995).

Paroxysmal Hypnogenic Dyskinesia

PHD is characterized by abnormal movements occurring during the non-rapid eye movement (REM) stage of sleep, particularly stages two and three. The movements include choreiform movements, dystonia, and ballism. Males are more often affected than females. This disorder is now thought of as a type of nocturnal frontal lobe epilepsy, together with paroxysmal arousals and episodic wandering. These attacks tend to occur in clusters, usually lasting 30–60 seconds, and consist of tonic movements of all limbs, automatism, vocalization, and sleep fragmentation. Insomnia is common (Demirkiran and Jankovic, 1995; Oldani et al., 1996; van Rootselaar et al., 2009).

EEG records may show evidence of epilepsy but are often normal. Polysomnography showed interictal abnormalities in frontal lobes in approximately 30% (Oldani et al., 1996). Nocturnal frontal lobe epilepsy is divided into three categories: paroxysmal arousal lasting less than 20 seconds, nocturnal paroxysmal dystonia lasting less than 2 minutes, and episodic nocturnal wandering lasting up to 3 minutes. These three seizure types may overlap in the same patient (Demirkiran and Jankovic, 1995; Oldani et al., 1996).

Forty percent of patients have a positive family history, and the autosomal dominant form has been called "autosomal dominant nocturnal frontal lobe epilepsy" (ADNFLE). This is a ligand channelopathy associated with an abnormality in the acetylcholine receptor subunits (CHRNA4 and CHRNB2), with loci found on chromosomes 15q24 and 20q13 (Combi et al., 2004; Marini and Guerrini, 2007).

Treatment includes carbamazepine as well as phenytoin and acetazolamide (Oldani et al., 1996).

Paroxysmal Choreoathetosis/Episodic Ataxia

The episodic ataxias are a heterogeneous group of disorders characterized by ion channel abnormalities. Episodic ataxia (EA) types 1 and 2 are autosomal dominant disorders characterized by the presence of intermittent cerebellar symptoms.

EA-1 manifests during infancy or early childhood, the hallmark of the disorder being continuous myokymia as well as brief, often kinesigenic episodes of ataxia. This disorder is linked to chromosome 12p, with point mutations in the voltage-dependent potassium channel KCNA1 (Browne et al., 1994; D'Adamo et al., 1999; Gancher and Nutt, 1986; Litt et al., 1994). D'Adamo and coworkers (1999) found that the EA-1 mutation markedly impairs the ion channels' ability to set the resting potential, suggesting that in affected patients axons and terminals may be hyperexcitable because their resting potential is shifted more to depolarized values.

EA-1 is characterized by short attacks of less than 15 minutes of generalized ataxia, slowing of movements, as well as shaking and trembling. There is usually a kinesigenic precipitant, associated with a short sensory warning. Precipitants are usually axial movements after a period of rest. Nystagmus is usually absent. This, as well as the kinesigenic triggering of the attacks, differentiates this disorder from familial periodic ataxia without myokymia (i.e., EA-2), where the attacks usually last for hours, have associated nystagmus both between and during attacks, and do not have a kinesigenic trigger (Browne et al., 1994; D'Adamo et al., 1999; Gancher and Nutt,1986; Litt et al., 1994).

EA-2 is characterized by longer episodes of ataxia (hours) with interictal nystagmus and mildly progressive baseline ataxia. EA-2 is the most common type of episodic ataxia, and half of patients meet the International Headache Society criteria for migraine. EA-2 is mapped to chromosome 19p (Kramer et al., 1995) and causes a mutation in the *CACNA1A* calcium channel gene (Ophoff et al., 1996). This study also found EA-2 to be allelic to familial hemiplegic migraine type 1.

Gancher and Nutt (1986) described the first association of episodic ataxia and paroxysmal choreoathetosis in 1986, in which a review of six kindreds revealed one family (kindred V) with paroxysmal dyskinesia as part of the symptomatology. The proband of this family was a 16-year-old boy with episodic ataxia since the age of 6, the attacks occurring in clusters with complete remission for months at a time. The attacks were characterized by dysarthria, a sensation of swollen tongue, vertigo, and generalized ataxia. Episodes usually lasted 15 minutes to several hours and were precipitated by exercise, sudden head movements, and postural changes, especially if startled or excited. At the age of 15 the proband started developing a second type of attacks, with the same precipitators, but now with brief dystonic posturing lasting approximately 15 seconds. A trial of acetazolamide was unsuccessful; however, phenytoin reduced the severity and frequency of both types of attack. The disease had a benign course, with resolution in early adulthood.

Lubbers and colleagues (1995) reported on acetazolamide response in patients with hereditary myokymia and paroxysmal ataxia (EA-1). Again, the authors describe a patient who had experienced attacks of dizziness since the age of 6, associated with limb ataxia and dysarthria. At the age of 15 the patient developed brief attacks of stereotypic dystonic movements lasting approximately 10 seconds and occurring up to 20 times per day. These attacks were also precipitated by movements. The dystonic attacks were controlled with carbamazepine, but this did not alleviate the ataxic episodes.

The association between episodic ataxia and PKD again emphasizes the possibility of a link between the two disorders, with ion channels as the most likely common link.

Paroxysmal Choreoathetosis/Spasticity

This disorder is characterized by episodes of involuntary movements, dystonic postures of the toes and limbs, imbalance, dysarthria, paresthesia periorally and sometimes on lower limbs, and diplopia. These symptoms are either preceded or accompanied by headache. Cerebellar ataxia is not observed during attacks. Symptoms usually last 20 minutes and can occur multiple times a day or as infrequently as twice a year. Age at onset is typically preschool; however, it can be anywhere between 2 and 15 years. The attacks are precipitated by physical exercise, stress, lack of sleep, and alcohol consumption. In contrast to the other disorders described, a proportion of these patients have an abnormal neurological exam between events, with pyramidal signs, increased deep tendon reflexes, and spasticity in the lower limbs. Therapeutic response was seen with acetazolamide and phenytoin. Linkage to chromosome 1q mapped to the vicinity of a potassium channel (Auburger et al., 1996).

Familial Dyskinesia and Facial Myokymia

This autosomal dominant disorder is characterized by childhood onset of choreiform movements and facial myokymia (Fernandez et al., 2001). The choreiform movements are initially paroxysmal in nature and worsened by anxiety but not by voluntary movements, exercise, alcohol, or caffeine. The movements progressively increase in both frequency and severity, until the third decade when they are almost constant. Life span is normal, as is intellect; and some patients experience improvement later in adulthood. The myokymia is most pronounced periorally and periorbitally. Patients responded to acetazolamide and propranolol. No genetic linkage study has been published as of yet, but it is again anticipated that this disorder is related to ion channel mutations.

SECONDARY CAUSES OF PAROXYSMAL DYSKINESIAS

As previously discussed, most cases of paroxysmal dyskinesias are either familial (often autosomal dominant) or idiopathic. However, in a review from 2002, an identifiable cause was found in 22% of cases (17 of 76 cases) (Blakeley and Jankovic, 2002). Such causes include multiple sclerosis, vascular lesions, trauma, and acquired metabolic abnormalities (Table 19–1).

Secondary forms of paroxysmal dyskinesias have variable age at onset, due to the many different underlying etiologies. The latency from initial insult to onset of paroxysmal dyskinesia was approximately 3 years but ranged from days (e.g., following trauma) to 18 years, as seen with a patient with secondary dyskinesias due to kernicterus. Dystonia was the most common abnormal movement, seen in 16 of 17 patients. Chorea, ballism, and athetosis usually occurred together with dystonia. Most patients have unilateral symptoms.

The secondary dyskinesias do not necessarily adhere to the standard classification, and 29% of patients experienced both kinesigenic and nonkinesigenic dyskinesia (Blakeley and Jankovic, 2002). It is notable that the patient group that experienced kinesigenic symptoms was most responsive to anticonvulsant therapy.

TABLE 19–1. Causes of Secondary Paroxysmal Dyskinesia

Demyelination
Vascular: ischemia, moyamoya, or bleed
Infectious: encephalitis, HIV, CMV
Trauma: peripheral and cerebral
Neurodegenerative disorders as well as kernicterus
Migraine
Neoplasm
Chiari malformation
Drug-induced: e.g., methylphenidate (see Chapter 14)

CMV, cytomegalovirus; HIV, human immunodeficiency virus.

The most frequently cited cause for secondary dyskinesia in the literature is multiple sclerosis, where the abnormal movements usually are described as "tonic spasms" (Bhatia et al., 2000). The spasms are characterized by being precipitated by voluntary movements or sensory stimulation and are often preceded by an aura.

Patients with a secondary cause often have an abnormal neurological exam between attacks—directing the examiner to further investigations, usually including neuroimaging and laboratory testing to rule out multiple sclerosis—and cerebral vascular insufficiency (see Chapter 16) as well as metabolic derangements (glucose, calcium; see Chapter 15). A history of prior head trauma should be obtained (Blakeley and Jankovic, 2002).

CONCLUSION

Paroxysmal dyskinesias are a rare group of movement disorders characterized by a normal neurological exam between events, making their diagnosis a challenge for the examiner. Progress has been made in determining the genetic cause of these disorders, and a hypothesis for the pathophysiology of these disorders is that they are related to ion channel dysfunction. An argument for a similarity in mechanism between the paroxysmal dyskinesias, the episodic ataxias, and the periodic paralyses is further suggested by the response to medications such as anticonvulsants which stabilize the neuronal membranes. Further research will certainly shed light on these rare and intriguing disorders.

REFERENCES

Auburger G, Ratzlaff T, Lunkes A, et al. (1996) A gene for autosomal dominant paroxysmal choreoathetosis/spasticity (CSE) maps to the vicinity of a potassium channel gene cluster on chromosome 1p, probably within 2 cM between D1S443 and D1S197. Genomics 31:90–94.

Bhatia KP, Griggs RC, Ptacek LJ (2000) Episodic movement disorders as channelopathies. Mov Disord 15:429–433.

Blakeley J, Jankovic J (2002) Secondary paroxysmal dyskinesias. Mov Disord 17:726–734.

Browne DL, Gancher ST, Nutt JG, et al. (1994) Episodic ataxia/myokymia syndrome is associated with point mutations in the human potassium channel gene, *KCNA1*. Nat Genet 8:136–140.

Bruno MK, Hallett M, Gwinn-Hardy K, et al. (2004) Clinical evaluation of idiopathic paroxysmal kinesigenic dyskinesia: new diagnostic criteria. Neurology 63:2280–2287.

Bruno MK, Lee HY, Auburger GW, et al. (2007) Genotype–phenotype correlation of paroxysmal nonkinesigenic dyskinesia. Neurology 68:1782–1789.

Combi R, Dalpra L, Tenchini ML, et al. (2004) Autosomal dominant nocturnal frontal lobe epilepsy—a critical overview. J Neurol 251:923–934.

D'Adamo MC, Imbrici P, Sponcichetti F, et al. (1999) Mutations in the *KCNA1* gene associated with episodic ataxia type-1 syndrome impair heteromeric voltage-gated K+ channel function. FASEB J 13:1335–1345.

del Carmen GM, Intruvini S, Vazquez S, et al. (2000) Ictal SPECT in paroxysmal non-kinesigenic dyskinesia. Case report and review of the literature. Parkinsonism Relat Disord 6:119–121.

Demirkiran M, Jankovic J (1995) Paroxysmal dyskinesias: clinical features and classification. Ann Neurol 38:571–579.

Fahn S (1994) The paroxysmal dyskinesias. In: Marsden CD, Fahn S (eds.) Movement Disorders 3. Butterworth-Heinemann, Oxford, pp 310–345.

Fernandez M, Raskind W, Wolff J, et al. (2001) Familial dyskinesia and facial myokymia (FDFM): a novel movement disorder. Ann Neurol 49:486–492.

Gancher ST, Nutt JG (1986) Autosomal dominant episodic ataxia: a heterogeneous syndrome. Mov Disord 1:239–253.

Ghezzi D, Viscomi C, Ferlini A, et al. (2009) Paroxysmal non-kinesigenic dyskinesia is caused by mutations of the MR-1 mitochondrial targeting sequence. Hum Mol Genet 18:1058–1064.

Goodenough DJ, Fariello RG, Annis BL, et al. (1978) Familial and acquired paroxysmal dyskinesias. A proposed classification with delineation of clinical features. Arch Neurol 35:827–831.

Guerrini R (2001) Idiopathic epilepsy and paroxysmal dyskinesia. Epilepsia 42(Suppl 3): 36–41.

Guerrini R, Bonanni P, Nardocci N, et al. (1999) Autosomal recessive rolandic epilepsy with paroxysmal exercise-induced dystonia and writer's cramp: delineation of the syndrome and gene mapping to chromosome 16p12-11.2. Ann Neurol 45:344–352.

Hofele K, Benecke R, Auburger G (1997) Gene locus FPD1 of the dystonic Mount-Reback type of autosomal-dominant paroxysmal choreoathetosis. Neurology 49:1252–1257.

Houser MK, Soland VL, Bhatia KP, et al. (1999) Paroxysmal kinesigenic choreoathetosis: a report of 26 patients. J Neurol 246:120–126.

Kertesz A (1967) Paroxysmal kinesigenic choreoathetosis. An entity within the paroxysmal choreoathetosis syndrome. Description of 10 cases, including 1 autopsied. Neurology 17:680–690.

Kluge A, Kettner B, Zschenderlein R, et al. (1998) Changes in perfusion pattern using ECD-SPECT indicate frontal lobe and cerebellar involvement in exercise-induced paroxysmal dystonia. Mov Disord 13:125–134.

Kramer PL, Yue Q, Gancher ST, et al. (1995) A locus for the nystagmus-associated form of episodic ataxia maps to an 11-cM region on chromosome 19p. Am J Hum Genet 57:182–185.

Lance JW (1977) Familial paroxysmal dystonic choreoathetosis and its differentiation from related syndromes. Ann Neurol 2:285–293.

Lee HY, Xu Y, Huang Y, et al. (2004) The gene for paroxysmal non-kinesigenic dyskinesia encodes an enzyme in a stress response pathway. Hum Mol Genet 13:3161–3170.

Litt M, Kramer P, Browne D, et al. (1994) A gene for episodic ataxia/myokymia maps to chromosome 12p13. Am J Hum Genet 55:702–709.

Lombroso CT, Fischman A (1999) Paroxysmal non-kinesigenic dyskinesia: pathophysiological investigations. Epileptic Disord 1:187–193.

Lubbers WJ, Brunt ER, Scheffer H, et al. (1995) Hereditary myokymia and paroxysmal ataxia linked to chromosome 12 is responsive to acetazolamide. J Neurol Neurosurg Psychiatry 59:400–405.

Margari L, Perniola T, Illiceto G, et al. (2000) Familial paroxysmal exercise-induced dyskinesia and benign epilepsy: a clinical and neurophysiological study of an uncommon disorder. Neurol Sci 21:165–172.

Marini C, Guerrini R (2007) The role of the nicotinic acetylcholine receptors in sleep-related epilepsy. Biochem Pharmacol 74:1308–1314.

Mount LA, Reback S (1940) Familial paroxysmal choreoathetosis: preliminary report on a hitherto undescribed clinical syndrome. Arch Neurol Psychiatry 44:841–847.

Oldani A, Zucconi M, Ferini-Strambi L, et al. (1996) Autosomal dominant nocturnal frontal lobe epilepsy: electroclinical picture. Epilepsia 37:964–976.

Ophoff RA, Terwindt GM, Vergouwe MN, et al. (1996) Familial hemiplegic migraine and episodic ataxia type-2 are caused by mutations in the Ca^{2+} channel gene *CACNL1A4*. Cell 87:543–552.

Rainier S, Thomas D, Tokarz D, et al. (2004) Myofibrillogenesis regulator 1 gene mutations cause paroxysmal dystonic choreoathetosis. Arch Neurol 61:1025–1029.

Smith LA, Heersema PH (1941) Periodic dystonia. Mayo Clin Proc 16:842–846.

Suls A, Dedeken P, Goffin K, et al. (2008) Paroxysmal exercise-induced dyskinesia and epilepsy is due to mutations in SLC2A1, encoding the glucose transporter GLUT1. Brain 131:1831–1844.

Szepetowski P, Rochette J, Berquin P, et al. (1997) Familial infantile convulsions and paroxysmal choreoathetosis: a new neurological syndrome linked to the pericentromeric region of human chromosome 16. Am J Hum Genet 61:889–898.

Tomita H, Nagamitsu S, Wakui K, et al. (1999) Paroxysmal kinesigenic choreoathetosis locus maps to chromosome 16p11.2-q12.1. Am J Hum Genet 65:1688–1697.

Valente EM, Spacey SD, Wali GM, et al. (2000) A second paroxysmal kinesigenic choreoathetosis locus (EKD2) mapping on 16q13-q22.1 indicates a family of genes which give rise to paroxysmal disorders on human chromosome 16. Brain 123:2040–2045.

van Rootselaar AF, van Westrum SS, Velis DN, et al. (2009) The paroxysmal dyskinesias. Pract Neurol 9:102–109.

Weber YG, Lerche H (2009) Genetics of paroxysmal dyskinesias. Curr Neurol Neurosci Rep 9:206–211.

Weber YG, Storch A, Wuttke TV, et al. (2008) GLUT1 mutations are a cause of paroxysmal exertion-induced dyskinesias and induce hemolytic anemia by a cation leak. J Clin Invest 118:2157–2168.

20

Psychiatric Aspects of the Neurodegenerative Choreas

Mark Walterfang, MBBS (Hons), FRANZCP;
Andrew Evans, MBBS, MD, FRANZCP; and
Dennis Velakoulis, MBBS, MPM, FRANZCP, DipCrim

INTRODUCTION

Role of the Striatum in Behavioral and Neuropsychiatric Illness

Choreiform disorders invariably involve pathological change to the basal ganglia. In addition to the abnormal movements, there are often behavioral and psychiatric abnormalities as well as cognitive impairment. Historically, neurologists have generally focused on the external, motor manifestations of disease as opposed to the psychological and neurocognitive aspects of illness. This is despite the fact that the psychiatric and cognitive impairments may be as disabling for the patients as the motor disturbances, and may be the most problematic aspect of the patient's care for relatives and carers (Rosenblatt and Leroi, 2000). As knowledge and understanding of the pathophysiology of these diseases has advanced in recent decades, so too has the understanding of the inextricable association of neurological and psychiatric impairments in choreiform disorders. It is increasingly recognized that many disorders present initially as behavioral changes or frank psychiatric illness prior to the onset of motor symptoms. Concomitantly, our understanding of the nonmotor functions of the basal ganglia has advanced considerably as our knowledge of the corticosubcortical circuitry of the brain—and the motor, cognitive, and emotional functions they subserve—has evolved.

The basal ganglia consist of the caudate nucleus and putamen (collectively known as the "striatum"), globus pallidus, subthalamic nucleus, substantia nigra, and nucleus accumbens (Alheld et al., 1990). Cortical association areas are linked by multiple loops that run through the basal ganglia and thalamus and then return to the cortex. Each of the five main loops or circuits (motor, oculomotor, cognitive, associative, and limbic) receives multiple cortical inputs, which are integrated and project to a restricted thalamic region and then to a single cortical region (Alexander et al., 1986). A significant proportion of these project to the prefrontal cortex (PFC), including motor, associative, and limbic cortical regions. These loops are not anatomically separate, and as a result, cognitive, motor, and emotional loops can interact in the striatum to modulate each other's output to the cortex (Kimura and Matsumoto, 1997). For this reason, disorders that affect the basal ganglia generally do not discriminate between these circuits and tend to present with comorbid cognitive, motor, and emotional disturbances.

Within the striatum, the putamen appears to be involved in simple motor behaviors of limited flexibility, such as habit learning and stimulus–response associations, whereas the caudate nucleus is involved in action–outcome contingencies (where behavioral selection is based on knowledge and expected outcome and reward of the behavior), thus subserving goal-directed decision making (Grahn et al., 2008). Disorders that affect the striatum as a whole are thus likely to lead to the combination of features that characterizes many of the choreiform disorders; the codevelopment of movement disorder, cognitive impairment, and neuropsychiatric illness.

HUNTINGTON DISEASE

Huntington disease (HD) is a well-characterized neuropsychiatric disorder that very frequently presents with psychiatric illness comorbidly with, or preceding, the neurological features of the disorder (Chapter 3). This autosomal dominant trinucleotide repeat disease affects the huntingtin (*HTT*) gene on the short arm of chromosome 4. The mutant form of HTT (*mHTT*) in HD causes loss of neurons in particular brain regions, especially the caudate and putamen and, to a lesser extent, the substantia nigra, hippocampus, cerebellum, and cerebral cortex. This results in the characteristic behavioral, cognitive, and motor symptoms of the disease. HD is the archetypal neuropsychiatric basal ganglia disorder. Not only does it present with significantly elevated rates of major psychiatric illness, but its autosomal dominant pattern of inheritance—and the resulting 50% likelihood of siblings and offspring of a proband being affected by an untreatable, degenerative, and highly penetrant genetic disorder—results in a devastating psychosocial burden on the HD patient and his or her family members.

The onset of HD (symptomatic HD) is generally accepted to be the point when the patient exhibits neurological symptoms or signs such as chorea or cognitive decline. Since the first description of HD by Dr. George Huntington, behavioral, emotional, and psychiatric symptoms have been seen as core features of the illness but are not considered to constitute illness onset–defining symptoms. A large clinical research literature has identified increased prevalence of depression, psychosis, and obsessive–compulsive disorder (OCD) in patients with HD; but it remains unclear whether the psychiatric symptoms seen in asymptomatic patients (i.e., without motor or cognitive features) are due to the illness or to psychosocial, family, and environmental factors. Following the identification of the genetic mutation in 1993, it has been possible to investigate the prevalence of psychiatric syndromes in asymptomatic and symptomatic gene carriers. An understanding of the prevalence of psychiatric syndromes in HD provides important clinical information for clinicians caring for patients with HD and may inform our understanding of the neurobiological correlates of psychiatric conditions.

It is important to appreciate that two methodological approaches have been used to examine psychiatric morbidity in HD—a categorical and a dimensional approach. The categorical approach aims to ascertain psychiatric diagnoses, while the dimensional approach is interested in psychiatric symptoms. These differing methods may account for differences between studies; for example, a study assessing patients for a major depressive disorder may find a different prevalence of major depression compared to a study assessing the same subjects on a depression rating scale or using self-report scales that rate depression and anxiety such as the Symptom Checklist-90 (SCL-90). This issue has been highlighted by van Duijn and colleagues (2007), who undertook a review of psychopathology in HD using defined criteria for study selection and could identify only seven studies which met their strict criteria. The findings of this review are discussed in the following sections on psychopathology in symptomatic patients.

The Psychiatric Sequelae of Predictive Testing

Prior to the introduction of predictive genetic testing for HD, there was anxiety within the HD community that such testing would lead to psychiatric illness and even suicide as people found out they were gene mutation–positive. It is now well-recognized that the development of international guidelines for the genetic testing process in HD (International Huntington Association, 1994) has contributed to the development of high-quality programs for those at risk and their families (Tibben, 2007) and has been important in minimizing adverse psychiatric morbidity. A 1999 study identified that 44 of 4,527 (0.97%) people who participated in predictive HD testing had either completed suicide ($n = 5$) or attempted suicide ($n = 21$) or had a psychiatric hospitalization ($n = 18$) following an HD predictive test result (Almqvist et al., 1999). The risk was greatest in those with a positive test result, symptoms at the time of diagnosis, or preexisting psychiatric illness and those who were unemployed. Since this original study, follow-up studies of predictive testing outcomes have identified higher rates of depression in asymptomatic carriers followed up for periods ranging 2–5 years (Almqvist et al., 2003; Gargiulo et al., 2009; Larsson et al., 2006), though it is difficult to tease out the effects of the testing result from the effects of illness progression as the follow-up period increases.

Psychopathology in Presymptomatic Gene Carriers

Do asymptomatic HD gene mutation–positive people exhibit a higher prevalence of psychiatric diagnoses or symptoms? If so, is this increased prevalence a function of their genetic carrier status, the effect of psychosocial factors, or a combination of the two? Studies have sought to disentangle these issues by examining subjects known to be at risk and comparing those who turn out to be gene mutation–positive (gene carriers) vs. those who are gene mutation–negative. This approach assumes that psychosocial factors equally affect both groups and that differences in symptom prevalence are attributable to genetic/biological factors rather than psychosocial or environmental factors. Given that early neurobiological changes are likely to be associated with subtle psychiatric, personality, or emotional changes, it might be predicted that such symptoms would predate neurological and cognitive symptoms and would become more prevalent as an individual nears the onset of neurological symptoms.

Several studies have compared gene carriers to at-risk noncarriers for psychiatric symptoms, to identify whether such symptoms increase the closer the gene carrier is to onset of neurological symptoms. In a study of 681 at-risk subjects (589 gene carriers), gene carriers exhibited more symptoms than gene-negative subjects on the SCL-90 (depression, anxiety, obsessive–compulsiveness). Additionally, gene-positive subjects with more neurological symptoms exhibited more psychiatric symptoms (Duff et al., 2007). A study of 254 subjects (83 gene carriers) identified more psychiatric symptoms in five domains of the SCL-90 (obsessive–compulsive, anxiety, psychoticism, paranoid ideation, interpersonal sensitivity) and more depressive symptoms on a self-reported depression rating (Marshall et al., 2007). Julien et al. (2007) studied 204 at-risk subjects (89 gene carriers) and followed up 51 gene carriers to ascertain the relationship between depressive symptoms and the onset of neurological symptoms. This study identified more depressive symptoms in gene carriers compared to noncarriers and an increase in depression as gene carriers approached the onset of neurological symptoms. A Dutch study which used a categorical approach to assess 210 at-risk Dutch subjects (154 gene carriers) for *Diagnostic and Statistical Manual of*

Mental Disorders, fourth edition (DSM-IV), diagnoses identified increased major depression and OCD in both presymptomatic and symptomatic carriers compared to the general population (van Duijn et al., 2008). Symptomatic carriers had a greater prevalence of nonaffective psychosis.

These studies suggest that HD gene carriers exhibit a greater prevalence of psychiatric symptoms, particularly affective disturbances, before the onset of neurological symptoms. The prevalence of such symptoms increases as the neurological onset is approached, and they appear more likely to be related to the presence of the mutation rather than psychosocial or environmental factors. The early onset of psychiatric symptoms, predating neurological or cognitive symptoms, can be conceptualized as a reflection of early subcortical pathology with involvement of nonmotor regions. While CAG repeat length has been posited as a marker of illness severity, no relationship has been identified between psychiatric symptoms and CAG repeats in subjects undertaking predictive testing (Berrios et al., 2001; Weigell-Weber et al., 1996; Zappacosta et al., 1996). Ongoing longitudinal studies of asymptomatic gene carriers will shed further light on the trajectory of psychiatric, neurological, cognitive, and neuroanatomical changes in HD (Duff et al., 2007).

Psychopathology in Symptomatic Gene Carriers

Possibly the most rigorous review of the literature regarding psychopathology in gene carriers concluded that "their results (of the studies to date in HD) are impossible to compare and . . . reliable prevalence estimates cannot be made" (van Duijn et al., 2007). As an example of the variation in estimates, it has been estimated that 35%–95% of HD patients will have a major psychiatric disorder (affective disorders, schizophrenia-like disorder, OCD, personality disorders) or psychiatric symptoms (e.g., apathy, irritability, aggression, lability) (Craufurd et al., 2001; Woodcock, 1999; Paulsen et al., 2001). Any review of this literature must therefore bear in mind the methodological pitfalls in comparing across different studies.

Psychiatric Hospital Admissions

A study of HD patients and their first- and second-degree relatives based on admissions to Danish psychiatric hospitals between 1969 and 1991 found that HD patients, but not their relatives, had higher rates of psychiatric admissions. 65% of HD patients had at least one psychiatric admission with the diagnoses falling into three main groups; psychoses (schizophreniform, paranoid, and delusional), alcoholism, and other (Jensen et al., 1993).

Depression and Suicide

The link between depression and subcortical disease has been in part based on the finding that depression is increased in patients with subcortical neurodegenerative disorders such as HD and Parkinson disease. One of the earliest studies in the modern era involved a survey of 88 patients in the United States using DSM-III criteria for diagnosis. This study identified that 41% of HD patients were diagnosed with a major affective disorder (32% major depression, 9% bipolar disorder), which had preceded the development of chorea in two-thirds of patients (Folstein and Folstein, 1983). Affective disorder appeared to run in certain families within this cohort. The authors estimated that an at-risk young adult with a history of severe depression within this cohort had "considerably more than 50% likelihood of developing manifest HD." A 2001 review of studies to that time included 16 studies and identified a prevalence of 30% for depression in HD, together with a high rate of suicide (Slaughter et al., 2001). Using strict criteria for the studies selected, a review of six studies identified a prevalence of depressed mood of 33%–69% (van Duijn et al., 2007).

A study of 2,835 HD gene carriers using the United Huntington's Disease Rating Scale (UHDRS) identified that sad mood, low self-esteem, and anxiety were present in 41%, 25%, and 41% of the sample, respectively (Paulsen et al., 2005). Half of the sample had sought treatment for depression, and one-tenth reported at least one suicide attempt. The sample was divided into five illness stages based on a functional capacity scale (stage 1, least functional capacity; stage 5, greatest functional capacity). The highest prevalence of depressive symptoms was identified in gene carriers at stage 2 of illness, with reducing depressive symptoms in stages 3–5. The authors put forward three explanations for this finding; (1) missing data in patients with advanced illness, (2) increased cognitive deficits and reduced insight in later stages, and (3) adaptation to illness. The use of caregiver ratings has been proposed as a complementary assessment method to patient ratings in advanced stages of illness (Chatterjee et al., 2005).

An Italian study of at-risk subjects used psychiatric rating scales to assess 40 symptomatic gene carriers, 17 asymptomatic gene carriers, and 28 non-gene carriers; symptomatic patients had the highest prevalence of psychiatric symptoms, including depression. There was, however, no relationship between illness duration or CAG repeat number and psychiatric symptoms in the symptomatic group. The asymptomatic patients were no different from the non-gene carrier group (Soliveri et al., 2002).

Not all studies have identified an increased rate of depressive symptoms in symptomatic gene carriers compared to non-gene carriers. Shiwach and Norbury (1994) studied 20 asymptomatic gene carriers and found no difference in psychiatric symptoms between the patient group, 33 at-risk non-gene carriers, and 43 control subjects. The same authors in a retrospective study of 30 HD families (75 patients alive, 35 dead) found a lifetime prevalence of depression of 39%, with schizophrenia in 9% and significant personality changes in 72% (Shiwach, 1994). These authors concluded that depression or schizophrenia without organic personality changes or neurological symptoms was unlikely to be part of the early prodrome of HD (Shiwach, 1994).

In a Swiss study of 79 HD patients, 63% of patients met author-defined criteria for a psychiatric diagnosis: depression (15%), psychosis (13%), and personality change (35%) (Weigell-Weber et al., 1996). Seven of the 10 patients with a psychotic illness had had psychotic symptoms prior to the development of chorea. Three of the 12 patients (3.8% of the entire sample) with severe depression had attempted suicide. CAG repeat length was not associated with the development or severity of psychiatric symptoms in two studies.

While many studies have relied on self-reported symptoms or rating scales, a Greek study assessed HD patients with a semistructured psychiatric assessment, the Structured Clinical Interview for DSM-IV Disorders (SCID), together with information collected from multiple sources, to arrive at lifetime psychiatric disorder diagnoses (Vassos et al., 2008). A lifetime diagnosis of affective disorder, psychotic disorder, or anxiety disorder was identified in 47%, 17%, and 17% of patients, respectively, with 61% of the total sample showing a lifetime history of a formal psychiatric disorder (14 cases had more than one lifetime diagnosis). There was no relationship between CAG repeat length and the probability of developing a psychiatric disorder or the severity of the disorder. A second study using DSM-IV criteria compared psychopathology in patients with neurodegenerative disorders and identified that 43% of HD patients were diagnosed with a mood disorder (Leroi et al., 2002).

While the literature is limited by the differing methods of assessment, the available evidence supports the idea that depression and depressive symptoms are prevalent in HD gene carriers and that gene carriers are more likely to exhibit such symptoms than at-risk noncarriers. The high prevalence of depression may thus be due to neurobiological vulnerability factors in gene carriers, interacting with psychological and psychosocial factors. The counterintuitive finding that depressive symptoms reduce with illness stage (Paulsen et al., 2005) would be consistent with a neurobiological basis for depression in that more severe neurodegeneration and cognitive decline is associated with greater cognitive deficits, more frontal disinhibition, and less insight.

The pathophysiology of depression in HD and related disorders may relate to a disrupted limbic circuit in HD, which connects the amygdala and anterior cingulate with the ventral striatum and the medial and ventral lateral PFC, and the cognitive circuit, which connects the caudate head with the lateral PFC (Lafer et al., 1997). Disrupted connections between the PFC and ventral striatum may be core to the functional impairments in major depression (Drevets, 1998; Elliot et al., 1997), and disruption to these loops in HD may produce the vulnerable substrate that interacts with psychosocial stressors to result in depressive illness.

Anxiety Disorders

Anxiety disorders have not been a major focus of research in HD and tend to be reported in the context of other psychopathology, particularly depression.

In six studies which have reported anxiety symptoms in HD gene carriers, the prevalence ranged 28%–61% (Craufurd et al., 2001; Kulisevsky et al., 2001; Murgod et al., 2001; Paulsen et al., 2001, 2005; Pflanz et al., 1991). It is unclear, however, whether these high prevalence rates relate to psychological and psychosocial consequences of the illness or to an underlying neurobiological vulnerability to anxiety states.

Obsessive–Compulsive Disorder/Symptoms

Most studies in HD have identified obsessional or compulsive symptoms in patients rather than clusters of symptoms which meet the diagnostic criteria for OCD. One of the earliest such reports identified obsessional symptoms in 7/102 HD patients (Dewhurst et al., 1969). A more recent study of 3,964 individuals at risk for HD found that the prevalence of obsessive–compulsive symptoms increased threefold by the later stages of illness compared to the prevalence in asymptomatic subjects (Beglinger et al., 2007). The same authors subsequently described an increase in obsessive–compulsive symptoms in asymptomatic HD gene carriers compared to at-risk non-gene carriers (Beglinger et al., 2008). In another large study nearly one-quarter of 960 patients had obsessional or compulsive symptoms on the original presentation to a specialist clinic (Marder, 2000). A study of 27 HD patients found that over half described obsessive or compulsive symptoms and that these patients had greater executive dysfunction on neuropsychological assessment (Anderson et al., 2001).

Cases of OCD in HD have been rarely reported. Cummings and Cunningham (1992) reported two cases of OCD in patients with HD, one with a cleaning compulsion and the other with a smoking compulsion. De Marchi et al. (1998) reported an Italian pedigree of 16 subjects in which three were diagnosed with OCD and one with pathological gambling.

Psychosis

Early studies from 1970–1987 identified prevalence rates for psychosis in patients with HD of 0%–12% within defined geographical populations in Scotland (Bolt, 1970), Sweden (Mattsson, 1974), the United Kingdom (Oliver, 1970), and the United States (Folstein et al., 1987). The review of four carefully selected studies by van Duijn et al. (2008) found a prevalence range of 3%–11% for psychotic symptoms but with small sample sizes in three of these four studies. The largest study included 52 HD gene carriers and used an inventory of neuropsychiatric symptoms to identify symptoms within the month prior to assessment. Delusions and hallucinations were identified in 12% and 2% of patients, respectively (Paulsen et al., 2001). Other, more recent studies have identified rates of psychosis of 9%–17%. Seventeen percent of patients had a lifetime diagnosis of a psychotic disorder in a study using the SCID (Vassos et al., 2008), 13% were defined as psychotic in a study using author-defined criteria (Weigell-Weber et al., 1996), and 9% were defined as psychotic in a study relying on retrospective diagnoses (Shiwach, 1994). Taking these studies together and acknowledging the variability in the methods for ascertainment of psychosis, the prevalence of psychosis in patients with HD (approximately 10%) is greater than that within the general population (about 1%).

The clustering of psychosis within HD families has been described in at least two studies. In an Italian pedigree, all known cases of HD ($n = 4$) developed a schizophrenia-like psychosis at least 5 years prior to the onset of neurological or cognitive features of HD (Correa et al., 2006). A North American study of 44 patients with HD found that 45% (9/20) of the gene carriers diagnosed with a psychosis had a first-degree relative with a psychotic illness compared to 9% (2/21) of the gene carriers who had no history of a psychotic illness. A younger onset of psychosis was correlated with a greater number of CAG repeats (Tsuang et al., 2000). These authors speculate on possible reasons for the association, including the possibility that modifying genes may interact with the HD gene to predispose to the development of psychosis in these families (Tsuang et al., 2000). Alternatively, the proposal has been put forward that the HD gene acts in some way to lower the threshold for the emergence of schizophrenia (Correa et al., 2006).

HUNTINGTON DISEASE-LIKE DISORDERS

The Huntington disease-like (HDL) disorders 1–4 present as phenocopies of HD and should be considered in patients who present with the clinical picture of HD but do not exhibit the HD mutation. HDL4 has been molecularly identified as spinocerebellar ataxia 17 and is discussed later (see "Spinocerebellar Ataxias").

HDL1

HDL1 has been described in one Swedish family as an autosomal dominant disorder associated with a 192-nucleotide repeat expansion in the prion protein (PRP) gene (Moore et al., 2001; Xiang et al., 1998) (Chapter 11). This was associated with depression, aggression, and personality change, as precursors to rigidity, chorea, dysarthria, and basal ganglia atrophy, which eventually progressed to dementia (Xiang et al., 1998). A similar PRP expansion–related illness presentation had previously been described in a French pedigree, with presentation of major psychiatric illness (schizophrenia or bipolar disorder) in the third decade, followed by dementia, dystonia, and ataxia (Laplanche et al., 1999). Chorea has been associated with PRP repeat expansions in other pedigrees (Collinge et al., 1992; Poulter et al., 1992).

HDL2

Like HD, HDL2 is an autosomal dominant, neurodegenerative condition with clinical features of chorea and cognitive decline (Chapter 5). HDL2 is due to a CTG expansion in the junctophilin-3 gene (*JPH3*) on chromosome 16q24.3 (Holmes et al., 2001; Margolis et al., 2001). The mutation has been identified in patients of black African ancestry (Holmes et al., 2001) and is estimated to account for up to 15% of patients with an HDL condition who do not carry the HD mutation (Margolis et al., 2004). Brain imaging reveals significant striatal atrophy, and neuropathologically patients demonstrate prominent neurodegeneration and gliosis in the caudate and putamen, with lesser degenerative changes in the substantia nigra and pallidum and little in the way of changes in the thalamus or cortex (Margolis et al., 2001; Rudnicki et al., 2008).

The pedigree described by Margolis et al. (2001) had psychiatric symptoms including depression, anxiety, and psychosis in addition to more dysexecutive behaviors including apathy, perseveration, irritability, and eventually dementia. All four cases described in a Brazilian series exhibited some psychiatric symptoms including depression ($n = 2$), aggression ($n = 2$), and hallucinations ($n = 1$) (Rodrigues et al., 2008). In all four cases the psychiatric symptoms became apparent years after the onset of a movement disorder. Two of the five cases in the series described by Walker et al. (2003) had depressive symptoms together with dementia, and a movement disorder. Neither of the two patients described in a French study exhibited psychiatric symptoms, though one was described as showing frontal behavior (Stevanin et al., 2003). One of the three patients described in a South African pedigree, with illness identified over three generations, exhibited psychotic symptoms late in the illness, having presented earlier with cognitive decline, aggression, and movement disorder; one other patient presented with disinhibition and aggression, and all three ultimately developed dementia (Bardien et al., 2007).

HDL3

HDL3 has been described in an Arabian family as an autosomal recessive disorder associated with an abnormality on chromosome 4p15.3. The onset is in childhood (3–4 years of age) and is associated with cognitive decline, dystonia, dysarthria, ataxia, and pyramidal signs, and frontostriatal atrophy on magnetic resonance imaging (MRI) (Al-Tahan et al., 1999; Kambouris et al., 2000). The juvenile onset of disease, as opposed to early adulthood, makes a psychiatric presentation unlikely in this disorder (Walterfang et al., 2006b).

BENIGN HEREDITARY CHOREA

Benign hereditary chorea (BHC) is an autosomal dominant disorder with typical onset before the age of 5 but extending into adolescence, which has been associated with a mutation in the *TITF-1* gene on chromosome 14 (Breedveld et al., 2002b) (Chapter 4). The symptoms of BHC are characteristically choreic jerks, although the spectrum of the phenotype varies considerably even within families (Kleiner-Fisman and Lang, 2007). Psychiatric symptoms are not prominent (Mahajnah et al., 2007; Breedveld et al., 2002a; Hageman et al., 1996; Devos et al., 2006), although anxiety and depression (Loosmore and Wood, 1988) and psychosis (Glik et al., 2008) have been described. The psychiatric symptoms have generally responded to symptomatic treatment.

More recently, two Japanese families with adult-onset, autosomal dominant chorea without dementia were identified and shown to exhibit linkage to chromosome 8q (Shimohata et al., 2007). The authors named this condition "BHC type 2" (BHC2). Only one of the 12 patients identified by the authors had a psychiatric history, a woman who developed depression at age 65.

CHOREA-ACANTHOCYTOSIS

The neuroacanthocytoses are a group of disorders that present with neurological and psychiatric manifestations and acanthocytes, spiculated red blood cells. Chorea-acanthocytosis (ChAc, MIM 200150) is an autosomal recessive disorder associated with mutations or deletions in the *VPS13A* gene on chromosome 9q, which codes for the membrane protein chorein (Rampoldi et al., 2002; Ueno et al., 2001) (Chapter 6). Chorein is strongly expressed in the brain (Dobson-Stone et al., 2002). Loss of chorein particularly affects the basal ganglia, especially the caudate nucleus and putamen but also the ventrolateral substantia nigra and globus pallidus (Hardie et al., 1991). Onset of neurological problems in ChAc is usually between ages 25 and 45, commonly with limb and orobuccal chorea.

Significant psychopathology is common in ChAc patients, occurring in up to 60% (Danek et al., 2004; Hardie et al., 1991; Walterfang et al., 2008); and frank psychiatric illness may precede the onset of frank neurological symptoms in some cases by up to a decade (Sorrentino et al., 1999; Walterfang et al., 2008). In the original series of 19 individuals described by Hardie et al. (1991), the most prominent psychiatric feature was behavioral and cognitive change (apathy, disinhibition, poor judgment and planning), consistent with hypofrontality, in more than half the patients who were later genetically confirmed to have ChAc. However, numerous authors have reported typical symptoms of OCD in ChAc patients, including recurrent intrusive thoughts (obsessions) and compulsions regarding checking, cleanliness, symmetry, and hoarding (Bohlega et al., 2003; Bruneau et al., 2003; Habermeyer et al., 2006; Lossos et al., 2005; Muller-Vahl et al., 2007; Robertson et al., 2008; Saiki et al., 2004; Walterfang et al., 2008). The characteristic mutilation of the lips and tongue has also been conceptualized along the OCD spectrum as a pure motor compulsion (Walker et al., 2006). We reviewed the published cases of ChAc up to 2006, and of 38 patients on whom data were available, 16 presented with psychiatric symptoms at the time of illness diagnosis, with eight of these presenting initially with psychiatric symptoms. Patients presenting initially with psychiatric diagnoses had a mean interval between psychiatric and neurological presentation of more than 10 years (Walterfang et al., 2008). Approximately half of these patients presented initially with OCD. Limited treatment data suggest that serotonergic medication can be effective in the treatment of OCD in ChAc patients (Habermeyer et al., 2006; Walterfang et al., 2008).

Schizophrenia-like psychosis presents less commonly than OCD-type illness in ChAc, with only a small number of reported cases (Bohlega et al., 2003; Bruneau et al., 2003; Muller-Vahl et al., 2007; Rodrigues et al., 2009; Takahashi et al., 1983; Yamada et al., 2009). In the majority of these, the psychotic illness predated the onset of neurological symptoms by months or years, usually with schizophrenia-like symptoms such as auditory hallucinations and bizarre and/or persecutory delusions, with the ultimate diagnosis becoming apparent as frank chorea, epilepsy, and dementia supervened. Significant executive dysfunction has been described as occurring in a majority of ChAc patients as the illness progresses (Hardie et al., 1991; Kartsounis and Hardie, 1996; Walterfang et al., 2008), in addition to impairments in speed of processing and memory (Danek et al., 2001b), eventually leading to a frontosubcortical dementia (Hardie et al., 1991; Kartsounis and Hardie, 1996).

Given that the most significant neuronal loss in ChAc occurs in the caudate and putamen, it is not surprising that the disruption of frontal–subcortical loops involving these two structures can largely explain the behavioral syndromes that occur in individuals with ChAc. Disruptions in three of the five main frontal–subcortical loops, which originate in the frontal lobe and project to the striatum (caudate and putamen), the globus pallidus, and substantia nigra and then to specific thalamic nuclei (with a final link back to the frontal lobe), are known to result in significant behavioral disturbance (Bonelli and Cummings, 2007). Disruption to the dorsolateral–prefrontal loop, which projects from Brodmann areas 9 and 10 to the dorsal head of the caudate nucleus, results in typical executive dysfunction, seen in >50% of ChAc cases. This is likely to correlate with impairment in planning, shifting behavioral set, reasoning, sustaining attention, and mental flexibility (Tekin and Cummings, 2002). Similarly, disruption to the orbitofrontal loop, projecting from areas 10 and 11 (orbitofrontal) to the ventromedial caudate nucleus, results in impaired behavioral inhibition, poor social judgment, and demonstration of utilization behavior (Tekin and Cummings, 2002). Finally, disruption to the anterior cingulate circuit, which originates from the cingulate cortex (Brodmann area 24) and projects to the ventromedial caudate and ventral putamen, results in apathy, lack of drive and initiative, and reduced spontaneous speech and movement (Tekin and Cummings, 2002). These three behavioral syndromes have been well-described in large ChAc series (Hardie et al., 1991; Walterfang et al., 2008).

The high rate of OCD in ChAc (Walterfang et al., 2008) suggests that disruption of these frontal–subcortical loops in ChAc plays a significant role in the genesis of OCD-like symptoms. The head of the caudate, particularly affected in ChAc (Henkel et al., 2007), plays a key role in the lateral orbitofrontal loop (LOFL), where it serves to integrate information from the anterior cingulate, orbitofrontal, and dorsolateral PFC to determine the behavioral and motor programs that occur to resolve conflict or facilitate decision making (Aouizerate et al., 2004; Chamberlain et al., 2005). The role of the basal ganglia in this loop may be to "allow incentive-related signals from the limbic system to help determine whether and when a movement (or nonmotor function) should be performed" (Graybiel and Kimura, 1995). Disruptions to this loop appear to relate to the symptoms in OCD patients, with impaired decision making due to alterations to LOFL transmission being at the core of this deficit in OCD patients (Cavedini et al., 2006; Sachdev and Malhi, 2005).

The pure motor compulsions seen in many ChAc cases (which may include the oral mutilation that occurs in many patients [Walker et al., 2006]) may result from direct caudate pathology, leading to a behavioral dysregulation of simple motor acts (as opposed to complex cognitive–motor acts). This may be akin to the behavioral dysregulation that is felt to be the basis for compulsions in primary OCD (Chamberlain et al., 2005). The magnitude of striatal volume loss seen at illness onset in ChAc patients and the number that present with OCD-like symptoms in adolescence and early adulthood suggest that caudate atrophy predates the onset of illness by a number of years and may interfere with the normal developmental maturation of the LOFL. Unlike some other prefrontal functions such as event anticipation and volitional execution of delayed responses—which have largely completed development by mid-childhood—the circuitry of response inhibition continues to develop through adolescence and early adulthood (Rosenberg and Keshavan, 1998). While the caudate reaches its maximal volumetric size by age 10 (Lenroot and Giedd, 2006), related frontostriatal circuits show increasing activation with age during tasks of cognitive control, including medial frontal–orbitofrontal–caudate circuit activation during selective motor response inhibition (Rubia et al., 2006). This age-related increase in activation (but not volume) of the caudate and connected structures may reflect the ongoing maturation of interconnections between frontostriatal structures. If the development of the underlying circuitry of this response inhibition is interrupted or slowed, then it is conceivable that reduced motor inhibition—and thus motor compulsions—could result.

Schizophrenia-like presentations have been less frequently reported, although psychotic depression has been observed (R. H. Walker, personal communication). It is likely that ChAc patients would be predisposed to psychosis as a result of frontostriatal pathology (Pantelis et al., 1992). While the striatal loss in ChAc cannot be directly compared to the neurochemical and microstructural changes observed in schizophrenia, loss of caudate neurons may disrupt crucial processing of striatal–limbic information (Parent and Hazrati, 1993) and lead to psychotic symptoms in some ChAc patients.

MCLEOD SYNDROME

Like ChAc, McLeod syndrome (MLS, MIM 314850) is one of the neuroacantho-cytoses. MLS is an X-linked multisystem disorder that results from mutations to the *XK* gene (Jung et al., 2001) (Chapter 7), characterized by absent Kx red blood cell antigens, weak expression of Kell red blood cell antigens, peripheral blood acanthocytosis, and elevated creatine kinase levels. Affecting predominantly males (although female carriers can show mild symptoms), onset is usually between the ages of 25 and 60, with a mean of 40, often significantly later than that in ChAc (Danek et al., 2001a; Rampoldi et al., 2002). In addition to other neurological and nonneurological features, MLS patients often develop a range of psychiatric symptoms (Danek et al., 2001a; Jung et al., 2001).

XK and Kell are both expressed in tissues affected by MLS, including the brain, heart, and muscle. Only a few neuropathological cases have been described, which report a ChAc-like neuronal loss in the basal ganglia, most dramatic in the caudate and putamen (Brin et al., 1993; Hardie et al., 1991; Rinne et al., 1994). Cell loss in the basal ganglia is reflected on neuroimaging, often with marked caudate atrophy and increased T2 signal intensity in the lateral putamen (Danek et al., 1994; Dotti et al., 2000; Jung et al., 2001; Miranda et al., 2007; Oeschner et al., 2001; Takashima et al., 1994; Zeman et al., 2005), reduced striatal D_2 binding (Danek et al., 1994; Oeschner et al., 2001), and hypometabolism of the basal ganglia and frontal lobes (Dotti et al., 2000), suggesting that striatal cell loss significantly impairs frontostri-atal circuitry. That cortical changes occur in MLS has been suggested by one mag-netic resonance spectroscopic study of cortical regions in five affected MLS patients (four with a psychiatric diagnosis) and five female carriers, which showed altered *N*-acetylaspartate to creatine/choline ratios in the frontal and medial temporal cortex and thalamus in affected patients (Dydak et al., 2006). However, limited neuro-pathological studies suggest an absence of cortical neuronal loss (Rinne et al., 1994), suggesting that functional cortical changes are secondary to striatal neuronal loss.

More than 80% of patients present with neuropsychiatric illness at some stage during their illness course (Danek et al., 2001a), and much like in ChAc, the two most common illness presentations are of schizophrenia-like psychosis and OCD. Neuropsychiatric presentations often predate chorea and other neurological mani-festations in MLS, which may occur later in the illness course (Danek et al., 2001a; Hewer et al., 2007). OCD-like syndromes have been reported by a number of authors (Miranda et al., 2007; Oeschner et al., 1996; Vazquez and Martinez, 2009; Zeman et al., 2005) and have been described as comorbid with both psycho-sis (Oeschner et al., 1996) and major depression (Vazquez and Martinez, 2009).

Psychotic disorders have been reported at the same, if not a greater, frequency in MLS compared to OCD, with cases of schizophrenia being reported where the typical thought disorder, persecutory delusions, and auditory hallucinations preceded the onset of chorea by some years (Danek et al., 2001a; Jung and Haker, 2004; Miranda et al., 2007). As with other basal ganglia disorders, there is a tendency to diagnose choreiform disorders after exposure to antipsychotic medication as tardive dyskinesia (TD), which potentially delays the diagnosis of MLS and has led some authors to suggest that patients with suspected TD be screened routinely for MLS (Jung and Haker, 2004). A number of other related psychotic disorders have been described, including schizoaffective disorder, bipolar disorder, and schizotypal personality disorder (Dydak et al., 2006; Jung et al., 2001). Schizophrenia-like psychosis in MLS has been reported to respond to both typical and atypical antipsychotics (Jung and Haker, 2004; Miranda et al., 2007).

The intimate relationship between the striatal pathology and both OCD and schizophrenia is best illustrated by the report of two MLS-affected brothers, one of whom presented with a psychotic illness and the other with typical OCD (Miranda et al., 2007). This suggests that the striatal changes that occur in MLS may interact with other biological diatheses for both OCD and schizophrenia to result in these disorders in susceptible individuals and may not be sufficient alone to cause major psychiatric illness. Other, more common psychiatric illnesses have also been reported in MLS, including depression and anxiety disorders (Jung et al., 2001). However, given the high base rate in the population for these disorders, at this stage there is no evidence that they represent more than a chance co-occurrence with MLS.

In common with other frontostriatal disorders such as ChAc and HD, executive dysfunction is common in MLS and often presents as behavioral dysfunction (Danek et al., 2001a; Jung et al., 2001). Impaired executive function has also been described in neurologically unaffected female carriers (Jung et al., 2001). One patient presented initially with a frontotemporal dementia–like syndrome, with significant hoarding of car parts, tools, and rubbish; increasing behavioral disorganization; and disinhibition with indifference prior to the onset of chorea (Zeman et al., 2005). The prevalence of significant dysexecutive syndromes in MLS patients, combined with neuroimaging evidence (Dotti et al., 2000), reinforces the crucial role of frontostriatal circuits in modulating behavior and the impact on this circuitry if one crucial node in the network is disrupted.

DENTATORUBROPALLIDOLUYSIAN ATROPHY

Dentatorubropallidoluysian atrophy (DRPLA) is a disease caused by triplet repeat expansion of the atrophin gene on chromosome 12p13.31 (Koide et al., 1994) (Chapter 12). The clinical features of this rare disorder are largely restricted to small case series and case reports, the majority from the Japanese literature. A 1987 publication cited by Koide et al. (1994) describes two siblings with schizophrenic symptoms, including delusions and hallucinations, described in the Japanese literature (Naito et al., 1987). Four cases of Japanese patients presenting with a psychotic illness have been described (Adachi et al., 2001) and represent 10%–15% of the total number of patients with DRPLA treated in two national psychiatric hospitals. The age range at presentation with psychotic symptoms was 28–46 years. All exhibited persecutory delusions, one exhibited auditory hallucinations, and another described a delusional mood. The psychotic symptoms generally disappeared with neuroleptic medication and progressive cognitive decline. A single Japanese case report describes a 59-year-old woman with a 31-year history of involuntary movement disorder, ataxia, and unspecified psychiatric disorders (English-only abstract available [Konagaya et al., 2002]). A review of cases within the Japanese literature concluded that psychosis is found in about 10% of patients with DRPLA (Adachi et al., 2001).

Cases of DRPLA outside the Japanese literature have come from the United States and Wales. A report of an American kindred (Potter et al., 1995) described the index case as a 43-year-old man presenting with dementia and psychiatric symptoms including delusions and hallucinations, diagnosed with an organic psychosis. While the kindred included 14 affected family members, the report provided clinical information on only four of the subjects. None of the other three family members was described as having psychiatric symptoms.

Haw River syndrome was reported in five generations of an African American North Carolina family and was caused by the same triplet repeat abnormality as is found in DRPLA (Burke et al., 1994). Psychiatric symptoms are noted as being common, but the nature of these symptoms is not detailed in the relevant publications.

Of 17 affected family members from four families in south Wales (Wardle et al., 2008), three presented with psychiatric features, although the details of only two are provided. One presented at age 42 with severe depression and overdoses, while a second patient presented at age 29 with a primary psychiatric diagnosis requiring hospitalization and developed progressive neurological symptoms over a 20-year period.

Overall, the literature suggests that patients with DRPLA may present with psychotic symptoms, though there are insufficient cases and clinical descriptions to be certain of the nature of the association.

WILSON DISEASE

Wilson disease (WD) is an autosomal recessive disorder affecting 1 to 4/100,000 people. It is caused by a mutation in the *ATP7B* gene, coding for a protein important for copper transport. The mutated gene leads to copper accumulation in the liver, brain, kidney, and skeletal system caused by reduced excretion of copper in the bile (Ala et al., 2007). Symptoms usually appear between the ages of 6 and 20 years, but cases in much older patients have been described. Free copper precipitates in the kidneys, eyes, and brain, particularly the putamen and globus pallidus (de Bie et al., 2007). In half of the patients, computerized tomography reveals characteristic hypodensity in the basal ganglia (Williams and Walshe, 1981); virtually all show abnormalities on MRI, including T2-weighted hyperintensity in the thalamus, brainstem, and lenticular nuclei (Roh and Lee, 1994). Functional imaging generally shows significant hypometabolism in the lenticular nuclei (Hawkins et al., 1987).

Approximately one-third of WD patients initially present with hepatic disease, one-third with neurological symptoms, and one-third with psychiatric symptomatology. Between one- and two-thirds of WD patients report psychiatric symptoms at the time of initial presentation (Akil et al., 1991; Dening, 1991; Schwartz et al., 1993)—the same proportion seen in the case series published by Wilson almost 100 years ago (Wilson, 1912). At any one time, up to one-half of patients have current psychiatric symptoms (Rathbun, 1996) and in up to one-half of patients seen initially by a psychiatrist, an organic cause for their presentation was not suspected (Dening and Berrios, 1989). In one cross-sectional study of treated and clinically stable patients, 72% were reported to have at least one neuropsychiatric symptom present on screening with the NeuroPsychiatric Inventory (NPI); anxiety, depression, and apathy were the most frequently reported symptoms (Svetel et al., 2001). Another prevalence study of 50 confirmed patients, using the SCID, found a prevalence of axis I illness of 24%; all patients suffered a mood disorder, two-thirds of these being bipolar disorder (Shanmugiah et al., 2008). Suicidal behavior, impulse-control disorders, and substance-use disorders can also occur (Akil et al., 1991). Psychiatric manifestations may significantly affect treatment compliance (Dening, 1991).

Four symptom clusters have been identified in WD; mood and affective change, behavior and personality change, psychosis, and cognitive impairment (Dening, 1985). Personality changes, particularly irritability and aggression, are very common (Akil et al., 1991; Portala et al., 2001b). Mood disturbance, including both depression and mania, appears to be the most common neuropsychiatric illness (Akil et al., 1991; Dening and Berrios, 1990; Medalia and Scheinberg, 1989; Srinivas et al., 2008). The high prevalence of depression, occurring in up to 20% of patients, is in keeping with McHugh's model of basal ganglia disorders as "triadic" and presenting with the "3 Ds": dyskinesia, dementia, and depression (McHugh, 1989; Rosenblatt and Leroi, 2000). Depressive symptoms in WD appear to correlate with regional serotonin transporter availability in the basal ganglia (Eggers et al., 2003; Hesse et al., 2003).

Psychosis, delusional states, and catatonia, while less frequent, can be extremely disabling (Akil et al., 1991; Dening, 1985, 1991; Dening and Berrios, 1989, 1990).

While delusions in WD have been noted to be uncommon (Dening and Berrios, 1989), more recently a number of psychotic presentations meeting the criteria for delusional disorder have been reported (Sagawa et al., 2003; Spyridi et al., 2008; Stiller et al., 2008; Wichowicz et al., 2006). Given the high rate of OCD in some other basal ganglia disorders, it is notable that this has been reported only once in association with WD (Kumawat et al., 2007).

Deteriorating academic performance or work function is a key feature of neurological WD due to a range of cognitive deficits. Neurologically symptomatic patients display a range of difficulties, including impairments of frontal–executive ability, aspects of memory, and visuospatial processing (Isaacs-Glaberman et al., 1989; Medalia et al., 1988; Rathbun, 1996). In contrast, no such deficits are found in neurologically asymptomatic patients (Seniow et al., 2002). Lesions within the basal ganglia seem to be of central importance in cognitive change (Portala et al., 2001a; Seniow et al., 2002), given their interruption of frontal–subcortical circuits, as previously described.

After initiating treatment with chelation therapy, the disease often stabilizes or improves; but disease progression under treatment is more likely for neuropsychiatric than for hepatic symptoms (Merle et al., 2007). Resolution of neuropsychiatric illness with chelation has been reported (Machado et al., 2008; Srinivas et al., 2008; Stiller et al., 2008; Walter and Lyndon, 1997).

Little evidence exists to guide the clinician treating neuropsychiatric illness in WD. The use of neuroleptic medication has been seen as problematic because of the increased risk of movement disorder side effects in the setting of degenerative basal ganglia disease (Chroni et al., 2001; Hoogenraad, 1996; Tu, 1981; Varghese et al., 2008). However, some reports suggest relatively safe use of atypical medications such as olanzapine, risperidone, quetiapine, and clozapine, which each have a low propensity to cause movement disorders (Chroni et al., 2001; Krim and Barroso, 2001; Kulaksizoglu and Polat, 2003; Spyridi et al., 2008). These agents should be used with caution because of the increased risk of agranulocytosis in the presence of hypersplenism or penicillamine treatment. Treatment of mania with mood stabilizers can be difficult as valproate and carbamazepine may be contraindicated in the presence of significant hepatic impairment (Varghese et al., 2008). Lithium may be contraindicated in the presence of renal tubular acidosis (Varghese et al., 2008), although successful lithium treatment without metabolic compromise has been reported (Kulaksizoglu and Polat, 2003; Longanathan et al., 2008). Electroconvulsive therapy (ECT) has been successfully used in cases of catatonia (Rodrigues et al., 2004), psychosis (Shah and Kumar, 1997), and depression (Chan et al., 2004; Negro and Louza Neto, 1995; Sechi et al., 2006). Depression has been reported to respond to both tricyclic antidepressants and selective serotonin reuptake inhibitors (Chan et al., 2004; Keller et al., 1999; Sechi et al., 2006), although treatment resistance to traditional antidepressants has been described (Sechi et al., 2006), as has a manic switch in response to antidepressant therapy in one patient (Keller et al., 1999).

SPINOCEREBELLAR ATAXIAS

The spinocerebellar ataxias (SCAs) include a group of autosomal dominant, neurodegenerative conditions causing cerebellar ataxia and a spectrum of associated features, including hyperkinetic movement disorders such as chorea (Chapter 12). SCA17 (HDL4) causes cognitive decline and neuropsychiatric features and is the most common cause of an HD phenocopy syndrome in European populations. The majority of SCAs present with neuropsychological impairment typical of a subcortical dementia (Bonelli and Cummings, 2008; Geschwind, 1999; Kish et al., 1994) or depression and personality change (Leroi et al., 2002). In a large series of 139 patients with cerebellar degeneration seen through a neurogenetics service, 75% of whom had a neurological diagnosis of SCA, 41% presented with psychopathology and 30% with cognitive impairment (Liszewski et al., 2004). Cognitive changes may reflect disruptions to cerebrocerebellar circuitry and corticostriatal–thalamocortical circuitry (Kawai et al., 2009). Psychopathology is likely reflective of the crucial role that the cerebellum plays in executive functioning and regulation of the mental state as there is evidence of abnormality of cerebellar functioning in affective and psychotic illness (Andreasen et al., 1999; Schmahmann, 2004). Additionally, because of their autosomal dominant inheritance, the psychological issues that relate to predictive testing also apply to the SCAs (Broadstock et al., 2000); adverse consequences are rare (Goizet et al., 2002), and patients may have both positive and negative responses to test results, with the nature of the response being often independent of the test result itself (Smith et al., 2004). A study of SCA1 patients found no increase in distress at 1-year follow-up (Abe and Itoyama, 1997); for SCA2 patients, both carriers and noncarriers were shown to have reduced anxiety and depression rates posttesting (Paneque et al., 2007a,b).

SCA1

SCA1 is an autosomal dominant, progressive, neurodegenerative disorder caused by the expansion of a CAG repeat in the *ATXN1* gene located on chromosome 6p22-p23 (Orr et al., 1993). Clinical features of SCA1 are ataxia, pyramidal signs, ophthalmoplegia, and variable degrees of brainstem dysfunction (Namekawa et al., 2001; Orr et al., 1993). The symptoms usually begin during the third or fourth decade of life, and then the disease gradually worsens, often resulting in complete disability and death 10–20 years after onset. Movement disorders, including chorea, are occasionally observed in SCA1 (Chung et al., 1993; Namekawa et al., 2001; Ranum et al., 1991; Skinner et al., 1997; Zoghbi et al., 1991).

Neuropathological findings in SCA1 include loss of Purkinje cells and variable loss of granule cells in the cerebellar cortex, neuron loss and moderate gliosis in the dentate nuclei, neuron loss and severe gliosis in the inferior olives and the pontine nuclei, loss of neurons and pigment deposition in the substantia nigra, and variable involvement of the putamen, globus pallidus, and subthalamic nucleus, while the cerebral cortex appears normal (Kawai et al., 2009). On metabolic neuroimaging, SCA1 patients exhibit hypoperfusion of the cerebral cortex, caudate nucleus, putamen, and thalamus, as well as cerebellum and brainstem.

The profile of cognitive impairment in SCA1 consists of prominent executive dysfunction and impairments of verbal memory consistent with a type of frontal–subcortical dementia and appears to be contingent on disruption of the cerebro-cerebellar circuitry. A comparison of cognitive dysfunction among SCA1, SCA2, and SCA3 patients indicates that executive dysfunction is most prominent in SCA1 patients (Burk et al., 2003). Depressive and memory symptoms have also been found in 25% and 42% of SCA1 patients, respectively. Variants in the SCA1 gene have been associated with schizophrenia, although schizophrenia itself has not been associated with confirmed SCA1. In 55 schizophrenia multiplex families there was linkage disequilibrium between schizophrenia and SCA1 CAG repeat alleles within the normal size range (Wang et al., 1996). The S186C amino acid variant was shown to be present in a number of schizophrenia cases in a small cohort, in addition to other variants and polymorphisms (Pujana et al., 1997). Additionally, a CAG repeat polymorphism was found to be overrepresented in schizophrenia in a case–control study (Joo et al., 1999). These preliminary findings suggested that variants in the SCA1 gene may be a susceptibility factor for developing schizophrenia, and this was borne out in a scan of 64 candidate genes in major mental illness (Fallin et al., 2005). This led to a model of schizophrenia being a trinucleotide repeat disorder (Vincent et al., 2000), but the search for a trinucleotide expansion cause has remained fruitless (Fortune et al., 2003).

SCA2

Mutations in the *ATXN2* gene cause SCA2 (Pulst et al., 1996). Individuals carrying an expanded CAG repeat show early truncal ataxia and dysarthria, and most exhibit slowed saccades. Chorea and supranuclear ophthalmoparesis were observed in individuals in three of six families (Geschwind et al., 1997). Dementia seems to represent an independent part of the SCA2 phenotype; one-quarter of SCA2 subjects in one series showed evidence of dementia. However, even in nondemented SCA2 subjects, verbal memory and executive function are impaired (Burk et al., 1999, 2003; Le Pira et al., 2002). Depression with psychotic features responsive to lithium has been reported in SCA2 (Hering et al., 2009).

One case was reported of a patient with SCA2 who developed schizophrenia 10 years before neurological presentation, including ataxia and chorea, suggesting basal ganglia involvement (Rottnek et al., 2008).

SCA17

SCA17 is an autosomal dominant disorder caused by a CAG/CAA expansion in the *TBP* gene on chromosome 6q27 (Stevanin and Brice, 2008). About 20% of SCA17 cases present with chorea, and it is the most common cause of an HD phenocopy (Wild and Tabrizi, 2007). SCA17 has a significant degree of phenotypic variability, presenting not just with ataxia but also with parkinsonism and HD-like presentations (Lasek et al., 2006; Stevanin and Brice, 2008). MRI reveals atrophy not just of medial cerebellar structures but also of the basal ganglia (Lasek et al., 2006).

In a review of the reported cases, psychiatric disorder was identified in 67% (36 of 54 cases). A U.K. study of patients with SCA17 identified psychiatric symptoms in 27% of cases (Craig et al., 2005). In a study of 1,318 patients with a spinocerebellar phenotype, 16 were identified with SCA17 (Rolfs et al., 2003). The authors identified psychiatric symptoms in seven patients, who exhibited a range of psychiatric symptoms including aggression ($n = 3$), psychosis ($n = 3$), depression ($n = 2$), and mania ($n = 1$). One patient presented with depression then hallucinations, diagnosed as schizophrenia, at age 40, while another family member presented at age 23 with hallucinations and manic symptoms, which were present over a 12-year period.

A family described by Bruni et al. (2004) consisted of 16 affected members who exhibited a frontal dementia–like picture prior to the onset of ataxia. The patients presented with a range of frontal behaviors—poor insight (100%), personality changes (100%), apathy (56%), poor personal hygiene (38%), reduced verbal fluency (88%), attentional deficits (44%), distractibility (44%), poor judgment (56%), irritability/violence (31%)—and psychiatric symptoms—anxiety (44%), depression (38%), delusions (19%), auditory hallucinations (12%). The authors noted some differences compared to other SCA17 families, including a slow course of illness, which on average lasted 30 years.

A series of smaller case reports and series have identified psychiatric symptoms in families with SCA17. A Belgian pedigree (Fujigasaki et al., 2001) of six affected family members included four who presented with paranoid psychosis, hypersexuality, aggression, or euphoria. One of the case reports detailed a 37-year-old man who presented with a paranoid psychosis, hypersexuality, and aggression and was admitted to a psychiatric hospital. The psychotic symptoms abated as cognitive and neurological decline progressed. Kanai et al. (2007) reported a patient who presented with a psychotic illness that responded to sodium valproate at age 58, 2 years after the onset of neurological symptoms. Three of nine patients in a study of German and Austrian patients with SCA17 were reported to have psychiatric symptoms, though the nature of these was not specified (Bauer et al., 2004). Other case series have identified three siblings presenting between the ages of 37 and 45 with depression and aggression or personality changes early in the course of illness (Schneider et al., 2006) and an Italian family with a high prevalence of psychiatric symptoms (Maltecca et al., 2003).

SCA27

A mutation in the fibroblast growth factor 14 gene (*FGF14*) on chromosome 13q34 has been shown in one large kindred to lead to early-onset tremor, orofacial dyskinesia, and slowly progressive cerebellar ataxia. Intelligence was below average in affected individuals, and anxiety and depressive symptoms were common (Brusse et al., 2006).

PANTOTHENATE KINASE–ASSOCIATED NEURODEGENERATION

Pantothenate kinase–associated neurodegeneration (PKAN) is a rare autosomal recessive disorder with iron accumulation in the basal ganglia, due to mutations in the *PANK2* gene (Chapter 8). *PANK2* encodes a pantothenate kinase, the key regulatory enzyme in coenzyme-A synthesis (Zhou et al., 2001). The neuroradiological hallmark of the "eye of the tiger sign" is characterized by bilateral areas of hyperintensity within a region of hypointensity in the median globus pallidus on T2-weighted brain MRI (Savoiardo et al., 1993). Two main phenotypes have been identified; classic PKAN manifests in the first decade, with severe hyperkinetic movements and progresses rapidly with loss of ambulation within 15 years from onset; and atypical PKAN, with onset in the second to third decade, a less severe movement disorder, slower progression, and maintenance of independent ambulation well after 15 years of disease (Hayflick et al., 2003). Other symptoms include dysarthria, dystonia, rigidity, and corticospinal signs.

   Cognitive decline is frequent in PKAN (Dooling et al., 1974; Pellecchia et al., 2005; Sachin et al., 2009; Thomas et al., 2003). Cognitive function can vary from normal to markedly impaired, with earlier-onset patients being more severely affected (Freeman et al., 2007). The pattern of cognitive impairment often implicates executive function and attention (Marelli et al., 2005), and impairment may predate motor signs (Cooper et al., 2000). Psychiatric signs, such as behavioral disturbances (Hayflick et al., 2003), OCD (Nardocci et al., 1994; Nicholas et al., 2005), tic disorders (Scarano et al., 2002), psychosis (Öner et al., 2003), and depression (Morphy et al., 1989), are common, occurring in up to half of patients (Thomas et al., 2003).

ACERULOPLASMINEMIA

In aceruloplasminemia (AC), an autosomal recessive disorder occurring in 1 in 2 million nonconsanguineous births (Miyajima et al., 1999), mutations in the ceruloplasmin (*CP*) gene result in absent ferroxidase activity of ceruloplasmin, leading to deposition of iron in the central nervous system (CNS), retina, pancreatic cells, liver, spleen, and ovaries (Hellman and a Gitlin, 2002; Yoshida et al., 1995) (Chapter 10). The major sites of CNS iron deposition in AC are the basal ganglia, cerebellar dentate nuclei, red nucleus, thalamus, and hippocampus (Miyajima, 2003).

In keeping with the known sites of iron deposition, the major clinical features of AC consist of retinal degeneration, diabetes mellitus, and a neurological disorder, usually presenting in the fifth or sixth decade. The neurological picture is characterized by dystonia and subcortical dementia (Nittis and Gitlin, 2002). MRI typically shows marked T2 hypointensity in the regions of maximal iron deposition (Daimon et al., 1999; Grisoli et al., 2005; Morita et al., 1995). Subtle posterior white matter tract hyperintensity may also be seen. When spin-echo sequences that are most sensitive to the magnetic susceptibility effects of iron are used, very subtle superficial cerebral and cerebellar cortical hypointensity may also be detectable (Grisoli et al., 2005). White matter tract changes may reflect a disconnection of projecting fibers from key relay nuclei such as the thalamic nuclei, with subsequent subtle cortical changes (Grisoli et al., 2005).

Cognitive impairment is the presenting feature in up to one-half of patients (McNeill et al., 2008), and ultimately most AC patients develop a subcortical dementia in the fifth decade or beyond (Miyajima, 2003). This is characterized by typical executive dysfunction, including difficulty in switching set, apathy, perseveration, and impulsivity (Fasano et al., 2008; Miyajima et al., 2005; Walterfang et al., 2006a), in addition to significant cognitive slowing (Walterfang et al., 2006a). This has been associated with frontal hypometabolism (Miyajima et al., 2005; Walterfang et al., 2006a). The executive impairment in AC may be the result of impairment to both frontostriatal and frontocerebellar circuitry, given the striatal and cerebellar locations of iron deposition and the possible loss of efferents from the basal ganglia and dentate nuclei of the cerebellum (Miyajima et al., 2005). Only one case of major psychiatric illness associated with AC has been reported, with a typical schizophrenia-like psychosis in a young, neurologically asymptomatic woman known to have AC, who presented with a decline in self-care, persecutory delusions, and auditory hallucinations (Walterfang et al., 2006a).

NEUROFERRITINOPATHY

Neuroferritinopathy (NF), also known as "neurodegeneration with brain iron accumulation type 2" (NBIA2), is due to mutations in the ferritin light chain gene

(*FTL1*) and presents in the fourth to sixth decades with chorea, dystonia, or rigidity-bradykinesia (Curtis et al., 2001) (Chapter 9). Affected regions of the brain—particularly the globus pallidus but also the striatum—contain iron- and ferritin-positive spherical inclusions, often colocalizing with microglia, oligodendrocytes, and particularly neurons (Hautot et al., 2007). Excess brain iron accumulation is apparent on MRI, with a characteristic loss of T2 signal initially within the red nucleus and substantia nigra and progressing to involve the dentate nucleus, putamen, globus pallidus, thalamus, caudate nucleus, and PFC (Chinnery et al., 2007).

Only a small number of NF cases have been described, making the true prevalence of neuropsychiatric abnormalities unclear. Cognitive impairment seems to occur in most patients and typically follows a frontostriatal pattern of impairments. Disinhibition and emotional lability often present in early stages, with other executive impairments such as reduced verbal fluency progressing over decades, ultimately resulting in a subcortical dementia (Chinnery et al., 2007; Willis et al., 2002), which may progress to akinetic mutism (Ohta et al., 2007). The psychiatric illnesses that have been associated with NF have been psychotic disorders. One adolescent patient presented with neuroleptic-responsive psychosis comorbid with ataxia and rigidity-bradykinesia, although he had a family history of schizophrenia in a nonaffected uncle (Maciel et al., 2005). One other patient presented with severe generalized dystonia at the age of 22 and in his mid-30s developed a delusional jealousy of his partner that did not respond to neuroleptics (Mir et al., 2005).

TREATMENT OF PSYCHIATRIC SYMPTOMS IN CHOREA

Treatment of psychiatric problems in choreiform disorders is relatively uncomplicated in that the treatments that are used for psychosis, mood disorders, OCD, and other illnesses are those used in primary psychiatric illness, with a few caveats (Rosenblatt and Leroi, 2000). The clinician dealing with choreiform disorders needs to be vigilant for the presence of psychiatric illness as untreated major mental disorders can add considerably to functional impairment of the patient and carer burden. While it occurs less commonly than psychosis or mania, depression is commonly underdiagnosed, particularly if the patient has difficulty in communicating or if the debilitating neurological symptoms result in clinicians and carers labeling a depressive illness as "understandable." Additionally, differentiation of depressive illness from apathy and social withdrawal can often be difficult; evaluation of accompanying symptoms that may be indicative of neurovegetative disturbance, such as changes in appetite, sleep or agitation, may be helpful.

Depressive illnesses generally respond well to antidepressant treatment, particularly with the more recent classes of antidepressants. These have increasing specificity for enhancing serotonergic transmission but less of the anticholinergic and antihistaminic effects of older antidepressants (which may worsen cognitive impairment), as well as a very wide therapeutic index. As in patients with a major depressive illness in the absence of a neurological condition, full remission is sometimes only effected with the addition of antipsychotic medication. ECT can be a very effective treatment for otherwise treatment-resistant illness in patients with choreiform disorders (Kennedy et al., 2003; Ranen et al., 1994). For patients with secondary mania, the use of sodium valproate or carbamazepine is preferred (Rosenblatt and Leroi, 2000).

The treatment of psychosis can be more problematic in choreiform disorders as these predominantly dopamine-blocking agents do not readily discriminate between motor and nonmotor aspects of the striatum. Small-dose, high-potency neuroleptics (usually those with a high dopamine D_2 receptor affinity such as haloperidol and risperidone) are useful in suppressing chorea and may also be effective antipsychotics; however, when dosages need escalation to control psychotic symptoms, worsening parkinsonism may cause significant motor problems, particularly in gait and mobility, increasing the risk of falls. Use of newer agents with less D_2 receptor blockade, in addition to 5-hydroxytryptamine 2 (5-HT2) receptor blockade, may be preferable (Fernandez and Friedman, 1999). Medications such as olanzapine and quetiapine (alone or occasionally in combination) can often be used to provide adequate treatment of psychosis without significant worsening of motor symptoms.

Limited evidence exists on the treatment of compulsive disorders, but the authors (in addition to scattered reports in the literature) have found that serotonergic medications are helpful in reducing compulsive behaviors and movements in some patients. There is an increased risk of worsening chorea and parkinsonism in patients with vulnerable basal ganglia circuitry (Jimenez-Jimenez and Molina, 2000), but this usually responds to careful dose titration. For irritability, agitation, and stereotyped behaviors, the use of antidepressants, antipsychotics, and mood stabilizers can be helpful. Treatment of apathy is much more problematic as stimulant medication often worsens motor symptoms in these disorders.

SUMMARY

For many of the disorders described in this chapter, only limited data exist as to the true rate of comorbid major psychiatric illness. However, the prevalence and rate of psychiatric problems in many of these disorders suggest that processes that significantly disrupt frontostriatal function in adulthood eventually progress to a subcortical dementia. In many cases, this is presaged by major psychiatric illness. Psychosis, depression, and OCD appear to be the most common presenting illnesses, with at least one of these being reported to occur at a greater-than-expected rate in each of the disorders described. Disruptions to particular frontostriatal loops, and the resultant disruptions to prefrontal function, appear to result not only in cognitive disturbances in the neurodegenerative choreas but also in elevated rates of neuropsychiatric illness.

REFERENCES

Abe K, Itoyama Y (1997) Psychological consequences of genetic testing for spinocerebellar ataxia in the Japanese. Eur J Neurol 4:593–600.

Adachi N, Arima K, Asada T, Kato M, Minami N, Goto Y, et al. (2001) Dentatorubralpallidoluysian atrophy (DRPLA) presenting with psychosis. J Neuropsychiatry Clin Neurosci 13:258–260.

Akil M, Schwartz JA, Dutchak D, Yuzbasiyan-Gurkan V, Brewer GJ (1991) The psychiatric presentations of Wilson's disease. J Neuropsychiatry Clin Neurosci 3:377–382.

Ala A, Walker AP, Ashkan K, Dooley JS, Schilsky ML (2007) Wilson's disease. Lancet 369:397–408.

Alexander G, de Long M, Strick P (1986) Parallel organisation of functionally segregated circuits linking basal ganglia and cortex. Annu Rev Neurosci 9:357–381.

Alheld G, Himer L, Switzer R (1990) Basal ganglia. In: Paxinos G (ed.) The Human Nervous System. Academic Press, New York, pp 483–582.

Almqvist EW, Bloch M, Brinkman R, Craufurd D, Hayden MR (1999) A worldwide assessment of the frequency of suicide, suicide attempts, or psychiatric hospitalization after predictive testing for Huntington disease. Am J Hum Genet 64:1293–1304.

Almqvist EW, Brinkman RR, Wiggins S, Hayden MR (2003) Psychological consequences and predictors of adverse events in the first 5 years after predictive testing for Huntington's disease. Clin Genet 64:300–309.

Al-Tahan A, Divakaran M, Kambouris M, Bohlega S, Salih M, Ogunniyi A, et al. (1999) A novel autosomal recessive "Huntington's disease-like" neurodegenerative disorder in a Saudi family. Saudi Med J 20:85–89.

Anderson KE, Louis ED, Stern Y, Marder KS (2001) Cognitive correlates of obsessive and compulsive symptoms in Huntington's disease. Am J Psychiatry 158:799–801.

Andreasen N, Nopoulos P, O'Leary D, Miller D, Wassink T, Flaum M (1999) Defining the phenotype of schizophrenia: cognitive dysmetria and its neural mechanisms. Biol Psychiatry 46:908–920.

Aouizerate B, Guehl D, Cuny E, Rougier A, Biolac B, Tignol J, et al. (2004) Pathophysiology of obsessive–compulsive disorder: a necessary link between phenomenology, neuropsychology, imagery and physiology. Prog Neurobiol 72:195–221.

Bardien S, Abrahams F, Soodyall H, van der Merwe L, Greenberg J, Brink T, et al. (2007) A South African mixed ancestry family with Huntington disease-like 2: clinical and genetic features. Mov Disord 22.

Bauer P, Laccone F, Rolfs A, Wullner U, Bosch S, Peters H, et al. (2004) Trinucleotide repeat expansion in SCA17/TBP in white patients with Huntington's disease-like phenotype. J Med Genet 41.

Beglinger LJ, Langbehn DR, Duff K, Stierman L, Black DW, Nehl C, et al. (2007) Probability of obsessive and compulsive symptoms in Huntington's disease. Biol Psychiatry 61:415–418.

Beglinger LJ, Paulsen JS, Watson DB, Wang C, Duff K, Langbehn DR, et al. (2008) Obsessive and compulsive symptoms in prediagnosed Huntington's disease. J Clin Psychiatry 69:1758–1765.

Berrios GE, Wagle AC, Markova IS, Wagle SA, Ho LW, Rubinsztein DC, et al. (2001) Psychiatric symptoms and CAG repeats in neurologically asymptomatic Huntington's disease gene carriers. Psychiatry Res 102.

Bohlega A, Al-Jishi A, Dobson-Stone C, Rampoldi L, Saha P, Murad H, et al. (2003) Chorea-acanthocytosis: clinical and genetic findings in three families from the Arabian peninsula. Mov Disord 18:403–407.

Bolt JM (1970) Huntington's chorea in the west of Scotland. Br J Psychiatry 116.

Bonelli R, Cummings J (2007) Frontal-subcortical circuitry and behavior. Dialog Clin Neurosci 9:141–151.

Bonelli R, Cummings J (2008) Frontal-subcortical dementias. Neurologist 14:100–107.

Breedveld GJ, Percy AK, MacDonald ME, de Vries BBA, Yapijakis C, Dure LS, et al. (2002a) Clinical and genetic heterogeneity in benign hereditary chorea. Neurology 59.

Breedveld GJ, van Dongen JWF, Danesino C, Guala A, Percy AK, Dure LS, et al. (2002b) Mutations in TITF-1 are associated with benign hereditary chorea. Hum Mol Genet 11.

Brin M, Hays A, Symmans W, Marsh W, Rowland L (1993) Neuropathology of McLeod phenotype is like chorea-acanthocytosis. Can J Neurol Sci 20:S234.

Broadstock M, Michie S, Marteau T (2000) Psychological consequences of predictive genetic testing: a systematic review. Eur J Hum Genet 8:731–738.

Bruneau M, Lesperance P, Chouinard S (2003) Schizophrenia-like presentation of neuro-acanthocytosis. J Neuropsychiatry Clin Neurosci 15:378–380.

Bruni AC, Takahashi-Fujigasaki J, Maltecca F, Foncin JF, Servadio A, Casari G, et al. (2004) Behavioral disorder, dementia, ataxia, and rigidity in a large family with TATA box-binding protein mutation. Arch Neurol 61.

Brusse E, de Koning I, Maat-Kievit A, Oostra BA, Heutink P, van Swieten JC (2006) Spinocerebellar ataxia associated with a mutation in the fibroblast growth factor 14 gene (SCA27): a new phenotype. Mov Disord 21:396–401.

Burk K, Globas C, Bosch S, Graber S, Abele M, Brice A, et al. (1999) Cognitive deficits in spinocerebellar ataxia 2. Brain 122:769–777.

Burk K, Globas C, Bosch S, Klockgether T, Zuhlke C, Daum I, et al. (2003) Cognitive deficits in spinocerebellar ataxia type 1, 2, and 3. J Neurol 250:207–211.

Burke JR, Wingfield MS, Lewis KE, Roses AD, Lee JE, Hulette C, et al. (1994) The Haw-River-syndrome—dentatorubropallidoluysian atrophy (DRPLA) in an African-American family. Nat Genet 7:521–524.

Cavedini P, Gorini A, Bellodi L (2006) Understanding obsessive–compulsive disorder: focus on decision-making. Neuropsychol Rev 16:3–15.

Chamberlain S, Blackwell A, Fineberg N, Robbins T, Sahakian B (2005) The neuropsychology of obsessive–compulsive disorder: the importance of failures in cognitive and behavioral inhibition as candidate endophenotypic markers. Neurosci Biobehav Rev 29:399–419.

Chan K, Cheung R, Au-Yeung K, Mak W, Cheng T, Ho S (2004) Wilson's disease with depression and parkinsonism. J Clin Neurosci 12:303–305.

Chatterjee A, Anderson KE, Moskowitz CB, Hauser WA, Marder KS (2005) A comparison of self-report and caregiver assessment of depression, apathy, and irritability in Huntington's disease. J Neuropsychiatry Clin Neurosci 17.

Chinnery P, Crompton D, Birchall D, Jackson M, Coulthard A, Lombes A, et al. (2007) Clinical features and natural history of neuroferritinopathy caused by the FTL1 460InsA mutation. Brain 130:110–119.

Chroni E, Lekka N, Tsirbri E, Economou A, Paschalis C (2001) Acute progressive akinetic-rigid syndrome induced by neuroleptics in a case of Wilson's disease. J Neuropsychiatry Clin Neurosci 13:531–532.

Chung MY, Ranum LP, Duvick LA, Servadio A, Zoghbi HY, Orr HT (1993) Evidence for a mechanism predisposing to intergenerational CAG repeat instability in spinocerebellar ataxia type I. Nat Genet 5:254–258.

Collinge J, Brown J, Hardy J, Mullan M, Rossor M, Baker H, et al. (1992) Inherited prion disease with 144 base pair gene insertion. 2. Clinical and pathological features. Brain 115:687–710.

Cooper G, Rizzo M, Jones R (2000) Adult-onset Hallervorden-Spatz syndrome presenting as cortical dementia. Alzheimer Dis Assoc Disord 14:120–126.

Correa BB, Xavier M, Guimaraes J (2006) Association of Huntington's disease and schizophrenia-like psychosis in a Huntington's disease pedigree. Clin Pract Epidemiol Ment Health 2.

Craig K, Keers SM, Walls TJ, Curtis A, Chinnery PF (2005) Minimum prevalence of spinocerebellar ataxia 17 in the north east of England. J Neurol Sci 239.

Craufurd D, Thompson JC, Snowden JS (2001) Behavioral changes in Huntington disease. Neuropsychiatry Neuropsychol Behav Neurol 14:219–226.

Cummings JL, Cunningham K (1992) Obsessive–compulsive disorder in Huntington's disease. Biol Psychiatry 31.

Curtis A, Fey C, Morris C, Bindoff L, Ince P, Chinnery P, et al. (2001) Mutation in the gene encoding ferritin light polypeptide causes dominant adult-onset basal ganglia disease. Nat Genet 28:350–354.

Daimon M, Moriai S, Susa S, Yamatani K, Hosoya T, Kato T (1999) Hypocaeruloplasminaemia with heteroallelic caeruloplasmin gene mutation: MRI of the brain. Neuroradiology 41:185–187.

Danek A, Rubio J, Rampoldi L, Ho M, Dobson-Stone C, Tison F, et al. (2001a) McLeod neuroacanthocytosis: genotype and phenotype. Ann Neurol 50:775–764.

Danek A, Sheesley L, Tierney M, Uttner I, Grafman J (2004) Cognitive and neuropsychiatric findings in McLeod syndrome and in chorea-acanthocytosis. In: Danek A (ed.) Neuroacanthocytosis Syndromes. Springer, Dordrecht, pp 95–116.

Danek A, Tierney M, Sheesley L, Grafman J (2001b) Cognitive findings in patients with chorea-acanthocytosis. Mov Disord 16:S30.

Danek A, Uttner I, Vogl T, Tatsch K, Witt T (1994) Cerebral involvement in McLeod syndrome. Neurology 44:117–120.

de Bie P, Muller P, Wijmenga C, Klomp LW (2007) Molecular pathogenesis of Wilson and Menkes disease: correlation of mutations with molecular defects and disease phenotypes. J Med Genet 44:673–688.

De Marchi N, Morris M, Mennella R, La Pia S, Nestadt G (1998) Association of obsessive–compulsive disorder and pathological gambling with Huntington's disease in an Italian pedigree: possible association with Huntington's disease mutation. Acta Psychiatr Scand 97.

Dening T (1985) Psychiatric aspects of Wilson's disease. Br J Psychiatry 147:677–682.

Dening T (1991) The neuropsychiatry of Wilson's disease: a review. Int J Psychiatry Med 21:135–148.

Dening TR, Berrios GE (1989) Wilson's disease. Psychiatric symptoms in 195 cases. Arch Gen Psychiatry 46:1126–1134.

Dening TR, Berrios GE (1990) Wilson's disease: a longitudinal study of psychiatric symptoms. Biol Psychiatry 28:255–265.

Devos D, Vuillaume I, de Becdelievre A, de Martinville B, Dhaenens C-M, Cuvellier J-C, et al. (2006) New syndromic form of benign hereditary chorea is associated with a deletion of *TITF-1* and *PAX-9* contiguous genes. Mov Disord 21.

Dewhurst K, Oliver J, Trick KL, McKnight AL (1969) Neuro-psychiatric aspects of Huntington's disease. Confin Neurol 31.

Dobson-Stone C, Danek A, Rampoldi L, Hardie R, Chalmers R, Wood N, et al. (2002) Mutational spectrum of the *CHAC* gene in patients with choreoacanthocytosis. Eur J Hum Genet 10:773–781.

Dooling E, Schoene W, Richardson EJ (1974) Hallervorden-Spatz syndrome. Arch Neurol 30:70–83.

Dotti M, Battisti C, Malandrini A, Federico A, Rubio J, Circiarello G, et al. (2000) McLeod syndrome and neuroacanthocytosis with a novel mutation in the XK gene. Mov Disord 15:1282–1284.

Drevets W (1998) Prefrontal cortical-amygdala metabolism in major depressions. Ann N Y Acad Sci 877:614–637.

Duff K, Paulsen JS, Beglinger LJ, Langbehn DR, Stout JC (2007) Psychiatric symptoms in Huntington's disease before diagnosis: the predict-HD study. Biol Psychiatry 62.

Dydak U, Mueller S, Sandor P, Meier D, Boesiger P, Jung H (2006) Cerebral metabolic alterations in McLeod syndrome. Eur Neurol 56:17–23.

Eggers B, Hermann W, Barthel H, Sabri O, Wagner A, Hesse S (2003) The degree of depression in Hamilton rating scale is correlated with the density of presynaptic serotonin transporters in 23 patients with Wilson's disease. J Neurol 250:576–580.

Elliot R, Baker S, Rogers R, O'Leary D, Paykel E, Frith C, et al. (1997) Prefrontal dysfunction in depressed patients performing a complex planning task: a study using positron emission tomography. Psychol Med 27:931–942.

Fallin M, Lasseter V, Avramopoulos D, Nicodemus K, Wolyniec P, McGrath J, et al. (2005) Bipolar I disorder and schizophrenia: a 440-single-nucleotide polymorphism screen of 64 candidate genes among Ashkenazi Jewish case-parent trios. Am J Hum Genet 77: 918–936.

Fasano A, Colosimo C, Miyajima H, Tonali P, Re T, Bentivoglio A (2008) Aceruloplasminemia: a novel mutation in a family with marked phenotypic variability. Mov Disord 23.

Fernandez H, Friedman J (1999) The role of atypical antipsychotics in the treatment of movement disorders. CNS Drugs 11:467–483.

Folstein SE, Chase GA, Wahl WE, McDonnell AM, Folstein MF (1987) Huntington disease in Maryland: clinical aspects of racial variation. Am J Hum Genet 41.

Folstein SE, Folstein MF (1983) Psychiatric features of Huntington's disease: recent approaches and findings. Psychiatr Dev 1.

Fortune M, Kennedy J, Vincent J (2003) Anticipation and CAG*CTG repeat expansion in schizophrenia and bipolar affective disorder. Curr Psychiatry Rep 5:145–154.

Freeman K, Gregory A, Turner A, Blasco P, Hogarth P, Hayflick S (2007) Intellectual and adaptive behavior functioning in pantothenate kinase–associated neurodegeneration. J Intell Disabil Res 51:417–426.

Fujigasaki H, Martin JJ, De Deyn PP, Camuzat A, Deffond D, Stevanin G, et al. (2001) CAG repeat expansion in the TATA box–binding protein gene causes autosomal dominant cerebellar ataxia. Brain 124.

Gargiulo M, Lejeune S, Tanguy M-L, Lahlou-Laforet K, Faudet A, Cohen D, et al. (2009) Long-term outcome of presymptomatic testing in Huntington disease. Eur J Hum Genet 17.

Geschwind D (1999) Focusing attention on cognitive impairment in spinocerebellar ataxia. Arch Neurol 56:20–22.

Geschwind DH, Perlman S, Figueroa CP, Treiman LJ, Pulst SM (1997) The prevalence and wide clinical spectrum of the spinocerebellar ataxia type 2 trinucleotide repeat in patients with autosomal dominant cerebellar ataxia. Am J Hum Genet 60:842–850.

Glik A, Vuillaume I, Devos D, Inzelberg R (2008) Psychosis, short stature in benign hereditary chorea: a novel thyroid transcription factor-1 mutation. Mov Disord 23.

Goizet C, Lesca G, Durr A (2002) Presymptomatic testing in Huntington's disease and autosomal dominant cerebellar ataxias. Neurology 59:1330–1336.

Grahn J, Parkinson J, Owen A (2008) The cognitive functions of the caudate nucleus. Prog Neurobiol 86:141–155.

Graybiel A, Kimura M (1995) Adaptive neural networks in the basal ganglia. In: Houk J, Davis J, Beiser D (eds.) Models of Information Processing in the Basal Ganglia. MIT Press, Cambridge, MA, pp 103–116.

Grisoli M, Piperno A, Chiapparini L, Mariani R, Savoirardo M (2005) MR imaging of cerebral cortical involvement in aceruloplasminemia. Am J Neuroradiol 26: 657–661.

Habermeyer B, Fuhr P, Hiss B, Alber C, Muller-Spahn F (2006) Obsessive–compulsive disorder due to neuroacanthocytosis treated with citalopram. Pharmacopsychiatry 39: 193–194.

Hageman G, Ippel PF, van Hout MS, Rozeboom AR (1996) A Dutch family with benign hereditary chorea of early onset: differentiation from Huntington's disease. Clin Neurol Neurosurg 98.

Hardie RJ. Pullon HW, Harding AE, Owen JS, Pires M, Daniels GL, et al. (1991) Neuroacanthocytosis. A clinical, haematological and pathological study of 19 cases. Brain 114(Pt 1A):13–49.

Hautot D, Pankhurst Q, Morris C, Curtis A, Burn J, Dobson J (2007) Preliminary observation of elevated levels of nanocrystalline iron oxide in the basal ganglia of neuroferritinopathy patients. Biochim Biophys Acta 1772:21–25.

Hawkins R, Mazziotta J, Phelps M (1987) Wilson's disease studied with FDG and positron-emission tomography. Neurology 37:1707–1711.

Hayflick SJ, Westaway SK, Levinson B, Zhou B, Johnson MA, Ching KH, et al. (2003) Genetic, clinical, and radiographic delineation of Hallervorden-Spatz syndrome. N Engl J Med 348:33–40.

Hellman N, Gitlin J (2002) Ceruloplasmin metabolism and function. Annu Rev Nutr 22:439–458.

Henkel K, Walterfang M, Velakoulis D, Danek A, Kassubek J (2007) Volumetric imaging in chorea-acanthocytosis. In: Danek A, Walker R, Saiki S (eds.) Neuroacanthocytosis Syndromes. Springer, Dordecht.

Hering S, Achmuller C, Kohler A, Poewe W, Schneider R, Boesch S (2009) Phenotype variability in spinocerebellar ataxia type 2: a longitudinal family survey and a case featuring an unusual benign course of disease. Mov Disord 24:774–777.

Hesse S, Barthel H, Hermann W, Murai T, Kluge R, Wagner A, et al. (2003) Regional serotonin transporter availability and depression are correlated in Wilson's disease. J Neural Trans 110:923–933.

Hewer E, Danek A, Schoser B, Miranda M, Reichard R, Castiglioni C, et al. (2007) McLeod myopathy revisited: more neurogenic and less benign. Brain 130:3285–3296.

Holmes SE, O'Hearn E, Rosenblatt A, Callahan C, Hwang HS, Ingersoll-Ashworth RG, et al. (2001) A repeat expansion in the gene encoding junctophilin-3 is associated with Huntington disease-like 2. Nat Genet 29.

Hoogenraad T (1996) Wilson's Disease. Saunders, London.

International Huntington Association and the World Federation of Neurology Research Group on Huntington's Chorea (1994) Guidelines for the molecular genetics predictive test in Huntington's disease. J Med Genet 31.

Isaacs-Glaberman K, Medalia A, Scheinberg I (1989) Verbal recall and recognition abilities in patients with Wilson's disease. Cortex 25:353–361.

Jensen P, Sorensen SA, Fenger K, Bolwig TG (1993) A study of psychiatric morbidity in patients with Huntington's disease, their relatives, and controls. Admissions to psychiatric hospitals in Denmark from 1969 to 1991. Br J Psychiatry 163.

Jimenez-Jimenez F, Molina J (2000) Extrapyramidal symptoms associated with selective serotonin reuptake inhibitors, epidemiology, mechanisms and management. CNS Drugs 14:367–379.

Joo E, Lee J, Cannon T, Price R (1999) Possible association between schizophrenia and a CAG repeat polymorphism in the spinocerebellar ataxia type 1 (SCA1) gene on human chromosome 6p23. Psychiatr Genet 9:7–11.

Julien CL, Thompson JC, Wild S, Yardumian P, Snowden JS, Turner G, et al. (2007) Psychiatric disorders in preclinical Huntington's disease. J Neurol Neurosurg Psychiatry 78.

Jung H, Haker H (2004) Schizophrenia as a manifestation of X-linked McLeod-neuroacanthocytosis syndrome. J Clin Psychiatry 65:722–723.

Jung H, Hergersberg M, Kneifel S, Alkadhi H, Schiess R, Weigell-Weber M, et al. (2001) McLeod syndrome: a novel mutation, predominant psychiatric manifestions, and distinct striatal imaging findings. Ann Neurol.

Kambouris M, Bohlega S, Al-Tahan A, Meyer BF (2000) Localization of the gene for a novel autosomal recessive neurodegenerative Huntington-like disorder to 4p15.3. Am J Hum Genet 66.

Kanai K, Sakakibara R, Uchiyama T, Liu Z, Yamamoto T, Ito T, et al. (2007) Sporadic case of spinocerebellar ataxia type 17: treatment observations for managing urinary and psychotic symptoms. Mov Disord 22:441–443.

Kartsounis L, Hardie R (1996) The pattern of cognitive impairments in neuroacanthocytosis. Arch Neurol 53:77–80.

Kawai Y, Suenaga M, Watanabe H, Sobue G (2009) Cognitive impairment in spinocerebellar degeneration. Eur Neurol 61:257–268.

Keller R, Torta R, Lagget M, Crasto S, Bergamasco B (1999) Psychiatric symptoms as late onset of Wilson's disease: neuroradiological findings, clinical features and treatment. Ital J Neurol Sci 20:49–54.

Kennedy R, Mittal D, O'Jile J (2003) Electroconvulsive therapy in movement disorders: an update. J Neuropsychiatry Clin Neurosci 15:407–421.

Kimura M, Matsumoto N (1997) Neuronal activity in the basal ganglia. Functional implications. Adv Neurol 74:111–118.

Kish S, el-Awar M, Stuss D, Nobrega J, Currier R, Aita J, et al. (1994) Neuropsychological test performance in patients with dominantly inherited spinocerebellar ataxia: relationship to ataxia severity. Neurology 44:1738–1746.

Kleiner-Fisman G, Lang AE (2007) Benign hereditary chorea revisited: a journey to understanding. Mov Disord 22.

Koide R, Ikeuchi T, Onodera O, Tanaka H, Igarashi S, Endo K, et al. (1994) Unstable expansion of CAG repeat in hereditary dentatorubral-pallidoluysian atrophy (DRPLA). Nat Genet 6.

Konagaya M, Sakai M, Kato T, Kuru S, Matsuoka Y, Sobue G, et al. (2002) An autopsied case of dentatorubropallidoluysian atrophy with atypical pathological lesions [in Japanese]. No To Shinkei 54.

Krim E, Barroso B (2001) Psychiatric disorders treated with clozapine in a patient with Wilson's disease. J Neuropsychiatry Clin Neurosci 13:531–532.

Kulaksizoglu I, Polat A (2003) Quetiapine for mania with Wilson's disease. Psychosomatics 44:438–439.

Kulisevsky J, Litvan I, Berthier ML, Pascual-Sedano B, Paulsen JS, Cummings JL (2001) Neuropsychiatric assessment of Gilles de la Tourette patients: comparative study with other hyperkinetic and hypokinetic movement disorders. Mov Disord 16.

Kumawat BL, Sharma CM, Tripathi G, Ralot T, Dixit S (2007) Wilson's disease presenting as isolated obsessive–compulsive disorder. Indian J Med Sci 61:607–610.

Lafer B, Renshaw P, Sachs G (1997) Major depression and the basal ganglia. Psychiatr Clin North Am 20:885–896.

Laplanche J, Hachimi K, Durieux I, Thuillet P, Defebvre L, Deslasnerie-Laupretre N, et al. (1999) Prominent psychiatric features and early onset in an inherited prion disease with a new insertional mutation in the prion protein gene. Brain 122:2375–2386.

Larsson MU, Luszcz MA, Bui T-H, Wahlin T-BR (2006) Depression and suicidal ideation after predictive testing for Huntington's disease: a two-year follow-up study. J Genet Couns 15.

Lasek K, Lencer R, Gaser C, Hagenah J, Walter U, Wolters A, et al. (2006) Morphological basis for the spectrum of clinical deficits in spinocerebellar ataxia 17 (SCA17). Brain 129:2341–2352.

Le Pira F, Zappala G, Saponara R, Domina E, Restivo D, Reggio A, et al. (2002) Cognitive findings in spinocerebellar ataxia type 2: relationship to genetic and clinical variables. J Neurol Sci 201:53–57.

Lenroot R, Giedd J (2006) Brain development in children and adolescents: insights from anatomical magnetic resonance imaging. Neurosci Biobehav Rev 30:718–729.

Leroi I, O'Hearn E, Marsh L, Lyketsos CG, Rosenblatt A, Ross CA, et al. (2002) Psychopathology in patients with degenerative cerebellar diseases: a comparison to Huntington's disease. Am J Psychiatry 159.

Liszewski C, O'Hearn E, Leroi I, Gourley L, Ross C, Margolis R (2004) Cognitive impairment with psychiatric symptoms in 133 patients with diseases associated with cerebellar degeneration. J Neuropsychiatry Clin Neurosci 16:109–122.

Longanathan S, Nayak R, Sinha S, Taly A, Math S, Varghese M (2008) Treating mania in Wilson's disease with lithium. J Neuropsychiatry Clin Neurosci 20:487–489.

Loosmore SJ, Wood K (1988) Benign hereditary chorea. A case report. Br J Psychiatry 152.

Lossos A, Dobson-Stone C, Monaco A, Soffer D, Rahamim E, Newman J, et al. (2005) Early clinical heterogeneity in choreoacanthocytosis. Arch Neurol 62:611–614.

Machado A, Deguti M, Caixeta L, Spitz M, Lucato L, Barbosa E (2008) Mania as the first manifestation of Wilson's disease. Bipolar Disord 10:447–450.

Maciel P, Cruz V, Constante M, Iniesta I, Costa M, Gallati S, et al. (2005) Neuroferritinopathy: missense mutation in FTL causing early-onset bilateral pallidal involvement. Neurology 65:603–605.

Mahajnah M, Inbar D, Steinmetz A, Heutink P, Breedveld GJ, Straussberg R (2007) Benign hereditary chorea: clinical, neuroimaging, and genetic findings. J Child Neurol 22.

Maltecca F, Filla A, Castaldo I, Coppola G, Fragassi NA, Carella M, et al. (2003) Intergenerational instability and marked anticipation in SCA-17. Neurology 61.

Marder K (2000) Rate of functional decline in Huntington's disease. Neurology 54: 1712–1712.

Marelli C, Piacentini S, Garavaglia B, Girotti F, Albanese A (2005) Clinical and neuro-psychological correlates in two brothers with pantothenate kinase–associated neuro-degeneration. Mov Disord 20:208–212.

Margolis R, O'Hearn E, Rosenblatt A, Willour V, Holmes S, Franz M, et al. (2001) A disorder similar to Huntington's disease is associated with a novel CAG repeat expansion. Ann Neurol 50:373–380.

Margolis RL, Holmes SE, Rosenblatt A, Gourley L, O'Hearn E, Ross CA, et al. (2004) Huntington's disease-like 2 (HDL2) in North America and Japan. Ann Neurol 56.

Marshall J, White K, Weaver M, Flury Wetherill L, Hui S, Stout JC, et al. (2007) Specific psychiatric manifestations among preclinical Huntington disease mutation carriers. Arch Neurol 64.

Mattsson B (1974) Huntington's chorea in Sweden. Acta Psychiatr Scand Suppl 255.

McHugh P (1989) The neuropsychiatry of basal ganglia disorders: a triadic syndrome and its explanation. Neuropsychiatry Neuropsychol Behav Neurol 2:239–247.

McNeill A, Pandolfo M, Kuhn J, Shang H, Miyajima H (2008) The neurological presentation of ceruloplasmin gene mutations. Eur Neurol 60:200–205.

Medalia A, Isaacs-Glaberman K, Scheinberg I (1988) Neuropsychological impairment in Wilson's disease. Arch Neurol 45:502–504.

Medalia A, Scheinberg I (1989) Psychopathology in patients with Wilson's disease. Am J Psychiatry 146:662–664.

Merle U, Schaefer M, Ferenci P, Stremmel W (2007) Clinical presentation, diagnosis and long-term outcome of Wilson's disease: a cohort study. Gut 56:115–120.

Mir P, Edwards M, Curtis A, Bhatia K, Quinn N (2005) Adult-onset generalized dystonia due to a mutation in the neuroferritinopathy gene. Mov Disord 20:243–245.

Miranda M, Castiglioni C, Frey B, Hergersberg M, Danek A, Jung H (2007) Phenotypic variability of a distinct deletion in McLeod syndrome. Mov Disord 22:1358–1361.

Miyajima H (2003) Aceruloplasminemia, an iron metabolic disorder. Neuropathology 23:345–350.

Miyajima H, Kohno S, Takahashi Y, Yonekawa O, Kanno T (1999) Estimation of the gene frequency of aceruloplasminemia in Japan. Neurology 53:617.

Miyajima H, Takahashi Y, Kono S, Hishida A, Ishikawa K, Sakamoto M (2005) Frontal lobe dysfunction associated with glucose hypometabolism in aceruloplasminemia. J Neurol 252:996–997.

Moore RC, Xiang F, Monaghan J, Han D, Zhang Z, Edstrom L, et al. (2001) Huntington disease phenocopy is a familial prion disease. Am J Hum Genet 69.

Morita H, Ikeda S, Yamamoto K, Morita S, Yoshida K, Nomoto S, et al. (1995) Hereditary ceruloplasmin deficiency with hemosiderosis: a clinicopathological study of a Japanese family. Ann Neurol 37:646–656.

Morphy M, Feldman J, Kilburn G (1989) Hallervorden-Spatz disease in a psychiatric setting. J Clin Psychiatry 50:66–68.

Muller-Vahl K, Berding G, Emrich H, Peschel T (2007) Chorea-acanthocytosis in monozygotic twins: clinical findings and neuropathological changes as detected by diffusion tensor imaging, FDG-PET and 123I-b-CIT-SPECT. J Neurol 254:1081–1088.

Murgod UA, Saleem Q, Anand A, Brahmachari SK, Jain S, Muthane UB (2001) A clinical study of patients with genetically confirmed Huntington's disease from India. J Neurol Sci 190.

Naito H, Ohama E, Nagai H (1987) A family of dentatorubropallidoluysian atrophy including two cases with schizophrenic symptoms. Pyschiatr Neurol Jpn 74:871–897.

Namekawa M, Takiyama Y, Ando Y, Sakoe K, Muramatsu SI, Fujimoto KI, et al. (2001) Choreiform movements in spinocerebellar ataxia type 1. J Neurol Sci 187:103–106.

Nardocci N, Rumi V, Combi M, Angelini L, Mirabile D, Bruzzone M (1994) Complex tics, stereotypies, and compulsive behavior as clinical presentation of a juvenile progressive dystonia suggestive of Hallervorden-Spatz disease. Mov Disord 9:369–371.

Negro P, Louza Neto M (1995) Results of ECT for a case of depression in Wilson disease. J Neuropsychiatry Clin Neurosci 7:384.

Nicholas A, Earnst K, Marson D (2005) Atypical Hallervorden-Spatz disease with preserved cognition and obtrusive obsessions and compulsions. Mov Disord 20:880–886.

Nittis T, Gitlin J (2002) The copper–iron connection: hereditary aceruloplasminemia. Semin Hematol 39:282–289.

Oeschner M, Buchert R, Beyer W, Danek A (2001) Reduction of striatal glucose metabolism in McLeod choreoacanthocytosis. J Neurol Neurosurg Psychiatry 70:517–520.

Oeschner M, Danek A, Winkler G (1996) McLeod-Neuroakanthozytose: ein zu selten diagnostiziertes syndrom? Akt Neurol 23:245–250.

Ohta E, Nagasaka T, Shindo K, Toma S, Nagasaka K, Ohta K, et al. (2007) Neuroferritinopathy in a Japanese family with a duplication in the ferritin light chain gene. Neurology 70:1493–1494.

Oliver JE (1970) Huntington's chorea in Northamptonshire. Br J Psychiatry 116.

Öner Ö, Öner P, Deda G, İçağasioğlu D (2003) Psychotic disorder in a case with Hallervorden–Spatz disease. Acta Psychiatr Scand 108:394–397.

Orr HT, Chung MY, Banfi S, Kwiatkowski TJ Jr, Servadio A, Beaudet AL, et al. (1993) Expansion of an unstable trinucleotide CAG repeat in spinocerebellar ataxia type 1. Nat Genet 4:221–226.

Paneque H, Lemos C, Escalona K, Prieto A, Reynaldo R, Velazquez P, et al. (2007a) Psychological follow-up of presymptomatic genetic testing for spinocerebellar ataxia type 2 (SCA2) in Cuba. J Genet Couns 16:469–479.

Paneque H, Prieto A, Reynaldo R, Cruz M, Santos F, Almaguer M, et al. (2007b) Psychological aspects of presymptomatic diagnosis of spinocerebellar ataxia type 2 in Cuba. Community Genet 10:132–139.

Pantelis C, Barnes T, Nelson H (1992) Is the concept of frontal-subcortical dementia relevant to schizophrenia? Br J Psychiatry 160:442–460.

Parent A, Hazrati L (1993) Anatomical aspects of information processing in primate basal ganglia. Trends Neurosci 16:111–116.

Paulsen JS, Nehl C, Hoth KF, Kanz JE, Benjamin M, Conybeare R, et al. (2005) Depression and stages of Huntington's disease. J Neuropsychiatry Clin Neurosci 17.

Paulsen JS, Ready RE, Hamilton JM, Mega MS, Cummings JL (2001) Neuropsychiatric aspects of Huntington's disease. J Neurol Neurosurg Psychiatry 71.

Pellecchia M, Valente E, Cif L, Salvi S, Albanese A, Scarano V, et al. (2005) The diverse phenotype and genotype of pantothenate kinase–associated neurodegeneration. Neurology 64:1810–1812.

Pflanz S, Besson JA, Ebmeier KP, Simpson S (1991) The clinical manifestation of mental disorder in Huntington's disease: a retrospective case record study of disease progression. Acta Psychiatr Scand 83.

Portala K, Levander S, Westermark K, Ekselius L, von Knorring L (2001a) Pattern of neuropsychological deficits in patients with treated Wilson's disease. Eur Arch Psychiatry Clin Neurosci 251:262–268.

Portala K, Westermark K, Ekselius L, von Knorring L (2001b) Personality traits in treated Wilson's disease determined by means of the Karolinska Scales of Personality (KSP). Eur Psychiatry 16:362–371.

Potter NT, Meyer MA, Zimmerman AW, Eisenstadt ML, Anderson IJ (1995) Molecular and clinical findings in a family with dentatorubral-pallidoluysian atrophy. Ann Neurol 37.

Poulter M, Baker H, Frith C, Leach M, Lofthouse R, Ridley R, et al. (1992) Inherited prion disease with 144 base pair insertion. I. Genealogical and molecular studies. Brain 115:675–685.

Pujana M, Martorell L, Volpini V, Valero J, Labad A, Vilella E, et al. (1997) Analysis of amino-acid and nucleotide variants in the spinocerebellar ataxia type 1 (SCA1) gene in schizophrenic patients. Hum Genet 99:772–775.

Pulst SM, Nechiporuk A, Nechiporuk T, Gispert S, Chen XN, Lopes-Cendes I, et al. (1996) Moderate expansion of a normally biallelic trinucleotide repeat in spinocerebellar ataxia type 2. Nat Genet 14:269–276.

Rampoldi L, Danek A, Monaco AP (2002) Clinical features and molecular bases of neuro-acanthocytosis. J Mol Med 80:475–91.

Ranen N, Peyser C, Folstein S (1994) ECT as a treatment for depression in Huntington's disease. J Neuropsychiatry Clin Neurosci 6:154–158.

Ranum LP, Duvick LA, Rich SS, Schut LJ, Litt M, Orr HT (1991) Localization of the autosomal dominant HLA-linked spinocerebellar ataxia (SCA1) locus, in two kindreds, within an 8-cM subregion of chromosome 6p. Am J Hum Genet 49:31–41.

Rathbun J (1996) Neuropsychological aspects of Wilson's disease. Int J Neurosci 85: 221–229.

Rinne J, Daniel S, Scaravilli F, Pires M, Harding A, Marsden C (1994) The neuropathological features of neuroacanthocytosis. Mov Disord 9:297–304.

Robertson B, Evans A, Walterfang M, Ng A, Velakoulis D (2008) Epilepsy, progessive movement disorder and cognitive decline. J Clin Neurosci 15:812.

Rodrigues A, Dalgalarrondo P, Banzato C (2004) Successful ECT in a patient with a psychiatric presentation of Wilson's disease. J ECT 20:55.

Rodrigues G, Walker R, Bader B, Danek A, Marques W Jr, Tumas V (2009) Chorea-acanthocytosis: report of two brazilian cases. Mov Disord 23:2090–2093.

Rodrigues GGR, Walker RH, Brice A, Cazeneuve C, Russaouen O, Teive HAG, et al. (2008) Huntington's disease-like 2 in Brazil—report of 4 patients. Mov Disord 23.

Roh J, Lee T (1994) Initial and follow-up brain MRI findings and correlation with the clinical course in Wilson's disease. Neurology 44:1064–1068.

Rolfs A, Koeppen AH, Bauer I, Bauer P, Buhlmann S, Topka H, et al. (2003) Clinical features and neuropathology of autosomal dominant spinocerebellar ataxia (SCA17). Ann Neurol 54.

Rosenberg D, Keshavan M (1998) Toward a neurodevelopmental model of obsessive–compulsive disorder. Biol Psychiatry 43:623–640.

Rosenblatt A, Leroi I (2000) Neuropsychiatry of Huntington's disease and other basal ganglia disorders. Psychosomatics 41:24–30.

Rottnek M, Riggio S, Byne W, Sano M, Margolis RL, Walker RH (2008) Schizophrenia in a patient with spinocerebellar ataxia 2: coincidence or a neurodegenerative cause of psychiatric disease. Am J Psychiatry 165(8):964–967.

Rubia K, Smith A, Woolley J, Nosarti C, Heyman I, Taylor E, et al. (2006) Progressive increase of frontostriatal brain activation from childhood to adulthood during event-related tasks of cognitive control. Hum Brain Mapp 27:973–993.

Rudnicki D, Pletnikova O, Vonsattel J, Ross C, Margolis R (2008) A comparison of Huntington disease and Huntington disease-like 2 neuropathology. J Neuropathol Exp Neurol 67:366–374.

Sachdev P, Malhi G (2005) Obsessive–compulsive behavior: a disorder of decision-making. Aust N Z J Psychiatry 39:757–763.

Sachin S, Goyal V, Singh S, Shukla G, Sharma M, Gaikwed S, et al. (2009) Clinical spectrum of Hallervorden-Spatz syndrome in India. J Clin Neurosci 16:253–258.

Sagawa M, Takao M, Nogawa S, Mizuno M, Murata M, Amano T, et al. (2003) Wilson's disease associated with olfactory paranoid syndrome and idiopathic thrombocytopenic purpura. Brain Nerve 55:899–902.

Saiki S, Hirose G, Sakai K, Matsunari I, Higashi K, Saiki M, et al. (2004) Chorea-acanthocytosis associated with tourettism. Mov Disord 19:833–836.

Savoiardo M, Halliday WC, Nardocci N, Strada L, D'Incerti L, Angelini L, et al. (1993) Hallervorden-Spatz disease: MR and pathologic findings. AJNR Am J Neuroradiol 14:155–162.

Scarano V, Pellecchia M, Filla A, Barone P (2002) Hallervorden-Spatz syndrome resembling a typical Tourette syndrome. Mov Disord 17:618–620.

Schmahmann J (2004) Disorders of the cerebellum: ataxia, dysmetria of thought, and the cerebellar cognitive affective syndrome. J Neuropsychiatry Clin Neurosci 16:367–378.

Schneider SA, van de Warrenburg BPC, Hughes TD, Davis M, Sweeney M, Wood N, et al. (2006) Phenotypic homogeneity of the Huntington disease-like presentation in a SCA17 family. Neurology 67.

Schwartz M, Feics S, Polak H, Sharf B (1993) Psychiatric manifestations in Wilson's disease. Harefuah 124:75–77.

Sechi G, Cocco G, Errigo A, Delana L, Rosati G, Agnetti V, et al. (2006) Three sisters with very-late-onset major depression and parkinsonism. Parkinsonism Relat Disord 13: 122–125.

Seniow J, Bak T, Gajda J, Poniatowska R, Czlonkowska A (2002) Cognitive functioning in neurologically symptomatic and asymptomatic forms of Wilson's disease. Mov Disord 17:1077–1083.

Shah N, Kumar D (1997) Wilson's disease, psychosis and ECT. Convuls Ther 13:278–279.

Shanmugiah A, Sinha S, Taly A, Prashanth L, Tomar M, Arundaya G, et al. (2008) Psychiatric manifestations in Wilson's disease: a cross-sectional analysis. J Neuropsychiatry Clin Neurosci 20:81–85.

Shimohata T, Hara K, Sanpei K, Nunomura J-i, Maeda T, Kawachi I, et al. (2007) Novel locus for benign hereditary chorea with adult onset maps to chromosome 8q21.3-q23.3. Brain 130.

Shiwach R (1994) Psychopathology in Huntington's disease patients. Acta Psychiatr Scand 90.

Shiwach RS, Norbury CG (1994) A controlled psychiatric study of individuals at risk for Huntington's disease. Br J Psychiatry 165.

Skinner PJ, Koshy BT, Cummings CJ, Klement IA, Helin K, Servadio A, et al. (1997) Ataxin-1 with an expanded glutamine tract alters nuclear matrix–associated structures. Nature 389:971–974.

Slaughter JR, Martens MP, Slaughter KA (2001) Depression and Huntington's disease: prevalence, clinical manifestations, etiology, and treatment. CNS Spectr 6.

Smith C, Lipe H, Bird T (2004) Impact of presymptomatic genetic testing for hereditary ataxia and neuromuscular disorders. Arch Neurol 61:875–880.

Soliveri P, Monza D, Piacentini S, Paridi D, Nespolo C, Gellera C, et al. (2002) Cognitive and psychiatric characterization of patients with Huntington's disease and their at-risk relatives. Neurol Sci 23(Suppl 2).

Sorrentino G, De Renzo A, Miniello S, Nori O, Bonavita V (1999) Late appearance of acanthocytes during the course of chorea-acanthocytosis. J Neurol Sci 163:175–178.

Spyridi S, Diakogiannis I, Michaelides M, Sokolaki S, Iacovides A, Kaprinis G (2008) Delusional disorder and alcohol abuse in a patient with Wilson's disease. Gen Hosp Psychiatry 30:585–586.

Srinivas K, Sinha S, Taly A, Prashanth L, Arunodaya G, Reddy J, et al. (2008) Dominant psychiatric manifestations in Wilson's disease: a diagnostic and therapeutic challenge! J Neurol Sci 266:104–108.

Stevanin G, Brice A (2008) Spinocerebellar ataxia 17 (SCA17) and Huntington's disease-like 4 (HDL4). Cerebellum 7:170–178.

Stevanin G, Fujigasaki H, Lebre A-S, Camuzat A, Jeannequin C, Dode C, et al. (2003) Huntington's disease-like phenotype due to trinucleotide repeat expansions in the *TBP* and *JPH3* genes. Brain 126.

Stiller P, Kassubek J, Schonfeldt-Leucona C, Connemann B (2008) Wilson's disease in psychiatric patients. Psychiatry Clin Neurosci 56:649.

Svetel M, Kozic D, Stefanova E, Semnic R, Dragasevic N, Kostic VS (2001) Dystonia in Wilson's disease. Mov Disord 16:719–723.

Takahashi Y, Kojima T, Atsumi Y, Okubo Y, Shimazono Y (1983) Case of chorea-acanthocytosis with various psychotic symptoms. Psychiatr Neurol Jpn 85:457–472.

Takashima H, Sakai T, Iwashita H, Matsuda Y, Tanaka K, Oda K, et al. (1994) A family of McLeod syndrome, masquerading as chorea-acanthocytosis. J Neurol Sci 124:56–60.

Tekin S, Cummings J (2002) Frontal-subcortical neuronal circuits and clinical neuro-psychiatry: an update. J Psychosom Res 53:647–654.

Thomas M, Hayflick S, Jankovic J (2003) Clinical heterogeneity of neurodegeneration with brain iron accumulation (Hallervorden-Spatz syndrome) and pantothenate kinase–associated neurodegeneration. Mov Disord 19:36–42.

Tibben A (2007) Predictive testing for Huntington's disease. Brain Res Bull 72.

Tsuang D, Almqvist EW, Lipe H, Strgar F, DiGiacomo L, Hoff D, et al. (2000) Familial aggregation of psychotic symptoms in Huntington's disease. Am J Psychiatry 157.

Tu J (1981) The inadvisability of neuroleptic medication in Wilson's disease. Biol Psychiatry 16:963–968.

Ueno S, Maruki Y, Nakamura M, Tomemori Y, Kamae K, Tanabe H, et al. (2001) The gene encoding a newly discovered protein, chorein, is mutated in chorea-acanthocytosis. Nat Genet 28:121–122.

van Duijn E, Kingma EM, Timman R, Zitman FG, Tibben A, Roos RAC, et al. (2008) Cross-sectional study on prevalences of psychiatric disorders in mutation carriers of Huntington's disease compared with mutation-negative first-degree relatives. J Clin Psychiatry 69.

van Duijn E, Kingma EM, van der Mast RC (2007) Psychopathology in verified Huntington's disease gene carriers. J Neuropsychiatry Clin Neurosci 19.

Varghese S, Narayanan D, Dinesh D (2008) Mania in a patient with Wilson's disease awaiting liver transplant. J Neuropsychiatry Clin Neurosci 20:501–502.

Vassos E, Panas M, Kladi A, Vassilopoulos D (2008) Effect of CAG repeat length on psychiatric disorders in Huntington's disease. J Psychiatr Res 42.

Vazquez M, Martinez M (2009) Electroconvulsive therapy in neuroacanthocytosis or McLeod syndrome. J ECT 25:72–73.

Vincent J, Paterson A, Strong E, Petronis A, Kennedy J (2000) The unstable trinucleotide repeat story of major psychosis. Am J Med Genet 97:77–97.

Walker R, Liu Q, Ichiba M, Muroya S, Nakamura M, Sano A, et al. (2006) Self-mutilation in chorea-acanthocytosis: manifestation of movement disorder or psychopathology? Mov Disord 21:2268–2269.

Walker RH, Jankovic J, O'Hearn E, Margolis RL (2003) Phenotypic features of Huntington's disease-like 2. Mov Disord 18.

Walter G, Lyndon B (1997) Depression in hepatolenticular degeneration (Wilson's disease). Aust N Z J Psychiatry 31:880–882.

Walterfang M, March E, Varghese D, Miller K, Simpson L, Tomlinson B, et al. (2006a) Schizophrenia-like psychosis and aceruloplasminemia. Neuropsychiatr Dis Treat 2: 577–581.

Walterfang M, Wood S, Velakoulis D, Copolov D, Pantelis C (2006b) Diseases of white matter and schizophrenia-like psychosis. Aust N Z J Psychiatry 39:746–756.

Walterfang M, Yucel M, Walker R, Evans A, Bader B, Ng A, et al. (2008) Adolescent obsessive compulsive disorder heralding chorea-acanthocytosis. Mov Disord 23:422–425.

Wang S, Detera-Wadleigh SD, Coon H, Sun CE, Goldin LR, Duffy DL, et al. (1996) Evidence of linkage disequilibrium between schizophrenia and the SCa1 CAG repeat on chromosome 6p23. Am J Hum Genet 59:731–736.

Wardle M, Majounie E, Williams NM, Rosser AE, Morris HR, Robertson NP (2008) Dentatorubral pallidoluysian atrophy in south Wales. J Neurol Neurosurg Psychiatry 79.

Weigell-Weber M, Schmid W, Spiegel R (1996) Psychiatric symptoms and CAG expansion in Huntington's disease. Am J Med Genet 67.

Wichowicz H, Cubala W, Slawek J (2006) Wilson's disease asociated with delusional disorder. Psychiatry Clin Neurosci 60:758–760.

Wild EJ, Tabrizi SJ (2007) Huntington's disease phenocopy syndromes. Curr Opin Neurol 20.

Williams J, Walshe J (1981) Wilson's disease: an analysis of the cranial computerized tomographic appearances found in 60 patients and the changes in response to treatment with chelating agents. Brain 104:735–752.

Willis A, Sawle G, Guilbert P, Curtis A (2002) Palatal tremor and cognitive decline in neuroferritinopathy. J Neurol Neurosurg Psychiatry 73:91–92.

Wilson S (1912) Progressive lenticular degeneration: a familial nervous disease associated with cirrhosis of the liver. Brain 34:295–507.

Woodcock JH (1999) Behavioral aspects of Huntington's disease. In: Joseph AB, Young RR (eds.) Movement Disorders in Neurology and Neuropsychiatry. Blackwell Science, Oxford.

Xiang F, Almqvist E, Huq M, Lundin A, Hayden M, Edstrom L, et al. (1998) A Huntington disease-like neurodegenerative disorder maps to chromosome 20p. Am J Hum Genet 63:1431–1438.

Yamada H, Ohji T, Sakurai S, Yamaguchi E, Uchimura N, Morita K, et al. (2009) Chorea-acanthocytosis presenting with schizophrenia symptoms as first symptoms. Psychiatry Clin Neurosci 63:253–254.

Yoshida K, Furihata K, Takeda S, Nakamura A, Yamamoto K, Morita H, et al. (1995) A mutation in the ceruloplasmin gene is associated with systemic hemosiderosis in humans. Nat Genet 9:267–272.

Zappacosta B, Monza D, Meoni C, Austoni L, Soliveri P, Gellera C, et al. (1996) Psychiatric symptoms do not correlate with cognitive decline, motor symptoms, or CAG repeat length in Huntington's disease. Arch Neurol 53.

Zeman A, Daniels G, Tilley L, Dunn M, Toplis L, Bullock T, et al. (2005) McLeod syndrome: life-long neuropsychiatric disorder due to a novel mutation of the XK gene. Psychiatr Genet 15:291–293.

Zhou B, Westaway SK, Levinson B, Johnson MA, Gitschier J, Hayflick SJ (2001) A novel pantothenate kinase gene (PANK2) is defective in Hallervorden-Spatz syndrome. Nat Genet 28:345–349.

Zoghbi HY, Jodice C, Sandkuijl LA, Kwiatkowski TJ Jr, McCall AE, Huntoon SA, et al. (1991) The gene for autosomal dominant spinocerebellar ataxia (SCA1) maps telomeric to the HLA complex and is closely linked to the D6S89 locus in three large kindreds. Am J Hum Genet 49:23–30.

21

Psychogenic Chorea

John C. Morgan, MD, PhD; Shyamal H. Mehta, MD, PhD; and Kapil D. Sethi, MD, FRCP

INTRODUCTION

Psychogenic movement disorders (PMDs) are not uncommon and comprise 3% or more of practice in movement disorder specialty clinics (Factor et al., 1995; Ertan et al., 2009; Thomas et al., 2006). Tremor, dystonia, myoclonus, and gait disorders are the most common phenomenologies (Factor et al., 1995; Feinstein et al., 2001; Hinson et al., 2005); however, psychogenic parkinsonism and pseudo-tics are also reported (Factor et al., 1995; Thomas et al., 2006; Lang et al., 1995). Chorea, athetosis, and ballism comprise a small percentage of PMDs in large published series (Factor et al., 1995; Feinstein et al., 2001; Hinson et al., 2005; Thomas et al., 2006; Anderson et al., 2007).

The diagnostic criteria for PMDs is broken into four major categories according to Fahn and Williams (1988); documented, clinically established, probable, and possible. Patients falling in the first two categories of "documented" and "clinically established" are considered to have "clinically definite" PMDs (Williams et al., 1995). "Documented" PMDs are involuntary movements that are persistently relieved by suggestion, psychotherapy, or placebos, or the patient is witnessed to be free of the involuntary movements when supposedly unobserved. "Clinically established" PMDs consist of movements that are incongruent or inconsistent with the classic description of recognized movement disorders, and the patient has other psychogenic signs on neurological examination, somatizations, or obvious psychiatric disturbance. "Probable" PMDs are inconsistent with typical movement disorders, or there are other psychogenic signs or multiple somatizations. "Possible" PMDs are inconsistent with typical movement disorders, and the patient has evidence of emotional disturbance. Most patients seen in practice fall into the category of "clinically established" or "probable." The "possible" category appears more difficult to apply in clinical practice.

Psychogenic chorea was perhaps first reported by Arthur Van Gehuchten in 1920 when his son posthumously published his work *Les Maladies nerveuses* (Giménez-Roldán and Aubert, 2007). He described a hysterical outbreak of chorea in an orphanage of boys and girls that was precipitated by a 15-year-old girl developing hysterical movements. He described the movement as *chorée salutatoire* (saluting chorea) in a girl with an unusual gait, but by today's phenomenology, the movement would be considered more consistent with dystonia (Giménez-Roldán and Aubert, 2007). These movements eventually involved over 13 teenagers in the orphanage between the ages of 13 and 18 and were cured by a promise to take the first to recover to the seaside.

PREVALENCE

The phenomenology of movement disorders has evolved into a unified framework since this first report of "psychogenic chorea," probably due to a combination of international meetings, wide dissemination of videos, and peer review. In any case, many patients with PMDs present with multiple phenomenologies, and some patients with complex movements that have chorea as a part of their PMD are probably labeled in reports as having a single dominant phenomenology (e.g., tremor). This may lead to the underrepresentation of "chorea" as a label in the PMD literature (Feinstein et al., 2001).

The prevalence of psychogenic chorea in large series of psychogenic neurological patients ranges from nonexistent in some series (Lempert et al., 1990; Factor et al., 1995; Feinstein et al., 2001) to a maximum of 9%–10% (Hinson et al., 2005; Anderson et al., 2007). Psychogenic chorea was not reported in a series of 842 consecutive patients with movement disorders (with 28 of these patients having other PMDs) (Factor et al., 1995).

Hinson et al. (2005) reported that eight of 88 patients, examined during the development of a PMD rating scale, were rated by trained movement disorder specialists as having chorea. In comparison, raters reported that 60% had gait dysfunction, >40% had tremor, and 32% had dystonia (Hinson et al., 2005). Anderson et al. (2007) reported chorea as being part of the phenomenology in 6% of 66 patients with PMDs. A report from a very large movement disorder practice (12,625 patients) found only three patients with psychogenic chorea out of 517 with PMDs (for a prevalence of 0.6%) (Thomas et al., 2006). In the same practice, psychogenic tremor (211, 40.8%), psychogenic dystonia (206, 40.2%), and psychogenic myoclonus (88, 17%) were the most common PMDs (Thomas et al., 2006). A report from Turkey identified chorea-ballism as a feature in 6% of their PMD patients (Ertan et al., 2009).

PSYCHIATRIC FEATURES OF PSYCHOGENIC CHOREA

It should be noted that many neuropsychiatric symptoms (irritability, mood swings, obsessive–compulsive features, etc.) accompany "organic" forms of chorea such as Sydenham chorea (Moore, 1996) (Chapter 17) and Huntington disease (Phillips et al., 2008) (Chapter 23). These signs and symptoms may also be a part of the underlying psychopathology in a patient with a PMD. We have seen several patients with psychogenic chorea in our experience (>20 years), and frequently these patients have concomitant phenomenology (dystonia, myoclonus, tremor). In addition, most PMD patients exhibit other psychogenic signs (unusual sensory deficits, give-way weakness, exaggerated startle, selective disabilities, unusual gait) that should provide clues to the diagnosis. Up to 15% of psychogenic patients can have an underlying "organic" movement disorder as well, so it is important to consider this in the differential diagnosis.

The vast majority of patients with PMDs are thought to have conversion disorder by treating psychiatrists (Feinstein et al., 2001). PMD patients in one large series (Feinstein et al., 2001) had a lifetime prevalence of anxiety disorders in 62%, major depression in 43%, both anxiety and depression in 29%, somatoform disorder in about 5%, and adjustment disorder in 10%, indicating significant psychiatric comorbidity. Many patients present with PMDs and have no prior psychiatric diagnoses, but they have evidence of somatization or other previous unexplained neurological symptoms when a comprehensive past medical history is obtained.

EVALUATION, TREATMENT, AND OUTCOME

Clinicians should be cautious to exclude all plausible causes of organic chorea in a patient with suspected psychogenic chorea, given the rarity of this PMD. However, excessive investigation in a patient with suspected PMDs may cause morbidity (if the tests are invasive) and may give the patient the false impression that the clinician believes the PMD to be organic. Clinicians evaluating a PMD should aim to tread the fine line between appropriate exclusion of other possible causes for a suspected PMD and the "kitchen sink" work-up.

While there are very little data on treatment and outcomes in patients with psychogenic chorea (given the rarity of this PMD), there are some data on treatment and outcomes in PMDs and conversion disorders in neurology in general. Multi-disciplinary treatment with intensive psychiatric care can yield good outcomes (Williams et al., 1995), but the majority of neurologists in practice lack the psychiatric and rehabilitative resources to be able to effectively and intensively treat patients with PMDs. We do know that a long duration of symptoms, multiple psychiatric comorbidities, and a gradual onset of symptoms are all poor prognostic factors for outcomes in patients with conversion disorders (Lempert et al., 1990; Couprie et al., 1995; Feinstein et al., 2001). Unfortunately, many patients with one conversion disorder may have remission with treatment, only to have the same conversion disorder recur; or they may develop a completely new phenomenology (e.g., stroke-like symptoms in a patient who previously had nonepileptic seizures).

Long-term outcomes in a large series of PMD patients ($n = 228$) were reported by Thomas et al. (2006). The mean age of patients in this series was 42, with a mean duration of symptoms of approximately 5 years. The mean duration of follow-up was over 3 years. Approximately 57% of patients had improvement of symptoms, 22% were worse, and 21% remained the same over time. The authors found that positive social life perceptions, good physical health, reduction or elimination of stress, patient perception of "effective treatment" by the physician, and treatment with a specific medication contributed to better outcomes (Thomas et al., 2006).

CONCLUSION

It is very important to consider all organic causes in a patient presenting with any movement disorder, but this is especially true of chorea. Illustrative of this, there are cases of Huntington disease mislabeled as conversion disorder (Teasell and Shapiro, 2002). Fortunately, there has been a decline in the mislabeling of organic disorders as conversion disorder. In the 1950s perhaps 29% of patients were improperly labeled compared with only 4% of patients estimated to be misdiagnosed in the past two decades (Stone et al., 2005).

In conclusion, psychogenic chorea should be a very rare diagnosis in any neurological practice. Further research is needed into the causes and treatments of PMDs as these disorders can cause significant disability and have a negative impact on quality of life for our patients (Anderson et al., 2007). Hopefully, neurologists, psychiatrists, and other health professionals can work together to address the needs of all PMD patients in the future to improve patient outcomes.

REFERENCES

Anderson KE, Gruber-Baldini AL, Vaughan CG, Reich SG, Fishman PS, Weiner WJ, Shulman LM (2007) Impact of psychogenic movement disorders versus Parkinson's on disability, quality of life, and psychopathology. Mov Disord 22:2204–2209.

Couprie W, Wijdicks EF, Rooijmans HG, van Gijn J (1995) Outcome in conversion disorder: a follow up study. J Neurol Neurosurg Psychiatry 58:750–752.

Ertan S, Uluduz D, Özekmekçi S, Kiziltan G, Ertan T, Yalçinkaya C, Özkara Ç (2009) Clinical characteristics of 49 patients with psychogenic movement disorders in a tertiary clinic in Turkey. Mov Disord 24:759–762.

Factor SA, Podskalny GD, Molho ES (1995) Psychogenic movement disorders: frequency, clinical profile, and characteristics. J Neurol Neurosurg Psychiatry 59:406–412.

Fahn S, Williams D (1988) Psychogenic dystonia. Adv Neurol 50:431–455.

Feinstein A, Stergiopoulos V, Fine J, Lang AE (2001) Psychiatric outcome in patients with a psychogenic movement disorder: a prospective study. Neuropsychiatry Neuropsychol Behav Neurol 14:169–176.

Giménez-Roldán S, Aubert G (2007) Hysterical chorea: report of an outbreak and movie documentation by Arthur van Gehuchten (1861–1914). Mov Disord 22:1071–1076.

Hinson VK, Cubo E, Comella CL, Goetz CG, Leurgans S (2005) Rating scale for psychogenic movement disorders: scale development and clinimetric testing. Mov Disord 20:1592–1597.

Lang AE, Koller WC, Fahn S (1995) Psychogenic parkinsonism. Arch Neurol 52:802–810.

Lempert T, Dieterich M, Huppert D, Brandt T (1990) Psychogenic disorders in neurology: frequency and clinical spectrum. Acta Neurol Scand 82:335–340.

Moore DP (1996) Neuropsychiatric aspects of Sydenham's chorea: a comprehensive review. J Clin Psychiatry 57:407–414.

Phillips W, Shannon KM, Barker RA (2008) The current clinical management of Huntington's disease. Mov Disord 23:1491–1504.

Stone J, Smyth R, Carson A, Lewis S, Prescott R, Warlow C, Sharpe M (2005) Systematic review of misdiagnosis of conversion symptoms and "hysteria." BMJ 331(7523):989.

Teasell RW, Shapiro AW (2002) Misdiagnosis of conversion disorders. Am J Phys Med Rehabil 81:236–240.

Thomas M, Vuong KD, Jankovic J (2006) Long-term prognosis of patients with psychogenic movement disorders. Parkinsonism Relat Disord 12:382–387.

Williams DT, Ford B, Fahn S (1995) Phenomenology and psychopathology related to psychogenic movement disorders. In: Weiner WJ, Lang AE (eds.) Behavioral Neurology of Movement Disorders. Raven Press, New York, pp 231–257.

22

Treatment of Chorea

Brandon Barton, MD and Kathleen M. Shannon, MD

INTRODUCTION

Pathophysiology of Chorea as Related to Current Treatment Strategies

The focus of this chapter is on primary choreas (idiopathic or genetic in origin), with emphasis on evidence-based treatments, commonly employed treatment protocols, and potentially efficacious treatments that should be tried in specific conditions. Treatment of secondary choreas or accompanying comorbid symptoms is specific to the underlying pathophysiology and may be determined by the context of the particular disorder.

Therapies for chorea may be understood in terms of current concepts of the pathophysiology of chorea, which itself is not fully elucidated. Chorea can be viewed as an imbalance between the indirect and direct circuits of the basal ganglia, resulting from pathology in any of several parts of the circuit (Figure 22–1) (Chapter 2). In the classic model of basal ganglia function, chorea is related to either underactivity of the indirect pathway or increased activity in the direct pathway. This imbalance is associated with loss of gamma-aminobutyric acid (GABA)-ergic inhibition in the globus pallidus internal segment (GPi) and subsequent increase in thalamocortical motor drive and motor cortical activation via

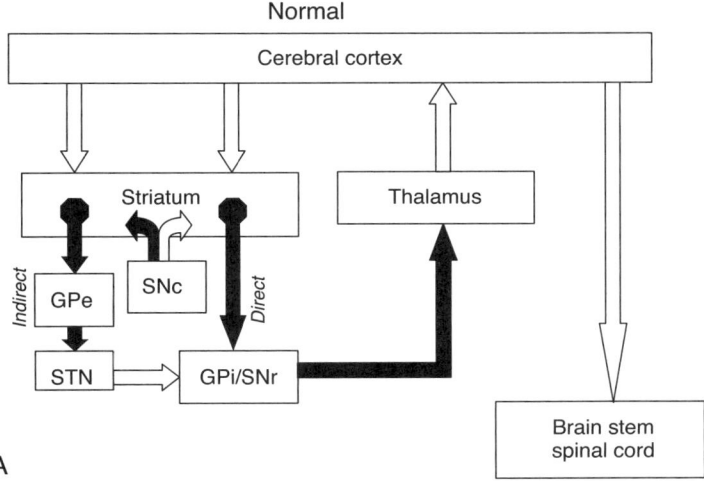

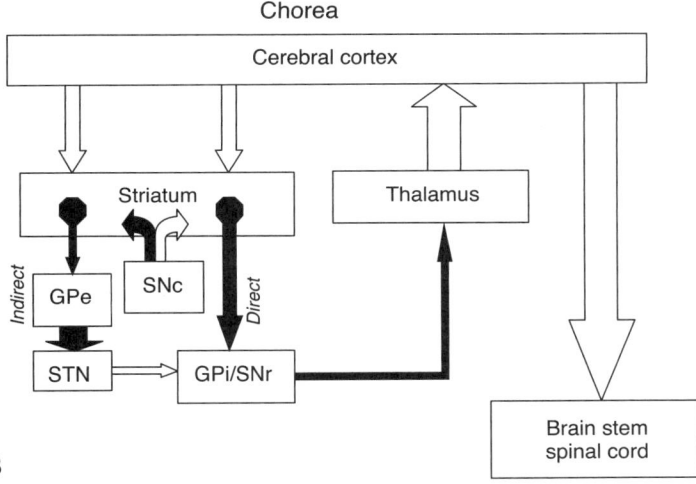

FIGURE 22–1. Circuit diagrams depicting normal basal ganglia physiology and presumed pathophysiology underlying chorea in Huntington disease. **A** Normal basal ganglia physiology. **B** Reduced inhibitory output from the striatum in the indirect pathway leads to excessive inhibition of the subthalamic nucleus by the globus pallidus externa. Excitatory outflow from the subthalamic nucleus to the globus pallidus interna/substantia nigra pars reticulata is reduced, so there is less inhibition of the thalamus by the globus pallidus interna/substantia nigra pars reticulata, leading ultimately to increased thalamocortical activity and, thus, an increase in extraneous movements. *Open arrows* indicate excitatory (glutamatergic) influences, while *filled arrows* indicate inhibitory (GABAergic) influences. GPe, globus pallidus externa; SNc, substantia nigra pars compacta; STN, subthalamic nucleus; GPi/SNr, globus pallidus interna/substantia nigra pars reticulata. From Shannon (2007), reproduced with permission of Lippincott Williams & Wilkins.

excitatory glutamatergic activity. The net result of these abnormalities is motor cortical disinhibition, resulting in hyperkinetic movements such as chorea (Cardoso et al., 2006). Based on this model, treatments that enhance GABAergic tone or reduce glutamatergic activity should therefore play a role in reducing chorea. In addition to GABA and glutamate, the established efficacy of dopamine-blocking or dopamine-depleting agents in treating chorea supports the prominent role of the dopaminergic system in modulating choreic movements. Since dopamine inhibits striatopallidal neurons of the indirect pathway and enhances the activity of neurons of the direct pathway, increased dopaminergic activity may increase chorea, while decreased dopaminergic activity should reduce chorea (Shannon, 2007). Additionally, cholinergic systems appear to be hypoactive since anticholinergic drugs may increase chorea and cholinergic agents have been reported to reduce chorea (Cubo et al., 2006).

This classic model of chorea pathogenesis is not perfect, particularly since surgical lesions of the GPi have been shown to abolish chorea, instead of worsening movements, as would be predicted by the model. Chorea is therefore likely a result of more complex abnormalities of spatial and temporal firing patterns of GPi neurons, modulated by the activity of multiple neurotransmitters (Obeso et al., 2002; Mink, 2003). This more complex etiology of chorea is also suggested by the antichoreic effects of various drugs with multiple mechanisms of action.

General Treatment Approach

A general strategy of treatment is proposed in Table 22–1. The first crucial step in treatment is to search for accompanying signs of common or treatable underlying conditions by performing a detailed medical history and physical examination as well as appropriate diagnostic testing. Time course, family history, drug history, associated signs and symptoms, and ancillary laboratory and imaging studies may give clues to the underlying cause. Chorea related to identified metabolic conditions, infections, drugs, or endocrine disorders may be transient and may improve or resolve with appropriate treatment of the underlying disorder. Important treatable factors to investigate include vitamin B_{12} levels, thyroid function, drug ingestion, and current or prior infections.

In cases of drug-induced chorea, withdrawal of the suspected provoking agent is the most important step. However, in certain cases, such as levodopa-induced chorea associated with Parkinson disease (PD) or psychiatric illness requiring antipsychotic medication, where the causative drug cannot readily be withdrawn, these conditions demand alternative management strategies. Chorea associated with autoimmune causes may benefit from immunomodulatory therapies, with use of these potent medications determined by the severity of the underlying autoimmune condition as well as the severity of the chorea and its response to more easily administered drugs (i.e., anticonvulsants, dopamine receptor antagonists).

TABLE 22–1. General Approach to Treatment of Chorea

Step 1	Careful medical history and physical examination: Identify and treat possible underlying, reversible, or treatable conditions, including • Correction of metabolic derangements • Removal of drugs known to cause chorea • Anti-infective treatments • Immunomodulatory therapy for autoimmune disease • Anticoagulation or revascularization for cerebrovascular disease
Step 2	Introduce symptomatic pharmacological therapy if chorea is significantly disabling (Tables 22–3, 22–4)
Step 3	Consider surgery for severe or refractory cases (Table 22–5)
Step 4	(Conjunctive with step 1 and beyond) Implement multidisciplinary, supportive, nonpharmacological treatments (Table 22–6), including • Physical therapy • Occupational therapy • Patient/caregiver education

Source: Adapted from Cardoso (2008a) by permission of Wiley-Blackwell.

Secondly, when treatment of the underlying condition does not adequately control chorea, antichoreic treatments may be initiated, most commonly with medications acting on the dopaminergic system (Cardoso, 2008a). The appropriate treatment for chorea should be selected with care for several reasons. The presence of chorea alone may not necessarily be reason enough to treat the movements as disability from chorea may be overshadowed by disease-related factors, including neuropsychiatric or other motor features; these other symptoms may be more amenable to treatment or may impair quality of life more than the chorea itself. For many patients, chorea is a "cosmetic" problem, and patients often are unaware of the presence or severity of chorea, especially when the movements themselves cause no adverse changes in functional status (Vitale et al., 2001). Moreover, reducing chorea severity does not necessarily result in improved function (Huntington Study Group, 2003). Both pharmacological and nonpharmacological therapies may be considered if the chorea is severe enough to interfere with functional ability or poses risk of injury, such as falling. Since no one drug is particularly effective and since adverse events related to pharmacological treatment have the potential to worsen overall disability, medication should be used sparingly and for specific functional or symptomatic purposes. Antichoreic medications which also have parallel effects on associated comorbidities (i.e., psychosis, seizures, or mood disorders) should be prioritized. Finally, if chorea is resistant to medical therapies or if there is intolerance to pharmacological treatments, surgical therapy may be considered.

PHARMACOLOGICAL THERAPIES

There are very few controlled studies for the treatment of chorea, with the majority related to Huntington disease (HD), the prototypical and most common genetic cause of chorea (Chapter 3). Treatment of chorea in conditions other than HD may be extrapolated from the results of HD trials or considered based on individual case reports or case series. A recent systemic, evidenced-based review of the literature for HD trials between 1969 and 2005 concluded that there is limited evidence to suggest a symptomatic treatment of high clinical relevance (Bonelli and Wenning, 2006). Several outcome measures for chorea improvement have been used (Table 22–2), making comparisons between trial outcomes difficult. There is therefore no standardized approach to the pharmacological treatment of chorea, with mixed treatment outcomes observed even in the same disease groups, emphasizing the need for an individualized and empirical treatment approach. Categories of pharmacological treatments and most common applications to disease are summarized in Table 22–3. Table 22–4 lists common dosing schemes and associated adverse effects of medications used for chorea. The remainder of the chapter discusses therapies grouped by primary mechanism of action; however, in some instances, as in the case of antiepileptic drugs, mechanisms are either poorly understood or multifactorial; in the latter situation, drugs will be described as a general class.

Antidopaminergic Drugs

The majority of patients with choreiform disorders improve with antidopaminergic agents, in the form of either postsynaptic dopamine receptor blockers (typical or

TABLE 22–2. Quantitative Measurements Used to Measure Chorea Improvement in Clinical Trials

NAME OF RATING SCALE	REFERENCE
Abnormal Involuntary Movement Scale (AIMS)	Munetz and Benjamin, 1988
Unified Huntington Disease Rating Scale (UHDRS)	Huntington Study Group, 1996
Chorea Severity Scale (CSS)	Marsden and Schachter, 1981
Quantitated Neurological Examination (QNE)	Folstein et al., 1983
HD Motor Rating Scale (HDMRS)	Young et al., 1986
UFMG (Federal University of Minas Gerais) Sydenham Chorea Rating Scale	Teixeira et al., 2005
Subjective chorea quantification	Not applicable

TABLE 22–3. Classes of Medications with Reported Efficacy for Chorea

CLASS OF DRUGS	EXAMPLES OF SPECIFIC AGENTS	DISEASES TREATED
Antidopaminergic agents	Pimozide, haloperidol, aripiprazole, quetiapine, ziprasidone, risperidone, clozapine	SC, HD, vascular, drug-induced
Dopaminergic agents	Carbidopa/levodopa, apomorphine	Benign hereditary chorea (*TITF-1*), HD
Dopamine-depleting agents	Reserpine, tetrabenazine	HD, drug-induced, vascular
NMDA/antiglutamatergic agents	Amantadine, riluzole, memantine, remacemide	HD
GABA agonists	Clonazepam, lorazepam, baclofen	HD
Anticonvulsants	Valproic acid, carbamazepine, levetiracetam, topiramate, lamotrigine	HD, SC, PKD, PNKD, vascular, CP
Acetylcholinesterase inhibitors	Galantamine, donepezil	HD

CP, cerebral palsy; HD, Huntington disease; PNKD, paroxysmal nonkinesigenic dyskinesia; PKD, paroxysmal kinesigenic dyskinesia; SC, Sydenham chorea.

atypical) or dopamine-depleting agents. These drugs remain the mainstay of chorea treatment irrespective of the underlying cause. In general, the stronger the anti-D_2 receptor–blocking ability of the drug, the more effective it is in treating chorea (Cardoso et al., 2006).

Dopamine Receptor Antagonists

This class of drugs may have the dual advantage of treating both the chorea and the behavioral or psychiatric symptoms such as irritability or outbursts when present, as is commonly seen in neurodegenerative choreas.

Typical Antipsychotics

Previous studies support the possible effectiveness of typical antipsychotics for chorea in HD, with stronger evidence for haloperidol and fluphenazine, although pimozide, sulpiride, and tiapride have been reported as effective. Despite their frequent use, no high-level, randomized, controlled trials exist to guide the clinical use of these agents (Bonelli and Wenning, 2006). Prevailing clinical wisdom suggests that lower doses of these medications are better tolerated, which may

TABLE 22–4. Typical Dose Ranges and Side Effects for Antichoreic Drugs

DRUG	DOSE RANGES	ADVERSE EVENTS
Dopamine-depleting drugs		
Tetrabenazine	Start 12.5 mg/day, increase by 12.5 mg/week to symptomatic effect, maximum of 100 mg/day, divided bid/tid	Sedation, parkinsonism (30%), depression, suicidal ideation, orthostatic hypotension, akathisia, anxiety, constipation, neuroleptic malignant syndrome
Atypical Antipsychotics		
Risperidone	Start 0.5 mg/day, increase to 3 mg/day; available in liquid form	Acute dystonic reactions, parkinsonism, sedation, tardive dyskinesia, prolonged Q–T interval, hyperglycemia, fatigue
Olanzapine	Start 2.5 mg/day, maximum 30 mg/day	Acute dystonic reactions, parkinsonism, sedation, tardive dyskinesia, prolonged Q–T interval, hyperglycemia, fatigue
Ziprasidone	Start 20 mg/day, maximum 160 mg/day	Acute dystonic reactions, parkinsonism, sedation, tardive dyskinesia
Clozapine	Start 12.5 mg/day, maximum 100 mg/day	Acute dystonic reactions, parkinsonism, sedation, tardive dyskinesia
Aripiprazole	Start 5 mg/day, maximum 30 mg/day	Acute dystonic reactions, parkinsonism, sedation, tardive dyskinesia
Quetiapine	Start 12.5 mg/day, maximum 100 mg/day	Acute dystonic reactions, parkinsonism, sedation, tardive dyskinesia, hypotension
Clozapine	Start 12.5 mg/day, maximum 100 mg/day	Drowsiness, fatigue, anticholinergic symptoms, hypotension
Typical antipsychotics		
Haloperidol	Start 0.5 mg/day, maximum 8 mg	Acute dystonic reactions, parkinsonism, sedation, tardive dyskinesia
Fluphenazine	Start 0.5 mg/day, maximum 8 mg/day	Acute dystonic reactions, parkinsonism, sedation, tardive dyskinesia

Pimozide	Start 2 mg/day, maximum 10 mg/day	Acute dystonic reactions, parkinsonism, sedation, cardiac block in children, tardive dyskinesia
Glutamatergic antagonists		
Amantadine	Start 100 mg/day, maximum 500 mg/day divided bid/tid	Peripheral edema, livedo reticularis, confusion
Antiepileptic drugs		
Valproic acid	Start 250 mg/day, increase to 1,500 mg/day or 20–25 mg/kg/day	Tremor, thrombocytopenia, liver toxicity, pancreatitis, parkinsonism
Levetiracetam	Start 500 mg bid, maximum 3,000 mg/day (adjust for renal function)	Behavioral or mood changes, somnolence, parkinsonism
Carbamazepine	Start 200 mg twice daily, maximum 1,600 mg/day or 35 mg/kg/day	Rash, neutropenia, liver toxicity
Topiramate	Start 25 mg/day, increase by 25 mg/week, maximum 400 mg/day or to effect	Weight loss, paresthesias, cognitive problems, nephrolithiasis, ataxia
GABAergic agonists		
Clonazepam	Start 0.5 mg/day, maximum 3 mg/day	Sedation, confusion
Diazepam	Start 1 mg/day, maximum 20 mg/day	Sedation, confusion

reduce the severity of chorea while limiting the risk of adverse events. Side effects can include worsening gait, oculomotor function, dexterity, cognitive function, and dysphagia or the development of tardive movement disorders, with resultant decline in functional state.

Pimozide is used for anticonvulsant-refractory chorea in Sydenham chorea (SC). Reports suggest that while it may not be as effective as haloperidol in SC, it may have a more tolerable side-effect profile (Shannon and Fenichel, 1990; Demiororen et al., 2007) (Chapter 17). Antipsychotics should be given with caution in SC as one study demonstrated a small but significant increased incidence (5.5%) of drug-induced parkinsonism in SC patients compared to matched patients with Tourette syndrome (Teixeira et al., 2003). Given the possible spontaneous remission of chorea in SC, antipsychotics should be weaned carefully after a chorea-free period of at least 1 month (Cardoso, 2008b). In rare cases of *chorea paralytica* (associated with severe decrease of muscle tone, seen in a minority [1%–2%] of SC cases), dopamine receptor–blocking agents are recommended (Cardoso, 2004).

Persistent, disabling chorea or more severe, acute chorea from vascular disease may be treated with an antipsychotic, usually with typical agents such as haloperidol. Because spontaneous resolution is common in patients with vascular or metabolic chorea, there should be periodic attempts to taper the drug in order to avoid complications of long-term antipsychotic use (Dewey and Jankovic, 1989).

Atypical Antipsychotics

While typical antipsychotics have been used to treat chorea from many causes for many years, the newer, atypical antipsychotics are being increasingly employed. Atypical antipsychotics are thought to block serotonin as well as dopamine receptors, which may in part explain their decreased side-effect profile, including a lower incidence of sedation or tardive movement disorders. Similar to the case of typical antipsychotics, published studies have not demonstrated high levels of evidence for efficacy in treating chorea in HD. Efficacy and risk for tardive syndromes may be similar between low- to mid-potency typical antipsychotics and most atypical antipsychotics (Bonham and Abbott, 2008). Of the proposed atypical drugs, only clozapine and quetiapine may be truly atypical; this may be explained more by their rapid dissociation from dopamine receptors at clinically effective doses, allowing more physiological dopamine transmission (Seeman, 2002).

Olanzapine.   Of the atypical antipsychotics, only olanzapine showed possible efficacy for treating chorea in an evidence-based review (Bonelli and Wenning, 2006). Olanzapine may be particularly useful in HD as it has also been shown to augment treatments for mood disorders, encourage weight gain, improve orolingual dysfunction, and improve gait (Phillips et al., 2008).

Clozapine. In one randomized trial, clozapine had antichoreic effects at higher doses in antipsychotic-naive subjects, but the high incidence of side effects and need for frequent blood count monitoring due to the risk of agranulocytosis make this drug less attractive (van Vugt et al., 1997). In one case of chorea-acanthocytosis, hyperkinetic movements refractory to other antipsychotics responded dramatically to clozapine, although the effect was short-lasting, with return to the previous state after 4–5 months (Wihl et al., 2001).

Aripiprazole. In a small study of six patients, aripiprazole, a partial dopamine D_2 receptor and 5-hydroxytryptamine 1A (5-HT1A) receptor agonist, showed a similar reduction of chorea compared to tetrabenazine, with less associated sedation and a trend toward improvement of depressive symptoms (Brusa et al., 2009).

Risperidone. There are a few studies that support the use of risperidone for chorea and psychosis in HD, suggesting that the drug may be effective (Erdemoglu and Boratav, 2002).

Ziprasidone, Quetiapine. While evidence is limited, both ziprasidone (Bonelli et al., 2003) and quetiapine (Bonelli and Niederwieser, 2002) have been shown to reduce chorea in HD in open-label case reports.

Dopamine-Depleting Medications

Tetrabenazine

Tetrabenazine (TBZ) is a benzoquinolizine derivative which functions as a high-affinity, reversible inhibitor of monoamine uptake into presynaptic vesicles by blocking human vesicular monoamine transporter type 2 (VMAT2). TBZ preferentially depletes dopamine over norepinephrine or serotonin and has weak postsynaptic D_2 receptor–blocking capability at higher doses (Paleacu et al., 2004). Long-term response to TBZ can be predicted by the first 6 weeks of treatment (Jankovic and Orman, 1988).

TBZ has demonstrated clinical benefit for a number of hyperkinetic movement disorders, with minimal incidence of extrapyramidal side effects. An open-label, blinded, video-rated trial for HD showed a significant improvement in Abnormal Involuntary Movement Scale (AIMS) scores without serious adverse events after an average of 6 months on TBZ therapy (Ondo et al., 2002). A retrospective review of 118 patients with hyperkinetic movement disorders treated with open-label TBZ showed that patients with chorea (from HD or other causes) had particularly effective therapeutic responses compared to other movement disorder classes. These outcomes were determined by the global impression of change obtained from patients and caregivers (Paleacu et al., 2004). A larger, multicenter, prospective, double-blind, placebo-controlled, dose-finding study with 84 patients demonstrated significant improvement in United Huntington's Disease Rating Scale (UHDRS) chorea scores in doses of up to 100 mg daily over 12 weeks. While there was a significant improvement in clinical global impression, the treatment group experienced more serious adverse events, including depression and one completed suicide (Huntington Study Group, 2006). Another trial assessed the degree of chorea worsening after withdrawal of TBZ over a 5-day period in a double-blind fashion. Subjects withdrawn from TBZ had a significant worsening of their UHDRS chorea scores compared to those kept on the drug (Frank et al., 2008). Despite the evidence for efficacy, serious side effects may limit the full dose or prolonged used of TBZ, with parkinsonism, depression, suicide, and risk of possible neuroleptic malignant syndrome being among the more serious adverse effects (Video 22-1: Chorea-Acanthocytosis treated with Tetrabenazine). In addition, despite increasing therapeutic doses of TBZ over time, long-term use may show decreased efficacy, as seen in one study with HD patients (Fasano et al., 2008a).

Reserpine

Reserpine is pharmacologically similar to TBZ but is now infrequently used for several reasons. These include decreased availability, pharmacological effects lasting days to weeks, less selective depletion of dopamine compared to other monoamines, and increased rate of peripheral side effects including gastrointestinal symptoms, bradycardia, and hypotension.

Dopaminergic Drugs

While increasing dopamine levels would theoretically worsen chorea, in some instances dopaminergic drugs (levodopa or dopamine agonists) may have an antichoreic effect.

Levodopa

Two subjects in one pedigree with benign hereditary chorea related to a novel *TITF-1* gene mutation (Chapter 4) showed a rapid, dose-dependent improvement of chorea and gait on relatively high doses of levodopa (20–30 mg/kg/day). One subject developed increased chorea with higher doses of levodopa (Asmus et al., 2005).

Apomorphine

Low-dose dopamine agonists may paradoxically result in inhibition of dopamine release by stimulation of presynaptic D_2 autoreceptors, with potential applications for hyperkinetic disorders. Previous studies using bromocriptine showed mixed results, and no significant studies have been done using newer dopamine agonists (Bonelli and Wenning, 2006). Several open-label studies using low-dose apomorphine showed effectiveness for treating chorea in HD, while studies using bromocriptine showed mixed results. A double-blind, randomized, crossover trial demonstrated improvement of oculomotor signs, bradykinesia, and chorea after 5 days of continuous subcutaneous apomorphine infusion in five HD patients. However, four other patients screened for this study had no response or worsening chorea when administered an acute apomorphine dose (Vitale et al., 2007).

NMDA Receptor Antagonist/Antiglutamatergic Drugs

N-Methyl-D-aspartate (NMDA) receptor antagonists are thought to reduce glutamatergic tone, which has been implicated in the production of chorea in HD and PD.

Amantadine

Amantadine is a well-tolerated, noncompetitive NMDA receptor antagonist commonly used for its antichoreic effect. It remains the only agent proven to reduce levodopa-induced choreic dyskinesias in PD without exacerbating parkinsonism (Verhagen Metman et al., 1998) (Chapter 14). Reduction of chorea in HD has been demonstrated immediately after intravenous infusion of the drug (Lucetti et al., 2003). However, placebo-controlled, randomized trials for amantadine in HD have shown mixed results. Despite subjective improvement, chorea scores did not improve in a crossover study of 12 subjects treated with amantadine 300 mg daily for 2 weeks (O'Suilleabhain and Dewey, 2003). In contrast, a similarly designed study with 24 subjects treated with up to 400 mg daily showed a median of 36% improvement in chorea, with some subjects improving even more dramatically (Verhagen Metman et al., 2002). Amantadine remains a useful option for patients with milder chorea who do not have severe behavioral symptoms warranting treatment with antipsychotics.

Riluzole

Riluzole is an antiglutamatergic agent that acts by retarding striatal glutamate release, as well as demonstrating multiple other mechanisms to diminish glutamatergic neurotransmission. One small, open-label study using 100 mg daily of riluzole in HD patients appeared promising, showing as much as 35% improvement in chorea scores (Rosas et al., 1999). A larger, 1-year open-label trial with the same medication dose demonstrated improvement in chorea, total functional capacity, and total motor scores after 3 months. The drug was well tolerated and led to significant improvement of psychomotor speed and behavioral dysfunction, but motor improvement was not sustained after 12 months (Seppi et al., 2001). A dosage effect study of treatment with placebo vs. 100 mg or 200 mg daily of riluzole for

8 weeks noted a mild but significant reduction of chorea at the 200 mg dose; however, functional benefit or change in other disease parameters was not observed (Huntington Study Group, 2003). In addition, there was a dose-dependent elevation of liver enzymes in the 200 mg–dosed groups, limiting potential use due to need for blood monitoring. Unfortunately, a larger, randomized, controlled study with 537 subjects on 100 mg daily for 3 years did not demonstrate any improvement of motor or functional HD scores compared to a placebo group. Many subjects dropped out of the study to start other antichoreic medications (Landwehrmeyer et al., 2007).

Memantine

A small open-label trial of memantine, a noncompetitive NMDA receptor antagonist, at a maximum dose of 20 mg daily, showed significant improvement in motor symptoms, particularly chorea scores, over 3–4 months. The drug was well tolerated, and there was no effect on cognitive function (Ondo et al., 2007).

Remacemide

Remacemide is a low-affinity NMDA antagonist with sodium channel–blocking properties. It was investigated in a randomized, double-blind, 2×2 factorial design with coenzyme Q_{10} for HD. No significant symptomatic or neuroprotective effects were noted after 30 months, although a rapidly appearing, sustained trend toward reduced chorea was noted (Huntington Study Group, 2001).

GABA Agonists

As might be predicted by the loss of GPi GABAergic inhibition in the pathogenesis of chorea, GABA agonists would be expected to have a significant place in the armamentarium of antichoreic drugs. However, the use of GABAergic drugs in HD is sparsely documented. The positive effects of GABA agonists may be nonspecific as they are employed in a wide range of hyperkinetic disorders. Patients with comorbid anxiety may benefit from this class of medications.

Benzodiazepines

Benzodiazepines, such as clonazepam, diazepam, and alprazolam, which act at $GABA_A$ receptors, have demonstrated benefit in open-label use, mainly in older case reports (Bonelli and Wenning, 2006).

Baclofen

Baclofen is an agonist at $GABA_B$ receptors. While some reports demonstrated an antichoreic effect of baclofen, in a larger, randomized study baclofen did not show positive symptomatic or neuroprotective effects in HD (Bonelli and Wenning, 2006).

Antiepileptic Drugs

Antiepileptic drugs (AEDs) in general have a broad spectrum of mechanisms of action, which in some cases are less well characterized or unknown. Known mechanisms include blockage of voltage-dependent ion channels (topiramate, lamotrigine, carbamazepine), enhancement of GABA-mediated inhibition (valproic acid, gabapentin, topiramate), and antiglutamatergic effects (lamotrigine, topiramate). Several AEDs have found roles in treating diverse etiologies of chorea. Given that a single drug may have multiple mechanisms, the efficacy of AEDs in treating chorea may result from either primary effects on one neurotransmitter system or acting on multiple pathways simultaneously.

Valproic Acid

While no controlled studies have been done, valproic acid is a commonly used drug as a first-line agent in SC (Cardoso, 2004). Open-label studies and expert opinion support the safe and effective use of valproic acid for this indication (Davutoglu et al., 2004; Cardoso et al., 2006). Valproic acid has also been employed as an effective treatment for chorea associated with posttraumatic or postanoxic brain injury and kernicterus (Cardoso et al., 2006). Clinical response with valproic acid in vascular hemichorea/hemiballism is not uniformly positive, but it may be effective in some patients (Sethi and Patel, 1990).

Carbamazepine

Carbamazepine has been used to treat SC, with comparable results to valproic acid (Genel et al., 2002; Hernandez-Latorre and Roig-Quilis, 2003). Paroxysmal kinesigenic dyskinesias (PKDs), although most commonly associated with dystonic movements, often manifest with chorea (Chapter 19). PKD is typically very sensitive to treatment with doses of anticonvulsants lower than those required for treating epilepsy, such that improvement after administration of carbamazepine or phenytoin has been proposed as a clinical criterion for diagnosis (Bruno et al., 2004). A variety of other AEDs have also shown efficacy in suppressing the paroxysmal movements of PKD (Mehta and Sethi, 2008).

Levetiracetam

While its mechanism of action is uncertain, levetiracetam appears to be effective in treating chorea secondary to a wide variety of etiologies. It has been demonstrated to reduce chorea in HD and to reduce levodopa-induced chorea in PD (Zesiewicz et al., 2005b, 2006d. There are also reports of levetiracetam improving recurrent, infection-related chorea associated with cerebral palsy (Recio et al., 2005), vascular chorea (D'Amelio et al., 2005), idiopathic/autoimmune chorea (Zesiewicz et al., 2006a), and paroxysmal kinesigenic choreoathetosis (Chatterjee et al., 2002). Caution must be observed, however, as levetiracetam induced reversible parkinsonism in one HD patient (Zesiewicz et al., 2005a).

Lamotrigine

Lamotrigine has been implicated as a cause of chorea in some case reports (Zesiewicz et al., 2006b). Despite this observation, significant subjective symptomatic improvement and a trend toward decreased chorea scores over a 30-month period were noted in a double-blind, placebo-controlled study of lamotrigine for HD (Kremer et al., 1999).

Topiramate

Topiramate was effective in resolving one case of vascular generalized chorea refractory to antipsychotics and clonazepam (Siniscalchi et al., 2007), in five cases of hemichorea/hemiballismus (Zesiewicz et al., 2006c), and as monotherapy for paroxysmal kinesigenic choreoathetosis (Huang et al., 2005).

Acetylcholinesterase Inhibitors

Despite observations that cholinergic dysregulation is involved in HD and reports of cholinergic medications modulating chorea severity in some cases, more rigorous examinations of cholinergic drugs in the treatment of chorea have been less promising.

Galantamine

One case report described considerable improvement of chorea and psychotic symptoms in a patient with HD after treatment with galantamine, a reversible acetylcholinesterase inhibitor. However, this observation has not been investigated in clinical trials (Petrikis et al., 2004).

Donepezil

A small, open-label trial of donepezil, a reversible acetylcholinesterase inhibitor, showed significant improvement on total motor scores in subjects who tolerated the medication. However, chorea did not specifically improve, only half of the subjects completed the protocol, and there was worsening of chorea in two subjects (Fernandez and Friedman, 2000). One randomized, double-blind treatment trial comparing donepezil and placebo did not show improvement in chorea, cognition, or quality of life (Cubo et al., 2006).

Chemodenervating Agents

Botulinum toxin works at the level of the neuromuscular junction, preventing the presynaptic docking and release of acetylcholine vesicles and resulting in muscle paralysis. While botulinum toxin injections are rarely used for chorea alone given the random, typically more diffuse nature of choreic movements, more specific disabling or repetitive movements in choreic syndromes may respond to this therapy. This treatment is usually reserved for more focal dystonic movements, such as genioglossus muscle injections for tongue protrusion dystonia related to chorea-acanthocytosis (Schneider et al., 2006) (Chapter 6).

Disease-Modifying/Neuroprotective Agents

Numerous agents have been investigated or have shown potential promise for neuroprotection in HD, but none has yet met the criteria for effectiveness in a clinical trial (Hersch and Rosas, 2008).

NONPHARMACOLOGICAL TREATMENTS

Surgical Treatments

Given the effectiveness of medical treatments for chorea, the transient nature of secondary or structurally induced chorea, the severity of comorbid symptoms, and the poor long-term prognosis of many choreiform disorders, surgery for chorea is rarely indicated. However, in selected patients who are refractory to conservative therapy and experience prolonged disability specifically attributed to choreiform movements, surgery may improve motor symptoms and quality of life. Surgical approaches vary from correcting abnormal structural lesions to inducing focal lesions in specific locations of the basal ganglia. The most common strategies involve stereotactic lesioning or deep brain stimulation (DBS). Table 22–5 summarizes the surgical approaches and diseases in which they have been applied, with indication of quality of outcomes.

Correcting Structural Lesions

Treatment of structural lesions suspected of causing chorea (Chapter 16) may occasionally result in dramatic improvement. More striking examples include refractory chorea related to moyamoya disease resolving after vascular bypass surgery (Kamijo and Matsui, 2008), resolution of chorea following both removal of a malpositioned ventriculoperitoneal shunt (VPS) (Alakandy et al., 2008), and VPS placement for chorea associated with normal-pressure hydrocephalus (Voermans et al., 2007). Chorea in these cases likely results from local compression or ischemia of basal ganglia structures.

DBS Surgery

DBS surgery has grown in popularity and has found widespread applications in the treatment of many movement disorders. Although mostly employed for the treatment of PD, dystonia, and essential tremor, DBS has been used in patients with chorea with varying levels of success. DBS leads are most commonly placed

TABLE 22–5. Surgical Treatment Options and Quality of Reported Outcomes

SURGICAL TREATMENTS	DISEASES TREATED	OUTCOME*	REFERENCES
Deep brain stimulation	HD	+/–	Moro et al., 2004; Hebb et al., 2006; Fasano et al., 2008b; Bilosi et al., 2008
	Choreoathetotic cerebral palsy	+/–	Thompson et al., 2000; Krauss et al., 2003
	Neuroacanthocytosis (chorea-acanthocytosis, McLeod syndrome)	+/–	Burbaud et al., 2002; Guehl et al., 2007; Wihl et al., 2001
	"Benign senile chorea"	+	Yianni et al., 2004
	Diabetes-related hemichorea/ hemiballismus	+	Nakano et al., 2005
Stereotactic lesioning	Vascular chorea	+	Cardoso et al., 1995; Goto et al., 2001; Choi et al., 2003
	DRPLA	+	Watarai et al., 2003
	HD	+/–	Fasano et al., 2008b
	Chorea-acanthocytosis	+	Fujimoto et al., 1997
Fetal cell transplants	HD	+/–	Hauser et al., 2002; Keene et al., 2007, 2009; Bachoud-Levi et al., 2006

DRPLA, dentatorubral-pallidoluysian atrophy; HD, Huntington disease; +, overall benefit; +/–, mixed results.

in the GPi for chorea as this location has been shown to alleviate the choreic dyskinesias associated with chronic treatment with levodopa in PD. In addition, DBS lead placement in the thalamus, which receives downstream signals from the GPi, has been effective. The following choreic syndromes have been treated with DBS surgery:

Cerebral Palsy. Unilateral thalamic DBS was reported to drastically reduce contralateral chorea in two children with choreiform movement disorders due to intracerebral hemorrhage and cerebral palsy up to 18 months postsurgery (Thompson et al., 2000). However, in another series, bilateral GPi DBS in four patients with choreoathetosis related to perinatal hypoxia/ischemia-related cerebral palsy failed to show statistical improvement on rating scales after 2 years of follow-up (Krauss et al., 2003).

Huntington Disease.   Since the first publication in 2004, case reports of bilateral GPi DBS for HD have shown variable results, often with significant improvement of chorea but worsening bradykinesia at higher stimulation frequencies (Moro et al., 2004; Hebb et al., 2006; Fasano et al., 2008b). This differential effect suggests separate pathophysiological processes for bradykinesia and chorea in HD. The long-term effects of DBS in HD are unknown, given the overwhelming effects of progressive cognitive decline, dysphagia, and other motor features such as rigidity and parkinsonism (Fasano et al., 2008b). However, one report of a patient with HD treated with bilateral GPi DBS demonstrated marked improvement of chorea and quality of life up to 4 years after surgery (Bilosi et al., 2008).

Neuroacanthocytosis Syndromes.   DBS has been performed in a limited number of patients with neuroacanthocytosis syndromes, with targets including the posterior ventral oral nucleus of the thalamus (Vop) and GPi. Vop stimulation improved truncal spasms in one patient with chorea-acanthocytosis (Burbaud et al., 2002). While reducing belching and dyskinetic breathing, high-frequency stimulation in the GPi (130 Hz) worsened chorea, dysarthria, palilalia, and drooling in some patients. Conversely, low-frequency stimulation (40 Hz) improved chorea at the expense of any improvement in dystonic symptoms (Guehl et al., 2007). One patient with McLeod syndrome demonstrated improvement of chorea with low (40 Hz) stimulation (Burbaud et al., 2005). Another report with GPi stimulation showed no benefit, emphasizing that the ideal surgical treatment for these patients is unclear, particularly given the broad spectrum of symptoms of the disease and its inevitably progressive nature (Wihl et al., 2001).

"Benign Senile Chorea".   One 68-year-old patient with severe "senile" chorea refractory to medical management underwent both left Vop and GPi lead placement, with significant reduction of chorea up to 18 months postoperatively (Yianni et al., 2004).

Hemichorea/Hemiballism.   Left thalamic DBS for one patient with striatal pathology related to poorly controlled diabetes mellitus and associated refractory contralateral hemichorea/hemiballism resulted in rapid and sustained improvement of the involuntary movements (Nakano et al., 2005).

Stereotactic Lesioning

While pallidotomy and thalamotomy had been reported as partially effective for chorea as early as 1950 (Goto et al., 2001), stereotactic lesioning surgery has been less commonly performed in recent years due to the popularity, safety, and reversibility of DBS. Regardless, recent reports demonstrate that posteroventral pallidotomy (Choi et al., 2003), thalamotomy (Cardoso et al., 1995; Goto et al., 2001), and combined thalamus/zona incerta lesions (Krauss and Mundinger, 1996) have successfully treated persistent hemichorea/hemiballism related to cerebrovascular disease over long periods of follow-up. However, in some cases improvement of chorea occurred at the expense of mild persistent deficits, including worsening paresis or tremor. One case of severe chorea associated with juvenile-onset dentatorubral-pallidoluysian atrophy responded well to bilateral pallidotomies (Watarai et al., 2003). Pallidotomy in HD led to only modest improvement in dystonia but with worsening of parkinsonism (Fasano et al., 2003b). Improvement of choreoballistic movements with chorea-acanthocytosis occurred in one case after bilateral posteroventral pallidotomy (Fujimoto et al., 1997).

Fetal Cell Transplants

Clinical trials examining the safety and efficacy of fetal neural transplants have shown mixed results. Open-label, bilateral, human fetal striatal cells were transplanted into seven HD patients, three of whom developed postoperative subdural hematomas. There was no significant worsening of overall motor function after 12 months of observation, and autopsy after one early death at 18 months showed integration and survival of grafted tissue (Hauser et al., 2002). After 6 years of follow-up posttransplant in another group of subjects, autopsy findings from two patients, while confirming prolonged survival of neural grafts, demonstrated poor integration with the host striatal cells, which was thought to account for the lack of long-term clinical improvement (Keene et al., 2007). In another subject, fetal neural transplants developed into bilateral mass lesions and ependymal cysts, causing mass effect upon the internal capsules with clinically related pathological upper motor neuron signs, highlighting the risk of graft overgrowth as a potential complication of transplant therapy (Keene et al., 2009). A 6-year follow-up in another group of five transplanted patients showed disease stability or improvement for 2–4 years before resumption of continued decline, albeit with subsequently slower progression of chorea severity as compared to dystonia (Bachoud-Levi et al., 2006).

Rehabilitation Therapies

Systematic reviews examining the effectiveness of physical, occupational, and speech therapies for HD patients find insufficient evidence to support their efficacy in treating any feature of HD, including chorea and falls (Bilney et al., 2003; Busse and Rosser, 2007). A pilot study in early- to mid-stage HD patients, recruited for periodic 3-week inpatient rehabilitation sessions over 2 years, showed improvements in overall motor performance. However, there was a high dropout rate and chorea scores were not specifically monitored (Zinzi et al., 2007). Techniques to improve gait parameters used in PD have not proven effective in HD, a finding which is attributed to more severe deficits in attention (Delval et al., 2008). Regardless, physical and occupational therapies may be employed to help reduce the risk of serious complications of choreic illnesses, such as self-injury or falling, and to provide training for use of assistive or mechanical protective devices.

Patient Education/Information Resources

Most choreic diseases have societies or patient support organizations that may provide further education, fellowship, and counseling for patients and their caregivers. Web sites or office locations may be found through appropriate sources including the Internet and international organizations. Knowledge of what to expect at each stage of the disease and the projected course of symptoms may reduce caregiver stress and help guide future therapies.

Multidisciplinary Care

Given the multiple comorbidities and relentless progression of many degenerative or genetic choreas, a coordinated, multidisciplinary approach is ideal (Table 22–6).

TABLE 22–6. Multidisciplinary Team Members for Management of Patients with Chorea

TEAM MEMBERS	ROLE/NEEDS TO BE ADDRESSED
Neurologist (movement disorders specialist)	Diagnose underlying condition, oversee therapeutic trials, quantify and track disease severity, coordinate medical management
Psychiatrist	Diagnose and treat psychiatric comorbidities, provide psychological support to patient and caregivers
General practitioner	Manage medical complications of chronic neurological disease and other concomitant medical problems
Neuropsychologist	Quantify degree of cognitive impairment, provide psychological support to patient and caregivers
Nurse	Coordinate medical care, serve as point of contact, support patients and caregivers

(continued)

TABLE 22–6. (continued)

TEAM MEMBERS	ROLE/NEEDS TO BE ADDRESSED
Physical/occupational therapist	Maintain safety in the home, prevent falls, prevent complications of disease progression, adaptive strategies for activities of daily living, improve mobility, plan for more physically active lifestyle
Dietician	Monitor weight, discuss needs for dietary changes and alternative feeding methods such as percutaneous endoscopic gastrostomy tube
Palliative care	Provide palliative treatments including pain control, respite care
Social worker	Assist in obtaining disability benefits, power of attorney, wills, advanced directives, and guide patients and caregivers to available community, organizational, and governmental resources; assist in financial and health insurance–related issues
Speech and language therapists	Improve communication skills, assess swallowing function to avoid aspiration
Genetic counselor	Guide family planning, interpret test results, guide testing of relatives

SUMMARY

The treatment of chorea remains challenging due to the imperfect understanding of its pathophysiology, general lack of pertinent evidence-based therapeutic guidelines, the diversity of underlying etiologies, individual patient factors, and the broad spectrum of reportedly effective options. Dopamine receptor–blocking and dopamine-depleting medications have demonstrated the most consistent antichoreic effects, although their prolonged use poses the risk of significant adverse events. Antiglutamatergic and GABA-agonist drugs also show varying degrees of efficacy in treating chorea. Surgery may help treat patients with chorea who fail trials of conventional medications. Multidisciplinary care teams can help address the varied needs of patients with choreiform disorders.

REFERENCES

Alakandy LM, Iyer RV, Golash A (2008) Hemichorea, an unusual complication of ventriculperitonial shunt. J Clin Neurosci 15(5):599–601.

Asmus F, Horber V, Pohlenz J, et al. (2005) A novel TITF-1 mutation causes benign hereditary chorea with response to levodopa. Neurology 64(11):1952–1954.

Bachoud-Levi AC, Gaura V, Brugieres P, et al. (2006) Effect of fetal neural transplants in patients with Huntington's disease 6 years after surgery: a long-term follow-up study. Lancet Neurol 5(4):303–309.

Bilney B, Morris M, Perry A (2003) Effectiveness of physiotherapy, occupational therapy, and speech pathology for people with Huntington's disease: a systematic review. Neurorehabil Neural Repair 17(1):12–24.

Bilosi B, Cif L, Fertit HE, Robles SG, Coubes P (2008) Long-term follow-up of Huntington disease treated by bilateral deep brain stimulation of the internal globus pallidus: Case report. J Neurosurg 109(1):130–132.

Bonelli RM, Wenning GK (2006) Pharmacological management of Huntington's disease: an evidence-based review. Curr Pharm Des 12(21):2701–2720.

Bonelli R, Mayr B, Niederwieser G, Reisecker F, Kapfhammer HP (2003) Ziprasidone in Huntington's disease: the first case reports. J Psychopharmacol 17(4):459–460.

Bonelli R, Niederwieser G (2002) Quetiapine in Huntington's disease: a first case report. J Neurol 249(8):1114–1115.

Bonham C, Abbott C (2008) Are second generation antipsychotics a distinct class? J Psychiatr Pract 14(4):225–231.

Bruno MK, Hallett M, Gwinn-Hardy K, et al. (2004) Clinical evaluation of idiopathic paroxysmal kinesigenic dyskinesia: new diagnostic criteria. Neurology 63(12):2280–2287.

Brusa L, Orlacchio A, Moschella V, et al. (2009) Treatment of the symptoms of Huntington's disease: preliminary results comparing aripiprazole and tetrabenazine. Mov Disord 24(1):126–129.

Burbaud R, Rougeir A, Ferrer X, et al. (2002) Improvement of severe trunk spasms by bilateral high-frequency stimulation of the motor thalamus in a patient with chorea-acanthocytosis. Mov Disord 17(1):204–207.

Burbaud P, Cuny E, Guehl D, et al. (2005) Deep brain stimulation in neuroacanthocytosis. Mov Disord 20(12):1681–1682.

Busse ME, Rosser AE (2007) Can directed activity improve mobility in Huntington's disease? Brain Res Bull 72(2–3):172–174.

Cardoso F (2004) Chorea: non-genetic causes. Curr Opin Neurol 17(4):433–436.

Cardoso F (2008a) Chorea. In: Hallet M, Poewe W (eds.) Therapeutics of Parkinson's Disease and Other Movement Disorders. John Wiley & Sons, LTD, West Sussex, UK, pp 317–330.

Cardoso F (2008b) Sydenham's chorea. Curr Treat Options Neurol 10(3):230–235.

Cardoso F, Jankovic J, Grossman RG, Hamilton WJ (1995) Outcome after stereotactic thalamotomy for dystonia and hemiballismus. Neurosurgery 36(3):501–507.

Cardoso F, Seppi K, Mair KJ, Wenning GK, Poewe W (2006) Seminar on choreas. Lancet Neurol 5(7):589–602.

Chatterjee A, Louis ED, Frucht S (2002) Levetiracetam in the treatment of paroxysmal kinesigenic choreoathetosis. Mov Disord 17(3):614–615.

Choi SJ, Lee SW, Kim MC, et al. (2003) Posteroventral pallidotomy in medically intractable postapoplectic monochorea: case report. Surg Neurol 59(6):486–490.

Cubo E, Shannon KM, Tracy D, et al. (2006) Effect of donepezil on motor and cognitive function in Huntington disease. Neurology 67(7):1268–1271.

D'Amelio M, Callari G, Gammino M, et al. (2005) Levetiracetam in the treatment of vascular chorea: a case report. Eur J Clin Pharmacol 60(11):835–836.

Davutoglu V, Kilinc M, Dinckal H, Soydinc S, Sezen Y (2004) Sydenham's chorea—clinical characteristics of nine patients. Int J Cardiol 96(3):483–484.

Delval A, Krystkowiak P, Delliaux M, et al. (2008) Effect of external cueing on gait in Huntington's disease. Mov Disord 23(10):1446–1452.

Demiororen K, Yavuz H, Cam L, et al. (2007) Sydenham's chorea: a clinical follow-up of 65 patients. J Child Neurol 22(5):550–554.

Dewey RB, Jankovic J (1989) Hemiballism-hemichorea: clinical and pharmacological findings in 21 patients. Arch Neurol 46(8):862–867.

Erdemoglu AK, Boratav C (2002) Risperidone in chorea and psychosis of Huntington's disease. Eur J Neurol 9(2):182–183.

Fasano A, Cadeddu F, Guidubaldi A, et al. (2008a) The long-term effect of tetrabenazine in the management of Huntington disease. Clin Neuropharmacol 31(6):313–318.

Fasano A, Mazzone P, Piano C, et al. (2008b) GPi-DBS in Huntington's disease: results on motor function and cognition in a 72-year-old case. Mov Disord 23(9):1289–1293.

Fernandez HH, Friedman JH (2000) Donepezil for Huntington's disease. Mov Disord 15(1):173–175.

Folstein SE, Jensen B, Leigh J, Folstein MF (1983) The measurement of abnormal movement: methods developed for Huntington's disease. Neurobehav Toxicol Teratol 5(6):605–609.

Frank S, Ondo W, Fahn S, et al. (2008) A study of chorea after tetrabenazine withdrawal in patients with Huntington disease. Clin Neuropharmacol 31(3):127–133.

Fujimoto Y, Isozaki E, Yokochi F, et al. (1997) A case of chorea-acanthocytosis successfully treated with posteroventral pallidotomy [in Japanese]. Rinsho Sinkeigaku 37(10):891–894.

Genel F, Arslanoglu S, Uran N, Saylan B (2002) Sydenham's chorea: clinical findings and comparison of the efficacies of sodium valproate and carbamazepine regimens. Brain Dev 24(2):73–76.

Goto S, Kunitoku N, Hamasaki T, Nishikawa S, Ushio Y (2001) Abolition of postapoplectic hemichorea by Vo-complex thalamotomy: long-term follow-up study. Mov Disord 16(4):771–774.

Guehl D, Cuny E, Tison F, et al. (2007) Deep brain stimulation for movement disorders in neuroacanthocytosis. Neurology 68(2):160–161.

Hauser RA, Furtado S, Cimino CR, et al. (2002) Bilateral human fetal striatal transplantation in Huntington's disease. Neurology 58(5):687–695.

Hebb MO, Garcia R, Gaudet P, Mendez IM (2006) Bilateral stimulation of the globus pallidus internus to treat choreathetosis in Huntington's disease: technical case report. Neurosurgery 58(2):E383.

Hernandez-Latorre MA, Roig-Quilis M (2003) The efficiency of carbamazepine in a case of post-streptococcal hemichorea [in French]. Rev Neurol 37(4):322–326.

Hersch SM, Rosas HD (2008) Neuroprotection for Huntington's disease: ready, set, slow. Neurotherapeutics 5(2):226–236.

Huang YG, Chen YC, Du F, et al. (2005) Topiramate therapy for paroxysmal kinesigenic choreoathetosis. Mov Disord 20(1):75–77.

Huntington Study Group (2001) A randomized, placebo-controlled trial of coenzyme Q_{10} and remacemide in Huntington's disease. Neurology 57(3):397–404.

Huntington Study Group (2003) Dosage effects of riluzole in Huntington's disease. Neurology 61(11):1551–1556.

Huntington Study Group (2006) Tetrabenazine as antichorea therapy in Huntington disease: a randomized controlled trial. Neurology 66(3):366–372.

Huntington Study Group (1996) Unified Huntington's disease rating scale: reliability and consistency. Mov Disord 11(2):136–142.

Jankovic J, Orman J (1988) Tetrabenazine therapy of dystonia, chorea, tics, and other dyskinesias. Neurology 38(3):391–394.

Kamijo K, Matsui T (2008) Dramatic disappearance of moyamoya disease–induced chorea after indirect bypass surgery: case report. Neurol Med Chir (Tokyo) 48(9):390–393.

Keene CD, Sonnen JA, Swanson PD, et al. (2007) Neural transplantation in Huntington disease: long-term grafts in two patients. Neurology 68(24):2093–2098.

Keene CD, Chang RC, Leverenz JB, et al. (2009) A patient with Huntington's disease and long-surviving fetal neural transplants that developed mass lesions. Acta Neuropathol 117(3):329–338.

Krauss JK, Loher TJ, Weigel R, et al. (2003) Chronic stimulation of the globus pallidus internus for treatment of non-DYT1 generalized dystonia and choreoathetosis: 2-year follow up. J Neurosurg 98(4):785–792.

Krauss JK, Mundinger F (1996) Functional stereotactic surgery for hemiballism. J Neurosurg 85(2):278–286.

Kremer B, Clark CM, Almqvist EW, et al. (1999) Influence of lamotrigine on progression of early Huntington's disease: a randomized clinical trial. Neurology 53(5):1000–1011.

Landwehrmeyer GB, Dubois B, de Yebenes JG, et al. (2007) Riluzole in Huntington's disease: a 3-year, randomized controlled study. Ann Neurol 62(3):262–272.

Lang AE, Koller WC, Fahn S (1995) Psychogenic parkinsonism. *Arch Neurol.* 52: 802–810.

Lucetti C, Del Dotto P, Gambaccini G, et al. (2003) IV amantadine improves chorea in Huntington's disease: an acute, randomized, controlled study. Neurology 60(12):1995–1997.

Marsden CD, Schachter M (1981) Assessment of extrapyramidal disorders. Br J Clin Pharmacol 11(2):129–151.

Mehta SH, Sethi KD (2008) Therapeutics of paroxysmal dyskinesias. In: Hallet M, Poewe W (eds.) Therapeutics of Parkinson's Disease and Other Movement Disorders. John Wiley & Sons, LTD, West Sussex, UK, pp 345–352.

Mink JW (2003) The basal ganglia and involuntary movements: impaired inhibition of competing motor patterns. Arch Neurol 60(10):1365–1368.

Moro E, Lang AE, Strafella AP, et al. (2004) Bilateral globus pallidus stimulation for Huntington's disease. Ann Neurol 56:290–294.

Munetz MR, Benjamin S (1998) How to examine patients using the Abnormal Involuntary Movements Scale. Hosp Community Psychiatry 39(11):1172–1177.

Nakano N, Uchiyama T, Okuda T, Kitano M, Taneda M (2005) Successful long-term deep brain stimulation for hemichorea-hemiballism in a patient with diabetes: a case report. J Neurosurg 102(6):1137–1141.

Obeso JA, Rodriguez-Oroz MC, Rodriguez M, Arbizu J, Gimenez-Amaya JM (2002) The basal ganglia and disorders of movement: pathophysiological mechanisms. News Physiol Sci 17:51–55.

Ondo WG, Mejia HI, Hunter CB (2007) A pilot study of the clinical efficacy and safety of memantine for Huntington's disease. Parkinsonism Relat Disord 13(7):453–454.

Ondo WG, Tintner R, Thomas M, Jankovic J (2002) Tetrabenazine treatment for Huntington's disease–associated chorea. Clin Neuropharm 25(6):300–302.

O'Suilleabhain P, Dewey RB (2003) A randomized trial of amantadine in Huntington disease. Arch Neurol 60(7):996–998.

Paleacu D, Giladi N, Moore O, et al. (2004) Tetrabenazine treatment in movement disorders. Clin Neuropharmacol 27(5):230–233.

Petrikis P, Andreou C, Piachas A, Bozikas VP, Karavatos A (2004) Treatment of Huntington's disease with galantamine. Int Clin Psychopharmacol 19:49–50.

Phillips W, Shannon KM, Barker RA (2008) The current clinical management of Huntington's disease. Mov Disord 23(11):1491–1504.

Recio MV, Hauser RA, Louis ED, et al. (2005) Chorea in a patient with cerebral palsy: treatment with levitiracetam. Mov Disord 20(6):762–765.

Rosas HD, Koroshetz WJ, Jenkins BG, et al. (1999) Riluzole therapy in Huntington's disease. Mov Disord 14(2):326–330.

Schneider SA, Aggarwal A, Bhatt M, et al. (2006) Severe tongue protrusion dystonia: clinical syndromes and possible treatment. Neurology 67(6):940–943.

Seeman P (2002) Atypical antipsychotics: mechanism of action. Can J Psychiatry 47(1): 27–38.

Seppi K, Mueller J, Bodner T, et al. (2001) Riluzole in Huntington's disease (HD): an open label study with one year follow up. J Neurol 248(10):866–869.

Sethi KD, Patel BP (1990) Inconsistent response to divalproex sodium in hemichorea/hemiballism. Neurology 40(10):1630–1631.

Shannon KM (2007) Treatment of chorea. Continuum Lifelong Learn Neurol 13(1): 72–93.

Shannon KM, Fenichel GM (1990) Pimozide treatment of Sydenham's chorea. Neurology 40(1):186.

Siniscalchi A, Gallelli L, Davoli A, De Sarro G (2007) Efficacy and tolerability of topiramate in vascular generalized chorea. Ann Pharmacother 41(11):1915.

Teixeira AL, Cardoso F, Maia DP, Cunningham MC (2003) Sydenham's chorea may be a risk factor for drug induced parkinsonism. J Neurol Neurosurg Psychiatry 74(9): 1350–1351.

Teixeira AL, Maia DP, Cardoso F (2005) UFMG Sydenham's chorea rating scale (USCRS): reliability and consistency. Mov Disord 20:585–591.

Thompson TP, Kondziolka D, Albright AL (2000) Thalamic stimulation for choreiform movement disorders in children. Report of two cases. J Neurosurg 92(4):718–721.

van Vugt JP, Siesling S, Vergeer M, van der Velde EA, Roos RA (1997) Clozapine versus placebo in Huntington's disease: a double blind randomized comparative study. J Neurol Neurosurg Psychiatry 63(1):35–39.

Verhagen Metman L, Morris M, Farmer C, et al. (2002) Huntington's disease: a randomized, controlled trial using the NMDA-antagonist amantadine. Neurology 59(5): 694–699.

Verhagen Metman L, Del Dotto P, van den Munckhof P, et al. (1998) Amantadine as treatment for dyskinesias and motor fluctuations in Parkinson's disease. Neurology 50(5): 1323–1326.

Vitale C, Marconi S, Di Maio L, et al. (2007) Short-term continuous infusion of apomorphine hydrochloride for treatment of Huntington's chorea: a double blind, randomized cross-over trial. Mov Disord 22(16):2359–2364.

Vitale C, Pellecchia MT, Grossi D, et al. (2001) Unawareness of dyskinesias in Parkinson's and Huntington's disease. Neurol Sci 22(1):105–106.

Voermans NC, Schutte PJ, Bloem BR (2007) Hydrocephalus induced chorea. J Neurol Neurosurg Psychiatry 78(11):1284–1285.

Watarai M, Hashimoto T, Yamamoto K, et al. (2003) Pallidotomy for severe generalized chorea of juvenile-onset dentatorubral-pallidoluysian atrophy. Neurology 61(10): 1452–1454.

Wihl G, Volkmann J, Allert N, et al. (2001) Deep brain stimulation of the internal pallidum did not improve chorea in a patient with neuro-acanthocytosis. Mov Disord 16(3): 572–575.

Yianni J, Nandi D, Bradley K, et al. (2004) Senile chorea treated by deep brain stimulation: a clinical, neurophysiological, and functional imaging study. Mov Disord 19(5): 597–602.

Young AB, Shoulson I, Penney JB, et al. (1986) Huntington's disease in Venezuela: neurologic features and functional decline. Neurology 36(2):244.

Zesiewicz TA, Pathak A, Sullivan KL, Shamayev M, Hauser RA (2006a) Treatment of chorea with levetiracitam. Eur J Clin Pharmacol 62(1):87.

Zesiewicz TA, Sanchez-Ramos J, Sullivan KL, Hauser RA (2005a) Levetiracetam-induced parkinsonism in a Huntington disease patient. Clin Neuropharmacol 28(4):188–190.

Zesiewicz TA, Sullivan KL, Hauser RA (2006b) Chorea induced by lamotrigine. J Child Neurol 21(4):357.

Zesiewicz TA, Sullivan KL, Hauser RA (2006c) Vascular hemichorea/hemiballismus and topiramate. Mov Disord 21(4):581.

Zesiewicz TA, Sullivan KL, Hauser RA, Sanchez-Ramos J (2006d) Open-label pilot study of levetiracetam (Keppra) for the treatment of chorea in Huntington's disease. Mov Disord 21(11):1998–2001.

Zesiewicz TA, Sullivan KL, Maldonado JL, Tatum WO, Hauser RA (2005b) Open-label pilot study of levetiracetam (Keppra) for the treatment of levodopa-induced dyskinesias in Parkinson's disease. Mov Disord 20(9):1205–1209.

Zinzi P, Salmaso D, De Grandis R, et al. (2007) Effects of an intensive rehabilitation programme on patients with Huntington's disease: a pilot study. Clin Rehabil 21(7): 603–613.

Video Legends*

Video 3-1 Huntington's disease

57 year old patient with 42/17 CAG repeats in the *huntingtin* gene. His mother had been affected, and he had developed gait problems 3 years prior to this video. The video shows mild chorea affecting all four limbs, face and trunk. His speech is dysarthric and he is unable to maintain protrusion of the tongue, demonstrating motor impersistence.

Video 6-1 chorea-acanthocytosis

Segments 1 and 2.

Dysarthria is obvious as this patient (case 1) reports about his movement disorder that started three years earlier. During the interview at the age of 30 he shows pronounced chorea of the trunk with sudden body flexions and extensions. Repeated head banging has caused a spot of hair loss on the back of his head. There is some choreoathetosis of his hands and fingers. Involuntary trunk movements severely interfere with his stance.

Segment 3.

Truncal instability, albeit milder, is also present in this 35 year old man (case 2). His gait is shuffling due to a dystonic foot posture.

Segments 4 and 5.

In this female patient (case 3, 30 years old), the equinovarus foot dystonia is so pronounced that it results in a high-stepping gait and mimics pareses. Unusual whole body movements appear to be initiated by the abnormal foot postures. Not surprisingly, walking backwards, running and skipping were performed with less effort. While walking, she also shows arm dystonia in flexion and shrugs her shoulders involuntarily. As she raises her arms, she displays right hand dystonia and choreoathetosis. A brief involuntary grunt can be heard.

Segments 6 and 7.

This patient (case 4) also displayed choreoathetosis of his arms (right hand flexion, shoulder shrugging) when seen at the age of 45 years, but had developed a hypokinetic syndrome when filmed again six years later (age 51). Arm movements are slow now and there is hypomimia with a dystonic, gaping mouth and drooling. Swallowing is impaired and anarthria had necessitated the use of an electronic communicator. Atrophy is obvious in the temporalis and small hand muscles.

Segment 8.

Case 5 (younger brother of case 4) was seen at the age of 42 years. To prevent oral mutilations, such as the ulcer visible on his lower lip, he used to keep a cotton bud in his mouth. His speech was dysarthric and his tongue movements were slowed.

Segment 9.

This 36 year old man (case 8) displays mutilations of his lower lip and his tongue. An episode of compulsive smacking and grunting occurred when he was asked to perform rapid tongue movements. He habitually stuck his fingers in his mouth and sucked on them. This behavior reduced perioral mutilation but caused bite marks on his fingers.

Segment 10.

Case 3 displays dysarthria while she was asked to write a self-proposed sentence ("the cow jumped over the moon"). There is drooling and slight hypomimia. In addition to the abnormal writing posture of her hand, several vocal tics (such as involuntary grunts) are documented.

Segments 11-13.

Case 1 was again seen at the age of 44 years. His face is masked. He has difficulty to initiate tongue movements and has developed severe dysphonia. Part of the earlier video (segment 1, taken 14 years before) is repeated to illustrate the development of the present hypokinetic state from his initial chorea.

Video 7-1 McLeod syndrome

This 48 year old man developed changes in behaviour at the age of 42, with neglect of his appearance and weight loss. He subsequently developed peripheral neuropathy, hepatomegaly, and weight loss. In the video he demonstrates mild generalized chorea and a shambling, wide-based gait.

Video 10-1 aceruloplasminemia

This 54 year-old woman presented with a 3-4 year history of depression and cognitive impairment (Skidmore et al., 2008). She developed generalised chorea, as seen in the video, and spasticity of the lower limbs. Evaluation found no detectable serum ceruloplasmin or ceruloplasmin ferroxidase actvitity, high ferritin, low serum iron, and iron-overloaded liver on biopsy. However, no brain iron deposition was found on neuroimaging, making this an atypical case. Genetic testing was not performed.

Video 12-1 apraxia with oculomotor ataxia I

Ataxia with oculomotor apraxia I. This 21 year- old patient presented at the age of 5 years with ataxia, and chorea, followed by peripheral neuropathy and mild mental retardation. In this video oculomotor apraxia, dysarthria, apendicular chorea and prominent ataxia are noted. Genetic testing demonstrated heterozygousmutationsc.837G>A;NM_175073intheAPTXgene(p.W279X;NP_778243.1) (Moreira et al. 2001; Le Ber et al. 2003) . Video courtesy of Esther Cubo, MD, Burgos, Spain.

Video 12-2 spinocerebellar ataxia 2

Chorea in SCA2. This 32 year old patient developed schizophrenia at the age of 22, and clumsiness and dysarthria at age 27, which were initially ascribed to his antipsychotic medications. Subsequent neurological examination, as seen in this video demonstrated mild-moderate generalized chorea, spasmodic dysphonia, dysdiadochokinesia – more pronounced on the left, and ataxia of gait. He also had areflexia and peripheral neuropathy. Eye movements were, unusually, normal. Genetic testing demonstrated an expansion in the ataxin-2 gene 39/22 repeats (normal <31) (Rottnek et al. 2008).

Video 16-1 post-stroke hemichorea

Patient with sudden onset of right hemi-chorea at the time of an ischemic stroke affecting the posterior limb of the left internal capsule. The video was taken at 5 months after this event, but the symptoms have gradually reduced over several years. Moderate chorea of the right arm and leg is seen which does not interfere with purposeful movements. There was some benefit from carbamazepline.

Video 17-1 Sydenham's chorea

The video shows a 7 year old boy with a 4 week history of involuntary movements, clumsiness, balance difficulty and falls. There was no history of recent infections or medication exposures. Developmental and medically history were negative. ASO titres were elevated. The video shows interrupted speech, motor impersistence, clumsiness, and generalized chorea. Video courtesy of Jennifer Goldman, MD, Chicago, USA.

Video 18-1 anti-NMDA receptor antibody syndrome

Patient with anti-NMDA receptors antibodies secondary to presumed ovarian teratoma.

A 14-year-old girl presented with four days of fever, headache, asthenia, and difficulty concentrating. This progressed to manic behavior and she was admitted to a psychiatric ward with a diagnosis of acute psychosis. A few days later she became encephalopathic and subsequently developed myoclonic and choreiform movements with oculogyric crises. Continuous video electroencephalographic monitoring did not reveal any seizure activity. An extensive evaluation, including brain MRI and a CT of the chest/abdomen/pelvis as well as abdominal ultrasound, was unrevealing. She received a course of intravenous steroids without clear improvement of her encephalopathy or movement abnormalities. She underwent a protracted rehabilitation course lasting eight months, during which time her hyperkinetic movements subsided and she became hypokinetic. Presence of an NMDA receptor antibody was confirmed with CSF.

The video shows semi-rhythmic repetitive movements of lips, trunk and limbs in this encephalopathic patient. The movement disorder of this syndrome is often hard to characterize but can include chorea in addition to bizarre repetitive movements.

Video 18-2 hyperthyroidism

A 67 year-old woman presented with a four year history of abnormal involuntary movements. She had also been noted to have personality changes such as increased anxiety, reclusiveness and fearfulness along with some increased thickness of speech. Her neurological examination revealed moderate generalized chorea (of which she was largely unaware), slight rigidity in the right hand, bradykinesia and difficulty on tandem walking. Her lab results revealed thyroglobulin < 0.5 (0.5 - 55.0) and presence of an elevated thyroglobulin antibody- 326 (0 – 35). Her family history was significant for two nieces with young-onset immune-related thyroid disorders.

Video 18-3 celiac disease

This 60 year-old man had a 1 year history of involuntary movements. The video shows chorea affecting face, trunk and limbs, which is reduced in the second segment, when he has been compliant with a gluten-free diet, with concomitant reduction in anti-gliadin antibodies

Video 22-1 Tetrabenazine for chorea-acanthocytosis.

This 48 year old woman with a 15 year history of partial epilepsy developed progressive oromandibular dyskinesias, eating dystonia, tongue pain, dysphagia, gait disorder, and impulsive behavior. Erythrocyte membrane testing for the presence of chorein revealed absent or markedly reduced chorein levels. Initial examination (video segment 1) demonstrated intermittent, moderate limb chorea, prominent orobuccolingual dyskinesias parkinsonism, and features of a dystonic gait. She also demonstrated (video segment 2) motor impersistance of voluntary tongue protrusion or jaw opening, difficulty with fine motor control of the jaw and tongue, left tongue deviation, and near continuous orobuccolingual dyskinesias associated with tongue pain, with pain and movements moderately relieved by placing her fingers within her mouth. As her tongue movements did not respond to quetiapine, she was titrated up to 75mg daily of tetrabenazine daily. At this dose (video segment 3) there was resolution of limb chorea and oromandibular chorea, but a marked increase of parkinsonism with increased postural instability. Reduction of tetrabenazine to 68.75mg daily resulted in improvement of parkinsonism and continued improvement of orobuccolingual movements including much improved fine motor control of the jaw and tongue without motor impersistence. At this dose, however, involuntary tongue protrusion became more prominent (video segment 4, first demonstrating involuntary followed by voluntary tongue movements), and while resulting in less dysphagia has led to greater cosmetic embarrassment for the patient. (There is no sound for this video.)

Video 22-2 Tetrabenazine for Huntington's disease.

This 37 year old man with genetically-confirmed HD was started on tetrabenazine for generalized chorea (video segment 1). His chorea was markedly reduced on tetrabenazine (video segment 2). Due to the patient's cognitive impairment the dose he was taking in the second segment was unclear, but was probably 37.5mg three times a day. Although he did not develop appreciable parkinsonism he became severely depressed on this dose, and it was decided to stop the medication completely due to safety concerns.

---

* Accompanying videos can be found at the following website: www.oup.com/us/chorea

Index